Radiotherapy in Managing Brain Metastases

Yoshiya Yamada • Eric Chang
John B. Fiveash • Jonathan Knisely
Editors

Radiotherapy in Managing Brain Metastases

A Case-Based Approach

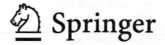
Springer

Editors
Yoshiya Yamada
Department of Radiation Oncology
Memorial Sloan Kettering Cancer
Center
New York, NY
USA

Eric Chang
Department of Radiation Oncology
University of Southern
California
Los Angeles, CA
USA

John B. Fiveash
Department of Radiation Oncology
University of Alabama at Birmingham
Birmingham, AL
USA

Jonathan Knisely
Weill Cornell Medicine
New York–Presbyterian Hospital
New York, NY
USA

ISBN 978-3-030-43742-8   ISBN 978-3-030-43740-4   (eBook)
https://doi.org/10.1007/978-3-030-43740-4

This Springer imprint is published by the registered company Springer Nature Switzerland AG
The registered company address is: Gewerbestrasse 11, 6330 Cham, Switzerland

Foreword

Galileo and Michelangelo. Hippocrates and the Beatles. There is science and there is art. There are scientists and there are artists. This textbook is the best of both. Much of the science is new, and the integrated application of that science is the art. The focus of their science and art is one of the most rapidly evolving topics in oncology today – brain metastases. This topic transcends any one type of cancer. While in the past this diagnosis was under-researched because of the incorrect conventional wisdom that all such patients held the same dismal prognosis, we now understand the vast heterogeneity among this patient population. We are now able to peek over the horizon at the dawn of a new era in which this heterogeneity holds clues that will lead us far beyond local control of an individual tumor to a future in which a systemic response may be ignited by the application of modern therapies in proper sequence and intensity.

This textbook is unique because of the case-based nature of each chapter which not only offers the reader practical guidance on the optimal management of patients today but also reveals trending topics of tomorrow within this burgeoning field. The editors and authors are the best in the world on their assigned topics and should be congratulated on this excellent textbook. It is an honor and a privilege to review this textbook. I have the utmost confidence that the students of this discipline will find this textbook an essential reference for years to come.

Minneapolis, MN, USA   Paul W. Sperduto, MD, MPP, FASTRO

Preface

If one were asked, "What is the most efficacious treatment in radiation oncology?", her answer might be stereotactic radiosurgery. If one were to assess a treatment by weighing the potential benefit against the potential harms, it would be difficult to find a treatment as effective in tumor control and safe in terms of the low incidence of treatment toxicity as stereotactic radiosurgery for brain metastases.

The consequences of uncontrolled brain metastases are devastating Radiosurgery can be performed as a painless, minimally invasive, highly effective treatment that maintains quality of life, with minimal impact upon neurocognition, even when multiple brain metastases are present.

The evolution of advanced neuroimaging and sophisticated treatment planning has allowed highly conformal radiation to be coupled with image-guided treatment delivery ushering in high-precision radiation treatment into the modern era. The result is a powerful yet safe and effective tool that can successfully treat an otherwise vexing clinical problem. As technology advances and our understanding of the biology of metastatic brain disease evolves, radiosurgical treatment will continue to adapt and complement systemic targeted therapies and immune checkpoint inhibitors.

This book is designed to be a very practical, case-based approach to the modern management of brain metastases from the point of view of a radiation oncologist. Clinical cases are presented to illustrate clinically based chapters, while key points are provided at the end of each chapter.

We dedicate this book to our families; without their support, none of this would have been possible.

Los Angeles, CA, USA   Eric Chang
Birmingham, AL, USA   John B. Fiveash
New York, NY, USA   Jonathan Knisely
                                                Yoshiya Yamada

Contents

Contributors

Anthony Asher, MD Department of Neurosurgery, Carolina Neurosurgery and Spine Associates, Charlotte, NC, USA

Ahmet F. Atik, MD Department of Neurosurgery, Rose Ella Burkhardt Neuro-Oncology Center, Cleveland Clinic Foundation, Cleveland, OH, USA

Åse Ballangrud, PhD Department of Medical Physics, Memorial Sloan Kettering Cancer Center, New York, NY, USA

Gene H. Barnett, MD Department of Neurosurgery, Rose Ella Burkhardt Neuro-Oncology Center, Cleveland Clinic Foundation, Cleveland, OH, USA
Cleveland Clinic Lerner College of Medicine of Case Western Reserve University, Cleveland, OH, USA

Jeremy Brownstein, MD, MSc Department of Radiation Oncology, Massachusetts General Hospital, Boston, MA, USA

Stuart Burri, MD Department of Radiation Oncology, Levine Cancer Institute, Carolinas Medical Center, Southeast Radiation Oncology Group, Charlotte, NC, USA

Marc Bussiere, MSc Stereotactic Physics, Department of Radiation Oncology, Massachusetts General Hospital, Boston, MA, USA

James Byrne, MD, PhD Department of Radiation Oncology, Harvard Radiation Oncology Program, Boston, MA, USA

Joycelin F. Canavan, MD, FRCPC Department of Radiation Oncology, Taussig Cancer Institute, Cleveland Clinic, Cleveland, OH, USA

Eric Chang, MD Department of Radiation Oncology, University of Southern California, Los Angeles, CA, USA

Samuel T. Chao, MD Department of Radiation Oncology, Rose Ella Burkhardt Brain Tumor and Neuro-Oncology Center, Cleveland Clinic, Cleveland, OH, USA

Mei Chin Lim, MBBS Department of Diagnostic Imaging, National University Hospital, National University Health System, Singapore, Singapore

Robert M. Conry, MD Division of Hematology & Oncology, University of Alabama at Birmingham, Birmingham, AL, USA

Elizabeth L. Covington, PhD Department of Radiation Oncology, The University of Alabama at Birmingham, Birmingham, AL, USA

Fabio Ynoe de Moraes, MD Department of Oncology, Division of Radiation Oncology, Kingston General Hospital, Queens University, Kingston, ON, Canada

Laura E. Donovan, MD Department of Neurology, Columbia University Irving Medical Center, New York, NY, USA

John B. Fiveash, MD Department of Radiation Oncology, University of Alabama at Birmingham, Birmingham, AL, USA

Matthew Foote, BSc, MBBS (Hons) FRANZCR School of Medicine, The University of Queensland, Brisbane, QLD, Australia

Department of Radiation Oncology, Princess Alexandra Hospital, Brisbane, Australia

Ermias Gete, PhD Medical Physics, BC Cancer, Vancouver Centre, Vancouver, BC, Canada

Michael Huo, MBBS, FRANZCR Radiation Medicine Program, Princess Margaret Cancer Centre, Toronto, ON, Canada

Department of Radiation Oncology, University of Toronto, Toronto, ON, Canada

School of Medicine, The University of Queensland, Brisbane, QLD, Australia

Krishna C. Joshi, MD Department of Neurosurgery, Rose Ella Burkhardt Neuro-Oncology Center, Cleveland Clinic Foundation, Cleveland, OH, USA

Diana A. R. Julie, MD, MPH Department of Radiation Oncology, NewYork-Presbyterian Hospital, Weill Cornell Medicine, New York, NY, USA

Kejia Teo, MBBS Department of Neurosurgery, National University Hospital, National University Health System, Singapore, Singapore

Jonathan Knisely, MD, FASTRO Department of Radiation Oncology, Weill Cornell Medicine, NewYork–Presbyterian Hospital, New York, NY, USA

Guang Li, PhD Department of Medical Physics, Memorial Sloan Kettering Cancer Center, New York, NY, USA

Eric Lis, MD Department of Radiology, Memorial Sloan Kettering Cancer Center, New York, NY, USA

Simon Lo, MBChB, FACR, FASTRO Department of Radiation Oncology, University of Washington School of Medicine, Seattle, WA, USA

Rajiv S. Magge, MD Department of Neurology, Weill Cornell Medicine, NewYork-Presbyterian Hospital, New York, NY, USA

Sean S. Mahase, MD Department of Radiation Oncology, NewYork-Presbyterian Hospital, Weill Cornell Medicine, New York, NY, USA

Lijun Ma, PhD Department of Radiation Oncology, University of California San Francisco, San Francisco, CA, USA

Shawn Malone, MD The Ottawa Hospital Regional Cancer Center, Ottawa, ON, Canada

Gustavo N. Marta, MD, PhD Department of Radiation Oncology, Hospital Sírio-Libanês and Instituto do Câncer de Estado de São Paulo (ICESP) – Faculdade de Medicina da Universidade de São Paulo (FMUSP), São Paulo, Brazil

Hooney D. Min, MD College of Medicine, Seoul National University, Seoul, South Korea

Giuseppe Minniti, MD, PhD Department of Medicine, Surgery and Neuroscience, University of Siena, Siena, Italy

Radiation Oncology Unit, UPMC Hillman Cancer Center, San Pietro Hospital, Rome, Italy

Alireza Mohammad Mohammadi, MD Department of Neurosurgery, Rose Ella Burkhardt Neuro-Oncology Center, Cleveland Clinic Foundation, Cleveland, OH, USA

Mihir Naik, DO Department of Radiation Oncology, Maroone Cancer Center, Cleveland Clinic Florida, Weston, FL, USA

Alan Nichol, MD Department of Radiation Oncology, BC Cancer, Vancouver, BC, Canada

Anatoly Nikolaev, MD, PhD Department of Radiation Oncology, University of Alabama at Birmingham, Birmingham, AL, USA

Kevin S. Oh, MD Department of Radiation Oncology, Massachusetts General Hospital, Boston, MA, USA

Peter C. Pan, MD Department of Neurology, Weill Cornell Medicine/NewYork-Presbyterian Hospital, New York, NY, USA

Mira A. Patel, MD Department of Radiation Oncology, Memorial Sloan Kettering Cancer Center, New York, NY, USA

David Peters, MD Department of Neurosurgery, Atrium Health, Carolinas Medical Center, Carolina Neurosurgery and Spine Associates, Charlotte, NC, USA

Mark B. Pinkham, BM BCh MA (Hons) (Oxon) FRANZCR School of Medicine, The University of Queensland, Brisbane, QLD, Australia

Department of Radiation Oncology, Princess Alexandra Hospital, Brisbane, Australia

Erqi L. Pollom, MD, MS Department of Radiation Oncology, Stanford University, Stanford, CA, USA

Richard A. Popple, PhD Department of Radiation Oncology, University of Alabama at Birmingham, Birmingham, AL, USA

Roshan Prabhu, MD Department of Radiation Oncology, Levine Cancer Institute, Carolinas Medical Center, Southeast Radiation Oncology Group, Charlotte, NC, USA

David Roberge, MD Département de Radiologie, Radio-Oncologie et Médecine Nucléaire, Université de Montréal, Montreal, QC, Canada

Clement Yong, MBBS Department of Diagnostic Imaging, National University Hospital, National University Health System, Singapore, Singapore

Mark Ruschin, PhD Department of Radiation Oncology, Sunnybrook Health Sciences Centre, Odette Cancer Centre, University of Toronto, Toronto, ON, Canada

Arjun Sahgal, MD, FRCPC Department of Radiation Oncology, Sunnybrook Health Sciences Centre, Odette Cancer Centre, University of Toronto, Toronto, ON, Canada

Anurag Saraf, MD Department of Radiation Oncology, Massachusetts General Hospital, Boston, MA, USA

Claudia Scaringi, MD, PhD Radiation Oncology Unit, UPMC Hillman Cancer Center, San Pietro Hospital, Rome, Italy

Helen A. Shih, MD, MS, MPH Proton Therapy Centers, Department of Radiation Oncology, Massachusetts General Hospital, Boston, MA, USA

Siyu Shi, BS Department of Radiation Oncology, Stanford University, Stanford, CA, USA

Scott G. Soltys, MD Department of Radiation Oncology, Stanford University, Stanford, CA, USA

John H. Suh, MD, FASTRO, FACR Department of Radiation Oncology, Taussig Cancer Institute, Cleveland Clinic, Cleveland, OH, USA

Anuradha Thiagarajan, MBBS Department of Radiation Oncology, National Cancer Centre Singapore, Singapore, Singapore

Evan M. Thomas, MD, PhD Department of Radiation Oncology, University of Alabama at Birmingham, Birmingham, AL, USA

Barbara Tolu, MD Radiation Oncology Unit, UPMC Hillman Cancer Center, San Pietro Hospital, Rome, Italy

Balamurugan A. Vellayappan, MBBS Department of Radiation Oncology, National University Cancer Institute Singapore, National University Health System, Singapore, Singapore

Lei Wang, PhD Department of Radiation Oncology, Stanford University, Palo Alto, CA, USA

Nancy Wang, MD, MPH Division of Neuro-Oncology, Department of Neurology, Massachusetts General Hospital, Boston, MA, USA

Tony J. C. Wang, MD Department of Radiation Oncology, Columbia University Irving Medical Center, New York, NY, USA

Yoshiya Yamada, MD Department of Radiation Oncology, Memorial Sloan Kettering Cancer Center, New York, NY, USA

Introduction

Eric Chang, John B. Fiveash, Jonathan Knisely, and Yoshiya Yamada

There is no question that technological innovation coupled with increased understanding of the biology of brain metastases has changed the modern management of this disease. Improved patient survival in stage IV cancer has mandated that even in those with brain metastases, treatment provides durable tumor control with minimal negative impact upon quality of life. These principles form the underpinnings of modern management of brain metastases.

Etymologically speaking, the term "stereotactic" is derived from the Greek "stereos," meaning solid, and the Latin "tactic," meaning touch. The mathematical basis of stereotactic radiosurgery was laid down in the seventeenth century by the great French mathematician Rene Descartes, who is credited with the development of Cartesian

E. Chang
Department of Radiation Oncology, University of Southern California, Los Angeles, CA, USA

J. B. Fiveash
Department of Radiation Oncology, University of Alabama at Birmingham, Birmingham AL, USA

J. Knisely
Department of Radiation Oncology, Weill Cornell Medicine, New York–Presbyterian Hospital, New York, NY, USA

Y. Yamada (✉)
Department of Radiation Oncology, Memorial Sloan Kettering Cancer Center, New York, NY, USA
e-mail: yamadaj@mskcc.org

geometry, which forms the basis of how brain tumors can be accurately mapped.

Cartesian coordinate geometry formed the basis of the Horsley Clarke apparatus, first described in 1908. This seminal paper described an apparatus designed to hold an electrode and guide it into the brain based on Cartesian coordinates, for electrical stimulation or ablation. They coined the phrase "stereotactic" [1]. Robert H Clarke was a British neurophysiologist and anatomist who first conceived the idea of applying Cartesian geometry to the brain. Sir Victor Horsley was a distinguished surgeon and neurophysiologist, who was the first to use intraoperative electrical stimulation of the cortex to find epileptic foci in humans (Fig. 1.1). The first device was made of brass in London in 1905 and used to map structures in the brains of cats and monkeys by attaching it to skull and probing the brain. The first stereotactic apparatus designed for human use was a modification of the Horsley–Clarke device and was built in 1918 by Abrey Mussen, a Canadian neuroanatomist at McGill University. His colleague Clarke also suggested that radium could be stereotactically implanted within brain tumors as a form of treatment [2]. Various versions of the frame would be used by neurophysiologists and anatomists to produce brain atlases of monkeys and other mammals, where landmark studies of stereotactic encephalography and evoked potentials were undertaken in the 1930s [3]. The device was first used in

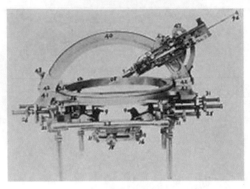

Plate XXX.

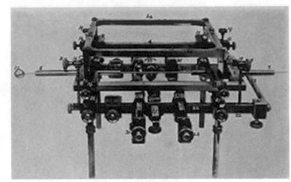

Plate XXXII.

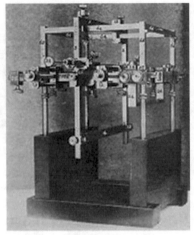

Plate XXXI.

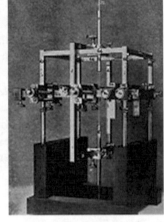

Plate XXXIII.

Fig. 1.1 Photographs of the Horsley–Clarke frame. (From: Pereira et al. [14]. Reprinted with permission)

humans in 1933 by Martin Kirschner, a German surgeon who is best known as the forefather of emergency medicine, and the "K" wire was also described as a stereotactic method to electrocoagulate the trigeminal ganglion in patients with trigeminal neuralgia [4]. A similar device was also described in 1947 by Spiegel and Wycisto to make electroencephalograms of epilepsy patients by incorporating pneumoencephalogram radiography into the localizing process, hence, the first efforts at image-guided neuronavigation in humans. Lars Leksell, commonly acknowledged as the father of Gamma Knife radiosurgery, developed an arc-based electrode carrier that attached to the skull with pins. The position of the arc was adjustable and the electrode pointed at the target of interest, regardless of the angle of attack, by placing the center of rotation of the arc

inside the target [5]. The device was first described in 1948 to treat craniopharyngioma by injecting the tumor with radioactive phosphorus. He continued animal experiments using high-energy proton beams, which were placed in a stereotactic fashion [6]. Because of the cumbersome nature of the synchrocyclotron technology needed to generate high-energy protons, Leksell settled on Co-60 sources as a radiation source. The first unit was commissioned in 1967 at the Karolinska Institute. The original intention of the device was to provide high precision functional noninvasive treatment with high-dose radiation-induced lesions, such as thalamotomy for the treatment of Parkinson's disease, and avoid the complications of surgery. The success of the original device led to a second unit with 179 Co-60 sources arrayed approximately in a half dome configuration, all aimed at a single point to produce spherical lesions at the central point. A newer version of the machine, named the "Gamma Knife" with 201 sources, began to proliferate around the world, and now more than 70,000 patients around the world are treated with Gamma Knife radiosurgery every year.

Godfrey Hounsfield, father of the computed tomography (CT) scanner, first used the device on a preserved human brain, and then, the first use in a patient was to diagnose a right frontal lobe cyst on October 1971 [7]. The CT scan could be mapped and registered in a three dimensional space and could directly provide the exact location of brain tumors, rendering pneumoencephalograms obsolete while ushering a new era of stereotactic radiosurgery as a viable treatment tool in neuro-oncology. CT imaging also provided an electron density map necessary for accurate radiation dose calculations, thus allowing for precision radiation therapy by using stereotactic localization relative to a fiducial frame attached to the skull and highly accurate dose calculations within the CT-defined space. The introduction of the MRI also enhanced the ability to accurately identify and delineate tumors in the brain and was quickly incorporated in the workflow of stereotactic radiosurgery.

In concert with the development of the Gamma Knife, the linear accelerator was also developed in which a single radiation beam was created by shooting a beam of accelerated electrons through a dense target such as tungsten to artificially produce X-rays which could be accurately aimed at central point from any angle. The device was first used to treat a human in 1953 at Hammersmith Hospital in London [8]. Neurosurgeon Osvaldo Betti and Victor Derechinsky, an engineer, first modified a linear accelerator for radiosurgery and treated a patient in 1982 [9]. Leading academic centers in Gainesville, Montreal, Boston, and Heidelberg began publishing their initial experience in the later 1980s. Commercial systems that provided the necessary mechanical accuracy had become available by the 1990s and Linac-based SRS began to be widely used. Initial systems used cylindrical collimators of varying diameters to produce spherical targets that would approximate the tumor in three dimensions. In the mid-1990s, the micro-multi leaf collimator, a device that was placed in the path of the radiation beam and could shape the radiation beam to the exact outline of the tumor, was a further enhancement, rather than depending on a multiple sphere shaped done clouds to approximate the three dimensional characteristics of the tumer [10]. This device was later used to modify the intensity of the radiation within the treatment field to allow even greater conformality. John Adler, a neurosurgeon at Stanford, developed the use of a portable Linac mounted on a robotic arm using orthogonal X-ray imaging to guide the treatment of brain tumors without depending on an isocenter. This device eventually became the CyberKnife and received FDA approval in 2001.

Recognizing the importance of robust immobilization of the skull for safe and accurate radiosurgery, neurosurgeons applied stereotactic frames to immobilize the skull and serve as a coordinate reference system for stereotactic navigation. The first suggestion that a frameless approach could be used was in reference to facilitating surgical applications in 1986, using the skull as a fiducial reference [11]. X-ray stereophotogrammetry, or orthogonal kV localization, was introduced to provide X-ray-image-based stereoscopy to verify positioning for radiosurgery in the early 1990s [12]. Yenice et al. described the use of CT imaging, which provided volumetric data, for stereotactic radiosurgery in 2003 [13]. Volumetric image-guided stereotactic radiosurgery, or frameless radiosurgery, is now available using either Gamma Knife or linear accelerator-based platforms.

Although stereotactic radiosurgery has its roots in the seventeenth century, it is a clear example of how incremental technological innovations have evolved into one of the most effective and safe cancer therapies available today. The subsequent chapters will describe, using case-based examples, the role of stereotactic and other forms of radiation therapy in the management of brain metastases in the twenty-first century. The intent of the book is to provide practical assistance from thought leaders and acknowledged experts in the field. We sincerely express our profound thanks for their willingness to contribute and sacrifice of their time to share their expertise. This book would not have been possible without them.

References

1. Horsley V, Clarke RH. The structure and functions of the cerebellum examined by a new method. Brain. 1908;31(1):45–124.
2. Jensen RL, Stone JL, Hayne RA. Introduction of the human Horsley-Clarke stereotactic frame. Neurosurgery. 1996;38:563–7.
3. Gerard RW, Marshall WH, Saul IJ. Electrical activity of the cat's brain. Arch Neurol Psychiatr. 1936;36:675–738.
4. Dick W. Martin Kirschner: 1879–1942—a surgeon in prehospital care. Resuscitation. 2006;68(3):319–21.
5. Gildenberg P. The history of stereotactic neurosurgery. Neurosurg Clin N Am. 1990;1:765–80.
6. Lozano AL, Gildenberg PL, Tasker RR. Textbook of stereotactic functional neurosurgery. 2nd ed. Berlin Heidelberg: Springer-Verlag; 2009. p. 67.
7. Beckmann EC. CT scanning the early days. Br J Radiol. 2006;79(937):5–8.
8. Thwaites DI, Tuohy JB. Back to the future: the history and development of the clinical linear accelerator. Phys Med Biol. 2006;51:R343–62.
9. Betti OO, Derechinsky YE. Irradiations stereotaxiques multifaisceaux. Neurochirurgie. 1982;28:55–6.
10. Schlegel W, Pastry O, Bortfeld T, et al. Computer systems and mechanical tools for stereotactically guided conformation therapy with linear accelerators. Int J Radiat Oncol Biol Phys. 1992;24:781–7.
11. Roberts DW, Strohbehn JW, Hatch JF, et al. A frameless stereotaxic integration of computerized tomographic imaging and the operating microscope. J Neurosurg. 1986;64:545–9.
12. Selvik G. Roentgen stereophotogrammetric analysis. Acta Radiol. 1990;31:113–26.
13. Yenice KM, Lovelock DM, Hunt MA, et al. CT image-guided intensity modulated therapy for paraspinal tumors using stereotactic immobilization. Int J Radiat Oncol Biol Phys. 2003;55:583–93.
14. Pereira EAC, Green AL, Nandi D, Aziz TZ. History of stereotactic surgery in Great Britain. In: Lozano AL, Gildenberg PL, Tasker RR, editors. Textbook of stereotactic functional neurosurgery. 2nd ed. Berlin Heidelberg: Springer-Verlag; 2009. p. 67.

Part I
Clinical Overview: Brain Metastases

Brain Metastases: Introduction

Mihir Naik, Joycelin F. Canavan,
and Samuel T. Chao

Case Vignette

A 54-year-old woman with a history of left-sided breast cancer, initial stage T1cN2M0, presented with dizziness and gait imbalance 4 years after treatment of her breast cancer. Her tumor originally was estrogen receptor (ER) positive, progesterone receptor (PR) positive, and Her2 amplified, and she was treated with chemotherapy, modified radical mastectomy with reconstruction, and postmastectomy chest wall radiation. She also was treated with 1 year of trastuzumab. Originally, her symptoms were thought to be due to hypertension, but because her symptoms became worse, she went to the emergency room. CT revealed a large right-sided cerebellar mass. Her diagnostic MRI is shown in Fig. 2.1. She underwent a gross total resection following her resection, confirming metastatic adenocarcinoma, but ER was negative, PR negative, and TTF-1 negative. Restaging CT was negative for any extracranial metastasis.

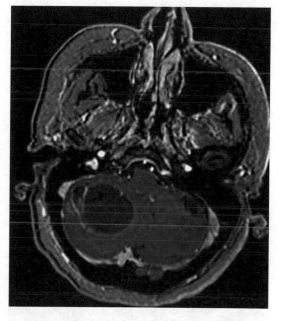

Fig. 2.1 Axial postcontrast T1 MRI showing right-sided cerebellar mass

M. Naik
Department of Radiation Oncology, Maroone Cancer Center, Cleveland Clinic Florida, Weston, FL, USA

J. F. Canavan
Department of Radiation Oncology, Taussig Cancer Institute, Cleveland Clinic, Cleveland, OH, USA

S. T. Chao (✉)
Department of Radiation Oncology, Rose Ella Burkhardt Brain Tumor and Neuro-Oncology Center, Cleveland Clinic, Cleveland, OH, USA
e-mail: CHAOS@ccf.org

Based on her original breast cancer histology, her median survival using the Diagnosis-Specific Graded Prognostic Assessment (DS-GPA) score is 25.3 months. Accounting for the loss of ER and PR positivity within her brain metastasis, it decreases to 15.1 months. Postoperative management of her resected brain metastasis was discussed, specifically stereotactic radiosurgery (SRS) to the resection cavity versus whole-brain radiation (WBRT). She elected to proceed with

WBRT and received 37.5 Gy over 15 fractions. Aside from some facial swelling post radiation, serous otitis, and hair loss, she did well without major long-term sequela from her WBRT, except mild imbalance, mild intermittent fatigue, and mild short-term memory and word finding difficulty. She was placed on anastrozole by her medical oncologist. She remains alive without evidence of systemic or intracranial progression 7 years after her diagnosis of brain metastasis. Figure 2.2 shows her follow-up MRI 7 years later. She continues to work as an interior decorator.

Although the diagnosis of brain metastasis typically portends a poor prognosis and well-established prognostic scales predicted her survival to be a few years at best, long-term survivors do exist. Despite this case being an outlier, prognostic scales do help predict, in general, who is likely to do well and who is likely to do poorly, which may help guide treatment. This chapter reviews the epidemiology and predictive scales that exist for brain metastases.

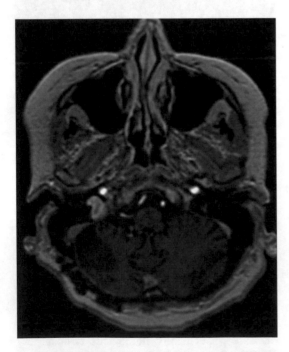

Fig. 2.2 Axial postcontrast T1 MRI showing stable resected cavity 7 years after her craniotomy and whole-brain radiotherapy

Epidemiology

Brain metastases are the most common intracranial tumors in adults, with the majority developing in the context of known primary or metastatic disease. In patients with solid tumors, brain metastases occur in 10–30% of adults and 3–13% of children [1–4].

The incidence may be increasing, due to both improved detection of small metastases by magnetic resonance imaging (MRI) which leads to early diagnosis and better control of extracranial disease resulting from improved systemic treatment regimens [3, 4].

The incidence of metastatic brain tumors which is estimated to be around 7–14 persons per 100,000 population is derived from population-based studies which typically underestimate the true incidence [5].

Risk Factors

In adults, the most common primary tumors responsible for brain metastases include lung, breast, kidney, colorectal cancers, and melanoma [4]. In children, the most common sources of brain metastases are sarcomas, neuroblastoma, and germ cell tumors [3, 6, 7].

Lung Cancer

Lung cancer is the most common primary malignancy that results in brain metastases, with adenocarcinomas accounting for over half of all brain metastases [3, 8]. Approximately 30–43% of patients develop brain metastases alone with no evidence of disease elsewhere [9]. In a large series of 975 patients with stage I/II non-small-cell lung cancer (NSCLC), the risk factors associated with developing brain metastases were younger age, larger tumor size, lymphovascular space invasion, and hilar lymph node involvement [8].

Small-cell lung cancer (SCLC) is characterized by early metastases with the brain being the most common site of metastases with a cumulative incidence of over 50% at 2 years [10]. At initial diagnosis, asymptomatic brain metastases are found in 15% of patients on MRI imaging [11]. With prophylactic cranial irradiation (PCI), the risk of developing brain metastases can be reduced from 59% to 33% at 3 years and is accompanied by a survival benefit (21% versus 15%) [10].

Breast Cancer

Among women with breast cancer, the incidence of brain metastasis is particularly high in patients with lung metastases, those with hormone receptor-negative tumors, and those who are positive for human epidermal growth factor receptor 2 (HER2) overexpression [12, 13]. In one series, 30% of patients presenting with lung metastases as first site of relapse subsequently developed a brain relapse [12].

In a cohort study of 1434 women treated with breast-conserving therapy plus systemic chemotherapy, the overall 5-year cumulative incidence of brain metastases differed by breast cancer subtype: 0.1% for luminal A, 3.3% for luminal B, 3.2% for luminal HER2, 3.7% for HER2, and 7.4% for triple negative/basal-like subtype [14].

A high incidence of central nervous system (CNS) metastases (34%) was found among patients treated with trastuzumab for stage 1V breast cancer [15]. It is felt that the higher rate of CNS events is probably related to increased survival of patients with improved systemic therapies and the lack of trastuzumab penetration into the central nervous system [16].

Renal Cell Cancer (RCC)

Brain metastases occur in 2–10% of patients with recurrent RCC and are often symptomatic in 80% or more of cases [3]. Brain metastases from RCC are also unique in the high incidence of associated hemorrhage, demonstrated by neurosurgical series from Memorial Sloan-Kettering Cancer

Center (MSKCC), showing that intratumoral hemorrhage was seen in 46% of all patients with brain metastases from RCC [17].

Colorectal Cancer

The incidence of brain metastases in metastatic colorectal cancer is around 2.3% in one series [18]. Brain metastases are usually a late-stage phenomenon, and the vast majority of patients have metastases in other sites, particularly lung [18]. Although tumors mostly metastasize to the supratentorial region, up to 40% of patients had cerebellar metastases, with isolated cerebellar metastases occurring in 23% of all patients [18].

Melanoma

Melanoma is the third most frequent cause of brain metastases, accounting for 6–11% of all metastatic brain lesions [3]. Cutaneous melanomas of the head and neck are more likely to develop brain metastases [19] and are also commonly associated with hemorrhage in up to 40% of patients [19, 20]. Eighty percent of melanoma brain metastases are supratentorial, while 15% are infratentorial or leptomeningeal, and 5% are located in the brainstem [21].

Pathophysiology

The most common mechanism of metastasis to the brain is by hematogenous spread because the CNS lacks lymphatic drainage [22]. Metastases are usually located at the junction of the gray/white matter and watershed areas where blood vessels decrease in diameter and act as a trap for clumps of tumor cells [23, 24]. This type of spread is referred to as parenchymal brain metastases and is the most common presentation of brain metastases. Figure 2.3 is an axial MRI with contrast consistent with parenchymal brain metastasis. The distribution of metastases generally parallels blood flow [23]:

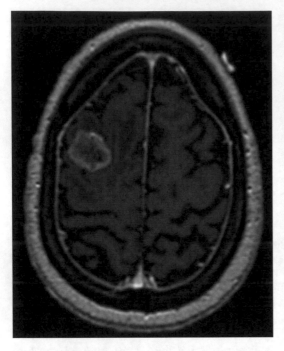

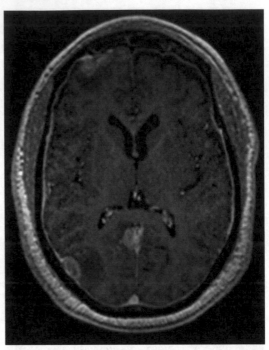

Fig. 2.3 Axial T1 MRI with contrast of parenchymal brain metastasis

Fig. 2.4 Axial T1 MRI with contrast of dural-based brain metastasis

- Cerebral hemispheres – approximately 80%
- Cerebellum – 15%
- Brainstem – 5%

Brain metastases can also develop on the dura (dural-based brain metastasis) and lepto-meninges (leptomeningeal brain metastases). Leptomeningeal brain metastasis is associated with poor prognosis, given limited treatment options. Figures 2.4 and 2.5 show axial MR imaging of a patient with dural-based metasta-ses and leptomeningeal disease, respectively.

Clinical Features

Although brain metastases should be suspected in any cancer patient who develops neurologic symptoms or behavioral abnormalities, multiple other causes can also be responsible. In an analysis of over 800 cancer patients evaluated for neurologic symptoms, only 16% had brain metastases [25].

The most common symptoms at presentation include headache (50%), focal weakness (40%), altered mental status (30%), seizures (15%), and

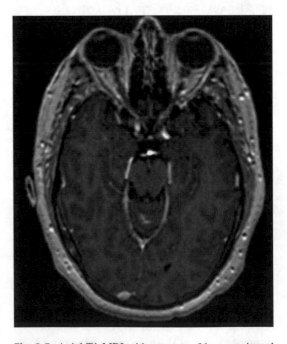

Fig. 2.5 Axial T1 MRI with contrast of leptomeningeal brain metastasis (see linear enhancement in cerebellum)

ataxia (10%), which tend to worsen with time as the tumor grows and the surrounding edema exerts a mass effect on nearby structures [26].

Symptoms usually evolve over a period of days or several weeks. In contrast to tension-type headaches, brain tumor headaches were worse with bending over in 32%, and nausea or vomiting was present in 40% [27]. Worsening headache may also follow maneuvers that raise intrathoracic pressure, such as coughing, sneezing, or the Valsalva maneuver, and metastases with associated hemorrhage can also contribute to acute neurologic symptoms [26, 27].

Diagnosis

Brain metastases are more commonly diagnosed in patients with known malignancy; however, up to 30% of brain metastases are diagnosed either at the time of or prior to primary tumor discovery [28]. While a CT brain is often used as initial screening examination in patients who present with acute neurologic symptoms, gadolinium-enhanced MRI is the best diagnostic test to detect brain metastases. Metastases are usually isodense or hypodense compared with brain tissue on non-contrast CT studies and demonstrate enhancement following administration of contrast [29]. Acute hemorrhage results in increased intensity on noncontrast CT studies [29]. However, the most common patterns observed on imaging are solid or rim enhancement with a central cystic nonenhancing region on a CT brain with contrast. The cystic areas may arise due to keratin deposits in squamous cell carcinoma, necrosis, or mucin secretion in adenocarcinoma [26].

Radiographic features that can help differentiate brain metastases from other CNS lesions include the presence of multiple lesions, localization at the junction of the gray and white matter, circumscribed margins, and ring enhancement with prominent peritumoral edema [28].

T1 precontrast MRI images can detect subacute hemorrhage, which is evident as a hyperintense signal. Melanin, fat, and protein can also demonstrate bright signal on noncontrast T1-weighted images [29]. T2-weighted sequences can detect hemorrhage or melanin, which appears as a decreased signal and is occasionally the only abnormality that brain metastasis from melanoma seen on MRI [29]. Peritumoral edema is also best evaluated on T2-weighted images, especially the fluid-attenuated inversion recovery (FLAIR) sequence, where the cerebrospinal fluid signal is suppressed, resulting in increased conspicuity of hyperintensity adjacent to ventricles and sulci.

Susceptibility-weighted imaging is a high-resolution gradient echo MRI sequence that has an increased ability to detect blood products and venous structures, and this technique is currently being explored for its ability to identify additional internal characteristics of brain tumors [28, 29].

Tissue biopsy confirmation should be performed when the diagnosis of brain metastases is in doubt, especially in patients with a solitary lesion. Positron emission tomography (PET) may also be useful in these patients, either by identifying the primary tumor or other sites of metastatic disease that can be biopsied more readily. Advanced MRI sequences such as diffusion, perfusion, and spectroscopy can also provide complementary information and help differentiate metastatic lesions from primary brain tumors or other nonneoplastic conditions, such as abscesses, ischemia, and radiation necrosis [28].

Prognostic Factors

While the development of brain metastases is common, there is tremendous heterogeneity in terms of prognosis for patients who develop brain metastases. Several prognostic systems have been designed and later refined for clinicians and patients to better understand their prognosis and help select and stratify patients for clinical trials [30].

One of the first prognostic factors for patients with brain metastases was the recursive partitioning analysis (RPA). This retrospective analysis of three Radiation Therapy Oncology Group (RTOG) trials conducted between 1979 and 1993 included 1200 patients, which used Karnofsky Performance Status (KPS), age, control of the primary tumor, and the status of extracranial disease to predict overall survival (Table 2.1) [31]. Patients were divided into three classes: class I included patients with a KPS score of ≥70, age

Table 2.1 Recursive partitioning analysis (RPA)

	RPA
Class I	Age <65, KPS ≥70
	Controlled primary tumor
	No extracranial metastases
Class II	All patients not in class I or III
Class III	KPS <70

From Sperduto et al. [37]. Reprinted with permission from Elsevier

Abbreviations: *RPA* recursive partitioning analysis, *KPS* Karnofsky Performance Status

<65 years, controlled primary tumor, and no extracranial metastases (ECM); class III included patients with a KPS score of <70; and class II included all other patients. Approximately 20%, 65%, and 15% of the patients were in classes I, II, and III, respectively. Notably although the trials used for analysis did not include patients with small-cell lung cancer (SCLC), there was a subsequent analysis of patients with SCLC confirming the validity of RPA in this patient population [32]. There were several limitations of the RPA classification for prognostication, including the definition of class III patients which included all patients with a KPS <70 but did not account for different patient characteristics, including extent of systemic disease, number of brain metastases, and different histologies.

In order to better understand prognostic factors for patients with brain metastases treated with stereotactic radiosurgery (SRS), a Score Index for Radiosurgery (SIR) was created. The SIR is the sum of scores (0–2) for each of five prognostic factors: age, KPS, extracranial disease status, number of brain lesions, and largest brain lesion volume [33]. However, the detailed workup needed to assess the systemic disease limited the wide spread use of this prognostic index [34]. Lorenzoni et al. published another prognostic index called the Basic Score for Brain Metastases (BSBM), which aimed to simplify the scoring system. The BSBM included only three factors: KPS, control of primary tumor, and presence of extracranial disease [35].

However, there were several limitations to the RPA, SIR, and BSBM to give an easy and less subjective prognosis in the setting of brain metastasis. For example, the RPA and BSBM did not

account for the number of metastases, and the RPA, BSBM, and SIR require an estimation of control of systemic disease which can be inconsistent. Furthermore, the SIR required treatment factors such as the volume of the largest lesion at the time of radiosurgery, making it difficult to use the prognostic index to predict outcome before any treatment decisions are made. Also around this time, the results of RTOG 9508 which was a randomized trial looking to evaluate patients treated with a SRS boost after whole-brain radiotherapy showed that the number of brain metastases was prognostic for survival [36].

Thus, in 2008, Sperduto et al. published a new prognostic index called the Graded Prognostic Assessment (GPA) that could eliminate components in the other indices that can be subjective such as the control of extracranial disease, as well as account for the number of metastases being prognostic for overall survival in patients with brain metastasis [36, 37]. The GPA used data from 1960 patients with brain metastases from five randomized trials and was found to be more prognostic than other indices. The GPA used four factors: age, KPS, number of metastases, and ECM that affect prognosis in brain metastases. Each factor was given a score of 0, 0.5, or 1.0, and GPA was calculated from a cumulative score of all four factors. The GPA had four different groups: a GPA of 0–1 was associated with a median survival of 2.6 months; GPA of 1.5–2.5 with a median survival of 3.8 months; GPA of 3.0 with a median survival of 6.9 months, and GPA of 3.5–4.0 with a median survival of 11 months. The GPA was less subjective, was easy to use, and became a commonly used prognostic index in clinical practice (Table 2.2).

It had long been suggested that prognostic systems will vary by primary diagnosis and that site-specific prognostic systems should be developed [38]. A multi-institutional retrospective analysis of patients from 11 institutions looked at 4259 patients treated with brain metastases from 1985 to 2007 with the aim to identify disease-specific prognostic factors [39]. This led to the development of the Diagnosis-Specific Graded Prognostic Assessment (DS-GPA) (Tables 2.3 and 2.4). This showed that prognostic factors

Table 2.2 Graded Prognostic Assessment (GPA)

Prognostic factor	GPA scoring criteria		
	0	0.5	1.0
Age	>60	50–60	<50
KPS	<70	70–80	90–100
ECM	Present	–	Absent
No. of BMs	>3	2–3	1

GPA	Median survival (months)
0–1.0	2.6
1.5–2.5	3.8
3	6.9
3.5–4	11.0

From Sperduto et al. [37]. Reprinted with permission from Elsevier

Abbreviations: *GPA* Graded Prognostic Assessment, *KPS* Karnofsky Performance Status, *ECM* extracranial metastases, *BMs* brain metastases

Table 2.4 Median survival stratified by diagnosis and Diagnosis-Specific GPA score for patients with newly diagnosed BMs

Diagnosis	DS-GPA median survival (months)				
	Overall	0–1.0	1.5–2.5	3.0	3.5–4.0
NSCLC	7	3.0	6.5	11.3	14.8
SCLC	4.9	2.8	5.3	9.6	17.1
Melanoma	6.7	3.4	4.7	8.8	13.2
Renal cell carcinoma	9.6	3.3	7.3	11.3	14.8
Breast cancer	11.9	6.1	9.4	16.9	18.7
GI cancer	5.4	3.1	4.4	6.9	13.5

From Sperduto et al. [39]. Reprinted with permission from Elsevier

Abbreviations: *NSCLC* non–small-cell lung cancer, *SCLC* small-cell lung cancer, *DS-GPA* Diagnosis-Specific Graded Prognostic Assessment, *GI* gastrointestinal, *BM* brain metastases

Table 2.3 Definition of Diagnosis-Specific Graded Prognostic Assessment indexes for patients with newly diagnosed brain metastases

	Prognostic factor	DS-GPA scoring criteria				
NSCLC/SCLC		0	0.5	1.0		
	Age	>60	50–60	<50	–	–
	KPS	<70	70–80	90–100	–	–
	ECM	Present	–	Absent	–	–
	No. of BM	>3	2–3	1	–	–
Melanoma/renal cell cancer						
		0	1	2		
	KPS	<70	70–80	90–100	–	–
	No. of BM	>3	2–3	1	–	–
Breast/GI cancer		0	1	2	3	4
	KPS	<70	70	80	90	100

From Sperduto et al. [39]. Reprinted with permission from Elsevier

looking at overall survival also varied by diagnosis. For example, non-small-cell lung cancer (NSCLC) and SCLC prognostic factors include KPS, age, ECM, and number of metastases. For melanoma and renal cell cancer, the only significant prognostic factors were KPS and number of brain metastases. For breast and gastrointestinal cancer, the only significant prognostic factor was the KPS.

Further studies were performed to better determine prognosis in patients with brain metastasis with different primary diagnosis. For example, it is well known that breast cancer patients with certain histological subtypes such as an overexpression of human growth factor receptor 2 (HER2) and estrogen receptor (ER) negativity

are more associated with the development of brain metastases [40–42]. While the original DS-GPA only found KPS to be a prognostic factor in patients with breast cancer, a refined analysis of the existing breast cancer-specific GPA index (Breast-GPA) was performed by analyzing a larger sample of patients with additional variables including HER2 and ER/PR status [43]. The study was significant in showing that genetic subtypes of breast cancer had significant prognostic implications in patients with breast cancer. The basal subtype (ER/PR negative and HER2 negative) patients were associated with the shortest survival, whereas patients with the luminal B subtype (ER/PR positive and HER2 positive) had the best survival. This study clearly demonstrated the variation in prognosis in different subgroups of patients with breast cancer and brain metastases. The median survival for patients with a Breast-GPA of 0.5–1.0 is only 3.4 months versus 25.3 months in patients with a Breast-GPA of 3.5–4.0. Also ECM and number of brain metastases were not determined to be prognostic (Table 2.5) [43]. Newer trials have also shown effectiveness of systemic therapies in the management of brain metastasis, for example, the LANDSCAPE trial showed an intracranial response of 66% when using lapatinib and capecitabine as first-line combination therapy prior to radiation [44]. Furthermore, other studies are looking at the activity of T-DM1 specifically in HER2-positive breast cancer and give clinicians additional treatment options offering clinical activity in brain metastases [45].

Given the high incidence of brain metastases in patients with NSCLC, efforts were made to refine prognosis in the setting of brain metastasis as studies showed that patients with gene alterations (epidermal growth factor receptor (EGFR) and anaplastic lymphoma kinase (ALK) alterations) have a markedly improved survival [46–48]. Sperduto et al. published an update of the DS-GPA for patients with lung cancer using molecular markers (Lung-molGPA) [49]. This new Lung-molGPA was associated with improved prognostic ability over both the RTOG RPA and the original DS-GPA by incorporating

the effect of EGFR and ALK gene alterations on survival in patients with NSCLC and brain metastases. For example, while only 4% of participants had a Lung-molGPA score of 3.5–4.0, the median survival in this group was nearly 4 years (Table 2.6). The results validating the Lung-molGPA were also validated in other large data sets in different patient populations [50]. Furthermore, better targeted therapies for EGFR mutation–positive NSCLC and ALK+ NSCLC are expected to continue to improve prognosis for selected NSCLC patients with brain metastasis. For example, while it is known that first-generation EGFR tyrosine kinase inhibitors (TKIs) have moderate activity in brain metastases, newer EGFR inhibitors such as afatinib and osimertinib show increased activity in patients with brain metastases as well as appear to reduce the risk of CNS metastasis [51]. For example, in a recent phase III study, osimertinib showed that in patients who were evaluable for CNS response, the CNS ORR was 70% with osimertinib and the drug has shown superior CNS efficacy vs chemotherapy (platinum pemetrexed in T790M-positive advanced NSCLC) [52]. Other studies have shown that in patients with ALK+

Table 2.5 Graded Prognostic Assessment (GPA) index for women with breast cancer and brain metastases

Prognostic factor	Breast-GPA scoring criteria				
	0.0	0.5	1.0	1.5	2
KPS	≤50	60	70–80	90–100	–
Genetic subtype	Basal	–	Luminal A	HER2	Luminal B
Age (yr)	≥60	<60	–	–	

Breast-GPA	Median survival (months)
0–1.0	3.4
1.5–2.0	7.7
2.5–3.0	15.1
3.5–4.0	25.3

From Sperduto et al. [43]. Reprinted with permission from Elsevier
Abbreviations: *Breast-GPA* Breast Graded Prognostic Assessment, *HER2* human growth factor receptor 2

Table 2.6 Graded Prognostic Assessment for lung cancer using molecular markers (Lung-molGPA)

Prognostic factor	Lung-molGPA scoring criteria		
	0	0.5	1.0
Age	≥70	<70	NA
KPS	<70	80	90–100
ECM	Present		Absent
No. of BM	>4	1–4	NA
Gene status	EGFR negative/ unknown	NA	EGFR positive or
	ALK Negative/unknown		ALK positive

GPA	Adenocarcinoma Median survival (months)	Nonadenocarcinoma Median survival (months)
0–1.0	6.9	5.3
1.5–2.0	13.7	9.8
2.5–3.0	26.5	12.8
3.5–4.0	46.8	

Data from Sperduto et al. [49]
Abbreviations: *KPS* Karnofsky Performance Status, *ECM* extracranial metastases, *BMs* brain metastases, *EGFR* epidermal growth factor receptor, *ALK* anaplastic lymphoma kinase

NSCLC, ALK inhibitors are effective in both pretreatment and previously treated patients with brain metastasis. In patients who are receiving ALK inhibitors in the first-line setting, the pooled intracranial overall response rate was 39.2% and pooled intracranial disease control rate was 70.3%. As CNS response rates for brain metastases continue to improve with targeted therapies, there has even been discussion in using these newer agents as an alternative to radiotherapy [53].

In a continued effort to improve prognostication of patients with different histological subtypes and brain metastases, a multi-institutional retrospective review of 711 patients with renal cell carcinoma (RCC) looked for clinical parameters to define evolving patterns of care and the effect of targeted therapies in a more contemporary group of patients. As was previously noted in the DS-GPA, the only prognostic factor for survival was KPS and number of brain metastases [43]. This study showed that while the existing renal GPA and the prognostic factors previously identified (KPS and number of BM) were confirmed, additional prognostic factors including age, ECM, and hemoglobin (Hgb) were found to refine prognostication in this larger more contemporary cohort.

Another common malignancy with a high incidence of brain metastases is malignant melanoma. Patients with a diagnosis of melanoma can have a lifetime incidence of developing metastases greater than 50% [54]. A study looking at the prognostic value of various mutations including BRAF, C-kit, and NRAS mutations in melanoma showed that BRAF-positive patients survive longer than BRAF-negative patients and overall survival has improved from 1985–2005 to 2006–2015 [55]. While the original melanoma-GPA found that only KPS and number of brain metastases were prognostic for survival [39], an updated melanoma-graded prognostic assessment (Melanoma-molGPA) showed that there were five significant prognostic factors for survival: age, KPS, ECM, number of brain metastases, and BRAF status (Table 2.7) [56]. This study showed that the median survival improved from 6.7 to 9.8 months between the two treatment eras,

Table 2.7 Graded Prognostic Assessment for Melanoma-molGPA

Prognostic factor	Melanoma-molGPA scoring criteria		
	0	0.5	1.0
Age	≥70	<70	
KPS	≤70	80	90–100
ECM	Present		Absent
No. of BM	>4	2–4	1
BRAF gene status	Negative/ unknown	Positive	

Melanoma-molGPA	Median survival (months)
0–1.0	4.9
1.5–2.0	8.3
2.5–3.0	15.8
3.5–4.0	34.1

From Sperduto et al. [56]. Reprinted with permission from Elsevier

Abbreviations: *BM* brain metastases, *ECM* extracranial metastases, *GPA* Graded Prognostic Assessment, *KPS* Karnofsky Performance Status, *MS* median survival by months

and the median survival times for patients with Melanoma-molGPA vary dramatically based on the Melanoma-molGPA. For example, those patients with a Melanoma-molGPA of 0–1.0 have a median survival of only 4.9 months vs nearly 34.1 months for patients with a Melanoma-molGPA of 3.5–4. Furthermore, given that nearly 50% of metastatic melanoma patients are BRAFV600 positive, it will be important to continue to refine prognosis as newer BRAF inhibitors, such as vemurafenib and dabrafenib, help improve intracranial response and get incorporated with radiation therapy to improve clinical outcomes [57, 58].

Given the complexities and variation in estimating prognosis for patients with brain metastasis, a user-friendly tool is available both online at www.brainmetgpa.com and as a smartphone app to provide clinicians a useful tool to accurately discuss and predict prognosis for patients. As our understanding of the biology behind brain metastasis continues to improve and novel agents with improved CNS penetration are being investigated, prognostic factors will continue to be refined and clinical outcomes will likely continue to improve for patients with brain metastases.

Areas of Uncertainty/Future Directions

As reviewed, molecular pathology is recognized to be important in predicting survival. EGFR, ALK, and BRAF gene alterations allow for additional targeted agents that lead to improved systemic and brain control, resulting in improved overall survival. As more molecular targets are identified and targeted agents are developed, these prognostic scales will need to be revised constantly. For instance, the use of TKIs increased overall survival, but when given concurrently, it may increase toxicity [59]. Thus, prognostication will continue to be a subject of ongoing investigation. Regardless, what we have learned historically will continue to serve as a guide moving forward.

Similarly, as will be discussed in future chapters, we need to understand how to use these prognostic scales and molecular factors to optimize how we manage brain metastases. Although crudely we may consider treatment like supportive care and WBRT for patients with poor prognoses, we will need to define how to manage patients with good prognoses, including consideration of systemic therapy options, along with the traditional options of surgery, SRS, and perhaps WBRT [59]. We may need to think beyond survival and consider the natural history of the disease, including local and distant recurrence. Ayala-Peacock and colleagues developed a nomogram to predict for distant brain failure (DBF) [60]. This is particularly important as the decision to add WBRT as opposed to SRS alone requires us to understand the likelihood of DBF; specifically, one may consider WBRT with patients at high risk of DBF. Interestingly, in this study by Ayala-Peacock et al., it is not just the number of brain metastases, histology, and status and burden of extracranial disease that predict for DBF, but also marginal dose. Total brain metastasis volume appears to be more predictive than number of brain metastases, as nicely shown by Routman et al. and other studies [61]. These results suggest that the choice of therapy should not be based on number as we have done historically but by intracranial burden of disease.

Also, how patients present with their disease may also impact their prognosis. For instance, someone with synchronous development of their brain metastases may have different prognoses compared to someone who developed brain metastases some time out from their cancer diagnosis. Synchronous disease may suggest more aggressive disease upfront. Woody and colleagues looked specifically at patients with synchronous brain metastases in NSCLC and were able to validate the DS-GPA for this group of patients [62]. We need to confirm that this is similar for other histologies.

Finally, prognostication may not just focus on natural history of disease, specifically overall survival and recurrence but also focus on the development of toxicity including neurocognitive changes and radiation necrosis. Molecular pathology may also predict the risk of radiation necrosis and Miller et al. showed that in their study of 1939 patients (5747 lesions). Her2-amplification, BRAF 600+ mutation, lung adenocarcinoma histology, and ALK rearrangement, which all typically are associated with improved survival, were also predictors of radiation necrosis [63]. The choice of therapy may also be influenced by predicting toxicity, in addition to overall survival and tumor control.

Kotecha and colleagues likewise suggested that for small brain metastases defined as <0.5 cm in diameter, dose may be reduced from 24 Gy, the prescription dose set forth by RTOG. Specifically, EGFR-mutated, luminal A breast, and BRAF-mutated melanoma may not have much a detriment in local control when dose is de-escalated. Here, prognostic factors may have an even more effect on just choice of therapy, but even radiation doses used. Radiogenomics and machine learning are at the forefront of this effort [64], and in time, we may use this to personalize the radiation doses used to treat our patients, which may lead to further improvements in overall survival or decreased toxicity for patients with brain metastases. Although rare, brain metastases patients can live 10 years or more from brain metastases [65].

Prognostication will need to go beyond standard clinical factors, and now consider molecular pathology, brain metastases volume, and treatment factors including systemic therapy and radiation dose. In doing so, we can move into an era of personalized medicine.

Conclusion

Brain metastasis is the most frequent neurological complication of cancer. The incidence is increasing due to more routine use of MRI for staging, as well as longer survival from their cancer. Prognostication, which historically has focused on clinical features, now needs to incorporate molecular features and treatment. Prognostic systems will constantly need updating and refining.

Key Points

- Brain metastasis is the most common intracranial tumor in adults.
- MRI is the best imaging technique for diagnosis.
- Diagnosis-Specific GPA is now incorporating molecular pathology, specifically with breast and non-small-cell lung cancer, and melanoma.
- Prognostic systems will continue to be refined by including other clinical data, treatment factors including the use of systemic agents, and additional molecular pathology.

References

1. Jyoti B, Alam A, Hofer S, Brada M. Brain metastases. In: Lisak R, Truong D, Carroll W, Bhidarasiri R, eds. International neurology. 2nd ed. Hoboken, NJ: Wiley; 2016.
2. Stelzer KJ. Epidemiology and prognosis of brain metastases. Surg Neurol Int. 2013;4(Suppl 4):S192–202.
3. Nayak L, Lee EQ, Wen P. Epidemiology of brain metastases. Curr Oncol Rep. 2012;14:48–54.
4. Tabouret E, Chinot O, Metellus P, et al. Recent trends in epidemiology of brain metastases: an overview. Anticancer Res. 2012;32:4655–62.
5. Fox BD, Cheung VJ, Patel AJ, Suki D, Rao G. Epidemiology of metastatic brain tumors. Neurosurg Clin N Am. 2011;22:1–6.
6. Graus F, Walker RW, Allen JC. Brain metastases in children. J Pediatr. 1983;103(4):558.
7. Bouffet E, Doumi N, Thiesse P, Mottolese C, Jouvet A, Lacroze M, et al. Brain metastases in children with solid tumors. Cancer. 1997;79(2):403–10.
8. Hubbs JL, Boyd JA, Hollis D, Chino JP, Saynak M, Kelsey CR. Factors associated with the development of brain metastases: analysis of 975 patients with early stage nonsmall cell lung cancer. Cancer. 2010;116(21):5038–46.
9. Shi AA, Digumarthy SR, Temel JS, Halpern EF, Kuester LB, Aquino SL. Does initial staging or tumor histology better identify asymptomatic brain metastases in patients with non–small cell lung cancer. J Thorac Oncol. 2006;1(3):205–10.
10. Aupérin A, Arriagada R, Pignon J-P, Le Péchoux C, Gregor A, Stephens RJ, et al. Prophylactic cranial irradiation for patients with small-cell lung cancer in complete remission. Prophylactic Cranial Irradiation Overview Collaborative Group. N Engl J Med. 1999;341(7):476–84.
11. Hochstenbag M, Twijnstra A, Wilmink J, Wouters E, Ten Velde GPM. Asymptomatic brain metastases (BM) in small cell lung cancer (SCLC): MR-imaging is useful at initial diagnosis. J Neuro-Oncol. 2000;48(3):243–8.
12. Slimane K, Andre F, Delaloge S, Dunant A, Perez A, Grenier J, et al. Risk factors for brain relapse in patients with metastatic breast cancer. Ann Oncol. 2004;15(11):1640–4.
13. Crivellari D, Pagani O, Veronesi A, Lombardi D, Nole F, Thurlimann B, et al. High incidence of central nervous system involvement in patients with metastatic or locally advanced breast cancer treated with epirubicin and docetaxel. Ann Oncol. 2001;12(3):353–6.
14. Arvold ND, Oh KS, Niemierko A, Taghian AG, Lin NU, Abi-Raad RF, et al. Brain metastases after breast-conserving therapy and systemic therapy: incidence and characteristics by biologic subtype. Breast Cancer Res Treat. 2012;136(1):153–60.
15. Pestalozzi BC, Zahrieh D, Price KN, Holmberg SB, Lindtner J, Collins J, et al. Identifying breast cancer patients at risk for central nervous system (CNS) metastases in trials of the International Breast Cancer Study Group (IBCSG). Ann Oncol. 2006;17(6):935–44.
16. Lin NU, Winer EP. Brain metastases: the HER2 paradigm. Clin Cancer Res. 2007;13(6):1648–55.
17. Wronski M, Arbit E, Russo P, Galicich JH. Surgical resection of brain metastases from renal cell carcinoma in 50 patients. Urology. 1996;47(2):187–93.
18. Mongan JP, Fadul CE, Cole BF, Zaki BI, Suriawinata AA, Ripple GH, et al. Brain metastases from colorectal cancer: risk factors, incidence, and the possible role of chemokines. Clin Colorectal Cancer. 2009;8(2):100–5.
19. Daryanani D, Plukker JT, de Jong MA, Haaxma-Reiche H, Nap R, Kuiper H, et al. Increased incidence of brain metastases in cutaneous head and neck melanoma. Melanoma Res. 2005;15(2):119–24.

20. Wronski M, Arbit E. Surgical treatment of brain metastases from melanoma: a retrospective study of 91 patients. J Neurosurg. 2000;93(1):9–18.
21. Sloan AE, Nock CJ, Einstein DB. Diagnosis and treatment of melanoma brain metastasis: a literature review. Cancer Control. 2009;16(3):248–55.
22. Gavrilovic IT, Posner JB. Brain metastases: epidemiology and pathophysiology. J Neuro-Oncol. 2005;75(1):5–14.
23. Delattre JY, Krol G, Thaler HT, Posner JB. Distribution of brain metastases. Arch Neurol. 1988;45(7):741–4.
24. Hwang TL, Close TP, Grego JM, Brannon WL, Gonzales F. Predilection of brain metastasis in gray and white matter junction and vascular border zones. Cancer. 1996;77(8):1551–5.
25. Clouston PD, DeAngelis LM, Posner JB. The spectrum of neurological disease in patients with systemic cancer. Ann Neurol. 1992;31(3):268–73.
26. Sneed PK, Kased N, Huang K, Rubenstein JL. Chapter 52: brain metastases and neoplastic meningitis. In: Abeloff MD, Armitage JO, Niederhuber JE, Kastan MB, WG MK, editors. Clinical oncology. Philadelphia: Churchill Livingstone; 2008. p. 827–41.
27. Forsyth PA, Posner JB. Headaches in patients with brain tumors: a study of 111 patients. Neurology. 1993;43(9):1678–83.
28. Nowosielski M, Radbruch A. The emerging role of advanced neuroimaging techniques for brain metastases. Chin Clin Oncol. 2015;4(2):23.
29. Bashour SI, William WN, Patel S, Rao G, Strom E, McAleer MF, et al. Brain metastasis from solid tumors. In: Brain Metastases from Primary Tumors: Epidemiology, Biology, and Therapy. Vol. 2. Cambridge, MA: Elsevier; 2015.
30. Venur VA, Ahluwalia MS. Prognostic scores for brain metastasis patients: use in clinical practice and trial design. Chin Clin Oncol. 2015;4(2):18.
31. Gaspar L, Scott C, Rotman M, Asbell S, Phillips T, Wasserman T, et al. Recursive partitioning analysis (RPA) of prognostic factors in three Radiation Therapy Oncology Group (RTOG) brain metastases trials. Int J Radiat Oncol Biol Phys. 1997;37(4):745–51.
32. Videtic GM, Adelstein DJ, Mekhail TM, Rice TW, Stevens GH, Lee SY, et al. Validation of the RTOG recursive partitioning analysis (RPA) classification for small-cell lung cancer-only brain metastases. Int J Radiat Oncol Biol Phys. 2007;67(1):240–3.
33. Weltman E, Salvajoli JV, Brandt RA, de Morais Hanriot R, Prisco FE, Cruz JC, et al. Radiosurgery for brain metastases: a score index for predicting prognosis. Int J Radiat Oncol Biol Phys. 2000;46(5):1155–61.
34. Nieder C, Mehta MP. Prognostic indices for brain metastases–usefulness and challenges. Radiat Oncol. 2009;4:10.
35. Lorenzoni J, Devriendt D, Massager N, David P, Ruiz S, Vanderlinden B, et al. Radiosurgery for treatment of brain metastases: estimation of patient eligibility using three stratification systems. Int J Radiat Oncol Biol Phys. 2004;60(1):218–24.
36. Andrews DW, Scott CB, Sperduto PW, Flanders AE, Gaspar LE, Schell MC, et al. Whole brain radiation therapy with or without stereotactic radiosurgery boost for patients with one to three brain metastases: phase III results of the RTOG 9508 randomised trial. Lancet. 2004;363(9422):1665–72.
37. Sperduto PW, Berkey B, Gaspar LE, Mehta M, Curran W. A new prognostic index and comparison to three other indices for patients with brain metastases: an analysis of 1,960 patients in the RTOG database. Int J Radiat Oncol Biol Phys. 2008;70(2):510–4.
38. Golden DW, Lamborn KR, McDermott MW, Kunwar S, Wara WM, Nakamura JL, et al. Prognostic factors and grading systems for overall survival in patients treated with radiosurgery for brain metastases: variation by primary site. J Neurosurg. 2008;109(Suppl):77–86.
39. Sperduto PW, Chao ST, Sneed PK, Luo X, Suh J, Roberge D, et al. Diagnosis-specific prognostic factors, indexes, and treatment outcomes for patients with newly diagnosed brain metastases: a multi-institutional analysis of 4,259 patients. Int J Radiat Oncol Biol Phys. 2010;77(3):655–61.
40. Bendell JC, Domchek SM, Burstein HJ, Harris L, Younger J, Kuter I, et al. Central nervous system metastases in women who receive trastuzumab-based therapy for metastatic breast carcinoma. Cancer. 2003;97(12):2972–7.
41. Gabos Z, Sinha R, Hanson J, Chauhan N, Hugh J, Mackey JR, et al. Prognostic significance of human epidermal growth factor receptor positivity for the development of brain metastasis after newly diagnosed breast cancer. J Clin Oncol. 2006;24(36):5658–63.
42. Tham YL, Sexton K, Kramer R, Hilsenbeck S, Elledge RJC. Primary breast cancer phenotypes associated with propensity for central nervous system metastases. Cancer. 2006;107(4):696–704.
43. Sperduto PW, Kased N, Roberge D, Xu Z, Shanley R, Luo X, et al. Effect of tumor subtype on survival and the graded prognostic assessment for patients with breast cancer and brain metastases. Int J Radiat Oncol Biol Phys. 2012;82(5):2111–7.
44. Bachelot T, Romieu G, Campone M, Dieras V, Cropet C, Dalenc F, et al. Lapatinib plus capecitabine in patients with previously untreated brain metastases from HER2-positive metastatic breast cancer (LANDSCAPE): a single-group phase 2 study. Lancet Oncol. 2013;14(1):64–71.
45. Bartsch R, Berghoff AS, Vogl U, Rudas M, Bergen E, Dubsky P, et al. Activity of T-DM1 in Her2-positive breast cancer brain metastases. Clin Exp Metastasis. 2015;32(7):729–37.
46. Sperduto PW, Yang TJ, Beal K, Pan H, Brown PD, Bangdiwala A, et al. The effect of gene alterations and tyrosine kinase inhibition on survival and cause of death in patients with adenocarcinoma of the lung and brain metastases. Int J Radiat Oncol Biol Phys. 2016;96(2):406–13.

47. Barnholtz-Sloan JS, Sloan AE, Davis FG, Vigneau FD, Lai P, Sawaya RE. Incidence proportions of brain metastases in patients diagnosed (1973 to 2001) in the Metropolitan Detroit Cancer Surveillance System. J Clin Oncol. 2004;22(14):2865–72.

48. Schouten LJ, Rutten J, Huveneers HA, Twijnstra A. Incidence of brain metastases in a cohort of patients with carcinoma of the breast, colon, kidney, and lung and melanoma. Cancer. 2002;94(10):2698–705.

49. Sperduto PW, Yang TJ, Beal K, Pan H, Brown PD, Bangdiwala A, et al. Estimating survival in patients with lung cancer and brain metastases: an update of the graded prognostic assessment for lung cancer using molecular markers (Lung-molGPA). JAMA Oncol. 2017;3(6):827–31.

50. Nieder C, Hintz M, Oehlke O, Bilger A, Grosu AL. Validation of the graded prognostic assessment for lung cancer with brain metastases using molecular markers (Lung-molGPA). Radiat Oncol. 2017;12(1):107.

51. Hochmair M. Medical treatment options for patients with epidermal growth factor receptor mutation-positive non-small cell lung cancer suffering from brain metastases and/or leptomeningeal disease. Target Oncol. 2018;13(3):269–85.

52. Wu YL, Ahn MJ, Garassino MC, Han JY, Katakami N, Kim HR, et al. CNS efficacy of osimertinib in patients with T790M-positive advanced non-small-cell lung cancer: data from a randomized phase III trial (AURA3). J Clin Oncol. 2018;36(26):2702–9.

53. Martinez P, Mak RH, Oxnard GR. Targeted therapy as an alternative to whole-brain radiotherapy in EGFR-mutant or ALK-positive non-small-cell lung cancer with brain metastases. JAMA Oncol. 2017;3(9):1274–5.

54. Davies MA, Liu P, McIntyre S, Kim KB, Papadopoulos N, Hwu WJ, et al. Prognostic factors for survival in melanoma patients with brain metastases. Cancer. 2011;117(8):1687–96.

55. Sperduto PW, Jiang W, Brown PD, Braunstein S, Sneed P, Wattson DA, et al. The prognostic value of BRAF, C-KIT, and NRAS mutations in melanoma patients with brain metastases. Int J Radiat Oncol Biol Phys. 2017;98(5):1069–77.

56. Sperduto PW, Jiang W, Brown PD, Braunstein S, Sneed P, Wattson DA, et al. Estimating survival in melanoma patients with brain metastases: an update of the graded prognostic assessment for melanoma using molecular markers (Melanoma-molGPA). Int J Radiat Oncol Biol Phys. 2017;99(4):812–6.

57. Long GV, Margolin KA. Multidisciplinary approach to brain metastasis from melanoma: the emerging role of systemic therapies. Am Soc Clin Oncol Educ Book. 2013;33(1):393–8.

58. Wolf A, Zia S, Verma R, Pavlick A, Wilson M, Golfinos JG, et al. Impact on overall survival of the combination of BRAF inhibitors and stereotactic radiosurgery in patients with melanoma brain metastases. J Neuro-Oncol. 2016;127(3):607–15.

59. Juloori A, Miller JA, Parsai S, Kotecha R, Ahluwalia MS, Mohammadi AM, et al. Overall survival and response to radiation and targeted therapies among patients with renal cell carcinoma brain metastases. J Neurosurg. 2019;1(aop):1–9.

60. Ayala-Peacock DN, Attia A, Braunstein SE, Ahluwalia MS, Hepel J, Chung C, et al. Prediction of new brain metastases after radiosurgery: validation and analysis of performance of a multi-institutional nomogram. J Neuro-Oncol. 2017;135(2):403–11.

61. Routman DM, Bian SX, Diao K, Liu JL, Yu C, Ye J, et al. The growing importance of lesion volume as a prognostic factor in patients with multiple brain metastases treated with stereotactic radiosurgery. Cancer Med. 2018;7(3):757–64.

62. Woody NM, Greer MD, Reddy CA, Videtic GMM, Chao ST, Murphy ES, et al. Validation of the disease-specific GPA for patients with 1 to 3 synchronous brain metastases in newly diagnosed NSCLC. Clin Lung Cancer. 2018;19(1):e141–e7.

63. Miller JA, Bennett EE, Xiao R, Kotecha R, Chao ST, Vogelbaum MA, et al. Association between radiation necrosis and tumor biology after stereotactic radiosurgery for brain metastasis. Int J Radiat Oncol Biol Phys. 2016;96(5):1060–9.

64. Kang J, Rancati T, Lee S, Oh JH, Kerns SL, Scott JG, et al. Machine learning and radiogenomics: lessons learned and future directions. Front Oncol. 2018;8:228.

65. Kotecha R, Vogel S, Suh JH, Barnett GH, Murphy ES, Reddy CA, et al. A cure is possible: a study of 10-year survivors of brain metastases. J Neuro-Oncol. 2016;129(3):545–55.

Radiobiology of Stereotactic Radiosurgery

3

Anuradha Thiagarajan and Yoshiya Yamada

Radiobiology of Stereotactic Radiosurgery

The advent of stereotactic radiosurgery (SRS) has revolutionized the practice of radiation oncology, perhaps nowhere more so than in the management of brain metastases. SRS is characterized by three key elements: (1) high doses per fraction (fraction sizes are typically 6 Gy or greater), (2) hypofractionation (1–5 fractions), and (3) high-precision targeting. The latter has been facilitated by technical advances in radiotherapy delivery with the advent of intensity-modulated radiation therapy (IMRT), which has the ability to create steep sculpted dose gradients between tumor and neighboring eloquent brain, as well as the development of sophisticated image-guided systems which assist in minimizing treatment errors associated with patient positioning.

In contrast to whole-brain radiation therapy which is associated with dismal local control rates, particularly in the setting of radioresistant tumors, SRS outcomes appear to be independent of the histologic subtype of the primary tumor. In fact, relatively radioresistant histologies (e.g.,

renal cell carcinoma, colorectal carcinoma, and melanoma) have control rates that are comparable to radiosensitive tumor types such as breast cancer. Studies evaluating SRS outcomes in radioresistant histologies have consistently shown excellent local control rates ranging between 70% and 90% at 12 months [1–4].

However, the radiobiology of SRS is not completely understood, and the radiobiologic targets that modulate the therapeutic response to Stereotactic Body Radiation Therapy (SBRT) remain the subject of ongoing debate. It is postulated that the greater biologically equivalent dose (BED) alone may not fully account for the superior local control rates observed with SRS. Additional biologic factors and/or cellular pathways are thought to be involved in the pathophysiology of the SRS response. These will be covered in the ensuing sections.

Microvascular Effects of SBRT

Seminal laboratory data by Fuks et al. have shown activation of the acid sphingomyelinase pathway at fraction sizes above 8–10 Gy, which, in turn, serves to activate tumor endothelial cell apoptosis, disrupt tumor vasculature, and increase tumor cell death [5]. This sequence of events is depicted diagrammatically in Fig. 3.1. The secretory form of the enzyme, acid sphingomyelinase (ASMase), is found in much higher

A. Thiagarajan (✉)
Department of Radiation Oncology, National Cancer Centre Singapore, Singapore, Singapore
e-mail: ntrat@nccs.com.sg

Y. Yamada
Department of Radiation Oncology, Memorial Sloan Kettering Cancer Center, New York, NY, USA

© Springer Nature Switzerland AG 2020
Y. Yamada et al. (eds.), *Radiotherapy in Managing Brain Metastases*,
https://doi.org/10.1007/978-3-030-43740-4_3

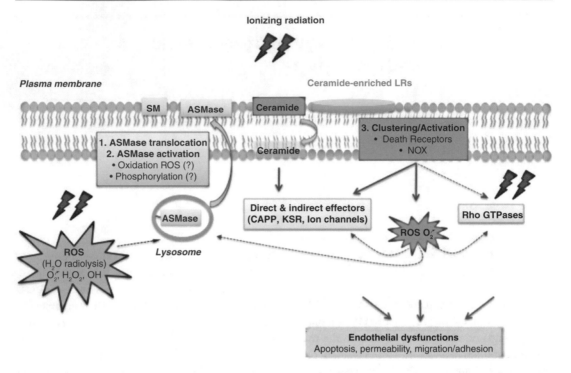

Fig. 3.1 Cell membrane signaling pathways in endothelial cells induced by stereotactic ablative radiotherapy. Abbreviations: *ASMase* acid sphingomyelinase, *CAPP* ceramide-activated protein phosphatase, *KSR* kinase suppressor of Ras, *LRs* lipid rafts, *NOX* nicotinamide adenine dinucleotide phosphate oxidase, *ROS* reactive oxygen species, *SM* sphingomyelin [48]. (From Corre et al. [48]. Open Access Creative Commons Attribution License)

concentrations in endothelial cells (approximately 20-fold higher) compared to any other cell within the body, making these cells particularly sensitive to radiation-induced apoptosis in vitro and in vivo via the ASMase pathway. High doses of radiation $\geq$ 8 Gy cause rapid translocation of ASMase from the cytosol to the glycosphingolipid- and cholesterol-enriched rafts in the cell membrane, where it hydrolyzes sphingomyelin to generate pro-apoptotic ceramide. Ceramide, in turn, acts as a second messenger, by stimulating the *Bax* pathway of pro-apoptotic signals and eventually triggering a mitochondrial-mediated apoptotic response with cytochrome C release from the mitochondria. In addition, ceramide can alter extracellular and intracellular signaling pathways by creating membrane rafts. Experimental data from Garcia-Barros et al. using transplanted melanoma and fibrosarcoma cell lines have demonstrated ceramide-mediated apoptosis in tumor endothelial cells 1–6 hours following receipt of single large radiation doses

of 15–20 Gy [6, 7]. In separate experiments involving ASMase and *Bax* knockout mice, this wave of apoptosis was not observed. The apparent radiotherapy dose threshold to induce the ASMase pathway was found to be 8–10 Gy, with a dose–response relationship being seen up to 20–25 Gy. The resulting microvascular dysfunction appeared to regulate the processing of radiation-induced tumor cell DNA damage with conversion of sublethal lesions within tumor cells into lethal ones through mechanisms that, at the time of publication, had yet to be elucidated. Interestingly, in recent experiments, Fuks et al. showed that massive, previously unrecognized ceramide-mediated ischemia/reperfusion injury occurring within 1 hour of receipt of a single large radiation dose and preceding detectable evidence of endothelial apoptosis dysregulated DNA damage response via generation of toxic reactive oxygen species in tumor cells [8]. Mechanistically, reactive oxygen species were demonstrated to trigger the evolutionarily conserved small ubiquitin modifier (SUMO) stress response, depleting unconjugated chromatin-associated SUMO3, a protein modifier which is considered to be a key component in the activation of multiple mediators of homology-directed repair. Chromatin-bound SUMO3 depletion renders global inactivation of homologous recombination to yield lethal chromosomal rearrangements, massive tumor clonogen lethality, and local tumor cure.

Although endothelial damage occurs with low-dose exposures (1.8–3 Gy) of conventionally fractionated radiotherapy as well, the endothelial cell apoptosis and microvascular dysfunction induced by low fraction sizes do not appreciably enhance tumor cell death, as the endothelial apoptotic response is suppressed by simultaneous activation of tumor cell hypoxia-inducible factor 1 (HIF-1). Reactive oxygen species generated by repeated waves of hypoxia/reoxygenation occurring after low-dose fractionated exposures lead to translation of HIF-1 mRNA transcripts stored in specialized cytosolic stress granules of hypoxic tumor cells. HIF-1, in turn, generates Vascular Endothelial Growth Factor (VEGF) and other proangiogenic factors that counteract and dampen radiation-induced endothelial apoptosis.

Oh et al. studied the effect of radiation on angiogenesis and relevant molecular pathways on endothelial cells of tumorous as well as normal breast tissue [9]. They demonstrated that there were distinct differences in the radiation responses between normal tissue-derived endothelial cells and cancer-derived endothelial cells. Importantly, they observed that tumor endothelial cells were significantly more radiosensitive than their normal tissue counterparts. That said, the difference in radioresponse between tumor vasculature and that of normal tissue may not be solely attributable to the intrinsic variance in the radiosensitivity of endothelial cells but also to the structural differences between the capillaries of tumors and normal tissues. Tumor capillaries typically consist of a poorly connected endothelial cell lining supported by an incomplete basement membrane sparsely covered by pericytes, rendering them leaky. In addition, the tumor microvessels are frequently tortuous, branched with dead ends, haphazard, and heterogeneously distributed. Endothelial cell swelling, a common feature following irradiation, further perturbs the sluggish and often interrupted passage of blood through narrow, immature capillaries. The structural deficiencies of these immature tumor capillaries render them extremely vulnerable to external stresses and amplify the effects of endothelial apoptosis induced by high-dose radiation [10, 11].

More recently, however, doubt has been cast on the validity of the endothelial cell apoptosis theory, as these data have not been independently confirmed by other laboratories, with the majority of publications showing only modest changes to the vasculature with a gradual loss of tumor endothelial cells after irradiation. In fact, the prevailing theory that the acid sphingomyelinase pathway and endothelial cell apoptosis are key contributors to the tumoral response to SRS has been further called into question by elegant laboratory data by Moding et al. Instead of utilizing transplanted tumor models which may not fully mimic the vasculature and immune surveillance of indigenous tumors, the authors used genetically engineered mouse models to develop tumors within the native microenvironment in immunocompetent mice in efforts to more faithfully recreate the tumor stroma and microenvironment of human cancers [12]. Using dual recombinase technology, they generated primary sarcomas in mice with targeted genetic mutations in tumor cells or endothelial cells. The proapoptotic gene *Bax* or the DNA damage response gene *ATM* was selectively mutated in efforts to genetically manipulate the radiosensitivity of endothelial cells in primary soft-tissue sarcomas, with the aim of either sensitizing the vasculature to radiation-induced cell death or protecting the vasculature from the proposed membrane damage-triggered apoptosis, respectively. Interestingly, following irradiation with 20 Gy in a single fraction, the authors did not observe a rapid wave of endothelial cell apoptosis in their primary sarcoma model. Similarly, they observed that *Bax* deletion from endothelial cells did not affect radiation-induced endothelial cell death or sarcoma response to radiation therapy. In contrast, deletion of *ATM* in endothelial cells successfully increased endothelial cell death at 24 hours after radiation treatment and prolonged tumor regrowth but did not translate into enhanced tumor eradication. Importantly, in complementary experiments, they demonstrated that *ATM* deletion from tumor cells augmented tumoral response to radiation therapy, putting forth the provocative argument that tumor cells, rather than endothelial cells, were the critical targets that regulated sarcoma eradication by radiation therapy. The authors conclude by acknowledging that their experiments primarily focused on soft-tissue sarcomas and that additional experiments were needed to determine the contribution, if any, of endothelial apoptosis to the radiation response in other tumor types.

Immunomodulatory Effects of SBRT

In addition to the acid sphingomyelinase pathway, it is increasingly being recognized that the immune system, which has long been known to play key roles in tumor surveillance and suppression, is also an integral component of the SRS response. While conventionally fractionated radiotherapy is often considered to be immunosuppressive because greater volumes of normal tissues such as the circulating blood pool of leukocytes and the hematopoietic bone marrow (comprising of radiosensitive lymphocytes) are incidentally irradiated, there is accumulating evidence to indicate that high-dose irradiation to tumors via the use of SRS acts as an in situ vaccine, eliciting or augmenting systemic antitumor immunity. It is thought that the extreme hypofractionation that characterizes SRS results in increased expression of immunomodulatory molecules, such as histocompatibility complex, adhesion molecules, heat shock proteins, cytokines, and death receptors on the surface of tumor cells. In addition, there a is massive release of tumor-specific antigens from the direct cytotoxic effects of SRS, leading to the priming of CD8+ T cells and a subsequent immune-mediated response, further enhancing tumor cell death (Fig. 3.2) [13].

Lugade et al. reported that irradiation of B16 melanoma of mice with 15 Gy in a single expo-

sure increased the generation of antitumor immune effector cells by facilitating antigen presentation and priming of antitumor T cells within draining lymph nodes [14]. Furthermore, radiation improved the trafficking of effector T cells into tumors. Compared to 15 Gy delivered in a single fraction, treating tumors with a fractionated regimen of 15 Gy in five daily fractions was less effective, underlining the importance of fraction size in eliciting antitumor immunity. However, there remains much debate over what the optimal fraction size is. In another preclinical mouse breast carcinoma model, mice were randomly assigned to eight groups receiving no radiotherapy or three different radiotherapy regimens (20 Gy × 1, 8 Gy × 3, or 6 Gy × 5 fractions) with or without a monoclonal antibody against CTLA-4 [15]. The mice were subsequently followed for tumor growth/regression both at primary and metastatic sites. The authors found that the combination of anti-CTLA-4 antibody and either fractionated radiotherapy regimens achieved enhanced tumor response at the primary site. Moreover, abscopal effects, defined as significant growth inhibition of the tumor outside the radiotherapy field, occurred only in mice treated with the immunotherapy and fractionated radiotherapy, with 8 Gy × 3 being the most effective dose-fractionation scheme.

Further evidence of enhanced antitumor immunity following SRS comes from another study by Lee et al., examining the effect of ablative radiotherapeutic doses in mouse melanoma models [16]. In this study, mice with B16 melanomas were subject to extreme hypofractionation, receiving a dose of 20 Gy in a single fraction. Histopathologic examination of the tumor microenvironment and lymphoid tissues 1–2 weeks posttreatment demonstrated tumor regression as well as an influx of T cells. By contrast, no significant decrease in tumor volume was noted when the experiment was repeated in athymic mice lacking T cells. Separate experiments utilizing CD8 depletion strategies in wild-type mice with B16 tumors have also documented diminished response to ablative radiation. Taken in combination, these studies suggest that CD8+ T cells play a critical role in radiation-induced

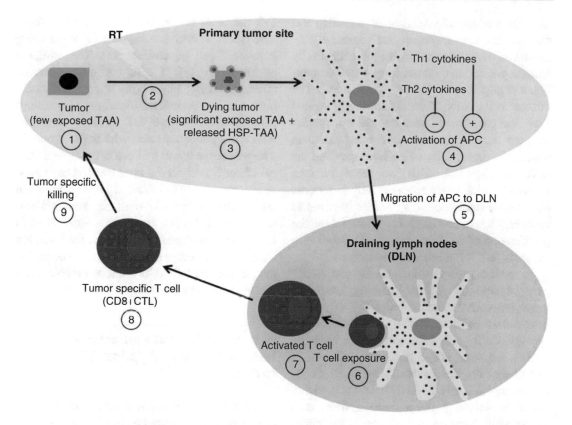

Fig. 3.2 Schematic representation for SBRT-induced antitumor immune regulation. (1) Within the primary tumor microenvironment (blue area), untreated tumors express limited exposed tumor-associated antigens (TAAs). (2) Exposure to RT induces the (3) dying tumors to express significantly more TAAs on their surface and to release DAMPS, (4) which are both taken up by antigen-presenting cells (APC) resulting in their activation. Activation of APC is enhanced (+) by the presence of Th1-type cytokines and suppressed (−) by the presence of Th2-type cytokine. (5) Activated APCs migrate to draining lymph nodes (DLN; gray area). (6) Within the DLN, T-cell exposure to APC is achieved by direct contact with activated APCs. (7) Activated T cells increase in size and granularity. (8) The activated T cells migrate from the DLN as tumor-specific T cells (CD8+ CTL) into the tumor microenvironment. (9) Within the tumor microenvironment, CD8+ CTL perform tumor-specific killing. (From Kaur and Asea [13]. Open Access Creative Commons Attribution License)

antitumor immune response following stereotactic ablative radiation therapy.

However, although these preclinical studies suggest that the immune system plays an integral role in tumor eradication following SBRT, the contribution of the immune response, relative to the contribution of the increased tumor cell kill from dose escalation, to the success of SBRT remains to be defined. At this juncture, it is important to note that the secondary tumor cell death that occurs after stereotactic ablative radiotherapy, as discussed in the earlier section, occurs within 1–3 days after irradiation, whereas the full development of radiation-induced tumor-specific

immunity typically takes 1–2 weeks. Further, this secondary wave of tumor cell death has been observed 2–3 days after a single fraction of 20-Gy irradiation even in human HT-1080 sarcoma xenografts grown in immune-compromised nu/nu mice [17]. Taken together, one can surmise that high-dose hypofractionated irradiation causes direct and indirect ablative cell death, leading to massive release of tumor antigens and, thereby, elevating antitumor immune response. It is also known that cell damage by high-dose radiation leads to the release of a variety of pro-oxidant and pro-inflammatory cytokines like TNF and interleukin IL-1 as well as adhesion molecules which initiate "danger" signaling and enhance immune response. Such inflammatory mediators facilitate the uptake of antigens by antigen-presenting cells and trigger their maturation and migration to draining lymph nodes. The effector cells (CD8 T cells) that are generated may then be recruited back into tumors by chemotactic factors. The effector cells will then assault the tumor cells which have survived the radiation exposure. This antitumor immune response, which peaks approximately 1–2 weeks after tumor irradiation, may not be involved in secondary tumor cell death, but it may inhibit the proliferation of surviving tumor cells, leading to suppression of recurrence and metastasis.

In addition to the hypothesis that SBRT may be able to, at least partially, overcome tumor-induced immunosuppression, there is tremendous excitement that SBRT could act synergistically with immunotherapies targeting various steps of antigen processing, generation of effector cells, and trafficking the effector cells into tumors [18, 19]. Several clinical approaches aimed at activating the immune system, such as the administration of cytokines, have previously been employed to treat tumors. The clinical response rates with these approaches have generally been low, although dramatic and durable disease regression has been observed in the minority of patients who do respond. More recently, there is mounting evidence that blocking inhibitory immune checkpoints using antibodies against cytotoxic T-lymphocyte-associated antigen 4 (CTLA-4) and programmed cell death protein 1 (PD-1)/PD-L1 may be a more potent method to trigger antitumor immunity [15, 20–22]. In addition, preclinical studies have shown the combination of immune checkpoint blockade and radiation treatment to be synergistic. Consequently, multiple clinical trials are currently underway combining SBRT with a variety of immunotherapies. Early results appear promising, and the abscopal effect on distant disease outside of the radiation field has been observed clinically in patients treated with a combination of immune checkpoint inhibition and SBRT. In a recent phase I clinical study, patients with metastatic melanoma or renal cell carcinoma were irradiated with SBRT (20 Gy in 1–3 fractions) and subsequently received high-dose IL-2, a cytokine capable of augmenting immune T-cell generation [23]. The levels of proliferating CD4+ T cells and early activated effector memory phenotypes were significantly higher in the peripheral blood of (responding) patients treated with SBRT and IL-2 compared with those patients treated with SBRT alone. In a separate case report by Postow et al., an abscopal effect was observed after treating metastatic melanoma with SBRT (28.5 Gy in 3 fractions) in combination with the immune checkpoint inhibitor, ipilimumab [24]. However, additional trials are required to determine the ideal fractionation schemes for immune system activation as well as to optimize the timing of immunotherapies relative to radiation treatment.

Biological Basis of Radiotherapeutic Response and Its Applicability to SRS – The 4 R's

The 4 R's – redistribution of cells within the cell cycle, repair of sublethal cellular damage, reoxygenation, and repopulation of surviving cells – are important components in the response of tumors to conventionally fractionated radiotherapy [25]. These factors may work in favor of or against tumor eradication depending on the particular context and whether they are applied to tumor cells or normal tissues. Traditionally, approaches to radiosensitize tumors and widen the therapeutic window have focused on these factors. In the ensuing section, we will consider the role, if any, these 4 R's play in the radiation response to SRS.

The biologically effective dose (BED) is a dose value that facilitates comparisons between the biologic effects of different dose-fractionation schemes and is based on the linear-quadratic (LQ) model. This model assumes that DNA double-strand break is primarily responsible for radiation-induced clonogenic cell death, that hypoxic cells are fully reoxygenated in the interfraction intervals of fractionated radiotherapy, and that complete repair of sublethal damage occurs between fractions. While it accurately describes the effects of conventionally fractionated radiation characterized by low doses per fraction, its validity in describing the effects of radiation in the ablative dose range (i.e., ≥8–10 Gy per fraction) as used in SRS is controversial and has been critically examined by many investigators [26–31]. Park et al. described the biologic effects of extreme hypofractionation using a universal survival curve (USC) model, which combined the LQ and multitarget models. Overall, the authors found that the LQ model significantly overestimated the effects of radiation in the ablative dose range and that the USC model better described measured data than the LQ model over a broad dose range. Others have demonstrated that the quantitative in vivo endpoints for both acute and late-responding tissues correlate well with the LQ model, over a wide range of doses per fraction up to 20 Gy [32–34]. In addition, in a recent analysis of local control rates for patients with early-stage non-small-cell lung cancer undergoing conventionally fractionated radiation therapy or SBRT, Mehta et al. observed that the clinical data could not distinguish between the LQ and USC models [35]. Proponents of the LQ model also question if alternative models which explicitly account for unique high-dose-specific tumoricidal mechanisms truly provide a statistically superior fit to laboratory and clinical data, given an increase in the number of adjustable parameters, and if there is any evidence, compelling or otherwise, that any these alternative models provide better estimates of clinically relevant endpoints [31, 36].

Redistribution or Reassortment

Cell cycle phase at the time of irradiation influences cellular radiosensitivity, being more radioresistant in the S-phase. Redistribution is the process by which, after transient cell cycle arrest due to the activation of cell cycle checkpoints by radiation, the surviving tumor cells become more sensitive to radiation because they progress through the cell cycle to more radiosensitive phases. Although the biological significance of this phenomenon, if any, is unknown in SRS, shortening the overall treatment time plays against redistribution of tumor cells into more radiosensitive phases of the cell cycle.

Reoxygenation

It is well recognized that hypoxic tumor cells are resistant to killing by ionizing radiation [37, 38]. In fact, an approximately threefold larger dose of radiation is required to produce an equivalent level of cell kill in a hypoxic cell population compared to one exposed to physiological oxygen conditions. Hypoxia is a phenomenon that has been observed in the vast majority of human cancers to varying degrees: Approximately 90% of all solid tumors have median oxygen concentrations less than 40–60 mmHg, the typical values found in normal tissues, and on average, hypoxic cells account for 10–20% of all tumors [39, 40]. Fractionation has traditionally been thought to mitigate the protection afforded by tumor hypoxia because of the phenomenon of reoxygenation, the process by which hypoxic tumor cells surviving a particular radiation dose become oxygenated prior to the next radiation dose. Reoxygenation of hypoxic tumor cells typically occurs when oxygen supply to the tumor is increased (due to fluctuations in tumor blood flow) or when oxygen consumption needs are reduced [41, 42]. Given that extensive vascular destruction within tumors is thought to be one of the cornerstones of SRS response, it is unlikely that reoxygenation of hypoxic tumor cells would occur following receipt of high-dose hypofractionated SRS. That said, significant reduction in oxygen consumption is probable after massive death of tumor cells, and hence, the surviving hypoxic tumor cells may be reoxygenated. The changes in oxygenation status within tumors following SRS remain to be elucidated.

There is some evidence to indicate that tumor hypoxia may have a more detrimental impact in SRS/SBRT compared with conventionally fractionated radiotherapy. In a preclinical study by Fowler et al. where control of transplanted mouse mammary tumors was measured for a given level of skin reaction for a variety of fractionation schemes, including large single fractions, the authors found that tumor control rates were inferior with single-dose radiation compared with fractionated radiation treatment and that this inferiority could be overcome if the resistance conferred by hypoxic tumor cells was eliminated by pretreatment of the mice with the hypoxic cell radiosensitizer misonidazole [43].

Similarly, a recent analysis by Brenner and colleagues of tumor control rates for brain metastases treated with single fraction or hypofractionated SRS demonstrated that tumor control probability was inferior with single fraction compared with fractionated SRS for the same BED, leading the authors to surmise that the observed results were consistent with the negative impact of tumor hypoxia on local control with single-dose radiation therapy [44].

Repopulation

Cellular depletion by ionizing radiation triggers compensatory repopulation of cells within tumors as well as normal tissues. It is known that in conventionally fractionated radiotherapy, tumor cell repopulation occurs 3–4 weeks following commencement of radiotherapy [45]. With the ablative doses used in SRS, it is conceivable that repopulation of tumor cells may start sooner. However, it is equally conceivable that given the short treatment duration of SRS and SBRT, typically less than 2 weeks, that tumor repopulation may not be a substantial issue.

Repair of Sublethal Damage

The half-time for repair of sublethal radiation damage in mammalian cells has been reported to be approximately 30 minutes [17, 46]. The occurrence of this phenomenon has been recognized as a potential drawback of the protracted dose delivery times required for SRS and SBRT, with a consequent decrease in cytotoxic effects and, hence, a detrimental impact on tumor control. This has been mitigated to a significant extent with the use of flattening filter-free photon beams which shorten the beam-on time considerably.

How the deterioration of the intratumor microenvironment due to vascular damage following SRS affects sublethal radiation damage repair remains to be elucidated. Along the same vein, an oft-cited objection about the generalizability of the LQ model at high doses is whether repair might saturate at high doses. However, there is ample evidence to suggest that this may not be the case. First, as discussed earlier, the dose–response curves fit the LQ model up to at least 20 Gy for both early- and late-responding tissues. Second, the rate and extent of double-strand repair are similar in cells after 1 Gy (determined by gamma-H2AX assay) and after 80 Gy (determined by pulsed field gel electrophoresis) [47]. Thus, concerns about the saturation of repair at high fraction sizes may not be warranted.

Conclusion

Stereotactic radiotherapy is increasingly being used in clinical practice in the management of cancers in both intracranial and extracranial sites, facilitated largely by significant technical advancements in radiotherapeutic delivery and image guidance over the last decade. However, the biological mechanisms underpinning the success of SRS have been poorly understood. There is accumulating evidence now to indicate that SRS with doses higher than about 8–10 Gy per fraction induces severe vascular damage within tumors, which in turn causes secondary or indirect tumor cell death. The resultant tumor cell degradation causes a massive release of tumor-specific antigens, triggering an antitumor immune response which, in turn, leads to suppression of tumor recurrence and metastasis. Further mechanistic understanding of the key cellular players mediating SRS response will be essential in designing targeted radiosensitizers ultimately aimed at potentiating antitumor efficacy of SRS and improving the therapeutic ratio. The role of the 4 R's and the validity of the LQ model in describing the biologic effects of SRS remain a matter of debate. As our understanding of critical molecular, cellular, and tissue effects produced at extreme hypofractionation increases, it is incumbent on us to continue to generate meaningful in vivo preclinical and clinical experimental data on the effect of radiosurgery on tumors and normal tissues alike, and in so doing, to develop or refine models that reflect the true underlying mechanisms governing tumor control, and to use and exploit these models to optimize tumor control. In addition, in spite of the mounting interest in combination therapies, in particular, the incorporation of SRS with immunotherapy, a significant proportion of patients show minimal or no response to treatment. Improving our understanding of the complex mechanisms of resistance, of the optimal timing and dosing of stereotactic radiation with immunotherapy, along with insights into the mechanisms that impair abscopal responses, is critical in determining the most reproducible efficacious strategy.

Key Points
- When delivering greater than 8 Gy, preclinical models and emerging clinical data suggest that endothelial apoptosis within the irradiated tumor mediated by ceramide generated in the cell membrane results in impaired double-strand break repair within tumor cells.
- Immune-mediated responses after high dose per fraction radiation may be important for ablation of brain metastases with radiosurgery.
- Classical radiobiology would suggest that high-dose, large-fraction radiation results in a high degree of lethal damage to irradiated cells.
- Stereotactic radiosurgery, utilizing very high-dose radiation, has radiobiologically unique mechanisms of response not seen in conventionally fractionated radiotherapy.

References

1. Muacevic A, et al. Stereotactic radiosurgery without radiation therapy providing high local tumor control of multiple brain metastases from renal cell carcinoma. Minim Invasive Neurosurg. 2004;47(4):203–8.
2. Shuto T, et al. Gamma knife surgery for metastatic brain tumors from renal cell carcinoma. J Neurosurg. 2006;105(4):555–60.
3. Wowra B, et al. Repeated gamma knife surgery for multiple brain metastases from renal cell carcinoma. J Neurosurg. 2002;97(4):785–93.
4. Auchter RM, et al. A multiinstitutional outcome and prognostic factor analysis of radiosurgery for resectable single brain metastasis. Int J Radiat Oncol Biol Phys. 1996;35(1):27–35.
5. Kolesnick R, Fuks Z. Radiation and ceramide-induced apoptosis. Oncogene. 2003;22(37):5897–906.
6. Garcia-Barros M, et al. Host acid sphingomyelinase regulates microvascular function not tumor immunity. Cancer Res. 2004;64(22):8285–91.
7. Garcia-Barros M, et al. Tumor response to radiotherapy regulated by endothelial cell apoptosis. Science. 2003;300(5622):1155–9.
8. Bodo S, et al. Single-dose radiotherapy disables tumor cell homologous recombination via ischemia/reperfusion injury. J Clin Invest. 2019;129(2):786–801.
9. Oh ET, et al. Radiation-induced angiogenic signaling pathway in endothelial cells obtained from normal and cancer tissue of human breast. Oncogene. 2014;33(10):1229–38.
10. Carmeliet P, Jain RK. Principles and mechanisms of vessel normalization for cancer and other angiogenic diseases. Nat Rev Drug Discov. 2011;10(6):417–27.
11. Song CW. Modification of blood flow. In: Mools M, Vaupel P, editors. Blood perfusion and microenvironment of human tumors, implications for clinical radio oncology. Berlin: Springer; 1998. p. 194–207.
12. Moding EJ, et al. Tumor cells, but not endothelial cells, mediate eradication of primary sarcomas by stereotactic body radiation therapy. Sci Transl Med. 2015;7(278):278ra34.
13. Kaur P, Asea A. Radiation-induced effects and the immune system in cancer. Front Oncol. 2012;2:191.
14. Lugade AA, et al. Local radiation therapy of B16 melanoma tumors increases the generation of tumor antigen-specific effector cells that traffic to the tumor. J Immunol. 2005;174(12):7516–23.
15. Dewan MZ, et al. Fractionated but not single-dose radiotherapy induces an immune-mediated abscopal effect when combined with anti-CTLA-4 antibody. Clin Cancer Res. 2009;15(17):5379–88.
16. Lee Y, et al. Therapeutic effects of ablative radiation on local tumor require CD8+ T cells: changing strategies for cancer treatment. Blood. 2009;114(3):589–95.
17. Song CW, et al. Is indirect cell death involved in response of tumors to stereotactic radiosurgery and stereotactic body radiation therapy? Int J Radiat Oncol Biol Phys. 2014;89(4):924–5.
18. Schoenhals JE, et al. Preclinical rationale and clinical considerations for radiotherapy plus immunotherapy: going beyond local control. Cancer J. 2016;22(2):130–7.
19. Bernstein MB, et al. Immunotherapy and stereotactic ablative radiotherapy (ISABR): a curative approach? Nat Rev Clin Oncol. 2016;13(8):516–24.
20. Callahan MK, Postow MA, Wolchok JD. CTLA-4 and PD-1 pathway blockade: combinations in the clinic. Front Oncol. 2014;4:385.

21. Postow MA, Callahan MK, Wolchok JD. Immune checkpoint blockade in cancer therapy. J Clin Oncol. 2015;33(17):1974–82.

22. Wang X, et al. Suppression of type I IFN signaling in tumors mediates resistance to anti-PD-1 treatment that can be overcome by radiotherapy. Cancer Res. 2017;77(4):839–50.

23. Seung SK, et al. Phase 1 study of stereotactic body radiotherapy and interleukin-2–tumor and immunological responses. Sci Transl Med. 2012;4(137):137ra74.

24. Postow MA, et al. Immunologic correlates of the abscopal effect in a patient with melanoma. N Engl J Med. 2012;366(10):925–31.

25. Steel GG, McMillan TJ, Peacock JH. The 5Rs of radiobiology. Int J Radiat Biol. 1989;56(6):1045–8.

26. Dutreix J, Cosset JM, Girinsky T. Biological equivalency of high single doses used in intraoperative irradiation. Bull Cancer Radiother. 1990;77(2):125–34.

27. Park C, et al. Universal survival curve and single fraction equivalent dose: useful tools in understanding potency of ablative radiotherapy. Int J Radiat Oncol Biol Phys. 2008;70(3):847–52.

28. Hanin LG, Zaider M. Cell-survival probability at large doses: an alternative to the linear-quadratic model. Phys Med Biol. 2010;55(16):4687–702.

29. Kirkpatrick JP, Meyer JJ, Marks LB. The linear-quadratic model is inappropriate to model high dose per fraction effects in radiosurgery. Semin Radiat Oncol. 2008;18(4):240–3.

30. Guerrero M, Li XA. Extending the linear-quadratic model for large fraction doses pertinent to stereotactic radiotherapy. Phys Med Biol. 2004;49(20):4825–35.

31. Brenner DJ. The linear-quadratic model is an appropriate methodology for determining isoeffective doses at large doses per fraction. Semin Radiat Oncol. 2008;18(4):234–9.

32. van der Kogel AJ. Chronic effects of neutrons and charged particles on spinal cord, lung, and rectum. Radiat Res Suppl. 1985;8:S208–16.

33. Douglas BG, Fowler JF. The effect of multiple small doses of x rays on skin reactions in the mouse and a basic interpretation. Radiat Res. 1976;66(2):401–26.

34. Peck JW, Gibbs FA. Mechanical assay of consequential and primary late radiation effects in murine small intestine: alpha/beta analysis. Radiat Res. 1994;138(2):272–81.

35. Mehta N, et al. Stereotactic body radiation therapy and 3-dimensional conformal radiotherapy for stage I non-small cell lung cancer: a pooled analysis of biological equivalent dose and local control. Pract Radiat Oncol. 2012;2(4):288–95.

36. Brown JM, Carlson DJ, Brenner DJ. The tumor radiobiology of SRS and SBRT: are more than the 5 Rs involved? Int J Radiat Oncol Biol Phys. 2014;88(2):254–62.

37. Brizel DM, et al. Oxygenation of head and neck cancer: changes during radiotherapy and impact on treatment outcome. Radiother Oncol. 1999;53(2):113–7.

38. Nordsmark M, Overgaard M, Overgaard J. Pretreatment oxygenation predicts radiation response in advanced squamous cell carcinoma of the head and neck. Radiother Oncol. 1996;41(1):31–9.

39. Gray LH, et al. The concentration of oxygen dissolved in tissues at the time of irradiation as a factor in radiotherapy. Br J Radiol. 1953;26(312):638–48.

40. Brown JM, Wilson WR. Exploiting tumour hypoxia in cancer treatment. Nat Rev Cancer. 2004;4(6):437–47.

41. Kallman RF, Dorie MJ. Tumor oxygenation and reoxygenation during radiation therapy: their importance in predicting tumor response. Int J Radiat Oncol Biol Phys. 1986;12(4):681–5.

42. Brown JM. Evidence for acutely hypoxic cells in mouse tumours, and a possible mechanism of reoxygenation. Br J Radiol. 1979;52(620):650–6.

43. Fowler JF, et al. Optimum fractionation of the C3H mouse mammary carcinoma using x-rays, the hypoxic-cell radiosensitizer Ro-07-0582, or fast neutrons. Int J Radiat Oncol Biol Phys. 1976;1(7–8):579–92.

44. Shuryak I, et al. High-dose and fractionation effects in stereotactic radiation therapy: analysis of tumor control data from 2965 patients. Radiother Oncol. 2015;115(3):327–34.

45. Bese NS, Hendry J, Jeremic B. Effects of prolongation of overall treatment time due to unplanned interruptions during radiotherapy of different tumor sites and practical methods for compensation. Int J Radiat Oncol Biol Phys. 2007;68(3):654–61.

46. Song CW, et al. Radiobiological basis of SBRT and SRS. Int J Clin Oncol. 2014;19(4):570–8.

47. Rothkamm K, et al. Pathways of DNA double-strand break repair during the mammalian cell cycle. Mol Cell Biol. 2003;23(16):5706–15.

48. Corre I, Guillonneau M, Paris F. Membrane signaling induced by high doses of ionizing radiation in the endothelial compartment. Relevance in radiation toxicity. Int J Mol Sci. 2013;14(11):22678–96.

Supportive Medical Management of Brain Metastases Patients Including Treatment Complications

4

Peter C. Pan, Laura E. Donovan, and Rajiv S. Magge

Scope

Between 6% and 30% of patients newly diagnosed with a primary systemic invasive cancer will develop metastases over their lifetime [1, 2]. Brain metastases from lung cancer are especially common, a combination of both its high volume and its predilection for the brain – with an incidence up to as high as 50% in some studies [3]. Melanoma, renal cell cancer, and breast cancer are also commonly metastatic to brain. The overall prevalence of brain metastases continues to rise with the improving outcomes of patients with systemic malignancy.

Metastases can arise anywhere in the brain. Tumor cells migrate from the bloodstream in a manner analogous to that of leukocyte extravasation, being guided by chemokines, rolling, adhering, and then transmigrating [4]. Epithelial-mesenchymal transition (EMT) is the classic model for metastasis; however, recent data support an alternative invasion model. In this alternative model, resident mesenchymal cells, such as microglia, act as both initiator and guide for invading tumor cells that then do not necessarily need to acquire mesenchymal features [5, 6]. The large size of tumor cells irreversibly injures the endothelial architecture in diapedesis [4], and vascular endothelial growth factor (VEGF), cytokines, and growth factors released by tumor cells lead to further increased vascular permeability [7–9]. VEGF not only leads directly to blood–brain barrier injury by downregulating zonula occludens-1 (ZO-1) in the tight junctions but also leads to microvascular proliferation by acting on VEGFR2 on endothelial cells [10]. Despite loss of blood–brain barrier integrity, the compromise of barrier function is partial [11] and only proportional to the size of the metastasis [12], thereby hindering efficient chemotherapy delivery into tumor tissue [13]. Furthermore, astrocytes engender chemotherapy resistance by gap junction communication with tumor cells and upregulation of survival genes, further frustrating chemotherapeutic approaches [13, 14]. Despite these barriers, a remarkable string of advances have made targeted and immunotherapeutic approaches to solid tumors gain traction in the clinic over the past decade.

The stereotypic appearance of a metastatic lesion is that of a punctate to round homogeneously gadolinium-enhancing lesion in the juxtacortical parenchyma. Peripherally enhancing cystic or large heterogeneously enhancing lesions

P. C. Pan
Department of Neurology, Weill Cornell Medicine/
New York-Presbyterian Hospital, New York, NY, USA

L. E. Donovan
Department of Neurology, Columbia University
Irving Medical Center, New York, NY, USA

R. S. Magge (✉)
Department of Neurology, Weill Cornell Medicine,
New York-Presbyterian Hospital, New York, NY, USA
e-mail: ram9116@med.cornell.edu

© Springer Nature Switzerland AG 2020
Y. Yamada et al. (eds.), *Radiotherapy in Managing Brain Metastases*,
https://doi.org/10.1007/978-3-030-43740-4_4

can also be seen. A measurable lesion is defined by the Response Assessment in Neuro-Oncology Brain Metastases (RANO-BM) working group as a contrast-enhancing lesion measurable to a minimum size of 10 mm in at least one dimension, and visible on two or more axial slices that are 5 mm or less apart [15], although it is recognized that many lesions are not well captured by this rubric – sub-centimeter lesions, predominantly cystic lesions, and lesions that are dural, calvarial, or leptomeningeal. Perfusion and glucose uptake on positron emission tomography (PET) are typically elevated [16].

As expected, the corresponding neurologic deficit can be accurately predicted by standard localization techniques, although examination findings are typically not as impressive as they are for analogous acute vascular lesions. Executive dysfunction, bradyphrenia, and personality changes are associated with frontal lobe lesions, while lateralizing motor or sensory deficits are commonly seen with a peri-Rolandic location. Temporoparietal and occipital lesions can cause homonymous visual field defects; infratentorial lesions often contribute to bulbar signs or ataxia.

Peritumoral cerebral edema increases the extent of tissue affected and thus the corresponding neurologic deficit. It appears as nonenhancing T2 hyperintensity surrounding the metastatic lesion, potentially with reduced diffusion restriction. While edema is commonly present, its absence does not reliably rule out metastasis, particularly for metastases smaller than 1 cm in size [17]. Interestingly, the same study suggests that in genitourinary (GU) cancers and skin cancers, the threshold for edema formation is even higher, at about 3 cm in size [17].

While hyperventilation, head of bed elevation, and osmotic therapy such as hypertonic saline and mannitol all have roles in managing elevated intracranial pressure [18], corticosteroids are the primary treatment of choice for peritumoral edema [19]. Corticosteroids are however associated with a number of undesirable side effects that complicate their long-term use.

The predilection of metastases for the juxtacortical parenchyma may explain the elevated seizure risk in this population. Prophylactic use of antiepileptics (AED) varied regionally until recently, with mounting evidence and recent guidelines advising against their prophylactic use. In those patients with symptomatic epilepsy, AEDs are carefully selected with attention to avoiding CYP450 inducers that may affect chemotherapy metabolism.

While radiotherapy is well tolerated, unintended collateral injury to normal tissues results in a range of adverse effects including postradiation fatigue and cerebral edema in the short term; more chronic issues include leukoencephalopathy, cognitive dysfunction, necrosis, and vasculopathy. The latter long-term complications are of particular concern in the pediatric cancer population.

As treatments improve and patients live longer, the prevalence of both brain metastases and treatment-related neurologic toxicity has increased. It is important to be familiar with their identification and management.

Evidence Base

Peritumoral Cerebral Edema

Peritumoral cerebral edema causes seizures, headaches, encephalopathy, and, if large enough in size, herniation. Edema preferentially accumulates in the white matter because of reduced resistance to bulk flow as compared to gray matter [20]. Despite the outsized way in which edema can contribute to symptoms, the literature is mixed regarding whether the degree of edema correlates with the outcome – in a study of patients operated on for a single brain metastasis, the extent of brain edema was found to independently correlate with prognosis [21]. However, another study of patients undergoing surgical resection for brain metastasis found no prognostic value to median edema volume or to ratio of edema to tumor volume [22]. The degree of edema may be more important in the space-constrained posterior fossa – another study supported the intuitive conclusion that peritumoral edema to tumor ratio is a strong predictor of overall survival specifically in posterior fossa metastases [23].

Corticosteroids

Corticosteroids have been used clinically to reduce peritumoral cerebral edema since the late 1950s [24, 25], and remain the standard of care [26]. Steroids are thought to exert their anti-edema effect by vasoconstriction [27], reduction of leukotriene formation [28], reduction of VEGF expression via glucocorticoid receptor activation [29], and restoration of cytoskeletal and tight junction proteins characterizing the intact blood–brain barrier [30, 31].

Potential adverse effects from steroids involve nearly every organ system, and include gastric irritation, weight gain, glucose intolerance, transaminitis, impaired wound healing, osteoporosis, avascular necrosis, myopathy, acne, hypertension, psychosis, hypoadrenalism, and glaucoma [20]. Prolonged treatment (greater than 3 weeks in duration) and hypoalbuminemia (less than 2.5 g/dL) are associated with greater toxicity [32]. For these reasons, corticosteroids are not recommended for an asymptomatic patient, and in symptomatic patients, the lowest effective dose should be used to manage symptoms.

Dexamethasone is favored for its relatively lower mineralocorticoid activity compared to other corticosteroids, and lower risk for infectious and neuropsychiatric effects [27]. For temporary relief of mild symptoms from cerebral edema, a total daily starting dose of 4–8 mg dexamethasone is typical, with higher doses of 16 mg daily reserved for more severe symptoms [19, 33, 34]. Although plasma half-life is on the order of 2 hours for dexamethasone, the biological half-life of 36–54 hours allows for a convenient dosing schedule – once to twice daily [34–36]. Doses are tapered to as low a dose as is necessary to maintain therapeutic benefit [37]. A typical steroid taper is completed over a period of 2 weeks. As adrenal suppression is possible after even just 2 weeks of corticosteroid treatment, a slower taper may be necessary in patients on extended steroid courses [36].

Corticosteroids: Gastrointestinal Prophylaxis

With the concern for peptic ulceration and upper gastrointestinal (GI) bleeding with corticosteroids, patients are often placed on histamine H2 receptor blockers or proton pump inhibitors. Early literature on the topic of whether steroids increased the risk for GI bleeding was conflicted [38–41]. A large recent review and meta-analysis by Narum et al. of over 30,000 patients found increased risk for GI bleeding or perforation in the hospitalized population only [42]. An increased, but not statistically significant, odds ratio was found in the ambulatory population; furthermore, few events were seen in the ambulatory population (0.13%).

In a Japanese study by Kondo et al. of rebleeding rates after hemostasis for peptic ulcer bleeding, those patients receiving prednisolone 20 mg or greater (equivalent roughly to dexamethasone 3 mg or greater) had higher rebleeding rates than the group on less corticosteroid [43]. However, it is unclear if 3 mg daily of dexamethasone represents the "safe" cutoff for GI bleeding risk. A convincing large retrospective analysis of nearly 9000 combined inpatient and outpatient cases from the Taiwan National Health Insurance Research Database by Tseng et al. found that short courses (7-day) at even lower doses (methylprednisolone 4 mg or greater, equivalent roughly to dexamethasone 0.8 mg or greater) were associated with elevated risks for peptic ulcer bleeding. Risk was found to be compounded for patients concurrently on aspirin or other NSAIDs [44], a finding echoed in earlier reports of elevated risk with this combination [45].

Beyond the direct mortality risk of a GI bleed, cancer patients may be at increased risk as they may already be receiving therapeutic anticoagulation for comorbid deep venous thrombus (DVT) or pulmonary embolism (PE), which will often need to be discontinued. Even after the GI bleed is stabilized, providers may be hesitant to resume anticoagulation, forcing consideration of less-effective alternatives such as inferior vena cava filters (which can expose the patient to further procedural morbidity without addressing clot burden in the extremities). The potential catastrophic morbidity and mortality risk of any single GI bleed event is far greater relative to the low morbidity of H2 blockers and proton pump inhibitors. Corticosteroids do seem to pose a threat of GI bleed – and, as noted earlier, data from Narum et al. did not convincingly prove a lack of threat [42]. Both Tseng et al. and Kondo et al. added to the body of literature demonstrating tangible risk of harm [43, 44]. The default clinical assumption, without definitive data otherwise, is that corticosteroids have the potential to increase the risk for GI bleeding and that patients should be placed on prophylaxis. In the inpatient setting, proton pump inhibitors such as pantoprazole should be administered (usual dose 40 mg daily), especially as they allow for intravenous (IV) dosing. In the ambulatory setting, despite the low overall incidence, prophylaxis with either an H2 receptor blocker or proton pump inhibitor is recommended (unless steroid doses are lower than equivalent of dexamethasone 0.8 mg daily).

Corticosteroids: Opportunistic Infections

The use of corticosteroids has long been known to be associated with opportunistic *Pneumocystis jirovecii* infection. The National Comprehensive Cancer Network guidelines suggest prophylaxis for patients on prednisone 20 mg daily (or dexamethasone 3 mg daily) for a period of 4 weeks or longer [46]. This is a reasonably conservative approach, based on a study of patients on dexamethasone who developed *P. jirovecii* pneumonia, where the median dose of patients infected was a total daily dexamethasone dose of 4.5 mg [47]. However, it is important to recognize that the limit of 3 mg daily dexamethasone is a guideline and does not represent a hard cutoff for risk. In the same study, doses as low as 2.4 mg of total daily dexamethasone were seen in 25% of those infected. Thus, there is no substitute for clinical judgment, and the treating provider should favor a stricter threshold in patients who have reason for immunocompromise, such as those with human immunodeficiency viral (HIV) infection, low T cell counts, or malnutrition.

It is important to consider also the biological half-life of corticosteroids when planning the period of prophylaxis, as the period of susceptibility to infection extends past the last date of corticosteroid treatment. This is true even for patients not on a daily corticosteroid. One study found that nearly half of patients with *P. jirovecii* pneumonia either took steroids intermittently (not daily) or not at all in a 4-week period prior to

discovery of the infection [48]. If the prophylactic antibiotic is well tolerated, we recommend considering the extension of prophylaxis to a period of 2 weeks [49] to 4 weeks [48] beyond the corticosteroid stop date. Typical prophylactic antibiotics include trimethoprim-sulfamethoxazole (160–800 mg) double-strength tabs, one tab three times a week, atovaquone 1500 mg daily, and dapsone 100 mg daily. Trimethoprim-sulfamethoxazole is generally well tolerated and considered first line, though it can cause hypersensitivity reactions, hepatic and renal dysfunction, and cytopenias; in the case of a sulfa allergy, atovaquone and dapsone can be considered [50].

Corticosteroids: Interactions with Immunotherapy

The advent of immune checkpoint inhibitors has expanded treatment options in many cancers including non-small-cell lung cancer, renal cell carcinoma, and melanoma. As many of these cancers commonly metastasize to the brain, the effect that corticosteroids have on immunotherapy is generating increased interest. Corticosteroids are used not only in the management of peritumoral cerebral edema, but also in the treatment of immune-related adverse effects secondary to immune checkpoint inhibitor use.

Naïve T-cell populations are particularly sensitive to corticosteroid exposure in a manner predominantly mediated by CTLA-4, while more differentiated effector memory T cells are relatively spared – suggesting that timing of corticosteroid administration is important. Administration of steroids after a successful antitumor immune response has developed is less likely to blunt the efficacy of immunotherapy [51]. This is supported by the observation in a large melanoma study that corticosteroid use for immune-related adverse events did not impact the response rate to nivolumab [52].

Cerebral Edema: VEGF Pathway Inhibition

Vascular endothelial growth factor (VEGF) secreted by tumor cells leads to vascular permeability and cerebral edema. Targeting the VEGF pathway helps normalize vessel morphology and reduces cerebral edema. Examples of VEGF pathway treatments include VEGF ligand inhibitors (bevacizumab), targeted VEGF receptor inhibitors such as cediranib and ramucirumab, and multiple tyrosine kinase inhibitors such as sorafenib, sunitinib, and nintedanib [53]. VEGF pathway inhibition, unlike corticosteroids, does not cause immunosuppression. This is an advantage in the setting of immunotherapy, especially as many cancers commonly metastatic to the brain are treated with immune checkpoint inhibitors, which can provide relatively durable responses.

Bevacizumab, a vascular endothelial growth factor A (VEGF-A) inhibitor, is the most commonly used steroid-sparing alternative for reduction of cerebral edema. Bevacizumab doses of 5–7.5 mg/kg, given on 2 3 week cycles, for up to 9 cycles, have been described in the literature for treatment of cerebral edema, used successfully on an off-label basis to reduce or eliminate corticosteroid need [54, 55].

Hypertension, constipation, and fatigue are common adverse effects and can typically be managed conservatively. The most concerning adverse events stem from the small but increased risk of thrombosis and bleeding that include (but are not limited to) myocardial infarction, acute ischemic stroke, deep venous thrombosis, pulmonary embolism, hemorrhage, and gastrointestinal bleeding. Gastrointestinal perforation, a rare complication appearing in less than 1% of patients on bevacizumab, is fatal in nearly a quarter of patients. A higher dose of bevacizumab (5 mg/kg per week, as opposed to 2.5 mg/kg per week) is a risk factor for perforation, but the ultimate cause is thought to be multifactorial [56]. The typical presentation of gastrointestinal perforation includes abdominal pain, constipation, and vomiting [57]; patients on bevacizumab should be closely monitored and constipation should be quickly treated.

Although theoretical concerns exist about VEGF blockade and increased risk of intracerebral hemorrhage, an extensive body of literature has found no increase in risk of intracranial hemorrhage over the baseline. A large retrospective by Khasraw et al. documenting the Memorial Sloan-Kettering experience with bevacizumab

reported frequencies of intracerebral hemorrhage as 3.7% versus 3.6% in treated and untreated patients, respectively [58]. Patients with glioblastoma, colon cancer, non-small-cell lung cancer, ovarian cancer, and angiosarcoma were included. Comprehensive reviews in 2008 and 2010 of anti-VEGF clinical trials by Carden et al. and Besse et al. arrived at a similar conclusion, and reported low and similar intracerebral hemorrhage incidence in bevacizumab-treated and untreated patients [59, 60]. Finally, the phase II PASSPORT study addressing the safety of bevacizumab in non-small-cell lung cancer reported no instances of CNS hemorrhage [61]. Two pulmonary hemorrhages were seen in PASSPORT however.

The safety of starting anti-VEGF therapy in patients with active intracranial or extracranial hemorrhage has not been well studied, and more data are necessary. The risk of exacerbating existing hemorrhages is a legitimate concern, and in practice, the presence of acute hemorrhage is considered a contraindication for initiation of bevacizumab.

Bevacizumab interferes with wound healing. This is especially important in hemiparetic or bed-bound patients at risk for decubitus ulcers, as well as patients with diabetes or peripheral vascular disease who often develop non-healing wounds. In the surgical patient, bevacizumab poses a risk of not just delayed wound healing but also bleeding and dehiscence. Bevacizumab has a long half-life of about 20 days. Various proposed washout periods before elective surgery range have been proposed, ranging from 4 to 8 weeks. Postoperative resumption is recommended to be delayed for at least 28 days after full wound healing [62].

The major limitations of the use of bevacizumab are its uncommon but severe adverse effects, prolonged half-life, the impact on timing of surgery, and the expense of treatment. There are also concerns about long-term effectiveness – chronic VEGF blockage may lead to angiogenesis via alternative pathways such as basic fibroblast growth factor or stromal cell-derived factor 1-α [63]. It is also unclear whether a VEGF-directed anti-edema strategy is generalizable across all metastatic tumor subtypes. The glioma literature has shown remarkable heterogeneity in both VEGF expression and the response of edema to anti-VEGF therapy [64, 65]. A comparison of histopathologic features of angiogenesis in brain metastases from non-small-cell lung cancer, small cell lung cancer, melanoma, renal cell carcinoma, and colorectal cancer found the highest microvascular proliferation in renal cell carcinoma and the lowest in melanoma [66].

Cerebral Edema: Experimental Treatments

Human Corticotropin-Releasing Factor (hCRF)

Human corticotropin-releasing factor (hCRF), an endogenous 41-residue peptide member of the corticoliberin superfamily, is a stimulator of the hypothalamic-pituitary axis (HPA). Evidence from the 1980s and early 1990s pointed to its role as an inhibitor of vascular leakage in various tissues [67]. Preclinical data in a rat glioma model showed reduction of contrast-enhancement on MRI and a dose-dependent reduction in tumor tissue water content [68]. The effect seen is not dependent on adrenal steroid release, as plasma corticosterone levels did not change following hCRF administration and adrenalectomy did not abolish the above effects of hCRF. The authors found that endothelial barrier antigen (EBA) stained most strongly in hCRF-treated animals, and posited that upregulation of blood–brain barrier-specific proteins such as EBA is a possible explanatory mechanism of action.

Despite promising preclinical evidence, clinical studies have been less impressive. A phase I study of hCRF given by intravenous (IV) infusion in 17 patients with brain metastases failed to convincingly demonstrate that hCRF reduces cerebral edema on MRI [69]. Adverse effects included flushing, headache, gastrointestinal disturbance, and hypotension. A prospective, randomized, double-blind study of 200 patients with peritumoral brain edema and primary or secondary malignancy found no statistically significant difference between corticorelin acetate, a synthetic formulation of hCRF administered subcutaneously (SC),

and placebo in reducing dexamethasone dosing [70, 71]. Corticorelin was compared with a dexamethasone increase (by 4 mg) in patients with subacute decline from peritumoral brain edema in another randomized trial – this study was terminated early for slow recruitment. Response rates were low in both groups – 3/20 in corticorelin, 3/17 with dexamethasone increase [72].

Corticorelin appears to be well tolerated [73], but it is unclear why the effectiveness seen in preclinical data have not translated into clinical effectiveness. Surrogate measures of reduced corticosteroid burden such as myopathy suggest that there is some degree of effect in the corticorelin treatments arms of the above studies; however, the effect size appears to be small. At present, while corticorelin may be considered as an adjunctive therapy to reduce corticosteroid burden, it has not demonstrated effectiveness to warrant replacing dexamethasone monotherapy.

Neurokinin 1 Receptor Antagonism

Neurokinin 1 (NK1) receptor antagonism is under investigation as a possible approach to treating cerebral edema. Recent data in the traumatic brain injury [74, 75] and ischemic stroke literature [76] have demonstrated a substance P and NK1 receptor-mediated pathway for vascular permeability and cerebral edema, responsive in each case to NK1 receptor inhibition. A preclinical study using fosaprepitant, a prodrug of aprepitant, in a mouse melanoma model of cerebral edema found increased substance P and NK1 receptor expression in the tumor, and reduction of brain water content as well as reduced extravasation of Evans Blue (indicative of blood–brain barrier permeability normalization) in animals that received fosaprepitant [77].

Nonsteroidal Antiinflammatory Drugs (NSAIDs)

Nonsteroidal antiinflammatory drugs have long been suggested as an alternative to corticosteroids. However, the available evidence is not convincing [78].

Indomethacin, a nonselective cyclooxygenase 1 and 2 inhibitor, readily crosses the blood–brain barrier [79] and reduces prostaglandin synthesis, but data on reduction of cerebral edema were mixed [80, 81]. This failure to reduce edema despite cyclooxygenase inhibition is attributed to a shift toward the lipoxygenase pathway and production of leukotrienes instead, which also induce cerebral edema [80]. A dual cyclooxygenase and lipoxygenase inhibitor, sodium meclofenamate [82], demonstrated impressive activity in one case report; however, the anti-edema effect was unable to be replicated in a rabbit brain tumor model [83].

Selective Cyclooxygenase-2 (COX-2) Inhibition

Tumor-infiltrating microglia in gliomas have long been known to produce prostaglandin E2 (PGE_2) in a cyclooxygenase-2 (COX-2)-dependent pathway that promotes tumorigenesis and cerebral edema [49, 84, 85]. Prostanoid synthesis is elevated in a variety of intracranial tumors, from primary gliomas to meningiomas to secondary metastatic cancers (lung, breast, gastric, melanoma), and increased expression in tumor tissue correlates with increased tumor grade. Thromboxane B2 (TXB_2) and prostaglandin E2 (PGE_2) are particularly elevated in metastases, supporting COX-2 inhibition as a promising approach for treating cerebral edema [86]. The intracerebral hemorrhage literature demonstrates evidence for inhibition of cycloxoxygenase-2 (COX-2). In a preclinical rat model of intracerebral hemorrhage, treatment with celecoxib, a COX-2 inhibitor, reduced prostaglandin E2 (PGE_2) production, reduced edema (measured by brain water content), and improved sensorimotor outcomes on the rotarod test [87]. The same group later demonstrated that celecoxib reduced perihematomal edema in acute intracranial hemorrhage in a small pilot multicenter randomized open-label trial [88]. In addition, preclinical evidence that celecoxib

also inhibits VEGF expression [89] made celecoxib a particularly attractive candidate for investigation of cerebral edema.

Penetration across the blood–brain barrier is an important consideration in determining the viability of targeting the COX-2 pathway of microglia. As a surrogate for concentration in brain tissue, the concentration in cerebrospinal fluid (CSF) is simpler to measure. Concentrations of COX-2 inhibitors celecoxib, rofecoxib, and valdecoxib in cerebrospinal fluid (CSF) are lower than in plasma by over two orders of magnitude [90]. Although the CSF concentrations of rofecoxib and valdecoxib are enough to exceed median COX-2 inhibitory concentration (IC50), celecoxib falls short of the CSF concentration of 6.3 nM – below IC50 39.3 nM – suggesting inadequate CSF penetration of celecoxib to inhibit COX-2. The variance in reported concentrations is high, however, and in a separate report of celecoxib given at 200 mg four times daily – published prior to the above study that demonstrated the superior blood–brain barrier penetration properties of rofecoxib and valdecoxib – a CSF concentration approaching the IC50 (40 nM) was achieved, in a patient being treated for posterior fossa glioblastoma [91].

Interestingly, in the case above of posterior fossa glioblastoma, the patient treated with celecoxib remained free of brain edema in the two MRI scans obtained during adjuvant therapy and in one scan obtained 2 months afterward in follow-up. It is tempting to ascribe this effect to celecoxib. However, the authors rightly point out that the patient may never have developed peritumoral edema in the first place even without celecoxib treatment. As it stands, clinical evidence for the effectiveness of celecoxib (and COX-2 inhibition at large) in cerebral edema remains scant and is restricted to case reports. Concerns regarding increased risk of cardiovascular events and the black box warnings issued by the US Food and Drug Administration in 2005 [92] have significantly tempered the enthusiasm for selective COX-2 inhibitors as a less toxic alternative to corticosteroids.

Boswellia

A German language preliminary report by Böker and Winking in 1997 documented the effectiveness of H15, a phytotherapeutic preparation derived from the gum resin (frankincense) of *Boswellia serrata*, in the reduction of brain edema in glioma patients. Similar observations of anti-edema effect were reported in a small series from 2001 of 11 glioma patients and 1 metastatic melanoma patient – 8 of the 12 patients had a clinical or a radiographic response, including the melanoma patient [93]. A small, placebo-controlled double-blinded randomized controlled trial of 44 primary and secondary malignant brain tumor patients undergoing radiation from 2010 found cerebral edema reduction of 75% or greater in 60% of treated patients (4200 mg/day of Boswellia) compared to 26% of placebo patients, with minor gastrointestinal discomfort being the only adverse effect [94]. The anti-edema effect of Boswellia is surmised to be a result of lipoxygenase inhibition [95]. Dosing Boswellia with fat-containing foods appears to improve the bioavailability [96]. While validation in larger randomized trials is needed, existing efficacy data are respectable and deserving of further studies.

Posttreatment Radiation Necrosis

White matter in the path of radiation suffers changes to its capillary structure and cerebrovascular permeability, potentially leading to acute cerebral edema in the weeks following treatment. This appears as nonenhancing T2 hyperintense lesions on MRI that may be transient and reversible in the acute form; if symptomatic, treatment with corticosteroids is often started [97].

Radiation injury to oligodendrocytes leads to transient disruption of myelin synthesis, and manifests in the so-called early-delayed reaction between the first few weeks and the first 3 months posttreatment [98]. The course, while at times prolonged, is self-limited with spontaneous recovery. Somnolence and fatigue are the most prominent clinical features.

Late-delayed radiation injury, usually composed of leukoencephalopathy and radiation necrosis, is often progressive and difficult to treat. The risk of a late-delayed radiation injury is greater with increasing total amount, fraction size, and volume of radiation – total dose over 60 Gy and fraction size over 1.8–2 Gy is associated with a higher risk [99, 100].

Two models exist for radiation-induced cerebral necrosis – vascular or glial injury. In the vascular model, radiotherapy injures the endothelium, stimulates the release of transforming growth factor-beta (TGF-β), and leads to microvasculopathy. Progressive vascular insufficiency leads to infarction and necrosis, with attendant disruption of blood–brain barrier integrity and infiltration of inflammatory T lymphocytes and macrophages. In the glial damage model, destruction of glial precursors leads to demyelinative necrosis and inflammatory infiltration. Proinflammatory cytokines such as tumor necrosis factor-alpha (TNF-α), interleukin-1 alpha (IL-1α), and interleukin-6 (IL-6) are released by infiltrating macrophages, which perpetuate chronic inflammation, further accelerating endothelial cell and CNS tissue injury [101]. The low proliferation rates of endothelial cells (on order of months) may explain why late radiation necrosis can appear after months or even years [102].

In the context of radiosurgery to metastases, the volume of tissue treated to 10 or 12 Gy with single-fraction radiosurgery is a risk factor for radiation necrosis [103]. Differentiating radiation necrosis from recurrent tumor can sometimes be difficult and require pathology confirmation. However, advanced imaging such as perfusion MR imaging and 2-[fluorine-18] fluoro-deoxy-D-glucose (FDG) positron emission tomography (PET) may help make the diagnosis.

Radiation Necrosis: Management

Clinical practice patterns for management of radiation necrosis revolve primarily around corticosteroids and, increasingly, bevacizumab. Surgery remains an option in medically refractory cases. Other modalities such as hyperbaric oxygen therapy and anticoagulation have garnered interest over the years. With only a few small randomized trials, the quality of data for management of radiation necrosis remains low overall [104].

The original mainstay of treatment for radiation necrosis was surgery. Its benefits include rapid debulking with reduction of mass effect. However, surgical risks can be high and the benefit can be short-lived. As a result, open microsurgical management for radiation necrosis has fallen out of favor as first-line management, and is relegated mainly to cases refractory to medical management [105].

Corticosteroids, useful not only in the role of retarding edema, have been identified as helpful in relieving radiation necrosis [106, 107]. In cases that do not respond to corticosteroids, bevacizumab has gained traction as a popular next-line therapy because of mounting evidence for its efficacy. VEGF appears to play a role in radiation necrosis pathophysiology and may explain bevacizumab's efficacy [108]. In an early retrospective study of eight patients with radiation necrosis, who were treated with bevacizumab at a dose of 5 mg/kg over 2 weeks (or 7.5 mg/kg every 3 weeks), all patients had a radiographic response, with average reduction in daily dexamethasone requirement by 8.6 mg [109]. In another retrospective study, 90% of patients with clinically symptomatic radiation necrosis improved on bevacizumab [110]. The most convincing data come from a randomized placebo-controlled double-blinded study in which 14 patients with radiation necrosis were treated with either IV saline or bevacizumab at 7.5 mg/kg at 3 week intervals; all patients randomized to placebo worsened by neurologic or radiographic criteria before 6 weeks, and all patients treated showed improvements clinically and by MRI at 6 weeks [111]. A regimen of 7.5 mg/kg every 3 weeks for 12 weeks (four doses) was suggested as a reasonable regimen for management, with no recurrence of radiation necrosis after a median follow-up of 10 months. However, in the 2013 report cited [110], over half of the patients relapsed at an average of 7.4 mg/kg and 5.4 doses. The appro-

priate dose and duration will likely become clear with increasing experience.

Hyperbaric oxygen therapy (HBOT), thought to promote tissue healing by improving angiogenesis and tissue perfusion, is a popular alternative to corticosteroids and bevacizumab. However, despite many anecdotal reports over the years, robust data are still elusive and no double-blind placebo-controlled studies exist [112]. In a report from 1976, a patient with "radiation encephalitis" was treated with two atmospheres absolute (ATA) HBOT for 2 hours daily but seemed to decline within the first five treatments. After coadministration of cyclandelate, a vasodilator, the patient gradually improved to ambulatory status by her 20th HBOT treatment [113]. In a more recent series from 1997, 10 pediatric cases of radiation necrosis were treated at 2.0–2.4 ATA for 90 minutes-2 hours daily for a minimum of 20 treatment sessions – all patients had stabilization of symptoms. However, as corticosteroids were administered before, during, and following HBOT, it was unclear how much of the effect was attributable to HBOT alone [114].

The combination of edaravone (an antioxidant free-radical scavenger approved by the FDA in 2017 for the treatment of amyotrophic lateral sclerosis) with corticosteroids against corticosteroid alone was investigated in a randomized open-label study. Although the authors concluded increased efficacy on the edaravone treatment arm by measure of reduction in area of nonenhancing T2 disease and on the Late Effects Normal Tissue Task Force (LENT)-Subjective, Objective, Management, Analytic (SOMA) scale, the data and their interpretation suffered from a number of problems [115]. The variance in the T2 lesion size reduction was large relative to the very small effect size, and the confidence intervals overlapped between treatment arms.

A number of other approaches have been described. Anticoagulation, thought to improve microcirculation, has been described in case reports. The typical treatment is heparin in the acute period followed by warfarin maintenance [116]. Pentoxifylline, thought to enhance circulation by decreasing red blood cell viscosity, has been studied preclinically and in small pilot studies in soft tissue radiation necrosis [117]. The combination of pentoxifylline and vitamin E appeared to demonstrate benefit in radiation necrosis in other organ systems. This inspired a small series from 2008 – patients with radiation necrosis after stereotactic radiosurgery or whole-brain radiation therapy were given pentoxifylline, 400 mg twice daily, and vitamin E, 400 international units (IU) twice daily. By volumetric measures of edema, there was improvement in all but one patient. However, in the majority of these patients, corticosteroids were used as adjunctive therapy to treat acute exacerbations [118]. Laser interstitial thermal therapy (LITT), used in the context of focal cerebral radiation necrosis in patients with rapidly worsening symptoms refractory to corticosteroids and contraindications to bevacizumab, has been described in at least two case reports with good success [119, 120]. LITT is discussed in greater depth in Chap. 7.

Seizures

Despite early evidence suggesting the benefit of prophylactic AEDs [121], it has not been well supported by later evidence. In the metastatic setting, there are two prospective randomized studies addressing the prophylactic use of AEDs in majority nonsurgical patients, and three studies addressing the prophylactic use of AEDs in postoperative patients. In the two studies addressing nonoperative prophylactic AEDs, the seizure occurrence was not found to be statistically different between nontreatment and treatment (in the first study, phenytoin or phenobarbital [122], and in the second study, valproate [123]). Of the three studies addressing postoperative prophylactic use of AEDs, two are prospective randomized studies. In the first, postoperative phenytoin for 7 days resulted in no statistically significant reduction at 30-day seizure incidence [124], while in the second, postoperative phenytoin or phenobarbital resulted in no statistically significant reduction in early (<1 week) or late (>1 week) seizure incidence [125]. The retrospective study similarly identified no reduction in

seizure incidence in those patients on prophylactic AEDs, over half of whom were on levetiracetam [126].

A Cochrane Reviews analysis in 2008 finds the evidence neutral, neither for nor against seizure prophylaxis with phenytoin, phenobarbital, or valproate [127]. The risk of an adverse event appeared to be higher in those treated prophylactically with AEDs; however, this cannot be extrapolated beyond phenytoin, phenobarbital, and valproate.

Clinical practice patterns vary, and the practice of temporary prophylactic courses of postoperative levetiracetam remains common. Levetiracetam is better tolerated than phenytoin, phenobarbital, and valproate, and it can be argued that the bulk of evidence in these other agents – for either lack of efficacy or higher rate of adverse effects – does not apply to levetiracetam. There is no question that levetiracetam is effective in seizure treatment, and that at least some number of these patients with metastases will have a first-time seizure. The brain metastasis population is a population at risk for seizures. Supposing a policy of starting all patients empirically on the maximum therapeutic dose of levetiracetam, it follows that first-seizure would be prevented in at least a proportion of those patients destined to have symptomatic epilepsy. However, clearly this is not an optimal policy as the burden of adverse effects imposed on all the patients who never would have had seizures anyway is high. Lowering the empiric dose may lower the burden of adverse effect, but it is unclear how much effectiveness is also lost with a lower empiric dose – how many epileptics who would have had seizure control at the higher dose, but not at the lower dose. The topic is not well studied and it is unknown what, if any, dose reaches the optimal ratio of adverse effect to effectiveness at the population level for brain metastasis. Current guidelines therefore do not support the practice of prophylaxis. The Congress of Neurological Surgeons in 2019 recommends against prophylaxis in the seizure-free patient, either in the postoperative or in the nonoperative setting [128]. This position is endorsed by the American Society of Clinical Oncology and the Society for

Neuro-Oncology [129], and echoes the similar position adopted in practice guidelines from the American Academy of Neurology [130].

Overview of Antiepileptic Drugs

Antiepileptics (AED) that are cytochrome P450 enzyme inducers are generally avoided because they may affect the metabolism of chemotherapy, influencing the efficacy of those treatments in unpredictable ways. Non-enzyme-inducing AEDs such as levetiracetam are generally favored over enzyme-inducing agents such as phenytoin, phenobarbital, and carbamazepine. An example of an enzyme-inhibiting agent is valproate.

Phenobarbital is one of the oldest AEDs used. A barbiturate with a relatively long half-life, phenobarbital, can be given both intravenously and by mouth, and prolongs opening of the γ-aminobutyric acid (GABA) receptor. While falling out of favor, it remains in widespread use in the acute setting for treatment of benzodiazepine-refractory status epilepticus. Sedation, teratogenicity, and osteoporosis are just some of its many adverse effects, and these along with induction of the cytochrome P450 enzyme system render it a poor choice in the brain tumor patient [131].

Phenytoin, similar to phenobarbital, is an older AED that is being used less commonly in general practice. Like many other AEDs, phenytoin acts on the sodium channel and interferes with high-frequency repetitive spike firing. Phenytoin is particularly poorly suited to the brain tumor patient not only because it is a P450 enzyme inducer but also because of its large adverse effect profile and kinetics. Two factors complicate phenytoin dosing and necessitate a slow measured approach to dose titration. The rise in plasma phenytoin concentration per unit increase in dose does not remain linear, but actually is lower at lower plasma concentrations and higher at higher plasma concentrations [132]. Small increases in dose are advised once the patient approaches therapeutic concentrations. Phenytoin is also highly protein-bound. In patients with hypoalbuminemia (elderly, pregnant, malnutrition, malignancy), the total phe-

nytoin level will underestimate the pharmacologically active free fraction of phenytoin. In patients on other protein-bound drugs, such as valproate, the competition for protein binding will complicate the overall regimen adjustment [133]. Phenytoin toxicity classically manifests as vertical nystagmus and ataxia. Sedation is less of a problem for phenytoin than it is for phenobarbital but teratogenicity remains a concern. Prolonged phenytoin use notably leads to a host of adverse effects including cerebellar atrophy, gingival hyperplasia, and osteoporosis. Its prodrug, fosphenytoin, is available in an intravenous formulation and has replaced phenytoin for management of status epilepticus, as it does not carry the risk of purple glove syndrome, a rare serious complication presenting with pain, edema, and discoloration at the injection site [134].

Carbamazepine is a sodium-channel blocker like phenytoin and lamotrigine. Similar to phenytoin and phenobarbital, carbamazepine is a cytochrome P450 enzyme inducer. Carbamazepine also induces its own metabolism; after the first several weeks of initiation, the dose may need to be increased to maintain the same plasma level. The same effect is seen during pregnancy, owing to a shortened half-life. Adverse effects include hyponatremia and, rarely, Stevens–Johnson syndrome and toxic epidermal necrolysis. There is an increased risk of toxic epidermal necrolysis in patients with the HLA-B1502 allele, common in the Asian population, which should be checked in this demographic before starting the medication [135]. Oxcarbazepine, a derivative of carbamazepine, does not inhibit cytochrome P450 enzymes as strongly but is more commonly associated with hyponatremia and typically requires three times daily dosing due to its shorter half-life. Eslicarbazepine, a prodrug of the active form of oxcarbazepine, has a longer half-life and allows for once daily dosing with a similar side-effect profile.

Lamotrigine is a sodium-channel blocker that is effective, well tolerated, and often a choice in the brain tumor patient. It is also known for its risk of Stevens-Johnson syndrome and toxic epidermal necrolysis if doses are titrated up too quickly. Started at a low dose and titrated at a gentle rate, lamotrigine is extremely effective and well tolerated. It has broad-spectrum activity, tends to have a lower rate of fatigue and cognitive adverse effects than do other AEDs, has one of the lowest rates of teratogenicity, and has mood-stabilizing effects. Furthermore, it has a convenient daily dosing schedule, and does not interfere significantly with the cytochrome P450 enzymes. Of note however, like carbamazepine, levels may fall during pregnancy [136]. The levels of lamotrigine have also been found to be lowered by oral contraceptive use [137] and bears monitoring.

Valproate is an inhibitor of the cytochrome P450 system. Its high teratogenicity limits its use in women of childbearing age. Outside this demographic, valproate is a very effective AED that remains in common use today for many epilepsy patients with a wide variety of seizure types. The therapeutic range is typically considered to be between 50 and 100 μg/mL [138]. The main adverse effects include fatigue, gastric irritation, liver toxicity, hyperammonemia, and weight gain. Both oral and intravenous formulations are available, and as it is an older medication, tends to be inexpensive. Valproate has mood-stabilizing activity, similar to lamotrigine, and is also effective in migraine prophylaxis.

Topiramate is an orally available broad-spectrum AED with activity on α-amino-3-hydroxy-5-methylisoxazole-4-proprionic acid (AMPA)/kainate receptors, GABA, and carbonic anhydrase. Adverse effects to consider include increased risk of kidney stones, weight loss, and severe cognitive effects. Topiramate is also used as a preventive agent in migraine and off-label in cluster headache as well as essential tremor. There are also data on its effectiveness as a mood stabilizer [139]. These effects may be an additional advantage in patients with frequent headaches, posture-kinetic tremors, or mood disorders, if there is already an indication for seizure control.

Zonisamide is a broad-spectrum AED that acts on sodium channels, T-type calcium channels, and, like topiramate, on carbonic anhydrase

[140]. It is similar to topiramate in its adverse effect profile. One unique advantage of zonisamide is its long half-life (in excess of 48 hours), mitigating the impact of missed doses.

Levetiracetam, the most widely used AED, is a broad-spectrum AED that binds to SV2A, a synaptic vesicle protein. It is typically the first choice in most patients. It is inexpensive, does not significantly bind protein, does not significantly affect the cytochrome P450 system, and can be administered both intravenously and orally. There is no hepatic metabolism. While clearance of levetiracetam may be hampered in severe renal disease and thus require gentler dosing, levetiracetam is not directly nephrotoxic. Its major adverse effects include fatigue, irritability, and depression, which are seen more commonly at higher doses. Brivaracetam, a second-generation derivative of levetiracetam, boasts higher affinity to SV2A and higher permeability into the brain [141]. It may be associated with fewer psychiatric effects compared to levetiracetam [142].

Lacosamide is a popular and often well-tolerated alternative to levetiracetam. It acts on the sodium channel like phenytoin, carbamazepine, and lamotrigine, but instead of affecting fast inactivation, lamotrigine enhances slow inactivation [143]. Adverse effects include nausea, fatigue, and a dose-dependent PR interval prolongation.

Clonazepam and clobazam, both long-acting benzodiazepines, act on the GABA receptor and increase the frequency of chloride channel opening. The main adverse effect, as expected, is sedation and dysarthria.

Other Antiepileptics

Perampanel, an AMPA receptor antagonist, has broad-spectrum activity, but owing to available alternatives, is not commonly used. It carries a warning for behavioral adverse effects. Gabapentin and pregabalin, calcium channel modulators, have limited activity and are used in adjunctive roles, rarely as monotherapy. Felbamate, an N-methyl-D-aspartate (NMDA) receptor antagonist and is reserved for severe epilepsy because of risk of aplastic anemia and liver toxicity [144]. Tiagabine and vigabatrin, inhibitors of GABA reuptake and degradation, respectively, play adjunctive roles and are typically avoided because of potential severe adverse effects. Rufinamide and ethosuximide have limited activity in focal seizures and limited utility in the brain metastasis patient with symptomatic epilepsy.

Headache

Headaches are a common symptom in patients with brain metastases. Neurologic deficits, positional headache, nausea, emesis, and meningismus should prompt further evaluation for secondary causes. Headache may be related to disease progression, cerebral edema, increased intracranial pressure, intracerebral hemorrhage, hydrocephalus, and wound infection or meningitis. Identifying and addressing the primary source should be the first step. For symptomatic relief, acetaminophen can be used as first-line therapy. Nonsteroidal antiinflammatory drugs (NSAIDs) can be used second line if acetaminophen is ineffective. The platelet inhibitory effects of NSAIDs should be taken into consideration in patients with myelosuppression from chemotherapy or hemorrhage. When pain is refractory to these more conservative measures, opioids are prescribed. It may be helpful to manage refractory headache with the assistance of a pain or headache specialist.

It is particularly important to counsel all patients on medication overuse headache, which develops in those patients that have prolonged analgesic use (inclusive of acetaminophen and NSAIDs) – typically, those at risk use the analgesic more than 2 days out of the week for more than a few weeks to months. Medication overuse headache manifests as a new or worsening headache, usually of different character than the prior headache, which develops and progressively worsens over the course of several months. Further analgesic use exacerbates the problem in a self-reinforcing cycle. Preventive daily agents – such as tricyclic antidepressants, select AEDs, and beta-blockers – reduce the burden of headache frequency, allowing for reduction in analgesic use and prevention of medication overuse headache. While the data for preventive daily agents are largely in the migraine and tension headache literature, they can be considered in the brain metastatic patient with frequent headaches in whom other treatable causes have been ruled out. It is important to identify and educate all at-risk patients early so that they can avoid finding themselves in the predicament in the first place.

Cognitive Impairment

Cognitive deficit after radiation therapy has long been an area of concern, and is growing in importance as patients live longer with their cancers. The sort of cognitive impairment seen typically involves higher-order functions such as attention or memory, and this is likely a result of white matter tract injury and has been found to be associated with preferential atrophy in areas of the cerebral cortex involved in higher-order cognition [145]. Increasing volume and dose of radiotherapy appears to be associated with increasing risk for cognitive decline.

Efforts at sparing neural stem cells in the subgranular zone of the hippocampal dentate gyrus have led to recent investigations of conformal hippocampal avoidance techniques. Hippocampal avoidance appeared to support improvement of cognitive function, in a multi-institutional phase II study (RTOG 0933) in which outcomes at 2, 4, and 6 months were compared to a historical control [146]. While this is a promising result, these findings await confirmation in a larger head-to-head trial. Furthermore, and perhaps more importantly, cognitive function relies not just on the hippocampus, but on the integrity of the Papez circuit – the entirety of which clearly cannot be spared treatment. The significant degree to which subcortical white matter leukoencephalopathy forms in the posttreatment brain may also limit any tangible advantage that hippocampal sparing may provide. It is clear that this topic requires significantly more investigation.

There are no proven effective agents for either preventing or treating radiotherapy-associated cognitive impairment. Donepezil, an anticholinesterase, and memantine, an NMDA-receptor antagonist, have been studied for treatment and prevention, respectively.

A phase III placebo-controlled randomized trial from 2015 of donepezil (5 mg for 6 weeks, then 10 mg for 18 weeks) in previously partial- or whole-brain-irradiated patients found significant improvement in memory and motor function in the treatment arm at 24 weeks, particularly in those who were more cognitively impaired prior to treatment [147]. There was no significant improvement in overall composite scores however. An earlier phase II study from 2006 with a similar course of treatment found improvements also in mood and health-related quality-of-life measures at 24 weeks, with minimal toxicities [148].

A large phase III placebo-controlled randomized trial from 2013 of memantine (20 mg daily, for 24 weeks) started within 3 days of initiating whole-brain radiotherapy found no statistically significant difference in most median cognitive scores at weeks 8, 16, and 24, but did find a significant extension in time to first failure on any of the neurocognitive tests [149]. Memantine was well tolerated. Additional phase III trials of memantine are being carried out in patients receiving whole-brain radiotherapy to clarify the role of this medication in decreasing neurocognitive toxicities.

Areas of Uncertainty and Future Directions

While corticosteroids have remained the mainstay of treatment for peritumoral edema, radiotherapy-associated edema, and radiation necrosis, the concern regarding its adverse effects and variable efficacy is driving research into better treatments. Central to future progress will be improved understanding of underlying tumoral pathophysiology and radiobiology. A better functional understanding of the biology and optimal targets will allow more effective treatments.

There are fortunately many options for management of seizures in patients with brain metastases. Improving seizure risk stratification with imaging or electrophysiologic testing may help identify those patients who are most likely to develop seizures and therefore benefit from prophylaxis.

Treatment options are unfortunately more limited for headaches and cognitive impairment. There has been a renaissance in the molecular understanding of the underlying mechanisms of headache, particularly in migraine, and it remains to be seen whether these new developments will translate into improved treatments.

Conclusions and Recommendations

Management of patients with brain metastases is complex and depends on a multidisciplinary approach. Accumulation of cerebral edema, whether tumoral or treatment-related, is the root of many symptoms and is best managed with corticosteroids, at the lowest dose needed to maintain symptom control. Bevacizumab, while effective in reducing cerebral edema and in managing cases of radiation necrosis unresponsive to steroids, may complicate surgical timing and is associated with a number of rare but potentially fatal adverse effects. Levetiracetam is the most commonly used drug for the management of seizures, but a number of effective and reliable alternatives exist. There is no blanket recommendation for seizure prophylaxis, although individual risk profiles should be considered. Further study is needed to establish evidence-based guidelines for headache and cognitive dysfunction management. Headaches may also be a warning sign for another underlying problem. The use of analgesics must be properly monitored, especially in the setting of potential medication overuse headache. Memantine and donepezil, though lacking large-scale evidence for efficacy, are well tolerated and can be trialed for prevention and treatment, respectively, of postradiation neurocognitive impairment.

Key Points

- Use dexamethasone in symptomatic cerebral edema, starting at 2 mg daily, dosed in the mornings, and increasing as needed to improve symptoms.
- Consider GI prophylaxis with a PPI or H2 receptor inhibitor in all patients on dexamethasone. In large retrospective studies, doses as low as dexamethasone 0.8 mg daily over a 7-day period have been associated with an elevated risk of peptic ulcer bleeding.
- Start *Pneumocystis* prophylaxis in all patients on dexamethasone 3 mg daily (or more) for a period of 4 weeks or longer. Consider initiating prophylaxis at lower doses in higher-risk patients (HIV infection, low T-cell counts, malnutrition).
- Radiation-induced injury is classified into acute, early-delayed, and late-delayed reactions, with the late-delayed reactions consisting of radiation necrosis and progressive leukoencephalopathy.
- Treat radiation necrosis with dexamethasone. If refractory, consider treating with bevacizumab 7.5 mg/kg every 3 weeks, continued to four doses to improve durability if there is a response. If surgically accessible and rapidly symptomatic, surgery may be more appropriate than bevacizumab in select cases.
- There is no recommendation for seizure prophylaxis in the seizure-free brain metastasis patient. However, the data are heavily influenced by adverse effects cited in studies using phenytoin and phenobarbital. Levetiracetam and other modern AEDs can be considered in patients who are at high risk for seizures.
- In the patient with symptomatic epilepsy, use levetiracetam first-line unless there is a specific contraindication. Lacosamide is a useful but often expensive alternative. Valproate is effective,

older, and likely inexpensive, but contra-indicated in women of childbearing age and not always well tolerated. Lamotrigine is exceptionally well tolerated but must be titrated gently to avoid rash.
- Topiramate and valproate have useful headache prophylactic properties in migraine.
- Lamotrigine, topiramate, and valproate have useful mood-stabilizing properties.
- Data for donepezil are limited; however, it is well tolerated, and at 5 mg daily increased to 10 mg daily after 6 weeks appears to improve memory, motor function, mood, and health-related quality-of-life measures at 24 weeks.
- Data for memantine are limited. However, it is well tolerated and when given at 20 mg daily for 24 weeks starting with initiation of radiotherapy may help delay and blunt the onset of cognitive decline.

Case Vignettes

Vignette 1: Seizures

A 59-year-old Asian gentleman, self-employed writer with hypertension, hyperlipidemia, paroxysmal supraventricular tachycardia, and well-controlled bipolar disorder, has metastatic melanoma and is found to have three sub-centimeter enhancing juxtacortical lesions with minimal surrounding edema in his right frontal, right parietal, and left parietal, suspicious for metastases. He has no symptoms and his neurologic examination is unremarkable. He has no personal or family history of seizures. Should seizure prophylaxis be started?

A: Seizure prophylaxis is not recommended.

The above patient is treated with stereotactic radiosurgery to each of the three lesions. His oncologist starts him on combination ipilimumab and nivolumab. He tolerates treatment well but returns four months later with a first-time seizure. There is no evidence of intracranial progression. What AEDs can be offered?

A: Levetiracetam is often the first choice, but may not be the best option in the setting of bipolar disease. Lacosamide can cause PR interval prolongation and may also not be the best choice in this patient with a heart arrhythmia. Topiramate's cognitive effects may interfere too much with his line of work and should be avoided. Valproate and lamotrigine each have mood-stabilizing effects and are both reasonable choices. However, with his vascular risk profile, lamotrigine is the better option of the two – avoiding the weight gain associated with valproate would be ideal. It is important to start low (at 25 mg daily) and titrate slowly (by 25–50 mg daily every 2 weeks).

Vignette 2: Radiation Necrosis

A 64-year-old Caucasian gentleman, never smoker, with hypertension and type 2 diabetes, has non-small-cell lung cancer with EML4-ALK fusion being treated with crizotinib. A solitary left peri-Rolandic metastasis is treated with stereotactic radiosurgery. Three months after treatment, he presents with a worsening headache and increased right-sided weakness, and a heterogeneously enhancing ill-defined spreading lesion with surrounding edema is seen at the site of prior treatment. There are no other sites of disease, and you suspect radiation necrosis. What is the treatment?

A: Corticosteroids should be tried first. Given the degree of symptomatology, (escalating headache, right-sided weakness), favor starting dexamethasone 4 mg twice daily.

The patient's headache and nausea improve, but his right-sided weakness continues to progress, despite escalating dexamethasone dose. What options can be considered?

A: In this instance, bevacizumab can be considered, given at a dose of 7.5 mg/kg every 3 weeks. In the trial by Levin et al., all the patients who were treated with four doses (12 weeks) had a durable response. Surgery, or possibly LITT, can be considered in place of bevacizumab if there is growth despite steroids and the lesion is surgically accessible.

References

1. Davis FG, Dolecek TA, McCarthy BJ, Villano JL. Toward determining the lifetime occurrence of metastatic brain tumors estimated from 2007 United States cancer incidence data. Neuro-Oncology. 2012;14(9):1171–7.
2. Noh T, Walbert T. Brain metastasis: clinical manifestations, symptom management, and palliative care. In: Handbook of clinical neurology [Internet]. Elsevier; 2018 [cited 2019 Apr 13]. p. 75–88. Available from: https://linkinghub.elsevier.com/retrieve/pii/B9780128111611000062.
3. Nayak L, Lee EQ, Wen PY. Epidemiology of brain metastases. Curr Oncol Rep. 2012;14(1):48–54.
4. Strell C, Entschladen F. Extravasation of leukocytes in comparison to tumor cells. Cell Commun Signal [Internet]. 2008 [cited 2019 Apr 13];6(1). Available from: https://biosignal.biomedcentral.com/articles/10.1186/1478-811X-6-10.
5. Pukrop T, Dehghani F, Chuang HN, Lohaus R, Bayanga K, Heermann S, et al. Microglia promote colonization of brain tissue by breast cancer cells in a Wnt-dependent way: microglia promote brain metastasis. Glia. 2010;58(12):1477–89.
6. Nguyen DX, Chiang AC, Zhang XH-F, Kim JY, Kris MG, Ladanyi M, et al. WNT/TCF signaling through LEF1 and HOXB9 mediates lung adenocarcinoma metastasis. Cell. 2009;138(1):51–62.
7. Senger DR, Van De Water L, Brown LF, Nagy JA, Yeo K-T, Yeo T-K, et al. Vascular permeability factor (VPF, VEGF) in tumor biology. Cancer Metastasis Rev. 1993;12(3–4):303–24.
8. Persidsky Y, Ramirez SH, Haorah J, Kanmogne GD. Blood–brain barrier: structural components and function under physiologic and pathologic conditions. J Neuroimmune Pharmacol. 2006;1(3):223–36.
9. Dobrogowska DH, Lossinsky AS, Tarnawski M, Vorbrodt AW. Increased blood–brain barrier permeability and endothelial abnormalities induced by vascular endothelial growth factor. J Neurocytol. 1998;27(3):163–73.
10. da Fonseca ACC, Matias D, Garcia C, Amaral R, Geraldo LH, Freitas C, et al. The impact of microglial activation on blood-brain barrier in brain diseases. Front Cell Neurosci [Internet]. 2014 [cited 2019 Apr 13];8. Available from: http://journal.frontiersin.org/article/10.3389/fncel.2014.00362/abstract.
11. Lockman PR, Mittapalli RK, Taskar KS, Rudraraju V, Gril B, Bohn KA, et al. Heterogeneous blood-tumor barrier permeability determines drug efficacy in experimental brain metastases of breast cancer. Clin Cancer Res. 2010;16(23):5664–78.

12. Fidler IJ. The biology of brain metastasis. Cancer J. 2015;21(4):10.
13. Lowery FJ, Yu D. Brain metastasis: unique challenges and open opportunities. Biochim Biophys Acta Rev Cancer. 2017;1867(1):49–57.
14. Kim S-J, Kim J-S, Park ES, Lee J-S, Lin Q, Langley RR, et al. Astrocytes upregulate survival genes in tumor cells and induce protection from chemotherapy. Neoplasia. 2011;13(3):286–98.
15. Lin NU, Lee EQ, Aoyama H, Barani IJ, Barboriak DP, Baumert BG, et al. Response assessment criteria for brain metastases: proposal from the RANO group. Lancet Oncol. 2015;16(6):e270–8.
16. Galldiks N, Langen K-J, Albert NL, Chamberlain M, Soffietti R, Kim MM, et al. PET imaging in patients with brain metastasis—report of the RANO/PET group. Neuro-Oncology [Internet]. 2019 [cited 2019 Apr 13]; Available from: https://academic.oup.com/neuro-oncology/advance-article/doi/10.1093/neuonc/noz003/5274178.
17. Schneider T, Kuhne JF, Bittrich P, Schroeder J, Magnus T, Mohme M, et al. Edema is not a reliable diagnostic sign to exclude small brain metastases. Ahmad A, editor. PLOS ONE. 2017;12(5):e0177217.
18. Walcott BP, Kahle KT, Simard JM. Novel treatment targets for cerebral edema. Neurotherapeutics. 2012;9(1):65–72.
19. Wen PY, Schiff D, Kesari S, Drappatz J, Gigas DC, Doherty L. Medical management of patients with brain tumors. J Neuro-Oncol. 2006;80(3):313–32.
20. Bebawy JF. Perioperative steroids for peritumoral intracranial edema: a review of mechanisms, efficacy, and side effects. J Neurosurg Anesthesiol. 2012;24(3):5.
21. Spanberger T, Berghoff AS, Dinhof C, Ilhan-Mutlu A, Magerle M, Hutterer M, et al. Extent of peritumoral brain edema correlates with prognosis, tumoral growth pattern, HIF1a expression and angiogenic activity in patients with single brain metastases. Clin Exp Metastasis. 2013;30(4):357–68.
22. Kerschbaumer J, Bauer M, Popovscaia M, Grams AE, Thomé C, Freyschlag CF. Correlation of tumor and peritumoral edema volumes with survival in patients with cerebral metastases. Anticancer Res. 2017;37(2):871–6.
23. Calluaud G, Terrier L-M, Mathon B, Destrieux C, Velut S, François P, et al. Peritumoral edema/tumor volume ratio: a strong survival predictor for posterior fossa metastases. Neurosurgery [Internet]. 2018 [cited 2019 Apr 13]; Available from: https://academic.oup.com/neurosurgery/advance-article/doi/10.1093/neuros/nyy222/5035747.
24. McClelland S, Long DM. Genesis of the use of corticosteroids in the treatment and prevention of brain edema. Neurosurgery. 2008;62(4):965–8.
25. Galicich JH, French LA, Melby JC. Use of dexamethasone in treatment of cerebral edema associated with brain tumors. J Lancet. 1961;81:46–53.
26. Ryken TC, Kuo JS, Prabhu RS, Sherman JH, Kalkanis SN, Olson JJ. Congress of Neurological Surgeons systematic review and evidence-based guidelines on the role of steroids in the treatment of adults with metastatic brain tumors. Neurosurgery. 2019;84(3):E189–91.
27. Batchelor T, DeAngelis LM. Medical Management of Cerebral Metastases. Neurosurg Clin N Am. 1996;7(3):435–46.
28. Black KL, Hoff JT, McGillicuddy JE, Gebarski SS. Increased leukotriene C4 and vasogenic edema surrounding brain tumors in humans. Ann Neurol. 1986;19(6):592–5.
29. Michinaga S, Koyama Y. Pathogenesis of brain edema and investigation into anti-edema drugs. Int J Mol Sci. 2015;16(12):9949–75.
30. Papadopoulos MC, Saadoun S, Binder DK, Manley GT, Krishna S, Verkman AS. Molecular mechanisms of brain tumor edema. Neuroscience. 2004;129(4):1009–18.
31. Murayi R, Chittiboina P. Glucocorticoids in the management of peritumoral brain edema: a review of molecular mechanisms. Childs Nerv Syst. 2016;32(12):2293–302.
32. Weissman DE, Dufer D, Vogel V, Abeloff MD. Corticosteroid toxicity in neuro-oncology patients. J Neuro-Oncol. 1987;5(2):125–8.
33. Ryken TC, McDermott M, Robinson PD, Ammirati M, Andrews DW, Asher AL, et al. The role of steroids in the management of brain metastases: a systematic review and evidence-based clinical practice guideline. J Neuro-Oncol. 2010;96(1):103–14.
34. Vecht CJ, Hovestadt A, Verbiest HBC, van Vliet JJ, van Putten WLJ. Dose-effect relationship of dexamethasone on Karnofsky performance in metastatic brain tumors: a randomized study of doses of 4, 8, and 16 mg per day. Neurology. 1994;44(4):675.
35. Weissman DE, Janjan NA, Erickson B, Wilson FJ, Greenberg M, Ritch PS, et al. Twice-daily tapering dexamethasone treatment during cranial radiation for newly diagnosed brain metastases. J Neuro-Oncol. 1991;11(3):235–9.
36. Ryan R, Booth S, Price S. Corticosteroid-use in primary and secondary brain tumour patients: a review. J Neuro-Oncol. 2012;106(3):449–59.
37. Hempen C, Weiss E, Hess CF. Dexamethasone treatment in patients with brain metastases and primary brain tumors: do the benefits outweigh the side-effects? Support Care Cancer. 2002;10(4):322–8.
38. Conn HO, Blitzer BL. Nonassociation of adrenocorticosteroid therapy and peptic ulcer. N Engl J Med. 1976;294(9):473–9.
39. Messer J, Reitman D, Sacks HS, Smith H, Chalmers TC. Association of adrenocorticosteroid therapy and peptic-ulcer disease. N Engl J Med. 1983;309(1):21–4.
40. Conn HO, Poynard T. Adrenocorticosteroid administration and peptic ulcer: a critical analysis. J Chronic Dis. 1985;38(6):457–68.

41. Gøtzsche PC. Steroids and peptic ulcer: an end to the controversy? J Intern Med. 1994;236(6):599–601.
42. Narum S, Westergren T, Klemp M. Corticosteroids and risk of gastrointestinal bleeding: a systematic review and meta-analysis. BMJ Open. 2014;4(5):e004587.
43. Kondo Y, Hatta W, Koike T, Takahashi Y, Saito M, Kanno T, et al. The use of higher dose steroids increases the risk of rebleeding after endoscopic hemostasis for peptic ulcer bleeding. Dig Dis Sci. 2018;63(11):3033–40.
44. Tseng C-L, Chen Y-T, Huang C-J, Luo J-C, Peng Y-L, Huang D-F, et al. Short-term use of glucocorticoids and risk of peptic ulcer bleeding: a nationwide population-based case-crossover study. Aliment Pharmacol Ther. 2015;42(5):599–606.
45. Piper JM. Corticosteroid use and peptic ulcer disease: role of nonsteroidal anti-inflammatory drugs. Ann Intern Med. 1991;114(9):735.
46. Baden LR, Swaminathan S, Angarone M, Blouin G, Camins BC, Casper C, et al. Prevention and treatment of cancer-related infections, version 2.2016, NCCN clinical practice guidelines in oncology. J Natl Compr Cancer Netw. 2016;14(7):882–913.
47. Yale SH, Limper AH. Pneumocystis carinii pneumonia in patients without acquired immunodeficiency syndrome: associated illnesses and prior corticosteroid therapy. Mayo Clin Proc. 1996;71(1):5–13.
48. Calero-Bernal ML, Martin-Garrido I, Donazar-Ezcurra M, Limper AH, Carmona EM. Intermittent courses of corticosteroids also present a risk for *Pneumocystis* pneumonia in non-HIV patients. Can Respir J. 2016;2016:1–7.
49. Wick W, Küker W. Brain edema in neurooncology: radiological assessment and management. Oncol Res Treat. 2004;27(3):261–6.
50. LoPiccolo J, Mehta SA, Lipson EJ. Corticosteroid use and pneumocystis pneumonia prophylaxis: a teachable moment. JAMA Intern Med. 2018;178(8):1106.
51. Giles AJ, Hutchinson M-KND, Sonnemann HM, Jung J, Fecci PE, Ratnam NM, et al. Dexamethasone-induced immunosuppression: mechanisms and implications for immunotherapy. J Immunother Cancer [Internet]. 2018 [cited 2019 Apr 13];6(1). Available from: https://jitc.biomedcentral.com/articles/10.1186/s40425-018-0371-5.
52. Weber JS, Hodi FS, Wolchok JD, Topalian SL, Schadendorf D, Larkin J, et al. Safety profile of nivolumab monotherapy: a pooled analysis of patients with advanced melanoma. J Clin Oncol. 2017;35(7):785–92.
53. Berghoff AS, Preusser M. Anti-angiogenic therapies in brain metastases. memo – Mag Eur Med Oncol. 2018;11(1):14–7.
54. Banks PD, Lasocki A, Lau PKH, Sandhu S, McArthur G, Shackleton M. Bevacizumab as a steroid-sparing agent during immunotherapy for melanoma brain metastases: a case series. Health Sci Rep. 2019;2(3):e115.
55. Wang Y, Wang E, Pan L, Dai J, Zhang N, Wang X, et al. A new strategy of CyberKnife treatment system based radiosurgery followed by early use of adjuvant bevacizumab treatment for brain metastasis with extensive cerebral edema. J Neuro-Oncol. 2014;119(2):369–76.
56. Hapani S, Chu D, Wu S. Risk of gastrointestinal perforation in patients with cancer treated with bevacizumab: a meta-analysis. Lancet Oncol. 2009;10(6):559–68.
57. Saif MW, Elfiky A, Salem RR. Gastrointestinal perforation due to bevacizumab in colorectal cancer. Ann Surg Oncol. 2007;14(6):1860–9.
58. Khasraw M, Holodny A, Goldlust SA, DeAngelis LM. Intracranial hemorrhage in patients with cancer treated with bevacizumab: the memorial Sloan-Kettering experience. Ann Oncol. 2012;23(2):458–63.
59. Carden CP, Larkin JMG, Rosenthal MA. What is the risk of intracranial bleeding during anti-VEGF therapy? Neuro-Oncology. 2008;10(4):624–30.
60. Besse B, Lasserre SF, Compton P, Huang J, Augustus S, Rohr U-P. Bevacizumab safety in patients with central nervous system metastases. Clin Cancer Res. 2010;16(1):269–78.
61. Socinski MA, Langer CJ, Huang JE, Kolb MM, Compton P, Wang L, et al. Safety of bevacizumab in patients with non–small-cell lung cancer and brain metastases. J Clin Oncol. 2009;27(31):5255–61.
62. Gordon CR, Rojavin Y, Patel M, Zins JE, Grana G, Kann B, et al. A review on bevacizumab and surgical wound healing: an important warning to all surgeons. Ann Plast Surg. 2009;62(6):707–9.
63. Gerstner ER, Duda DG, di Tomaso E, Ryg PA, Loeffler JS, Sorensen AG, et al. VEGF inhibitors in the treatment of cerebral edema in patients with brain cancer. Nat Rev Clin Oncol. 2009;6(4):229–36.
64. Eichler AF, Loeffler JS. Multidisciplinary management of brain metastases. Oncologist. 2007;12(7):884–98.
65. Pope WB, Lai A, Nghiemphu P, Mischel P, Cloughesy TF. MRI in patients with high-grade gliomas treated with bevacizumab and chemotherapy. Neurology. 2006;66(8):1258–60.
66. Berghoff AS, Ilhan-Mutlu A, Dinhof C, Magerle M, Hackl M, Widhalm G, et al. Differential role of angiogenesis and tumour cell proliferation in brain metastases according to primary tumour type: analysis of 639 cases. Neuropathol Appl Neurobiol. 2015;41(2):e41–55.
67. Wei ET, Gao GC. Corticotropin-releasing factor: an inhibitor of vascular leakage in rat skeletal muscle and brain cortex after injury. Regul Pept. 1991;33(2):93–104.
68. Tjuvajev J, Uehara H, Desai R, Beattie B, Matei C, Zhou Y, et al. Corticotropin-releasing factor decreases vasogenic brain edema. Cancer Res. 1996;56(6):1352–60.
69. Villalona-Calero MA, Eckardt J, Burris H, Kraynak M, Fields-Jones S, Bazan C, et al. A phase I trial of human corticotropin-releasing factor (hCRF) in patients with peritumoral brain edema. Ann Oncol. 1998;9(1):71–7.

70. Recht L, Mechtler LL, Wong ET, O'Connor PC, Rodda BE. Steroid-sparing effect of corticorelin acetate in peritumoral cerebral edema is associated with improvement in steroid-induced myopathy. J Clin Oncol. 2013;31(9):1182–7.

71. Recht LD, Mechtler L, Phuphanich S, Hormigo A, Hines V, Milsted R, et al. A placebo-controlled study investigating the dexamethasone-sparing effects of corticorelin acetate in patients with primary or metastatic brain tumors and peritumoral edema. J Clin Oncol. 2009;27(15_suppl):2078.

72. Shapiro WR, Mechtler L, Cher L, Wheeler H, Hines V, Milsted R, et al. A randomized, double-blind study comparing corticorelin acetate with dexamethasone in patients with primary malignant glioma who require increased dexamethasone doses to control symptoms of peritumoral brain edema. J Clin Oncol. 2009;27(15_suppl):2080.

73. Mechtler L, Wong ET, Hormigo A, Pannullo S, Hines V, Milsted R, et al. A long-term open-label extension study examining the steroid-sparing effects of corticorelin acetate in patients with cerebral tumors. J Clin Oncol. 2009;27(15_suppl):2079.

74. Donkin JJ, Nimmo AJ, Cernak I, Blumbergs PC, Vink R. Substance P is associated with the development of brain edema and functional deficits after traumatic brain injury. J Cereb Blood Flow Metab. 2009;29(8):1388–98.

75. Gabrielian L, Helps SC, Thornton E, Turner RJ, Leonard AV, Vink R. Substance P antagonists as a novel intervention for brain edema and raised intracranial pressure. In: Katayama Y, Maeda T, Kuroiwa T, editors. Brain edema XV [Internet]. Vienna: Springer Vienna; 2013 [cited 2019 Apr 16]. p. 201–4. Available from: http://link.springer.com/10.1007/978-3-7091-1434-6_37.

76. Turner RJ, Helps SC, Thornton E, Vink R. A substance P antagonist improves outcome when administered 4 h after onset of ischaemic stroke. Brain Res. 2011;1393:84–90.

77. Harford-Wright E, Lewis KM, Ghabriel MN, Vink R. Treatment with the NK1 antagonist emend reduces blood brain barrier dysfunction and edema formation in an experimental model of brain tumors. Alonso MM, editor. PLoS ONE. 2014;9(5):e97002.

78. Rutz HP. Effects of corticosteroid use on treatment of solid tumours. Lancet. 2002;360(9349):1969–70.

79. Bannwarth B, Netter P, Lapicque F, Péré P, Thomas P, Gaucher A. Plasma and cerebrospinal fluid concentrations of indomethacin in humans: relationship to analgesic activity. Eur J Clin Pharmacol. 1990;38(4):343–6.

80. Cotev S, Shapira Y, Davidson E, Wiedenfeld Y, Icu ES. Indomethacin reduces cerebral prostaglandin synthesis but not edema after experimental head injury. Crit Care Med. 1987;15(4):370.

81. Deluga KS, Plötz FB, Betz AL. Effect of indomethacin on edema following single and repetitive cerebral ischemia in the gerbil. Stroke. 1991;22(10):1259–64.

82. Ambrus JL, Halpern J, Baerwald H, Johnson RJ. Cyclo-oxygenase and lipo-oxygenase inhibitors may substitute for steroid treatment in brain oedema. Lancet. 1985;2(8447):148–9.

83. Weissman DE, Stewart C. Experimental drug therapy of peritumoral brain edema. J Neuro-Oncol [Internet]. 1988 [cited 2019 Apr 17];6(4). Available from: http://link.springer.com/10.1007/BF00177429.

84. Nathoo N. The eicosanoid cascade: possible role in gliomas and meningiomas. J Clin Pathol. 2004;57(1):6–13.

85. Badie B, Schartner JM, Hagar AR, Prabakaran S, Peebles TR, Bartley B, et al. Microglia cyclooxygenase-2 activity in experimental gliomas: possible role in cerebral edema formation. Clin Cancer Res. 2003;9(2):872–7.

86. Castelli MG, Chiabrando C, Fanelli R, Martelli L, Butti G, Gaetani P, et al. Prostaglandin and thromboxane synthesis by human intracranial tumors. Cancer Res. 1989;49(6):1505–8.

87. Chu K, Jeong S-W, Jung K-H, Han S-Y, Lee S-T, Kim M, et al. Celecoxib induces functional recovery after intracerebral hemorrhage with reduction of brain edema and perihematomal cell death. J Cereb Blood Flow Metab. 2004;24(8):926–33.

88. Lee S-H, Park H-K, Ryu W-S, Lee J-S, Bae H-J, Han M-K, et al. Effects of celecoxib on hematoma and edema volumes in primary intracerebral hemorrhage: a multicenter randomized controlled trial. Eur J Neurol. 2013;20(8):1161–9.

89. Wei D, Wang L, He Y, Xiong HQ, Abbruzzese JL, Xie K. Celecoxib inhibits vascular endothelial growth factor expression in and reduces angiogenesis and metastasis of human pancreatic cancer via suppression of Sp1 transcription factor activity. Cancer Res. 2004;64(6):2030–8.

90. Dembo G, Park SB, Kharasch ED. Central nervous system concentrations of cyclooxygenase-2 inhibitors in humans. Anesthesiology. 2005;102(2):409–15.

91. Rutz HP, Hofer S, Peghini PE, Gutteck-Amsler U, Rentsch K, Meier-Abt PJ, et al. Avoiding glucocorticoid administration in a neurooncological case. Cancer Biol Ther. 2005;4(11):1186–9.

92. Lenzer J. FDA advisers warn: COX 2 inhibitors increase risk of heart attack and stroke. BMJ. 2005;330(7489):440.

93. Streffer JR, Bitzer M, Schabet M, Dichgans J, Weller M. Response of radiochemotherapy-associated cerebral edema to a phytotherapeutic agent, H15. Neurology. 2001;56(9):1219–21.

94. Kirste S, Treier M, Wehrle SJ, Becker G, Abdel-Tawab M, Gerbeth K, et al. Boswellia serrata acts on cerebral edema in patients irradiated for brain tumors: a prospective, randomized, placebo-controlled, double-blind pilot trial. Cancer. 2011;117(16):3788–95.

95. Glaser T, Winter S, Groscurth P, Safayhi H, Sailer E-R, Ammon HPT, et al. Boswellic acids and malignant glioma: induction of apoptosis but

no modulation of drug sensitivity. Br J Cancer. 1999;80(5–6):756–65.

96. Sterk V, Büchele B, Simmet T. Effect of food intake on the bioavailability of boswellic acids from a herbal preparation in healthy volunteers. Planta Med. 2004;70(12):1155–60.

97. Burger PC, Mahaley MS, Dudka L, Vogel FS. The morphologic effects of radiation administered therapeutically for intracranial gliomas. A Postmortem study of 25 cases. Cancer. 1979;44(4):1256–72.

98. Fink J, Born D, Chamberlain MC. Radiation necrosis: relevance with respect to treatment of primary and secondary brain tumors. Curr Neurol Neurosci Rep. 2012;12(3):276–85.

99. Constine LS, Konski A, Ekholm S, McDonald S, Rubin P. Adverse effects of brain irradiation correlated with MR and CT imaging. Int J Radiat Oncol Biol Phys. 1988;15(2):319–30.

100. Shah R, Vattoth S, Jacob R, Manzil FFP, O'Malley JP, Borghei P, et al. Radiation necrosis in the brain: imaging features and differentiation from tumor recurrence. Radiographics. 2012;32(5):1343–59.

101. Eissner G, Kohlhuber F, Grell M, Ueffing M, Scheurich P, Hieke A. Critical involvement of transmembrane tumor necrosis factor-cu in endothelial programmed cell death mediated by ionizing radiation and bacterial endotoxin. Blood. 1995;86(11):4184–93.

102. Yoshii Y. Pathological review of late cerebral radionecrosis. Brain Tumor Pathol. 2008;25(2):51–8.

103. Lawrence YR, Li XA, el Naqa I, Hahn CA, Marks LB, Merchant TE, et al. Radiation dose–volume effects in the brain. Int J Radiat Oncol Biol Phys. 2010;76(3 Suppl):S20–7.

104. Chung C, Bryant A, Brown PD. Interventions for the treatment of brain radionecrosis after radiotherapy or radiosurgery. Cochrane Gynaecological, Neuro-oncology and Orphan Cancer Group, editor. Cochrane Database Syst Rev [Internet]. 2018 [cited 2019 Apr 13]; Available from: http://doi.wiley.com/10.1002/14651858.CD011492.pub2.

105. McPherson CM, Warnick RE. Results of contemporary surgical management of radiation necrosis using frameless stereotaxis and intraoperative magnetic resonance imaging. J Neuro-Oncol. 2004;68(1):41–7.

106. Eyster EF, Nielsen SL, Sheline GE, Wilson CB. Cerebral radiation necrosis simulating a brain tumor. J Neurosurg. 1974;40(2):267–71.

107. Shaw PJ, Bates D. Conservative treatment of delayed cerebral radiation necrosis. J Neurol Neurosurg Psychiatry. 1984;47(12):1338–41.

108. Furuse M, Nonoguchi N, Kawabata S, Miyatake S-I, Kuroiwa T. Delayed brain radiation necrosis: pathological review and new molecular targets for treatment. Med Mol Morphol. 2015;48(4):183–90.

109. Gonzalez J, Kumar AJ, Conrad CA, Levin VA. Effect of bevacizumab on radiation necrosis of the brain. Int J Radiat Oncol Biol Phys. 2007;67(2):323–6.

110. Deibert CP, Ahluwalia MS, Sheehan JP, Link MJ, Hasegawa T, Yomo S, et al. Bevacizumab for refractory adverse radiation effects after stereotactic radiosurgery. J Neuro-Oncol. 2013;115(2):217–23.

111. Levin VA, Bidaut L, Hou P, Kumar AJ, Wefel JS, Bekele BN, et al. Randomized double-blind placebo-controlled trial of bevacizumab therapy for radiation necrosis of the central nervous system. Int J Radiat Oncol Biol Phys. 2011;79(5):1487–95.

112. Bennett MH, Feldmeier J, Hampson NB, Smee R, Milross C. Hyperbaric oxygen therapy for late radiation tissue injury. Cochrane Gynaecological, Neuro-oncology and Orphan Cancer Group, editor. Cochrane Database Syst Rev [Internet]. 2016 [cited 2019 Apr 13]; Available from: http://doi.wiley.com/10.1002/14651858.CD005005.pub4.

113. Hary GB, Mainous EG. The treatment of radiation necrosis with hyperbaric oxygen (OHP). Cancer. 1976;37(6):2580–5.

114. Chuba PJ, Aronin P, Bhambhani K, Eichenhorn M, Zamarano L, Cianci P, et al. Hyperbaric oxygen therapy for radiation-induced brain injury in children. Cancer. 1997;80(10):2005–12.

115. Tang Y, Rong X, Hu W, Li G, Yang X, Yang J, et al. Effect of edaravone on radiation-induced brain necrosis in patients with nasopharyngeal carcinoma after radiotherapy: a randomized controlled trial. J Neuro-Oncol. 2014;120(2):441–7.

116. Rizzoli HV, Pagnanelli DM. Treatment of delayed radiation necrosis of the brain. J Neurosurg. 1984;60(3):589–94.

117. Dion MW, Hussey DH, Doornbos JF, Vigliotti AP, Wen B-C, Anderson B. Preliminary results of a pilot study of pentoxifylline in the treatment of late radiation soft tissue necrosis. Int J Radiat Oncol Biol Phys. 1990;19(2):401–7.

118. Williamson R, Kondziolka D, Kanaan H, Lunsford LD, Flickinger JC. Adverse radiation effects after radiosurgery may benefit from oral vitamin E and pentoxifylline therapy: a pilot study. Stereotact Funct Neurosurg. 2008;86(6):359–66.

119. Rahmathulla G, Recinos PF, Valerio JE, Chao S, Barnett GH. Laser interstitial thermal therapy for focal cerebral radiation necrosis: a case report and literature review. Stereotact Funct Neurosurg. 2012;90(3):192–200.

120. Fabiano AJ, Alberico RA. Laser-interstitial thermal therapy for refractory cerebral edema from post-radiosurgery metastasis. World Neurosurg. 2014;81(3–4):652.e1–4.

121. North JB, Hanieh A, Challen Robert G, Penhall Robert K, Hann Christopher S, Frewin DB. Postoperative epilepsy: a double-blind trial of phenytoin after craniotomy. Lancet. 1980;315(8165):384–6.

122. Forsyth PA, Weaver S, Fulton D, Brasher PMA, Sutherland G, Stewart D, et al. Prophylactic anticonvulsants in patients with brain tumour. Can J Neurol Sci. 2003;30(02):106–12.

123. Glantz MJ, Cole BF, Friedberg MH, Lathi E, Choy H, Furie K, et al. A randomized, blinded, placebo-

controlled trial of divalproex sodium prophylaxis in adults with newly diagnosed brain tumors. Neurology. 1996;46(4):985–91.

124. Wu AS, Trinh VT, Suki D, Graham S, Forman A, Weinberg JS, et al. A prospective randomized trial of perioperative seizure prophylaxis in patients with intraparenchymal brain tumors. J Neurosurg. 2013;118(4):873–83.

125. Franceschetti S, Binelli S, Casazza M, Lodrini S, Panzica F, Pluchino F, et al. Influence of surgery and antiepileptic drugs on seizures symptomatic of cerebral tumours. Acta Neurochir. 1990;103(1–2): 47–51.

126. Ansari SF, Bohnstedt BN, Perkins SM, Althouse SK, Miller JC. Efficacy of postoperative seizure prophylaxis in intra-axial brain tumor resections. J Neuro-Oncol. 2014;118(1):117–22.

127. Tremont-Lukats IW, Ratilal BO, Armstrong T, Gilbert MR. Antiepileptic drugs for preventing seizures in people with brain tumors. Cochrane Database Syst Rev [Internet]. 2008 [cited 2019 Apr 20];(2). Available from: https://www.cochranelibrary.com/cdsr/doi/10.1002/14651858.CD004424.pub2/abstract.

128. Chen CC, Rennert RC, Olson JJ. Congress of Neurological Surgeons systematic review and evidence-based guidelines on the role of prophylactic anticonvulsants in the treatment of adults with metastatic brain tumors. Neurosurgery. 2019;84(3):E195–7.

129. Chang SM, Messersmith H, Ahluwalia M, Andrews D, Brastianos PK, Gaspar LE, et al. Anticonvulsant prophylaxis and steroid use in adults with metastatic brain tumors: summary of SNO and ASCO endorsement of the Congress of Neurological Surgeons guidelines. Neuro-Oncology. 2019;21(4):424–7.

130. Glantz MJ, Cole BF, Forsyth PA, Recht LD, Wen PY, Chamberlain MC, et al. Practice parameter: anticonvulsant prophylaxis in patients with newly diagnosed brain tumors: report of the quality standards Subcommittee of the American Academy of Neurology. Neurology. 2000;54(10):1886–93.

131. Waxman DJ, Azaroff L. Phenobarbital induction of cytochrome P-450 gene expression. Biochem J. 1992;281(3):577–92.

132. Jusko WJ, Koup JR, Alván G. Nonlinear assessment of phenytoin bioavailability. J Pharmacokinet Biopharm. 1976;4(4):327–36.

133. Monks A, Boobis S, Wadsworth J, Richens A. Plasma protein binding interaction between phenytoin and valproic acid in vitro. Br J Clin Pharmacol. 1978;6(6):487–92.

134. Chokshi R, Openshaw J, Mehta NN, Mohler E. Purple glove syndrome following intravenous phenytoin administration. Vasc Med. 2007;12(1): 29–31.

135. Ferrell PB, McLeod HL. Carbamazepine, HLA-B∗1502 and risk of Stevens–Johnson syndrome and

toxic epidermal necrolysis: US FDA recommendations. Pharmacogenomics. 2008;9(10):1543–6.

136. Tran TA, Leppik IE, Blesi K, Sathanandan ST, Remmel R. Lamotrigine clearance during pregnancy. Neurology. 2002;59(2):251–5.

137. Sabers A, Buchholt JM, Uldall P, Hansen EL. Lamotrigine plasma levels reduced by oral contraceptives. Epilepsy Res. 2001;47(1–2):151–4.

138. Turnbull DM, Rawlins MD, Weightman D, Chadwick DW. Plasma concentrations of sodium valproate: their clinical value. Ann Neurol. 1983;14(1):38–42.

139. Marcotte D. Use of topiramate, a new antiepileptic as a mood stabilizer. J Affect Disord. 1998;50(2–3):245–51.

140. Leppik IE. Zonisamide: chemistry, mechanism of action, and pharmacokinetics. Seizure. 2004;13:S5–9.

141. Rosenstiel P. Brivaracetam (UCB 34714). Neurotherapeutics. 2007;4(1):84–7.

142. Biton V, Berkovic SF, Abou-Khalil B, Sperling MR, Johnson ME, Lu S. Brivaracetam as adjunctive treatment for uncontrolled partial epilepsy in adults: a phase III randomized, double-blind, placebo-controlled trial. Epilepsia. 2014;55(1):57–66.

143. Doty P, Rudd GD, Stoehr T, Thomas D. Lacosamide. Neurotherapeutics. 2007;4(1):145–8.

144. Kaufman DW, Kelly JP, Anderson T, Harmon DC, Shapiro S. Evaluation of case reports of aplastic anemia among patients treated with felbamate. Epilepsia. 1997;38(12):1265–9.

145. Seibert TM, Karunamuni R, Kaifi S, Burkeen J, Connor M, Krishnan AP, et al. Cerebral cortex regions selectively vulnerable to radiation dose-dependent atrophy. Int J Radiat Oncol Biol Phys. 2017;97(5):910–8.

146. Gondi V, Pugh SL, Tome WA, Caine C, Corn B, Kanner A, et al. Preservation of memory with conformal avoidance of the hippocampal neural stem-cell compartment during whole-brain radiotherapy for brain metastases (RTOG 0933): a phase II multi-institutional trial. J Clin Oncol. 2014;32(34):3810–6.

147. Rapp SR, Case LD, Peiffer A, Naughton MM, Chan MD, Stieber VW, et al. Donepezil for irradiated brain tumor survivors: a phase III randomized placebo-controlled clinical trial. J Clin Oncol. 2015;33(15):1653–9.

148. Shaw EG, Rosdhal R, D'Agostino RB, Lovato J, Naughton MJ, Robbins ME, et al. Phase II study of donepezil in irradiated brain tumor patients: effect on cognitive function, mood, and quality of life. J Clin Oncol. 2006;24(9):1415–20.

149. Brown PD, Pugh S, Laack NN, Wefel JS, Khuntia D, Meyers C, et al. Memantine for the prevention of cognitive dysfunction in patients receiving whole-brain radiotherapy: a randomized, double-blind, placebo-controlled trial. Neuro-Oncology. 2013;15(10):1429–37.

Neuroimaging of Brain Metastases

5

Mira A. Patel, Eric Lis, and Yoshiya Yamada

Imaging of the Brain: An Overview

Magnetic resonance imaging (MRI) performed with intravenous gadolinium contrast is the most useful imaging modality to evaluate brain metastases. The advantage of MR imaging lies in its ability to differentiate between tissues of the central nervous system (CNS) in a way that computed tomography (CT) cannot, as MR can produce much better soft tissue contrast. The standard MR sequences for evaluating brain metastases are T1 (longitudinal relaxation time)- and T2 (transverse relaxation time)-weighted images.

T1-weighted images allow detection of abnormality in normal brain architecture; gray matter appears hypointense on T1-weighted images and white matter appears mildly hyperintense. Cerebrospinal fluid (CSF) appears hypointense on T1-weighted MRI, and in the presence of gadolinium, often vessels become apparent as hyperintense structures and brain metastases typically appear as roughly spherical structures that enhance with the accumulation of gadolinium. If there is no perfusion to the center of a metastasis, it will appear to be ring-enhancing. Notably, inflammation or edema will appear hypointense on T1 [1].

T2-weighted images are ideal for assessing the extent of vasogenic edema associated with brain tumors. CSF is characteristically very hyperintense on T2-weighted imaging, with white matter appearing hypointense and gray matter appearing mildly hyperintense. Edema will appear bright on T2 imaging. Fluid attenuated inversion recovery (FLAIR) imaging is similar to T2-weighted imaging except that there is suppression of CSF; this type of imaging is most useful for identifying peri-ventricular enhancing lesions and visualization of vasogenic edema separate from CSF.

Brain metastases are typically found at the gray-white matter junction and are often well-circumscribed structures that may cause mass effect on surrounding brain parenchyma. Metastases may or may not be hemorrhagic, and they may or may not be associated with significant edema depending upon the primary disease histology.

Neuroanatomy

The anatomic lobes of the brain are separated by deep sulci. The anterior to posterior interhemispheric fissure divides the cerebrum into two hemispheres. The central sulcus defines the boundary between the frontal and parietal lobes [2] (Fig. 5.1). The central sulcus comes all the way to the midline at the vertex and may be identified as an "omega" sign on axial imaging, both of which may be used to identify the precentral and postcentral gyri (Fig. 5.1). Additionally, the

M. A. Patel · Y. Yamada (✉)
Department of Radiation Oncology, Memorial Sloan
Kettering Cancer Center, New York, NY, USA
e-mail: yamadaj@mskcc.org

E. Lis
Department of Radiology, Memorial Sloan Kettering
Cancer Center, New York, NY, USA

© Springer Nature Switzerland AG 2020
Y. Yamada et al. (eds.), *Radiotherapy in Managing Brain Metastases*,
https://doi.org/10.1007/978-3-030-43740-4_5

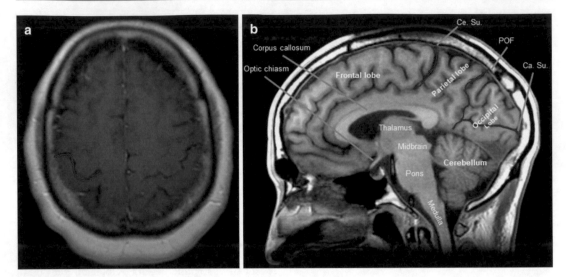

Fig. 5.1 (**a**) Axial T1-weighted image indicating characteristic "omega" sign in red that identifies the central sulcus separating the frontal and parietal lobes. (**b**) Sagittal T1 weighed image showing normal brain anatomy with major sulci indicated in red. Ce.Su. Central sulcus, POS parieto-occipital fissure, Ca. Su. calcarine sulcus

precentral gyrus (motor strip) is not split by a sulcus. The sagittal sulcus of the frontal lobe terminates in front of the motor strip and never transects it. The lateral, or Sylvian, fissure separates the parietal and frontal lobes from the temporal lobe and contains the middle cerebral artery. The parietal and occipital lobes are separated by the parieto-occipital fissure.

Frontal and Parietal Lobes

The frontal lobe is responsible for executive function and associational behaviors including judgment, reason, creativity, and social inhibition. The motor cortex is the most posterior gyrus of the frontal cortex and is located directly anterior to the central sulcus [3, 4]. The olfactory tract lies on the orbital surface of the frontal lobe.

The parietal lobe lies posterior to the frontal lobe and anterior to the occipital lobe. Important cortical structures in the parietal lobe include the sensory cortex at the postcentral gyrus, which is immediately posterior to the central sulcus.

Clinical Correlate

Brain metastases of the frontal lobe may result in motor deficit if the tumor is involving the precen-

tral gyrus or causing significant vasogenic edema at this location. Broca's area is an important language production center located in the anteroinferior frontal lobe and if affected may result in expressive aphasia. Brain metastases at the frontal lobe do not typically result in significantly disinhibited behavior or cognitive dysfunction, but a large frontal brain metastasis may result in contralateral midline shift (Fig. 5.2).

Parietal lobe lesions typically do not present with pathognomonic neurologic deficits, but they may be associated with sensory issues if there is postcentral gyrus involvement. Just as for the frontal lobe, large brain metastases in the parietal lobe with associated vasogenic edema may result in midline shift or increased intracranial pressure (ICP), resulting in headache, nausea, vomiting, or, in rare cases, downward herniation of the cerebellar tonsils.

Temporal Lobe

The temporal lobe is located inferior to the frontal and parietal lobes and houses important language and memory centers of the brain. The left posterior temporal lobe contains Wernicke's area, which is responsible for speech comprehension.

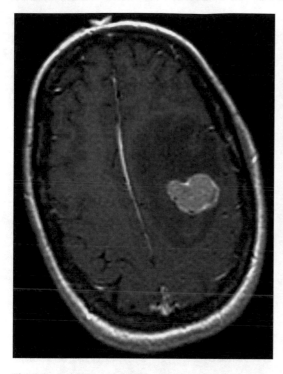

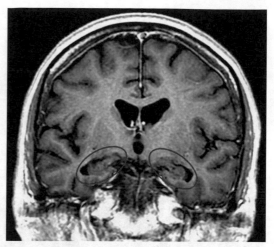

Fig. 5.3 Axial T1-weighted coronal image demonstrating bilateral hippocampi located within the medial temporal lobe, indicated with red ovals

Fig. 5.2 Axial T1-weighted image post gadolinium contrast demonstrating a large enhancing left frontal brain metastasis with surrounding hypointense vasogenic edema resulting in rightward midline shift

The hippocampus is located in the medial temporal lobe and is best seen on coronal imaging [5] (Fig. 5.3). The hippocampus is a vital structure of the limbic system that mediates long-term memory and emotion.

Clinical Correlate

Brain metastases in the temporal lobe may present with speech and language difficulty or memory deficit, depending upon the location of the tumor. Patients typically have issues with speech comprehension and display a receptive aphasia. Seizures are most frequently observed in patients with temporal lobe metastases. Small temporal lobe metastases may not present with any symptoms.

Diencephalon and Basal Ganglia

The diencephalon is composed of the thalamus and hypothalamus. The thalami bilaterally relay sensory information to the cortex and mediate

audio and visual reflexes [6]. The hypothalamus mediates endocrine function and communicates with the pituitary gland via the pituitary stalk. The basal ganglia include the internal capsules, the claustrum, the globus pallidus, the cauda nucleus, the amygdala, and the putamen and are responsible for emotion and cognition, as well as integration of motor and sensory information [7, 8] (Fig. 5.4). The insula is also a part of the limbic system responsible for emotional experience; it is a part of the cerebral cortex folded within the lateral sulcus (Fig. 5.4).

Clinical Correlate

If large, metastases of the diencephalon and basal ganglia may impede CSF flow and result in hydrocephalus and associated symptoms. Metastases of the thalamus or internal capsule that result in significant edema may disrupt the relay of information between the periphery and the cortex, resulting in somatosensory deficits.

Cerebellum

The cerebellum is located in the posterior fossa inferior to the cerebrum and is divided into four lobes: the flocculonodular lobe, the vermis, and the anterior and posterior lobes. The cerebellum

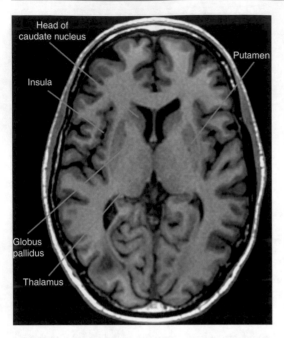

Fig. 5.4 Axial T1-weighted image indicating the basal ganglia

regulates balance and coordinated movements via interactions between the inferior vermis and flocculonodular lobes and the vestibular system. Inferolaterally, the cerebellar tonsils are small medial inferior projections of the cerebellum (Fig. 5.5). In the setting of suspected leptomeningeal disease, careful evaluation of the cerebellum and posterior fossa with a T1 gadolinium-enhanced multiplanar MRI study is warranted.

Clinical Correlate

A brain tumor in the posterior fossa may become quickly symptomatic, particularly because of the proximity of adjacent structures—such as the brainstem and cerebral aqueduct—that are rapidly affected by local mass effect in the posterior cranial fossa (Fig. 5.5).

A brain metastasis in the cerebellum may present as ataxic gait or difficulty with balance or coordination. Patients may complain of headache that is relieved by being supine, nausea, or vomiting if

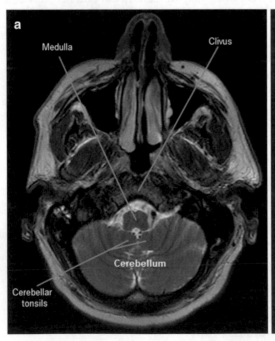

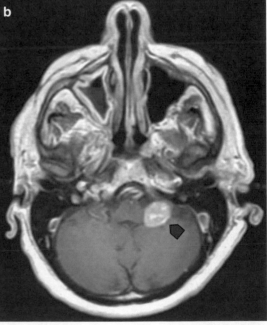

Fig. 5.5 (**a**) Axial T2-weighted image indicating key structures of the posterior fossa. (**b**) Axial T1-weighted image post gadolinium contrast demonstrating an enhanc- ing left cerebellar metastasis indicated by red arrowhead. Note abutment of medulla

there is compression of the fourth ventricle or cerebral aqueduct and subsequent increased ICP.

In cases of significant or acute changes in ICP—such as a large cerebral tumor with associated edema—the cerebellar tonsils may herniate inferiorly through the foramen magnum. Such a clinical finding signals a medical emergency, and intracranial decompression must be performed quickly.

Optic Apparatus and Sella Turcica

The anterior optic structures are composed of the orbits, optic nerves, and optic chiasm. Within the orbits are the extraocular muscles and lacrimal apparatus. Important structures of the globe include the cornea, lens, sclera, and retina [9]. The optic nerves meet at the optic chiasm, which is most easily visible on T2-weighted axial imaging (Fig. 5.6). The decussation of optic fibers occurs immediately superior to the pituitary gland and sella turcica, and anterior to the pituitary stalk, third ventricle, and mammillary bodies. The optic chiasm may be most easily identified using axial T2 imaging and cross-referencing the anatomy on sagittal and coronal imaging (Fig. 5.6). When contouring the optic chiasm on axial imaging, unless the imaging plane is parallel to the plane of the chiasm, it will be contoured on multiple axial slices. The nerve fibers from the retina project to the lateral geniculate nucleus and thence to the calcarine sulcus, which houses the primary visual cortex. The calcarine cortex begins near the occipital pole and continues anteriorly to a point inferior to the splenium of the corpus callosum, where it meets the medial portion of the parietooccipital fissure at an acute angle (see Fig. 5.1).

The pituitary stalk arises from the third ventricle's infundibular recess and gives rise to the pituitary gland, which is located in the sella turcica. The anterior pituitary gland appears isointense on T1- and T2-weighted images, whereas the posterior pituitary gland is hyperintense on T1. The pituitary gland is responsible for secre-

tion of several hormones regulating growth, fluid balance, metabolism, and sexual function.

Clinical Correlate

Metastases to the optic structures are not typically seen, but local mass effect upon the optic apparatus may cause visual disturbances depending upon the location of the lesion. Tumors compressing the chiasm may cause bilateral visual field deficits if affecting the proximal chiasm or unilateral deficits if affecting the distal chiasm or optic nerve (Fig. 5.6). A lesion at the calcarine sulcus may also result in complex visual disturbances. When performing radiosurgery near the calcarine sulcus, the treating physician should be aware of the potential consequences of treatment sequelae such as radionecrosis and the potential impact upon vision. This is particularly important when treating bilateral metastases near the calcarine sulci.

A metastatic lesion in the pituitary gland may present with endocrinopathy, but more commonly would present with bitemporal hemianopsia from compression of the optic chiasm.

Brainstem

The brainstem is composed of three segments: the midbrain (or mesencephalon), pons, and medulla oblongata, and it is responsible for maintaining basic life functions, including breathing and heartbeat (Fig. 5.1) [10]. The midbrain connects the diencephalon to the pons and on axial imaging appears as a "W." The midbrain gives rise to the fourth cranial nerve. The pons lies between the midbrain and the medulla, contains a large anterior convexity, and divides the cerebral hemispheres. The nuclei of the fifth, sixth, seventh, and eighth cranial nerves are located in the pons. The posterior aspect of the pons is the roof of the fourth ventricle. The medulla lies between the pons and the spinal cord. The ninth, tenth, eleventh, and twelfth cranial nerves emerge from the medulla. When contouring the brainstem, the superior aspect of the brainstem is defined by the cerebral aqueduct, and the inferior aspect of the

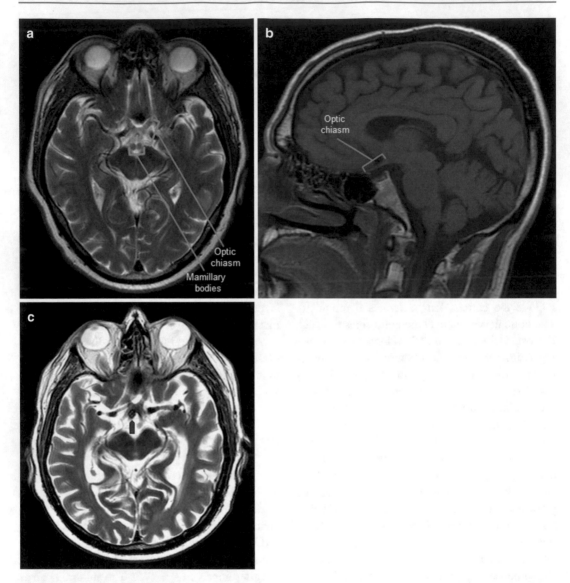

Fig. 5.6 (**a**) Axial T2-weighted MR image demonstrating the optic chiasm and mammillary bodies posteriorly. (**b**) Sagittal T1-weighted MR image localizing optic chiasm. (**c**) Axial T2-weighted MR image showing a right sided metastasis at the optic chiasm (red arrowhead); this patient presented with blurred vision, headache, nausea, and right-sided homonymous hemianopia

brainstem is defined by the C1 nerve root, or the foramen magnum.

Clinical Correlate

Brain metastases uncommonly occur within the brainstem. They may be asymptomatic or may cause symptoms related to local edema near cranial nerve nuclei or the ventricular system. Patients may present with cranial neuropathy or headache associated with elevated ICP.

Skull Base: Middle Cranial Fossa

The cavernous sinus is a dural venous sinus bound by the temporal and sphenoid bones and lies lateral to the pituitary gland [11]. It contains important structures including cranial nerves III, IV, V1, V2, and V3 as well as the internal carotid artery. On axial imaging, it is important not to mistakenly contour the vasculature of the cavernous sinus as the optic chiasm. The cavernous

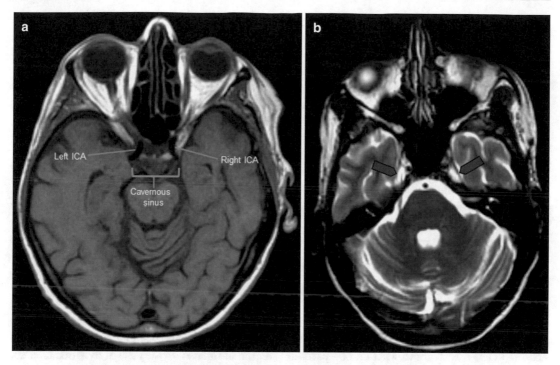

Fig. 5.7 (**a**) Axial T1-weighted MR image demonstrating the right and left internal carotid arteries (ICA), as well as the cavernous sinus. (**b**) Axial T2-weighted MR image demonstrating bilateral Meckel's cave (trigeminal cave), red arrows

sinus lies just inferior to the optic chiasm, and it is identifiable on axial imaging by the bilateral internal carotid arteries as they course anteriorly through the sinus (Fig. 5.7).

Meckel's cave, or the trigeminal cave, is another important neuroanatomic landmark, as it can be a route of disease spread to the extracranial portion of cranial nerve V. Meckel's cave is a dural pouch in the middle cranial fossa located lateral to the cavernous sinus bilaterally (Fig. 5.7). In reality, it appears like a truncated three-fingered glove, with the "fingers" reaching anteriorly and containing branches of cranial nerve V [12].

The cochlea is a structure that is important to identify and protect during radiation therapy for brain metastases. The cochlea is best visualized on T2 sequence in the middle cranial fossa located between the cerebellum and temporal lobe, just lateral to the brainstem (Fig. 5.8). If the cochlea is damaged, the patient may experience permanent sensorineural hearing loss and/or tinnitus. It is

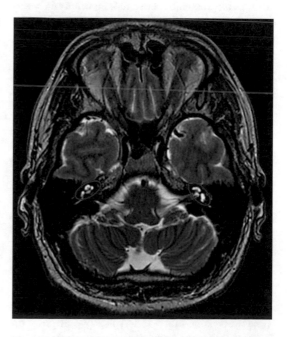

Fig. 5.8 Axial T2-weighted MR image demonstrating bilateral signal enhancing cochlea, indicated by red ovals

also easily identified on a simulation CT scan using bone window settings.

Clinical Correlate

Lesions of the cavernous sinus are of high risk, as it is a small structure containing several critical structures, and thrombosis may become life-threatening and is associated with significant morbidity. Patients may present with visual deficit, proptosis, unilateral or bilateral periorbital edema, photophobia, palsy of extraocular movements, facial numbness, and headache.

Imaging Brain Metastases

Parenchymal brain metastases are best identified on contrast-enhanced MRI imaging. Contrast is vital for identifying small lesions. Thin-slice (2 mm slice thickness) spoiled gradient recalled echo (SPGR) post-contrast MRI can be particularly useful to identify brain metastases. A 3D thin-slice study should be used for planning cranial radiosurgery. The most common site of brain metastases is the white matter/gray matter junction. Brain metastases are most commonly well-circumscribed enhancing lesions that may be heterogeneously enhancing. Although a brain metastasis does not have a formal capsule around it, many do form pseudocapsules and do not infiltrate beyond the enhancing rim of the tumor into the brain parenchyma. Many brain metastases, even small lesions, are accompanied with increased vasogenic edema, often manifested as hyperintensity on FLAIR imaging. However, in the case of a solid tumor metastasis, the surrounding edema does not contain tumor cells, and for the purposes of contouring and treatment planning, the gross tumor volume defined by the contrast-enhancing lesion and the clinical target volume are considered the same volume. Highly vascular metastases, such as melanoma, thyroid carcinoma, or renal cell carcinoma, may also exhibit hemorrhagic findings. On MRI, recent or subacute bleeding is typically bright on T1-weighted sequences, and hemorrhagic lesions may appear to be contrast enhanced in the absence of intravenous contrast. Alternatively, metastases that fail to enhance may be seen on susceptibility-weighted image sequences, which are very sensitive to the presence of iron in hemoglobin (Fig. 5.9).

Up to 11% of enhancing mass lesions in patients with cancer are not metastases [13]. Primary brain tumors can be mistaken for metastases. Nonmalignant space occupying lesions that can masquerade as brain metastases include abscesses, granulomas, and even parasitic infections in patients with appropriate travel histories. Acute demyelinating disease and intravascular thrombosis can also mimic a brain metastasis.

Radiation necrosis in patients who have been previously irradiated can be difficult to differentiate from active malignancy. MR perfusion is useful in helping to distinguish between active cancer and radionecrosis. Perfusion imaging is performed during the administration of intravenous contrast while sampling signal from the region of interest. In the case of dynamic contrast enhancement (DCE), T1-weighted sequences are used. Since brain metastases are often vascular, a useful perfusion metric is the relative cerebral blood volume, or plasma volume. This is calculated by comparing the cerebral blood volume in a tumor with a region of the brain that is not diseased, based upon the volume of contrast that passes through the region of interest. The plasma volume and estimation of capillary permeability can be calculated. In the setting of radionecrosis, plasma volume would be restricted, while capillary permeability may be elevated (Fig. 5.10). In the setting of an active metastasis, plasma volume would be expected to be high.

Special Cases

Leptomeningeal disease (LMD), or leptomeningeal carcinomatosis, is seeding of the subarachnoid space and arachnoid and pia mater by solid tumor. This occurs in 5–8% of patients with solid tumors and often has a very poor prognosis due to limitations in the ability to treat such secondary disease spread. On MR imaging, LMD is best visualized on post-contrast T1-weighted images, and leptomeningeal deposits appear as

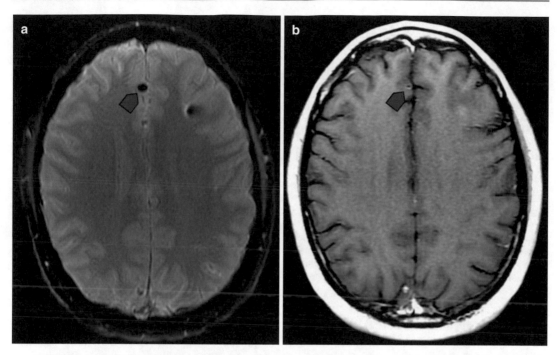

Fig. 5.9 In a patient with a right frontal lobe metastasis, susceptibility-weighted imaging (SWI) (**a**) shows increased signal at the site of metastasis, whereas the T1 post-contrast image (**b**) does not demonstrate contrast enhancement of the same metastatic lesion. The lesion is indicated by an arrowhead on both images

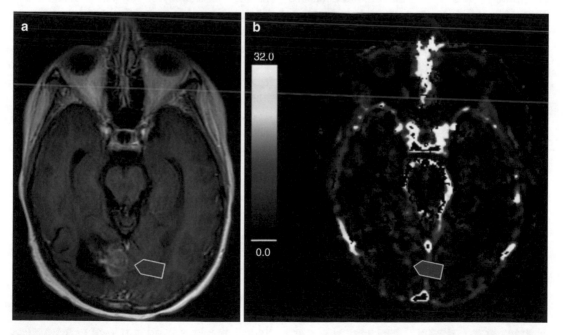

Fig. 5.10 Elevated enhancement of a right occipital lobe lesion on T1-weighted post-contrast imaging in (**a**), without associated elevated plasma volume on perfusion imaging in (**b**), presumably a site of radiation necrosis. Location of enhancement indicated by arrowhead

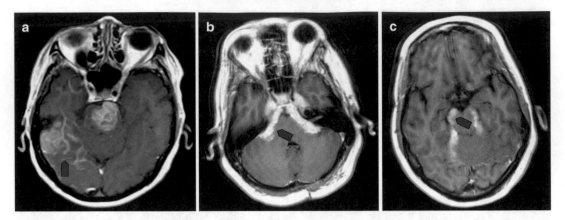

Fig. 5.11 (a) Axial T1-weighted MR image post-contrast demonstrating right inferior temporal leptomeningeal enhancement. Note characteristic sulcal enhancement. (b, c) Axial T1-weighted MR images post-contrast demonstrating pachymeningeal enhancement, not leptomeningeal enhancement. Note enhancement at the meningeal surface

enhancing, irregular nodularity at the brain parenchymal surface, most notable at the sulci [14] (Fig. 5.11). T1 FLAIR hyperintensity along the involved sulci can also accompany leptomeningeal disease. In cases of diffuse leptomeningeal disease, the involved sulci are brightly enhancing and a gadolinium-enhanced T1-weighted scan can look as bright as CSF in a T2-weighted image. Clinically, LMD may present with nonspecific signs and symptoms, such as mixed cranial neuropathies, increased ICP, or irritation of the meninges. The most commonly involved cranial nerves are the sixth, seventh, and eighth nerves, and as such patients present with visual disturbance, facial weakness, and issues with hearing. Patients may also present with headache, nausea, or vomiting.

Pachymeningeal disease is tumor involvement of the dura mater and often appears as enhancing dural thickening [15]. Patients may present with postural headache, meningeal irritation, or be asymptomatic. It is important not to confuse pachymeningeal disease with leptomeningeal disease, as they involve different layers of the meninges.

Hydrocephalus occurs when there is an obstruction in CSF flow. Under normal circumstances, CSF is produced by the choroid plexus and flows from the lateral ventricles, through the interventricular foramen (foramen of Monroe), to the third ventricle, through the cerebral aqueduct (aqueduct of Sylvius), to the fourth ventricle, through the median aperture (foramen of Magendie) and lateral aperture (foramen of Luschka), to the subarachnoid space where it is circulated throughout the space delimited by the meninges, including the surfaces of the brain and spinal cord and is reabsorbed by the arachnoid villi to merge with venous blood in the dural sinuses. Any external or internal obstruction along this path, including tumor, hemorrhage, or leptomeningeal deposits, may lead to ventricular dilation and clinical symptoms of increased intracranial pressure including postural headache, nausea, vomiting, and ataxia (Fig. 5.12) [16]. Patients will also present with papilledema due to elevated ICP. MR imaging demonstrates enlarged ventricular size and increased periventricular FLAIR signal abnormality in cases of acute decompensated hydrocephalus.

Conclusions

MR imaging with gadolinium contrast is a vital tool for localizing intracranial metastases. Symptomatology is often related to mass effect on adjacent neurologic structures, particularly if there is significant vasogenic edema. Patients may present with pathognomonic neurologic

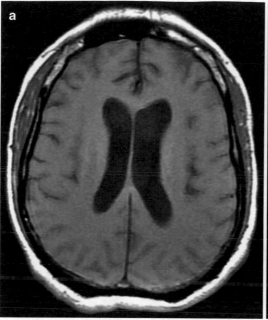
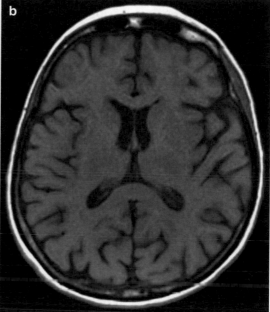

Fig. 5.12 (**a**) Axial T1-weighted image demonstrating enlarged lateral ventricles in a case of acute hydrocephalus in a patient with metastatic follicular thyroid cancer with previously known lumbar spinal metastasis presenting with severe headache and papilledema. (**b**) Normal lateral ventricles without hydrocephalus, for comparison

deficits, or they may be asymptomatic. A full workup involving imaging and neurologic exam will aid in diagnosis and management.

Key Points

- Although cranial radiosurgery and stereotactic radiation therapy can be performed without MRI imaging, MRI with and without gadolinium provides a degree of soft tissue definition that CT imaging cannot.
- Take advantage of the 3D characteristics of cranial MRI imaging and view the studies cross-referencing axial, sagittal, and coronal planes to identify important anatomic structures and to confirm that structures have been contoured correctly.
- T1 post-contrast SPGR images are particularly useful to identify metastases.
- Additional special sequences such as perfusion studies can be helpful to differentiate between necrosis and active metastases.

References

1. Dolgushin M, Kornienko V, Pronin I. Magnetic resonance imaging (MRI). Brain metastases: advanced neuroimaging. New York: Springer International Publishing; 2018. p. 51–83.
2. Erbil M, Onderoglu S, Yener N, Cumhur M, Cila A. Localization of the central sulcus and adjacent sulci in human: a study by MRI. Okajimas Folia Anat Jpn. 1998;75(2–3):155–62.
3. Berger MS, Cohen WA, Ojemann GA. Correlation of motor cortex brain mapping data with magnetic resonance imaging. J Neurosurg. 1990;72(3):383–7.
4. Kido DK, LeMay M, Levinson AW, Benson WE. Computed tomographic localization of the precentral gyrus. Radiology. 1980;135(2):373–7.
5. Naidich TP, Daniels DL, Haughton VM, Williams A, Pojunas K, Palacios E. Hippocampal formation and related structures of the limbic lobe: anatomic-MR correlation. Part I. Surface features and coronal sections. Radiology. 1987;162(3):747–54.
6. Lambiase LA, DiBella EM, Thompson BB. Neuroanatomy. In: White JL, Sheth KN, editors. Neurocritical care for the advanced practice clinician. New York: Springer International Publishing; 2018. p. 5–28.
7. Pukenas B. Normal brain anatomy on magnetic resonance imaging. Magn Reson Imaging Clin N Am. 2011;19(3):429–37, vii.

8. Choi CY, Han SR, Yee GT, Lee CH. Central core of the cerebrum. J Neurosurg. 2011;114(2):463–9.

9. Wichmann W, Muller-Forell W. Anatomy of the visual system. Eur J Radiol. 2004;49(1):8–30.

10. Angeles Fernandez-Gil M, Palacios-Bote R, Leo-Barahona M, Mora-Encinas JP. Anatomy of the brainstem: a gaze into the stem of life. Semin Ultrasound CT MR. 2010;31(3):196–219.

11. Rhoton AL. The middle cranial base and cavernous sinus. In: VVR D, Larry, editors. Cavernous sinus: developments and future perspectives. Austria: Springer-Verlag/Wien; 2009.

12. Sabanci PA, Batay F, Civelek E, Al Mefty O, Husain M, Abdulrauf SI, et al. Meckel's cave. World Neurosurg. 2011;76(3–4):335–41. Discussion 266–7.

13. Patchell RA, Tibbs PA, Walsh JW, Dempsey RJ, Maruyama Y, Kryscio RJ, et al. A randomized trial of surgery in the treatment of single metastases to the brain. N Engl J Med. 1990;322(8):494–500.

14. Wang N, Bertalan MS, Brastianos PK. Leptomeningeal metastasis from systemic cancer: review and update on management. Cancer. 2018;124(1):21–35.

15. Antony J, Hacking C, Jeffree RL. Pachymeningeal enhancement-a comprehensive review of literature. Neurosurg Rev. 2015;38(4):649–59.

16. Ammar A. Hydrocephalus: what do we know? And what do we still not know? Cham: Springer; 2017.

The Evolution of Combination Therapies Involving Surgery and Radiosurgery

6

David Peters, Roshan Prabhu, Stuart Burri, and Anthony Asher

Case Vignette

Case 1

A 37-year-old female presented with a 1-week history of severe headache, nausea, and intractable vomiting. Imaging of her brain revealed a solitary enhancing right frontal mass, approximately 3 × 3 × 3 cm, with surrounding edema measuring 7.6 × 6.8 cm and with 1.4 cm of right to left midline shift (Fig. 6.1).

Her past medical history was significant for BRCA gene positive, triple negative breast cancer (T2 N3b M0, stage IIIC) that was diagnosed 15 months prior. Her primary disease was treated with chemotherapy, radiation, and bilateral mastectomy with no signs of residual disease following completion of therapy up until her current presentation.

D. Peters (✉)
Department of Neurosurgery, Atrium Health, Carolinas Medical Center, Carolina Neurosurgery and Spine Associates, Charlotte, NC, USA
e-mail: david.peters@cnsa.com

R. Prabhu · S. Burri
Department of Radiation Oncology, Levine Cancer Institute, Carolinas Medical Center, Southeast Radiation Oncology Group, Charlotte, NC, USA

A. Asher
Department of Neurosurgery, Carolina Neurosurgery and Spine Associates, Charlotte, NC, USA

She was evaluated by the neurosurgical service, placed on high-dose dexamethasone, and admitted to the ICU. A CT of her chest, abdomen, and pelvis with contrast was performed, which showed no extracranial disease. She continued to suffer from nausea and vomiting despite high-dose steroids while in the hospital. Given the large size of her tumor, extensive surrounding edema, severe mass effect with profound midline shift, and persistent symptoms with well-controlled extracranial disease, she underwent a craniotomy for resection. A gross total resection was achieved (Fig. 6.2). Pathology confirmed metastatic breast cancer.

She was discharged and followed up for adjuvant radiotherapy. After discussion of risks and benefits, adjuvant stereotactic radiosurgery (SRS) was chosen over whole brain radiotherapy (WBRT). She was treated with 27 Gy over three fractions 5 weeks after the craniotomy based on a new MRI scan within a week of the treatment. The cavity was targeted with a 2 mm margin, and the planning target volume (PTV) measured 21.5 cm³. No systemic therapy was recommended by her medical oncologist.

She was reevaluated 6 weeks after receiving adjuvant radiotherapy with repeat CT of chest, abdomen, and pelvis and MRI of brain, both of which showed no signs of active disease. She was asymptomatic and doing well. Six weeks thereafter, she again returned to the ED with headaches and vomiting. Brain imaging revealed multiple

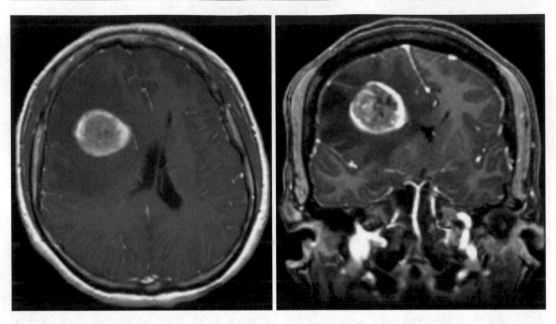

Fig. 6.1 MRI T1 with contrast showing solitary right frontal enhancing lesion with perilesional edema

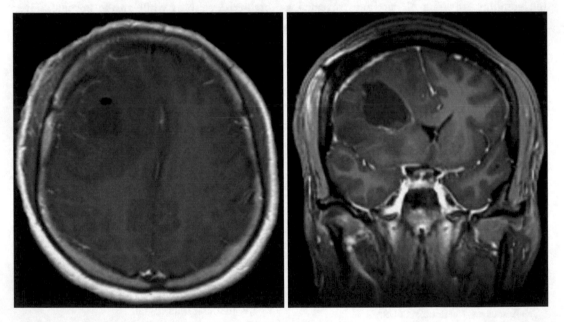

Fig. 6.2 Postoperative MRI T1 with contrast showing gross total resection

right-sided extra axial masses with leptomeningeal enhancement and a partially enhancing cyst within the surgical cavity. Midline shift from right to left measures 7 mm (Fig. 6.3).

She was again evaluated by both neurosurgery and radiation oncology, who recommend palliative WBRT, 30 Gy in 10 fractions. Her symptoms partially improved with dexamethasone and anti-emetics. She was discharged and immediately started on WBRT in the outpatient setting.

Two weeks later, she returned to the ED for intractable vomiting and confusion. CT of her head showed progression of her intracranial disease, now with 13 mm of right to left midline shift. She was admitted to the ICU where her symptoms were treated medically. While in the

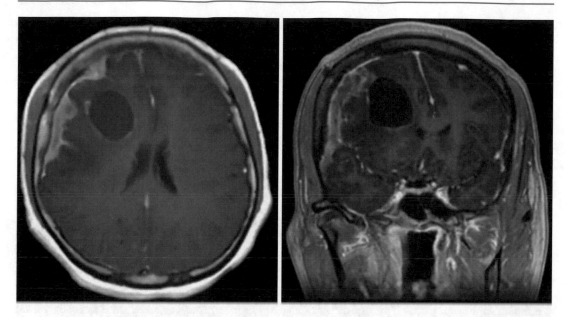

Fig. 6.3 MRI T1 with contrast 4 months postoperatively showing tumor recurrence and leptomeningeal disease

ICU, she abruptly deteriorated, becoming unresponsive with a fixed and dilated right pupil. She was given 50 g of mannitol, and her neurologic condition rapidly improved to the point where she was again awake and alert. After a discussion with the patient and her husband, she was offered an emergent craniotomy to prevent the herniation and rapid neurological death that would occur once the hyperosmolar therapy wears off. She was taken to the operating room where the right frontal cyst was drained. Resection of the leptomeningeal disease was not attempted due to the significant extent of her disease involving much of her right hemisphere and associated dura. The risk of stroke or neurologic injury secondary to resection of the leptomeningeal disease was felt to be higher than the potential benefit. Postoperatively, she was alert but still suffered from persistent nausea, vomiting, and confusion. The patient and her family elect to pursue hospice care. She was discharged to hospice and expired 1 month later.

Case 2

A 74-year-old male presented with insidious onset of confusion and word finding difficulty that acutely worsened to severe expressive apha-

sia, prompting hospitalization at a rural facility without neurosurgical coverage. Imaging of his brain revealed a solitary enhancing left frontal mass, approximately 3 × 3 × 4 cm, with a moderate amount of surrounding edema and with 2 mm of left to right midline shift (Fig. 6.4).

His past medical history was significant for diabetes, coronary artery disease, 50 pack-year smoking, chronic obstructive pulmonary disease, and atrial fibrillation treated chronically with rivaroxaban. He had no known history of cancer. A CT of his chest, abdomen, and pelvis with contrast was performed, revealing a 3.2 × 1.2 cm pulmonary mass. He was placed on high-dose dexamethasone and levetiracetam for suspected focal seizures. His speech improved significantly after receiving these medications. He was discharged from the hospital with planned outpatient neurosurgical follow-up 3 days later. An outpatient pulmonary biopsy was also arranged, which revealed the pulmonary mass to be squamous cell carcinoma.

Given the large size of his tumor, isolated symptomatic lesion, and limited extracranial disease, he was determined to be a good candidate for surgical treatment. After discussion of risks and benefits, the decision was made to treat the lesion with preoperative SRS. He was treated with 14 Gy to the 80% isodose line with 6MV

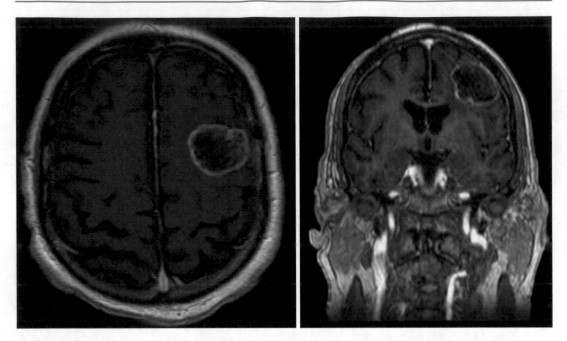

Fig. 6.4 MRI T1 with contrast showing ring enhancing left frontal mass at the gray-white junction

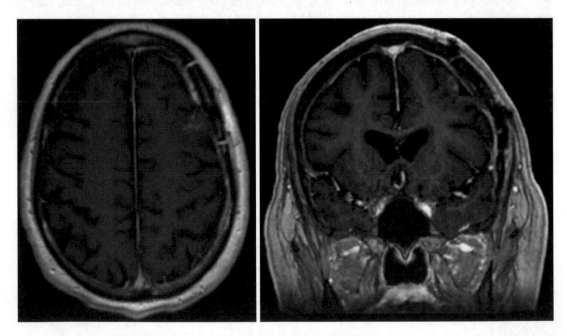

Fig. 6.5 Postoperative MRI T1 with contrast showing gross total resection

photons. The lesion maximum diameter was 38.7 mm, and there was no additional margin added to the tumor. Hence, the gross tumor volume equaled the planning target volume and measured 22.4 cm³. Prescription isodose volume was 29.46 cm³. The following day he underwent

a left frontal craniotomy for resection of the lesion. A gross total resection was achieved (Fig. 6.5).

Pathology confirmed squamous cell carcinoma of the lung. He spent one night in the ICU and was discharged home the next morning, neurologically intact. His levetiracetam was continued on discharge, and he was placed on a 2-week dexamethasone taper. His family noted that his confusion was significantly improved following surgery.

He was evaluated by cardiothoracic surgery, medical oncology, and radiation oncology. He underwent a PET scan which showed no other sites of metastasis. His pulmonary function was determined to be too poor to tolerate surgical removal of the pulmonary mass. Instead, his lung mass was treated with radiation therapy, which he tolerated well. No systemic chemotherapy or immunotherapy was recommended by his medical oncologist.

He was followed closely with brain MRIs every 3 months. PET scan of his entire body 6 months posttreatment of his lung lesion identifies a new liver lesion. This was subsequently treated with radiation therapy, and he tolerated it well. Currently, he is 1 year since his original diagnosis and has no residual or recurrent brain disease, well-controlled extracranial disease, and minimal symptoms with a Karnofsky score of 80%.

Introduction

Radiotherapy and surgical resection are the two most powerful and well-studied tools at a physician's disposal today for the treatment of patients with cerebral metastases. While these treatments can clearly provide great benefit when applied appropriately, the difficulty in management of these patients lies in determining the best patient-specific plan. Current generally accepted treatment combinations include whole brain radiotherapy (WBRT) alone, WBRT with stereotactic radiosurgery (SRS) boost, SRS alone, surgical resection followed by observation, surgical resection followed by WBRT, surgical resection followed by postoperative SRS, and preoperative SRS followed by surgical resection. Approaches that incorporate hippocampal avoidance and memantine administration to try to minimize the neurocognitive sequelae of WBRT are increasingly being employed, and brain metastases of

certain histologies are responsive enough to newly developed systemic therapies that deferring irradiation is often considered, as set out elsewhere in this book.

The wide clinical variability of patients presenting with cerebral metastases underscores the need for decision makers to have a thorough understanding of all treatment options. Guidelines for how to best integrate surgery and radiotherapy continue to evolve, and recent promising research has led to data that may help establish a new treatment standard for patients requiring surgical resection of brain metastases. The purpose of this chapter is to review existing treatment options and provide evidence-based recommendations for how to best integrate surgery and radiotherapy for the treatment of resected cerebral metastases.

Evidence Base

The use of radiotherapy for the treatment of cerebral metastases was first reported in the 1950s [1, 2]. Early use of radiotherapy involved WBRT without surgery and was generally used for symptom palliation, as overall survival (OS) remained poor [1, 3, 4]. Two landmark studies in the 1990s by Patchell et al. showed that for selected patients with a single brain metastasis, surgery in addition to WBRT could provide significant benefit over either surgery or WBRT alone [5, 6]. The first study included patients with a single brain metastasis and randomized them to either surgery followed by WBRT or WBRT alone. The group that received surgery had a median OS of 40 weeks compared to 15 weeks for the group that did not receive surgery ($p < 0.01$). The follow-up study randomized patients with a single brain metastasis to surgical treatment alone or surgical treatment followed by WBRT. This analysis did not show a significant survival benefit with the addition of WBRT (median OS of 43–48 weeks, for surgery versus surgery plus WBRT, respectively, $p = 0.39$), but it did show that surgery and WBRT was associated with significantly lower rates of intracranial tumor recurrence and neurological death. The group who received surgical treatment alone had a local cavity recurrence rate of 46% compared to 10% in the surgery and WBRT group [5]. Subsequent studies have confirmed a high rate of local recurrence within the surgical cavity for patients treated with surgery alone (47–59% at 1–2 years) [7, 8]. To reduce this high risk of local recurrence, adjuvant radiotherapy is usually recommended for patients treated with surgical resection.

For many years, WBRT was the standard radiotherapy treatment following surgical resection. However, concern developed over its strong link to neurocognitive decline and decreased overall quality of life [9–11]. This concern led to the investigation of the efficacy of adjuvant SRS. In multiple studies, SRS alone was compared to SRS + WBRT for nonsurgical patients with up to three or four metastases. These trials consistently showed worse tumor control with SRS alone, but with no significant decrease in OS survival compared to SRS + WBRT [9, 10, 12]. Furthermore, the SRS alone groups had significantly lower rates of neurocognitive decline at 3–4 months postoperatively [9, 10]. Multiple trials also examined quality of life (QOL) using validated QOL assessments and found that adding WBRT to SRS significantly decreased patient QOL compared to SRS alone [9, 11]. This data led to that SRS alone is becoming the preferred radiotherapy treatment for patients with a limited number of brain metastases and good performance status [13].

This information was then extrapolated and applied to patients undergoing surgical resection, based on the assumption that the data for radiotherapy treatment of intact brain metastases could be applied to postoperative patients as well. It was hypothesized that postoperative adjuvant SRS could lower the high risk of local recurrence seen with surgical resection alone, while also avoiding much of the risk of neurocognitive decline and worsened QOL seen with WBRT. SRS gradually became favored in clinical practice over WBRT for postoperative adjuvant radiotherapy in patients with a limited number of brain metastases. Initially, there were only limited retrospective data to support this approach, and only a single-arm prospective trial [14].

Recently, multiple prospective trials have been published that provide high-level evidence in support of SRS over WBRT for adjuvant therapy in this patient population. Adjuvant SRS has improved local control compared to surgical resection alone and is associated with significantly reduced risk of neurocognitive decline compared to adjuvant WBRT [8, 14, 15]. In addition, two recent retrospective studies have investigated surgery plus postoperative SRS versus SRS alone, both showing significantly reduced local recurrence and improved OS in the arm receiving surgery plus postoperative SRS [16, 17]. Both of these studies included patients with 1–4 metastases, although most enrolled patients had single lesions. In the study by Prabhu et al., all patients had at least one metastasis that had a volume of ≥ 4 cm^3.

Retrospective studies report a 1-year local recurrence (LR) rate of 0–39% for postoperative SRS, although these studies have high variability in the treatment methods, patient populations, statistical methods, and follow-up periods [18]. See Table 6.1 for list of best trials to date for postoperative SRS.

These retrospective studies also suffer from bias in that all of the patients were treated with post-op SRS without consideration of those lost to follow-up or to those who could not be treated with post-op SRS for technical or other factors. One prospective trial randomized surgical resection followed by observation to surgical resection followed by SRS. Postoperative SRS had a cavity LR rate of 28% at 1 year compared to 57% for the surgical resection and observation group ($p = 0.015$) [8]. No significant differences were seen in OS, other intracranial disease control rates, neurologic death, leptomeningeal disease (LMD) relapse, or use of subsequent WBRT. This is the strongest evidence supporting the efficacy of postoperative SRS in reducing cavity LR.

As the clinical practice of postoperative adjuvant SRS has increased and multiple high-quality prospective trials have been published, several key principles and observations have emerged related to this treatment paradigm. First, an important technical note is that postoperative

Table 6.1 Summary of postoperative SRS data [8, 14, 15, 19–22]

Institution	Study design	# of patients	Median marginal SRS dose (Gy)	Overall survival	1 year local recurrence (%)	1 year radiation necrosis	1 year LMD (%)
Atalar (Stanford) 2013	Retrospective	165	NR	1 year: 66%	10	7 (grade 2+, crude)	11
Iorio-Morin (Canada) 2014	Retrospective	110	16	Median: 11 months	27	6	NR
Patel (Emory) 2014	Retrospective	96	18	1 year: 56%	17	13	NR
Ojerholm (UPenn) 2014	Retrospective	91	16	Median: 22 months	19	7 (grade 2+, crude)	14 (crude)
Brennan (MSKCC) 2014	Prospective	39	18	Median: 12 months	22	18	NR
Mahajan (MDACC) 2017	Prospective	63 (SRS arm)	16	Median: 17 months	28	0	28
Brown (N107C) 2017	Prospective	98 (SRS arm)	NR	Median: 12 months	39	4 (grade 2+, crude)	7

adjuvant SRS target requires a margin expansion of 1–2 mm around the resection cavity. Without this 1–2 mm margin, the risk of local recurrence is higher, likely due to difficulty in precisely contouring the edge of the resection cavity, leading to incomplete targeting of residual cancer cells [23, 24]. Second, the rate of leptomeningeal disease (LMD) relapse is likely higher with postoperative SRS compared to WBRT [19, 21, 25, 26]. LMD is defined as metastasis to the meninges surrounding the brain (Fig. 6.6).

One retrospective study comparing postoperative SRS to postoperative WBRT showed that at 18 months, the rate of LMD was 31% to 13%, respectively ($p = 0.045$) [21]. Another retrospective study showed that SRS alone has an LMD rate of 5.2% at 1 year, compared to 16.9% for surgical resection followed by SRS ($p < 0.01$) [25]. It is believed that this observation is explained by surgical resection causing tumor dissemination into the leptomeningeal spaces and cerebrospinal fluid (CSF). WBRT after surgery may limit, or control, tumor dissemination through CSF pathways and subsequent LMD because the entire intracranial compartment is treated. SRS alone is likely associated with lower rates of LMD than postoperative SRS because there is no iatrogenic intraoperative dissemination of cells.

Preoperative SRS is a new approach to combining surgery and radiotherapy that has emerged. Like postoperative SRS, it provides adequate local control while minimizing neurocognitive damage compared to WBRT. However, this treatment sequence also provides advantages relative to some of the perceived and observed drawbacks of postoperative SRS.

From a theoretical perspective, preoperative SRS has several advantages. First, it is easier to contour an intact metastasis for SRS target delineation compared to a surgical resection cavity. Unlike a surgical resection cavity, an intact brain metastasis has well-defined borders and, therefore, a margin expansion around the target is not necessary. As previously mentioned, optimal postoperative SRS requires at least a 1–2 mm margin around the irregular borders of a resection cavity in order to ensure complete targeting of all residual tumor cells, but this also leads to a larger area of normal brain being subjected to radiation [23, 24] (Figs. 6.7 and 6.8).

It is well known that increasing the amount of normal brain tissue receiving high-dose radiation will increase the rate of radiation necrosis [27–29]. Thus, preoperative SRS would theoretically reduce the rate of RN observed with postoperative treatment. Second, it has been shown that

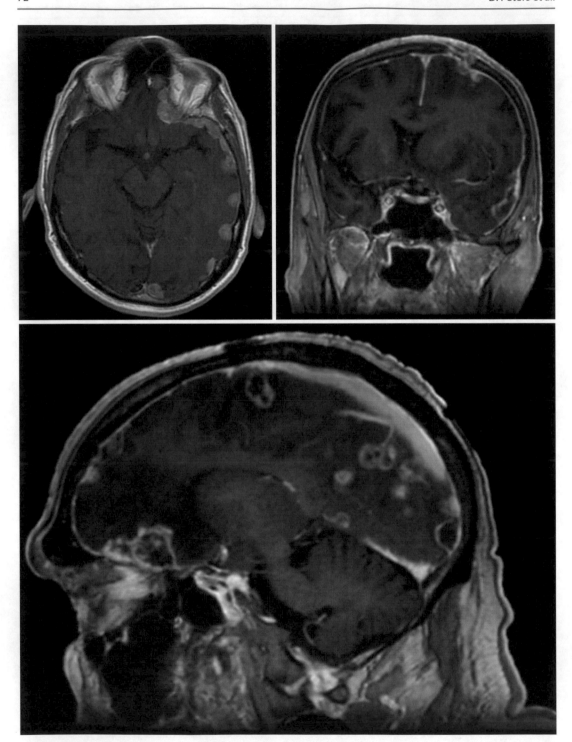

Fig. 6.6 MRI T1 with contrast in a patient who previously had a left posterior frontal solitary metastasis treated with surgery and postoperative SRS. Local recurrence in the left posterior frontal cavity is seen on the sagittal and coronal views. In addition, he has extensive leptomeningeal disease including subfrontal, posterior falcine, left temporal, and left parietal convexity dural metastases

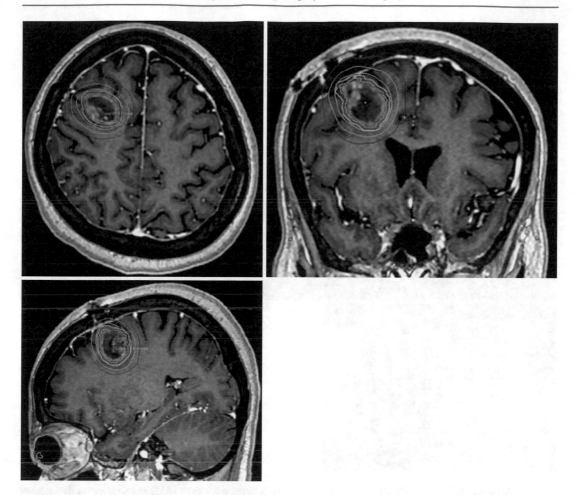

Fig. 6.7 A 54-year-old female who presented with a symptomatic 5 cm solitary brain mass after gross total resection. Pathology confirmed lung adenocarcinoma. Postoperative stereotactic radiosurgery treatment was to 15 Gy in one fraction. Orange = gross tumor volume (GTV), Cyan = 1.5 mm expansion to create planning target volume (PTV), Green = 80% isodose line (prescription isodose), Light blue = 50% isodose line, Dark blue = 30% isodose line

radiation therapy is more effective at killing tumor cells when the tumor has an intact blood supply and is oxygenated. It is therefore possible that lower doses of radiation are needed to treat an intact tumor preoperatively compared to a hypoxic tumor resection cavity with a compromised blood supply. Third, iatrogenic dissemination of viable tumor cells into the CSF should be reduced following preoperative SRS as these tumors would have been already exposed to radiation; thus, the rates of LMD developing would be much lower. Finally, compliance is likely to be higher with preoperative SRS than postoperative

SRS, as the surgery typically takes place 48 hours or less after SRS compared to a delay of what is often many weeks for SRS following surgery. This delay opens the door for other barriers to treatment including early CNS progression, systemic progression, and failure to follow-up. This is reflected in a single-arm prospective phase II study in which 20% of patients enrolled in a surgical resection plus postoperative SRS arm actually did not receive the planned postoperative SRS [14].

To date, no prospective randomized trials have been completed comparing preoperative SRS to

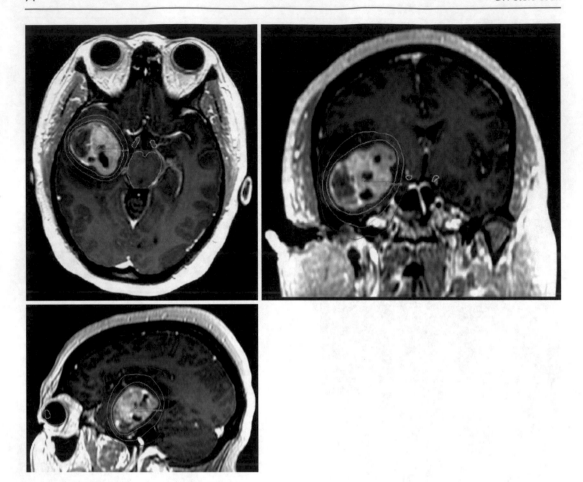

Fig. 6.8 A 34-year-old female with history of undifferentiated pleomorphic sarcoma, who presented with solitary right anterior temporal lobe metastasis. She was treated with preoperative SRS that was followed by surgical resection the next day. Preoperative stereotactic radiosurgery treatment was to 13 Gy in one fraction. Red = gross tumor volume (GTV), GTV = planning target volume (PTV) with no additional margin. Green = 80% isodose line (prescription isodose), Light blue = 50% isodose line, Dark blue = 30% isodose line

postoperative SRS, although trials are currently underway. A retrospective study of 180 patients comparing preoperative SRS versus postoperative SRS showed no significant difference in overall survival, local recurrence, or distant brain recurrence. However, at 2 years follow-up, postoperative SRS did have significantly higher rates of LMD (16.6% vs 3.2%, $p = 0.01$) and symptomatic radiation necrosis (16.4% vs 4.9%, $p = 0.01$) [30]. See Table 6.2 for a list of significant preoperative SRS studies.

Proposed drawbacks of preoperative SRS compared to postoperative SRS include lack of pathological confirmation of CNS disease prior to SRS, theoretical concerns for wound healing complica-

tions, management of subtotal resection after SRS, and an inability to perform if a patient is neurologically unstable or emergent surgery is required [34]. The lack of pathological confirmation of CNS disease is a real but low risk, as false positive rates have been shown to be approximately 2–3% for nonmetastatic pathology, and the vast majority of patients receiving SRS or WBRT without surgery do not require CNS pathological confirmation prior to treatment. Although quite rare, a few patients present with severe, life-threatening mass effect and require emergent surgery. These patients may not be able to obtain SRS prior to surgery. Wound-healing problems are mostly theoretical, as no increased risk with wound healing has yet

Table 6.2 Summary of preoperative SRS data [30–33]

	Design	Patients	Cavity local recurrence	Symptomatic RN	LMD
Asher et al. (2014)	Combined prospective and retrospective single arm	47 with 51 cavities	1 year: 14%	NR	1 year: 0%
Patel et al. (2016)	Retrospective pre-op SRS vs. post-op SRS	66 pre-op/114 post-op SRS	2 year: 23% vs. 16% ($p = 0.33$)	2 year: 5% vs. 16% ($p = 0.02$)	2 year: 3% vs. 17% ($p = 0.01$)
Patel et al. (2017)	Retrospective pre-op SRS vs. post-op WBRT	66 pre-op/36 post-op WBRT	2 year: 25% vs. 25% ($p = 0.81$)	Crude: 6% vs. 0% ($p = 0.29$)	2 year: 4% vs. 9% ($p = 0.66$)
Prabhu et al. (2018)	Combined prospective and retrospective single arm	117 with 125 cavities	2 year: 25%	1 year: 4.8%	1 year: 4.3%

been observed compared to postoperative SRS or WBRT. Subtotal resection (STR) after SRS has come up as a potential downside of preoperative SRS. The initial published reports of preoperative SRS only included patients' status post gross total resection, but a recent updated report by Prabhu et al. included six patients (5% of the cohort) who underwent preoperative SRS followed by STR. Four of the six patients experienced local recurrence. STR resection was a significant predictor of higher risk of cavity LR and mortality in multivariable analysis compared with gross total resection (GTR) [31]. The authors concluded that patient selection is important and patients who are likely to undergo a STR should not receive preoperative SRS and that those who experience an unexpected STR should be evaluated for re-resection or additional RT to limit the risk of local recurrence. However, the optimal management of this small minority of patients is the subject of ongoing studies.

Diagnosis and Management

A treatment plan involving some combination of radiotherapy with or without surgery should be considered for all patients with cerebral metastases. Thus, both the radiation oncology and neurosurgery services should be consulted to evaluate all of these patients. There is often significant variation from patient to patient when it comes to developing the optimal treatment plan. Factors to

consider when developing a treatment plan include age, symptomatology, total disease burden, overall prognosis, tumor histology, performance status, as well as the number, size, and location of brain metastases.

A thorough history and physical exam should be conducted first. Approximately 2–14% of patients with brain metastases present with no known cancer diagnosis [35]. If not recently performed (<8 weeks prior), a CT of chest, abdomen, and pelvis, with contrast or fluorodeoxyglucose positron emission tomography (FDG-PET) scan, is recommended to estimate the total disease burden and the cancer stage. For patients with no known cancer history, this can also help identify the tissue of origin, and any sites of extracranial disease are evaluated for potential biopsy. Further testing may be needed as directed by the history (e.g., mammogram, colonoscopy) to establish a diagnosis or to reevaluate a patient for progression of known disease. If there is no clear extracranial site to biopsy, a craniotomy may need to be performed to establish a tissue diagnosis. Generally, extracranial tumor tissue is both a more efficacious and safer target for biopsy than intracranial tumor tissue.

Once a tissue diagnosis has been established, a patient should be evaluated for potential benefit from surgical resection. Approximately 67–80% of all brain metastases are either non-small-cell lung cancer, breast cancer, or melanoma [13, 35]. A few types of cancer, most notably small-cell lung cancer, lymphoma, and some germ cell tumors, are exquisitely radiosensitive and do not benefit from surgical resection. This underscores the importance of establishing a tissue diagnosis prior to craniotomy, if possible. A tissue diagnosis also allows evaluation for potential targeted therapy, an emerging field that is beyond the scope of this chapter.

Surgery is a valuable tool in select patients, but the risk–benefit profile must be carefully considered. Indications for surgery include need for a tissue diagnosis, large brain metastases (>2 cm), significant mass effect or perilesional edema, and neurological symptoms refractory to steroids that would benefit from decompression. The goal of surgery may be increased survival, tissue diagnosis, and/or palliation of symptoms. Contraindications of varying strength to surgery include poor performance status, coagulopathy, leptomeningeal disease, high systemic disease burden with expected prognosis <3 months, multiple small lesions, and tumor histology exquisitely sensitive to radiotherapy, chemotherapy, or immunotherapy (see Table 6.3). Figures 6.9, 6.10, 6.11, and 6.12 give

Table 6.3 Surgical decision making

Good surgical candidate	Poor surgical candidate
Less tumors (preferably solitary lesion)	Multiple tumors (>3)
Large tumors (>2 cm)	Small tumors (<2 cm)
Easily accessible tumor location	High-risk location of tumor (eloquent brain)
Extensive perilesional edema or mass effect	Leptomeningeal disease
Neurologic symptoms refractory to medications	Coagulopathy
High-performance status	Low-performance status
Low extracranial disease burden	High extracranial disease burden (prognosis <3 months)
Recurrence following failed radiotherapy	Tumor histology exquisitely sensitive to radiotherapy, chemotherapy, or immunotherapy
Need for tissue diagnosis	

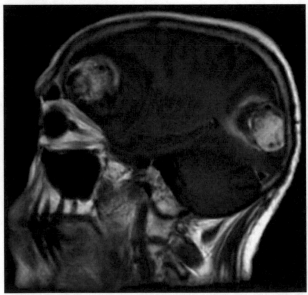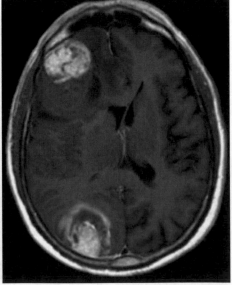

Fig. 6.9 68M with two large hepatocellular carcinoma metastases. These were removed in a single surgery with two separate incisions

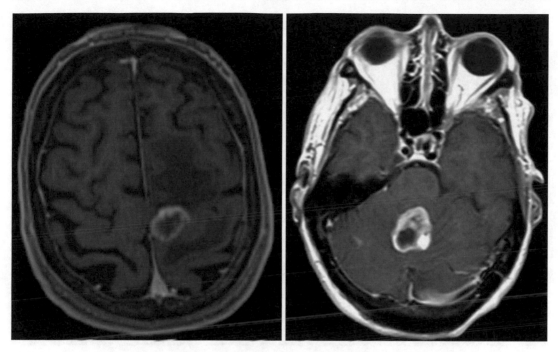

Fig. 6.10 Two examples of small, solitary, symptomatic metastases that were treated surgically. The left is a 76M with colorectal carcinoma presenting with right arm weakness and slurred speech. The right is a 72F with breast carcinoma presenting with dizziness, nausea, severe ataxia

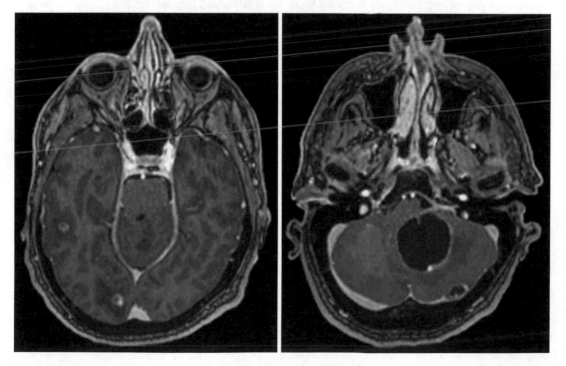

Fig. 6.11 56M with a large, cystic cerebellar esophageal adenocarcinoma metastasis and three other small metastases. The large cerebellar lesion was surgically removed and the others were treated with SRS

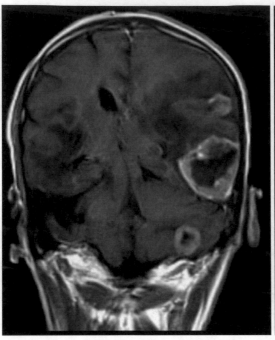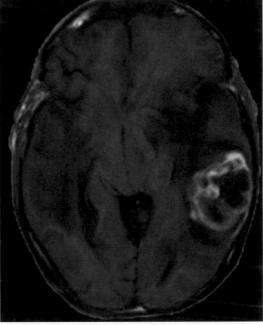

Fig. 6.12 64M with six total lung adenocarcinoma brain metastases. The dominant left temporal lesion was the only lesion removed. Palliation of symptoms was the goal of surgery, and this lesion was felt to be the one generating most of his symptoms given its large mass effect. He received WBRT postoperatively

examples of patients who are likely to benefit from surgery in addition to radiotherapy, while Figs. 6.13, 6.14, and 6.15 give examples of patients who are not likely to benefit from surgical resection.

For patients undergoing surgery, current evidence supports superior outcomes for OS and time to local recurrence if a gross total resection is achieved compared to subtotal resection [17, 22, 36–38]. Level III evidence also supports that an *en bloc* resection technique may have lower rates of developing LMD compared to piecemeal resection of solitary lesions [36, 39–41]. In a patient who has received a craniotomy, tumor recurrence locally in the resection cavity or distant brain recurrence should not be a contraindication to repeat surgery. These patients should be re-evaluated using the same criteria listed in Table 6.3 to determine whether they are a good surgical candidate or not, and they may benefit from repeat craniotomy. Level III evidence supports that craniotomy for resection of recurrent metastases after either surgery or SRS is associated with improved overall survival [36, 42, 43].

Ultimately, the risk-benefit profile of surgery must be assessed on a case-by-case basis by both the neurosurgical and radiation oncology teams, including input from the patient's medical oncologist and the patient's goals of care.

At the authors' institution, a multidisciplinary board of providers evaluates and collectively makes decisions on treatment plans for difficult cases where the patient does not have strong indications for or against surgery. For the patient described in the first case vignette, initially she was an ideal surgical candidate given her young age, large solitary lesion, extensive edema and mass effect, well-controlled extracranial disease, easily accessible location, refractory neurologic symptoms, high-performance status, and need for a tissue diagnosis. She experienced a large and immediate improvement postoperatively. Unfortunately, she developed LMD recurrence approximately 4 months after her initial surgery. Her second surgery was controversial. Leptomeningeal disease should generally be considered a contraindication to surgery given its extremely poor prognosis, and in this case, her

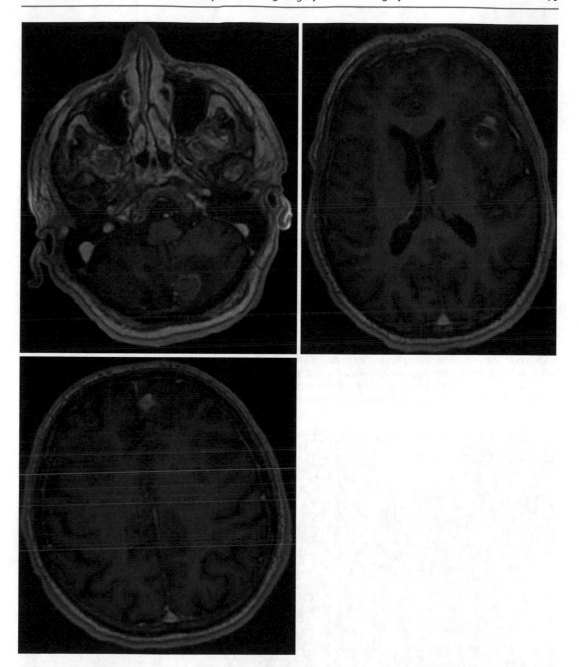

Fig. 6.13 66M with at least eight BRAF+ melanoma metastases. He was treated with combined therapy of WBRT and targeted immunotherapy

overall prognosis was known to be less than 3 months. However, she had an abrupt neurological decline with just as rapid improvement after receiving hyperosmolar therapy. Had she not have been offered surgery, she almost certainly would have progressed to neurologic death in the hospital within the next 24 hours since hyperosmolar ther-apy is only a temporary measure for treating elevated intracranial pressure. Surgery was offered emergently by the on-call surgeon after thorough discussion with the family, and only the frontal cyst was drained. If a patient with leptomeningeal disease and an additional metastasis is taken for surgery, resection of leptomeningeal disease

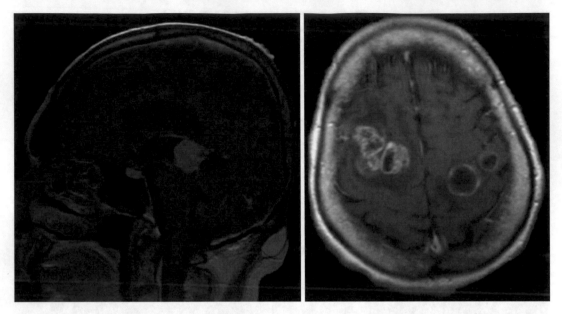

Fig. 6.14 Left: 84M presenting with solitary pineal mass causing obstructive hydrocephalus. He first received an endoscopic third ventriculostomy to treat his hydrocephalus with concurrent biopsy that showed melanoma metastasis. His surgical risk for resection was felt to be high given his age, functional status, and high-risk location of the lesion, so he was instead treated with SRS and immunotherapy. Right: 63F with bilateral frontoparietal non-small-cell lung carcinoma metastases. She had a high burden of extracranial disease and comorbidities. She received palliative WBRT and expired 3 months later

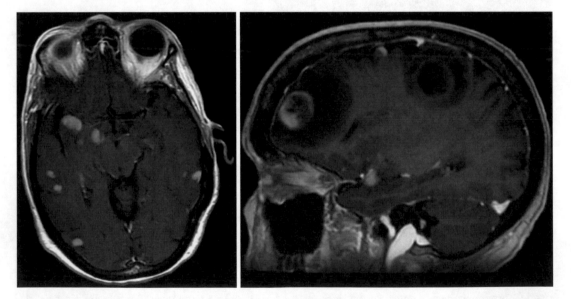

Fig. 6.15 72F with many melanoma metastases including dominant right frontal and right frontoparietal lesions. She was not a candidate for surgery given her overall burden of disease and poor prognosis

should rarely, if ever, be attempted given its significant risk with minimal benefit. Ultimately, surgery allowed her to transition to hospice care, leave the hospital, and survive for one more month.

The patient in the second case vignette was also an ideal surgical candidate with a large, symptomatic, solitary tumor in an easily accessible location with limited extracranial disease. He did not have nearly as much mass effect or edema as the first patient, and his symptoms significantly improved with medical therapy. His radiation and medical oncology plans were arranged in short order, and he was able to receive preoperative SRS for his brain lesion followed by surgery 1 day later. He has had a great response with no local recurrence and no LMD thus far and is doing well 1 year postoperatively. His case was chosen to help highlight the pros and cons of preoperative vs postoperative SRS.

If a patient is found to be a surgical candidate, the decision for how to provide adjuvant radiotherapy must be made. The risks and benefits of each option are discussed with the patient, and a joint decision is made. Generally speaking, SRS is preferred over WBRT for adjuvant therapy in patients with 1–4 (or more) brain metastases. The higher risk of recurrence is worth the benefit gained from lower rates of neurocognitive decline, and the rates of overall survival are similar. For surgical candidates with more than four lesions, WBRT may still be the preferred adjuvant of choice, but SRS to many individual metastases beyond four is often employed. Although definitive prospective, randomized trials are lacking at this time, we believe that preoperative SRS is preferable to postoperative SRS. This is generally performed 48 hours before planned resection, but may be as much as 1 week prior. For preoperative SRS, our preference is to use frameless SRS, and no margin expansion is used during target delineation. Thus, PTV is equivalent to gross tumor volume (GTV). We use a 10–20% dose reduction from the RTOG 90-05 based dosing, given in a single fraction. Brain metastases that are not resected are treated with standard SRS protocols. For patients with profound edema and mass effect and/or severe refractory symptoms, immediate surgery followed by SRS may be a safer option, although

most patients with cerebral metastases can safely undergo preoperative SRS prior to resection.

Areas of Uncertainty/Future Directions

Prospective randomized trials are currently underway to validate early limited retrospective evidence that suggests a higher risk of LMD and radiation necrosis with postoperative SRS compared to preoperative SRS. Additionally, work is being done to better characterize LMD recurrence after surgery and SRS, identify optimal management of postsurgical LMD, and determine outcomes in this setting. Lastly, it is known that radiation can induce increased surface tumor antigen expression, which can increase the effectiveness of immunotherapy agents. The patterns of surface tumor antigen expression in response to SRS and the timing of surgery are

Key Points

- All patients with cerebral metastases should have radiation oncology, medical oncology, and neurosurgical consultation. Factors favoring for or against surgery are listed in Table 6.3.
- For patients undergoing surgical resection, adjuvant radiotherapy is recommended to decrease the risk of local recurrence.
- Maximal safe resection should be the goal of surgery. Recurrent lesions after surgery can benefit from repeat craniotomy.
- Compared to adjuvant SRS, adjuvant WBRT has higher rates of neurocognitive decline, decreased quality of life, higher rates of intracranial tumor control, and equivalent overall survival. For these reasons, SRS is usually favored over WBRT in surgical patients with a limited number of brain metastases.
- Preoperative SRS has similar rates of tumor recurrence with lower rates

of radiation necrosis and leptomeningeal spread compared to postoperative SRS.

• Patients with subtotal resection after preoperative SRS should be strongly considered for re-resection or additional radiation therapy.

• Although definitive studies are still in progress, our recommendation is that preoperative SRS should be favored over postoperative SRS in surgical patients unless a patient has life-threatening mass effect requiring urgent intervention.

largely unknown, and studies are being planned with the hopes of identifying an ideal timing of surgery after SRS in order to maximize the benefit of surface tumor antigen expression for immunotherapy.

References

1. Chao JH, Phillips R, Nickson JJ. Roentgen-ray therapy of cerebral metastases. Cancer. 1954;7:682–9.
2. McTyre E, Scott J, Chinnaiyan P. Whole brain radiotherapy for brain metastasis. Surg Neurol Int. 2013;4(Suppl 4):S236–44.
3. Borgelt B, Gelber R, Kramer S, et al. The palliation of brain metastases: final results of the first two studies by the Radiation Therapy Oncology Group. Int J Radiat Oncol Biol Phys. 1980;6(1):1–9.
4. Gaspar L, Scott C, Rotman M, et al. Recursive partitioning analysis (RPA) of prognostic factors in three Radiation Therapy Oncology Group (RTOG) brain metastases trials. Int J Radiat Oncol Biol Phys. 1997;37(4):745–51.
5. Patchell RA, Tibbs P, Regine WF, et al. Postoperative radiotherapy in the treatment of single metastases to the brain. JAMA. 1998;280(17):1485–9.
6. Patchell RA, Tibbs P, Walsh JW, et al. A randomized trial of surgery in the treatment of single metastases to the brain. N Engl J Med. 1990;322(8):494–500.
7. Kocher M, Soffietti R, Abacioglu U, et al. Adjuvant whole-brain radiotherapy versus observation after radiosurgery or surgical resection of one to three cerebral metastases: results of the EORTC 22952-26001 study. J Clin Oncol. 2011;29(2):134–41.
8. Mahajan A, Ahmed S, McAleer MF, et al. Postoperative stereotactic radiosurgery versus observation for completely resected brain metastases, a single-

centre randomised, controlled, phase 3 trial. Lancet Oncol. 2017;18(8):1040–8.
9. Brown PD, Jaeckle K, Ballman KV, et al. Effect of radiosurgery alone vs radiosurgery with whole brain radiation therapy on cognitive function in patients with 1 to 3 brain metastases: a randomized clinical trial. JAMA. 2016;316(4):401–9.
10. Chang EL, Wefel J, Hess KR, et al. Neurocognition in patients with brain metastases treated with radiosurgery or radiosurgery plus whole-brain irradiation: a randomised controlled trial. Lancet Oncol. 2009;10(11):1037–44.
11. Soffietti R, Kocher M, Abacioglu UM, et al. A European Organisation for Research and Treatment of Cancer phase III trial of adjuvant whole-brain radiotherapy versus observation in patients with one to three brain metastases from solid tumors after surgical resection or radiosurgery: quality-of-life results. J Clin Oncol. 2013;31(1):65–72.
12. Aoyama H, Shirato H, Tago M, et al. Stereotactic radiosurgery plus whole-brain radiation therapy vs stereotactic radiosurgery alone for treatment of brain metastases. JAMA. 2006;295(21):2483–91.
13. Prabhu RS, Patel KR, Press RH, et al. Preoperative vs postoperative radiosurgery for resected brain metastases: a review. Neurosurgery. 2019;84(1):19–29.
14. Brennan C, Yang TJ, Hilden P, et al. A phase 2 trial of stereotactic radiosurgery boost after surgical resection for brain metastases. Int J Radiat Oncol Biol Phys. 2014;88(1):130–6.
15. Brown PD, Ballman K, Cerhan JH, et al. Postoperative stereotactic radiosurgery compared with whole brain radiotherapy for resected metastatic brain disease (NCCTG N107C/CEC3): a multicentre, randomised, controlled, phase 3 trial. Lancet Oncol. 2017;18(8):1049–60.
16. Prabhu RS, Press R, Patel KR, et al. Single-fraction stereotactic radiosurgery (SRS) alone versus surgical resection and SRS for large brain metastases: a multi-institutional analysis. Int J Radiat Oncol Biol Phys. 2017;99(2):459–67.
17. Quigley MR, Bello N, Jho D, et al. Estimating the additive benefit of surgical excision to stereotactic radiosurgery in the management of metastatic brain disease. Neurosurgery. 2015;76(6):707–13.
18. Roberge D, Parney I, Brown PD. Radiosurgery to the postoperative surgical cavity: who needs evidence? Int J Radiat Oncol Biol Phys. 2012;83(2):486–93.
19. Atalar B, Modlin LA, Choi CY, et al. Risk of leptomeningeal disease in patients treated with stereotactic radiosurgery targeting the postoperative resection cavity for brain metastases. Int J Radiat Oncol Biol Phys. 2013;87(4):713–8.
20. Iorio-Morin C, Masson-Cote L, Ezahr Y, Blanchard J, Ebacher A, Mathieu D. Early Gamma Knife stereotactic radiosurgery to the tumor bed of resected brain metastasis for improved local control. J Neurosurg. 2014;121(Suppl):69–74.
21. Patel KR, Prabhu RS, Kandula S, et al. Intracranial control and radiographic changes with adjuvant radia-

tion therapy for resected brain metastases: whole brain radiotherapy versus stereotactic radiosurgery alone. J Neuro-Oncol. 2014;120(3):657–63.

22. Ojerholm E, Lee J, Thawani JP, et al. Stereotactic radiosurgery to the resection bed for intracranial metastases and risk of leptomeningeal carcinomatosis. J Neurosurg. 2014;121(2):75–83.

23. Soltys SG, Adler J, Lipani JD, et al. Stereotactic radiosurgery of the postoperative resection cavity for brain metastases. Int J Radiat Oncol Biol Phys. 2008;70(1):187–93.

24. Choi CY, Chang S, Gibbs IC, et al. Stereotactic radiosurgery of the postoperative resection cavity for brain metastases: prospective evaluation of target margin on tumor control. Int J Radiat Oncol Biol Phys. 2012;84(2):336–42.

25. Johnson MD, Avkshtol V, Baschnagel AM, et al. Surgical resection of brain metastases and the risk of leptomeningeal recurrence in patients treated with stereotactic radiosurgery. Int J Radiat Oncol Biol Phys. 2016;94(3):537–43.

26. Huang AJ, Huang KE, Page BR, et al. Risk factors for leptomeningeal carcinomatosis in patients with brain metastases who have previously undergone stereotactic radiosurgery. J Neuro-Oncol. 2014;120(1):163–9.

27. Blonigen BJ, Steinmetz R, Levin L, et al. Irradiated volume as a predictor of brain radionecrosis after linear accelerator stereotactic radiosurgery. Int J Radiat Oncol Biol Phys. 2010;77(4):996–1001.

28. Minniti G, Clarke E, Lanzetta G, et al. Stereotactic radiosurgery for brain metastases: analysis of outcome and risk of brain radionecrosis. Radiat Oncol. 2011;6(1):48.

29. Sneed PK, Mendez J, Vemer-van den Hock JG, et al. Adverse radiation effect after stereotactic radiosurgery for brain metastases: incidence, time course, and risk factors. J Neurosurg. 2015;123(2):373–86.

30. Patel KR, Burri S, Asher AL, et al. Comparing preoperative with postoperative stereotactic radiosurgery for resectable brain metastases. Neurosurgery. 2016;79(2):279–85.

31. Prabhu RS, Miller KR, Asher AL, et al. Preoperative stereotactic radiosurgery before planned resection of brain metastases: updated analysis of efficacy and toxicity of a novel treatment paradigm. J Neurosurg. 2018:1–8.

32. Patel KR, Burri SH, Boselli D, et al. Comparing preoperative stereotactic radiosurgery (SRS) to postoperative whole brain radiation therapy (WBRT) for resectable brain metastases: a multi-institutional analysis. J Neuro-Oncol. 2017;131(3):611–8.

33. Asher AL, Burri SH, Wiggins WF, et al. A new treatment paradigm: neoadjuvant radiosurgery before surgical resection of brain metastases with analysis of local tumor recurrence. Int J Radiat Oncol Biol Phys. 2014;88(4):899–906.

34. Routman DM, Yan E, Vora S, et al. Preoperative stereotactic radiosurgery for brain metastases. Front Neurol. 2018;9:959.

35. Nayak L, Lee EQ, Wen PY. Epidemiology of brain metastases. Curr Oncol Rep. 2012;14(1):48–54.

36. Nahed BV, Alvarez-Breckenridge C, Brastianos PK, et al. Congress of neurological surgeons systematic review and evidence-based guidelines on the role of surgery in the management of adults with metastatic brain tumors. Neurosurgery. 2019;84(3):E152–5.

37. Lee CH, Kim D, Kim JW, et al. The role of surgical resection in the management of brain metastasis: a 17-year longitudinal study. Acta Neurochir. 2013;155(3):389–97.

38. Obermueller T, Schaeffner M, Gerhardt J, Meyer B, Ringel F, Krieg SM. Risks of postoperative paresis in motor eloquently and non-eloquently located brain metastases. BMC Cancer. 2014;14(1):21.

39. Suki D, Hatiboglu M, Patel AJ, et al. Comparative risk of leptomeningeal dissemination of cancer after surgery or stereotactic radiosurgery for a single supratentorial solid tumor metastasis. Neurosurgery. 2009;64(4):664–76.

40. Patel AJ, Suki D, Hatiboglu MA, Rao VY, Fox BD, Sawaya R. Impact of surgical methodology on the complication rate and functional outcome of patients with a single brain metastasis. J Neurosurg. 2015;122(5):1132–43.

41. Patel AJ, Suki D, Hatiboglu MA, et al. Factors influencing the risk of local recurrence after resection of a single brainmetastasis. J Neurosurg. 2010;113(2):181–9.

42. Stark AM, Stöhring C, Hedderich J, Held-Feindt J, Mehdorn HM. Surgical treatment for brain metastases: prognostic factors and survival in 309 patients with regard to patient age. J Clin Neurosci. 2011;18(1):34–8.

43. Kano H, Kondziolka D, Zorro O, Lobato-Polo J, Flickinger JC, Lunsford LD. The results of resection after stereotactic radiosurgery for brain metastases. J Neurosurg. 2009;111(4):825–31.

Laser Interstitial Thermal Therapy for Brain Metastasis

7

Ahmet F. Atik, Krishna C. Joshi,
Alireza Mohammad Mohammadi,
and Gene H. Barnett

Case Vignettes

Case 1

Λ 75-year-old male smoker was diagnosed with stage IIIB squamous carcinoma of the lung. He underwent carboplatin/docetaxel chemotherapy. Six months later, the patient started to have clumsiness with his right hand and problems with fine motor movements; subsequently, he started to drag his right leg. MRI revealed two intracranial lesions (left frontal and left cerebellar) consistent with metastases due to existing lung cancer. Both lesions were treated with Gamma Knife radiosurgery (GKRS) The left frontal 16-mm diameter metastasis was treated with 24 Gy at 68% isodose, and the left frontal 25.3-mm diameter metastasis received staged treatment with 18 Gy and then with 12 Gy at 57% isodose. Both frontal and cerebellar lesions disappeared over the course of 2 years. At the end of the second year, the cerebellar lesion started to regrow with new dysmetria and inability to perform rapid alternating movements on the left side. MRI studies showed increased cerebral blood volume (CBV) on a perfusion study, and our tumor board recommended Laser Interstitial Thermal Therapy (LITT) for this recurrent lesion. One trajectory was used for treatment (Fig. 7.1). The patient was followed up for over 2 years with disappearance of the cerebellar lesions as shown in Fig. 7.2. His neurological complaints diminished gradually. Unfortunately, the patient died 3 years after LITT due to progression of his primary disease.

Case 2

A 44-year-old woman was diagnosed with triple negative breast carcinoma with metastases to regional lymph nodes. She underwent modified radical mastectomy followed by chemotherapy at an outside medical center. She was diagnosed with two intracranial metastatic lesions 8 months after initial diagnosis and received staged GKRS (18 + 12 Gy at 50% isodose). The smaller lesion showed a good response to treatment, but the large right thalamic tumor persisted. Four months after GKRS this lesion started to grow, and the patient was subsequently referred to our clinic. We performed perfusion MRI imaging, which revealed an elevated CBV, suggesting that this lesion was most likely to be regrowing metastasis

A. F. Atik (✉) · K. C. Joshi · A. M. Mohammadi
Department of Neurosurgery, Rose Ella Burkhardt
Neuro-Oncology Center, Cleveland Clinic
Foundation, Cleveland, OH, USA
e-mail: ATIKA@ccf.org

G. H. Barnett
Department of Neurosurgery, Rose Ella Burkhardt
Neuro-Oncology Center, Cleveland Clinic
Foundation, Cleveland, OH, USA

Cleveland Clinic Lerner College of Medicine of Case
Western Reserve University, Cleveland, OH, USA

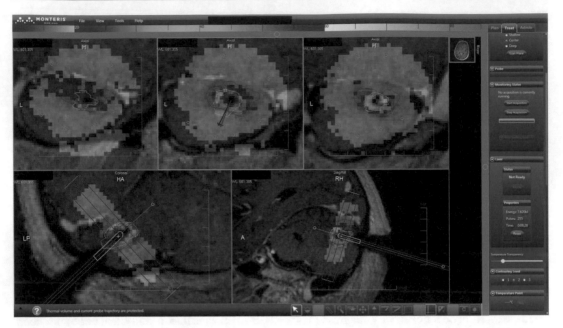

Fig. 7.1 Screenshot during the LITT procedure for a cerebellar metastatic lesion. Blue line: coagulation necrosis, turquoise line: tumor borders, green zone: MR thermometry zone, yellow circles in green zone: MR thermometry readings, blue arrow: planned direction, red arrow: actual location (red will move to blue subsequently). Yellow straight line depicts the probe tract, and yellow circle at the end demonstrates the maximum length the probe can reach

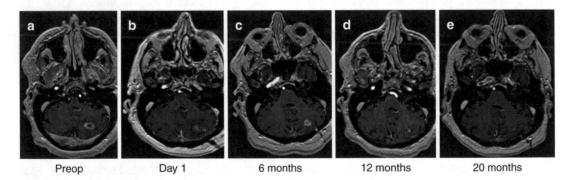

| Preop | Day 1 | 6 months | 12 months | 20 months |

Fig. 7.2 Magnetic resonance imaging (MRI) showing recurrent cerebellar metastasis from squamous cell carcinoma of the lung. (**a**) T1-weighted MRI with gadolinium showing preoperative lesion. (**b**) Post-op day 1, (**c**) post-op month 6, (**d**) post-op month 12, (**e**) post-op month 20

and not radiation injury. At the time of presentation, patient had no neurological deficit. Her past medical history did not include any other pathology than her breast cancer.

She underwent stereotactic biopsy that confirmed recurrent cancer followed by LITT with three trajectories from the same burr hole (Fig. 7.3) during the same procedure. The tumor diameter at the time of diagnosis was 41 mm, and the entire tumor was ablated. Her postoperative course was uneventful, and she was discharged 2 days after the surgery without any complications. On subsequent follow-up, the edema around the tumor diminished significantly and almost disappeared at 6 months (Fig. 7.4). There was also a volumetric response to LITT, and tumor shrunk from 18.9 to 14.7 cm^3 in 6 months (Fig. 7.5). Despite a significant decrease in

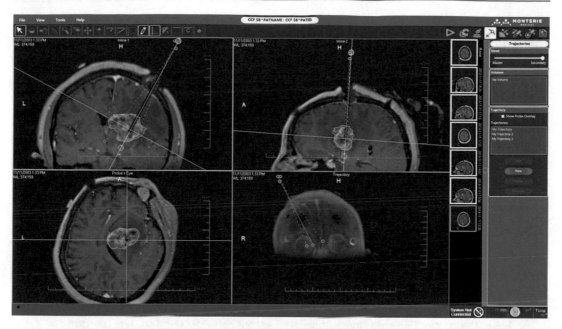

Fig. 7.3 Intraoperative screenshot of LITT with four inline windows. Three straight lines show the trajectories for each treatment

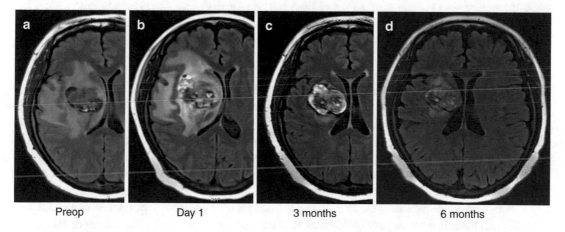

Preop   Day 1   3 months   6 months

Fig. 7.4 Magnetic resonance imaging (MRI) showing thalamic metastasis from squamous cell carcinoma of the lung. (**a**) T2 Flair MRI showing preoperative recurrent lesion. (**b**) Post-op day 1, (**c**) post-op month 3, (**d**) post-op month 6

edema, new contrast enhancing areas appeared on the posterior border of the tumor, which were positive for recurrence (Fig. 7.5d).

Introduction

Advances in cancer diagnosis and the advent of newer treatment modalities have increased the prevalence of brain metastasis. The last two decades have seen a paradigm shift in the treatment of these lesions. Although previously patients with brain metastasis are commonly considered incurable, more and more patients now are being treated, and the average treated lesion size is getting smaller. This can largely be attributed to the evolution and development of newer treatment approaches, with increasing recent emphasis on focal therapies whenever possible. MRI-guided laser interstitial thermal therapy (LITT) is one of

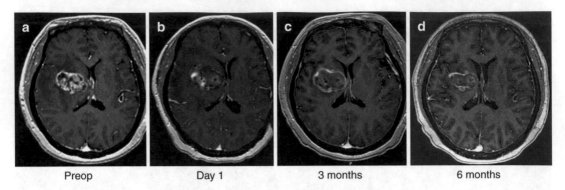

Fig. 7.5 Magnetic resonance imaging (MRI) showing recurrent thalamic metastasis from squamous cell carcinoma of the lung. (**a**) T1 weighted MRI with gadolinium showing preoperative lesion. (**b**) Post-op day 1, (**c**) post-op month 6, (**d**) post-op month 12, (**e**) post-op month 20

the newest tools in the neurosurgical armamentarium and can be used for minimally invasive treatment of a variety of intracranial tumors.

A laser (light amplification by stimulated emission of radiation) probe is directed to the desired area for thermal coagulation of the surrounding structures [1]. The mechanism of laser ablation relies on thermal energy (bioheat) transferral to the tissue surrounding the laser probe [2]. The overall effect is coagulation necrosis and blood vessel sclerosis by photocoagulation [3]. Similarly, microwave or ultrasound waves can be used as a heat-producing source for targeted lesioning purposes in the human body [4]. Two out of these three methods are currently being used in neurosurgery. Ultrasound ablation is mainly used for ablation purposes for neurodegenerative diseases such as essential tremor [5]. LITT was first employed in surgery by Bown et al. [6] and then in neurosurgery by Kahn et al. [7] for various intracranial tumors with the help of real-time MR imaging. The method is frequently used as an alternative treatment model for tumors that are not good candidates for surgery [8]. The inherent minimally invasive nature of the procedure promotes shorter hospital stay and decreased morbidity compared to conventional surgical procedures [9].

Unwanted side effects of LITT are carbonization and vaporization both of which happen as tissue reaches 100 °C temperature. Monitoring the temperature inside the thermal lesion as it is generated is a key step in the procedure and is accomplished by using MR thermometry.

Different types of lasers differ importantly in the depth of tissue penetration. For example, it is 4 mm for neodymium-doped yttrium aluminum garnet (Nd-YAG) lasers but 0.4 mm for argon laser. One of the most frequently used lasers is the CO_2 laser, and its tissue penetration is 30 μm. The best tissue penetration is with the Nd-YAG laser because it has a longer wavelength. Shorter wavelength lasers produce more heat, but less tissue penetration, and therefore carry a greater risk of thermal tissue necrosis.

Historically, Q-switched ruby lasers were first used in medicine to remove tattoos in the 1960s [10]. A ruby laser has a short wavelength (694 nm) that has been effectively used in dermatological procedures since its first application. Bown et al. used CO_2 lasers for the treatment of tumors in the early 1980s and reported that although long-wavelength laser can penetrate deeper distances and can be used for larger lesions, this type of laser reaches maximum temperature very quickly (in seconds), and it can cut and vaporize tissue instead of creating coagulation necrosis, and therefore, it is not practical to use in deep tissues [6].

Currently, lasers in the near-infrared (in Nd-YAG laser range) are used for LITT. Due to their long wavelength, they can be safely used for deeply located tumors and can stay in one position during the procedure for an extended period of time because they only slowly reach the maximum temperature [6]. Currently, both the technologies used in neurosurgery – Neuroblate (Monteris Co, Plymouth, MN, USA) and

Visualase (Medtronic, Minneapolis, MN, USA) use solid-state lasers in the near-infrared range (1064 nm at 12 W), but the cooling systems they use differ. The Neuroblate system uses a CO_2 gas-cooled laser probe, whereas the Visualase system uses a saline-based system that circulates around the probe and cools it [11].

Laser use in neurosurgery dates back to 1990 when Sugiyama et al. demonstrated the safe use of an Nd-YAG laser in intracranial tumors [12]. This long-wavelength laser was utilized with tomography with successful lesioning. Even though this long-wavelength and low-power lasers were utilized in the 90s, unsophisticated laser probes and a lack of intraoperative real-time monitoring posed difficulties for LITT use in neurosurgery. The Nd-YAG laser is, however, very suitable to use in well perfused soft tissues such as brain white matter [13].

The groundbreaking factor for utilization of LITT is the development of MRI thermography. Before this technology, lasers were used in 1980s with a surge in interest but subsided in a decade due to difficulty of monitoring or predicting the degree of thermal damage. The publication rate on LITT shows us that after introduction of MR thermography (1994), the number of publications on LITT has exponentially increased (Fig. 7.6). MR ther-

mography provides real-time monitoring of thermal damage inside the tissue, thereby maximizing lesion ablation while minimizing damage to nearby healthy structures [14]. Laser energy increases the temperature in the targeted area and breaks hydrogen bonds inside the cell, while at the same time increases the number of free water molecules. MR thermography can measure temperature in this tissue using a method called Proton Resonance Frequency Shift (PRFS) [15]. MR thermography is not restricted to LITT; it can also be used with intracranial ultrasound [16] and radiofrequency ablation in other parts of the body [17].

Tissue optical properties depend on multiple factors such as the level of parenchymal hyaluronic acid that is present. It has been shown that the penetration of laser energy in gray matter is much higher than in white matter [18]. Also, laser penetration/absorbance in abnormal tissue differs from that achieved in healthy parenchyma. Low-grade gliomas absorb less laser energy than high-grade gliomas, but it has been shown that low-grade glial tumors exhibit much more absorption than normal gray matter [18].

There are three zones of thermal effect inside the target area. The first zone around the probe absorbs maximum energy and creates true coagulation necrosis, along with carbonization and/or

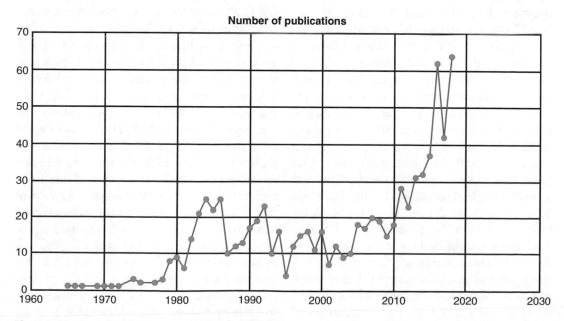

Number of publications

Fig. 7.6 Number of publications that are listed on PubMed about laser ablation of brain tumors since 1965

vaporization, depending on the degree of temperature that LITT achieved. Coagulation necrosis occurs when tissue temperature goes above 50 °C. Carbonization and vaporization occur when tissue temperatures pass 100 °C. The second zone also undergoes coagulation necrosis, and the third zone may receive a certain degree of thermal damage, but cells in this zone would be theoretically viable [19].

In this chapter, we discuss the current indications and review the literature in an effort to shed light on the current role of LITT in the treatment of brain metastases.

Operative Technique

At our institution, the LITT procedure is performed with the NeuroBlate System which uses a solid-state diode laser in the Nd-YAG range (1064 nm at 12 W). This laser energy is transferred to the target tissue via a CO_2 gas-cooled side-firing (directional) laser probe. The trajectory planning and insertion of the laser probe into the tumor are completed through the use of surgical navigation devices and a variety of tools specific to the NeuroBlate System. The location of the laser probe within the tumor is confirmed by intraoperative MRI. The lasing portion of the treatment is planned and controlled via the NeuroBlate System computer workstation utilizing proprietary M°Vision™ (Monteris Medical Corporation, Plymouth, MN) software under real-time MR-thermography guidance. The real-time extent of thermal ablation is calculated by the company's proprietary M°Vision software, which is based on the algorithm of heat-kill of cells (a relationship between time and temperature) and demonstrated as thermal damage threshold (TDT) lines which include distinct yellow, blue, and white TDT lines. The yellow TDT line represents the area of tissue that has been heated to the equivalent of 43 °C for at least 2 minutes; the blue TDT line represents heating to the equivalent of 43 °C for at least 10 minutes; and the white TDT line represents the equivalent of 43 °C for 60 minutes or heated to a higher temperature for a shorter interval. These TDT lines are true indicators of treatment effect on tumor tissue (Fig. 7.4) [20].

Diagnosis and Management

Metastatic brain tumors derive from a variety of different systemic cancers, most commonly of lung origin, regardless of gender, followed by breast and gastrointestinal in females and gastrointestinal and melanoma origins in males [21]. An intracranial lesion can be considered a brain metastasis without doing a biopsy if it has radiological features suggestive of metastasis in a patient with a primary cancer which has a predilection to spread to the brain. In case of ambiguity, due to atypical radiological features of absence of a known primary, stereotactic biopsy of the brain lesion is to be considered.

Recent clinical trials demonstrated that stereotactic radiosurgery (SRS) is comparable with or superior to whole brain radiotherapy (WBRT) in the management of brain metastasis. It can be used for multiple metastatic lesions, can be combined with WBRT or can be applied to a surgical-resection cavity. It is often considered a first-line treatment for patients with 1–3 brain metastases identified at the time of their diagnosis [22]. Radiation necrosis is a common posttreatment effect of SRS that can be very difficult to diagnose and treat. Advanced imaging modalities like perfusion MRI or fluorodeoxyglucose positron emission tomography (FDG-PET) can help differentiate radiation necrosis from tumor recurrence or progression [23, 24].

Surgery for brain metastases should be considered when there is diagnostic uncertainty or if the tumor is growing rapidly and causing neurological symptoms despite steroids [25]. LITT can be a good alternative for recalcitrant metastatic tumors, which have not been controlled by other therapeutic modalities, and it is often considered a last resort treatment modality for brain metastasis. Ahluwalia et al. showed that LITT can demonstrate complete response in 75% of the patients when total tumor ablation was achieved although 62.5% of the tumors progressed when ablation was subtotal [26]. Ali et al. reported that the use of hypo-fractionated stereotactic radiosurgery after LITT for recurrent metastatic tumors resulted in a lesion control rate as high as 100% compared to 57% for LITT alone [27].

Evidence

The first application of lasers to intracranial metastatic lesions goes back to 1986 when Tobler et al. reported a successful treatment of midbrain metastasis with laser ablation [28]. At that time, LITT was still in its infancy and was not coupled with MRI thermography. Since then, multiple new treatment methods for metastatic diseases have emerged, especially the use of stereotactic radiosurgery (SRS). Despite the substantial success rate of SRS, ~15% of the brain metastases are resistant to radiation [29], and LITT can be a good alternative to conventional surgery for these cases. The type of the primary source of the metastatic lesion can be an important predictor of SRS failure. Renal cell carcinoma [30], colorectal adenocarcinoma [31], BRAF wild-type melanoma [32], and triple negative breast carcinoma [33] have all been identified as SRS-resistant histologies [34]. LITT may be a good alternative or post-SRS salvage treatment for these patients.

Reports of successful utilization of LITT on metastatic lesions are sparse. An early noteworthy study by Carpentier et al. included patients who failed previous treatments such as chemotherapy, radiosurgery, radiotherapy, or immunotherapy. These studies excluded radiation necrosis from the study and worked on only recurrent metastatic lesions. Hawasli et al. reported on the use of LITT on a number of different pathologies prospectively. Among these, five metastatic tumors that were in surgically unresectable areas showed robust responses to laser ablation [35–37].

Areas of Uncertainty in LITT for Treatment of Brain Metastasis

Stereotactic radiosurgery (SRS) is widely considered the initial treatment of choice for many patients with intracranial metastases [38]. However, the treatment of lesions which recur after initial SRS can be challenging. These lesions are either recurrent metastatic disease, radiation necrosis, or a combination of the two. There are no clear imaging characteristics to differentiate between these two entities, and re-irradiation may exacerbate injury from the first treatment that is masquerading

as progressive tumor. Various treatment options have been utilized for cerebral radiation necrosis including observation, hyperbaric oxygen, pentoxifylline, Vitamin E, steroids, and bevacizumab, but none of them have shown a clear benefit over the other. Surgical resection is often undertaken to confirm diagnosis and reduce mass effect. In patients refractory to drug therapy with steroids, VEGF inhibitors like bevacizumab have shown some promise [39]. However, it is not FDA approved for treatment of post-radiosurgical enhancing lesions.

LITT has gained much interest in the recent years for treatment of post-SRS enhancing lesions. It has the distinct advantage of being both diagnostic and therapeutic, and at the same time, it is minimally invasive and can help prevent major cranial surgeries in patients who already have other systemic comorbidities [40, 41]. Patient selection is key to successful treatment with LITT. It is well suited for deep-seated and difficult to access lesions. However, it can also be used for patients who have superficial lesions, but are otherwise too ill for craniotomy, have a thin scalp due to prior radiation or multiple surgeries, or who prefer a minimally invasive approach.

Another concern in the treatment of a post-SRS enhancing lesion is delayed recurrence of the enhancing lesion *after* treatment with LITT. One possible reason for delayed failure after LITT may be that lesion was really a recurrent tumor, rather than radiation necrosis. Most of the previously published literature does not clearly describe the pathological findings in their series of treated cases [42, 43]. In cases of radiation necrosis, transient resolution of cerebral edema and suspension of the cytokine cascade promoting tissue injury may be sufficient for long-term control. In contrast, LITT used for treatment of recurrent tumor may require a more extensive ablation to prevent recurrence and the addition of post-LITT fractionated SRS [44].

Complications in LITT

Previous publications regarding the use of LITT have suggested that it is safe and well-tolerated modality of treatment for a variety of intracranial lesions, including malignant tumors and metastasis. However, the complication and technical malfunctions of LITT have been less frequently discussed. Review of literature on LITT treatment, including 25 clinical reports and treatment of 243 patients, reported a 20% rate of complication [45] including four (1.6%) catheter malpositions, which resulted in subdural hematoma [46], hemorrhage from arterial injury [47] and sub arachnoid hemorrhage [48], and one instance of tumor seeding along the track [49]. However, recent improvements in localization technologies, especially the skull anchoring devices, provide high degree of accuracy in catheter placement. Hemorrhage risks can be further reduced by using CT angiogram fused with the MRI while planning, especially in cases requiring long trajectories. Various complications related to tissue hyperthermia have also been described previously, which include new or worsening neurological deficits (like dysphasia [36, 37], homonymous hemianopia [50], seizure [51]), infection (cerebral abscess [52]), malignant cerebral edema [47], and CSF leak [51]. These can be minimized using smaller diffuser tips when possible [45] and by using tractography for planning and treatment of lesions close to eloquent structures [53].

Key Points

- There is currently insufficient evidence to recommend LITT as first-line therapy for brain metastases.
- It can be a very useful *adjunct* to SRS, especially in metastatic lesions which prove refractory to SRS or when radiation necrosis develops after SRS.
- It may also be considered an alternate to surgical resection in patients with deep seated and difficult to access lesions which are otherwise unsuitable for SRS.
- Further prospective trials studying SRS versus LITT are needed to assess its full safety and efficacy profile, particularly as a first-line therapy.

References

1. Gologorsky Y, Ben-Haim S, Moshier EL, Godbold J, Tagliati M, Weisz D, et al. Transgressing the ventricular wall during subthalamic deep brain stimulation surgery for Parkinson disease increases the risk of adverse neurological sequelae. Neurosurgery. 2011;69(2):294–9; discussion 9–300.
2. Fuentes D, Walker C, Elliott A, Shetty A, Hazle JD, Stafford RJ. Magnetic resonance temperature imaging validation of a bioheat transfer model for laser-induced thermal therapy. Int J Hyperth. 2011;27(5):453–64.
3. Ryan RW, Spetzler RF, Preul MC. Aura of technology and the cutting edge: a history of lasers in neurosurgery. Neurosurg Focus. 2009;27(3):E6.
4. Skinner MG, Iizuka MN, Kolios MC, Sherar MD. A theoretical comparison of energy sources—microwave, ultrasound and laser—for interstitial thermal therapy. Phys Med Biol. 1998;43(12):3535–47.
5. Quadri SA, Waqas M, Khan I, Khan MA, Suriya SS, Farooqui M, et al. High-intensity focused ultrasound: past, present, and future in neurosurgery. Neurosurg Focus. 2018;44(2):E16.
6. Bown SG. Phototherapy in tumors. World J Surg. 1983;7(6):700–9.
7. Kahn T, Bettag M, Ulrich F, Schwarzmaier HJ, Schober R, Furst G, et al. MRI-guided laser-induced interstitial thermotherapy of cerebral neoplasms. J Comput Assist Tomogr. 1994;18(4):519–32.
8. Stafford RJ, Fuentes D, Elliott AA, Weinberg JS, Ahrar K. Laser-induced thermal therapy for tumor ablation. Crit Rev Biomed Eng. 2010;38(1):79–100.
9. Leuthardt EC, Voigt J, Kim AH, Sylvester P. A single-center cost analysis of treating primary and metastatic brain cancers with either brain laser interstitial thermal therapy (LITT) or craniotomy. Pharmacoecon Open. 2017;1(1):53–63.
10. Goldman L, Wilson RG, Hornby P, Meyer RG. Radiation from a Q-switched ruby laser. Effect of repeated impacts of power output of 10 megawatts on a tattoo of man. J Invest Dermatol. 1965;44:69–71.
11. Mohammadi AM, Hawasli AH, Rodriguez A, Schroeder JL, Laxton AW, Elson P, et al. The role of laser interstitial thermal therapy in enhancing progression-free survival of difficult-to-access high-grade gliomas: a multicenter study. Cancer Med. 2014;3(4):971–9.
12. Sugiyama K, Sakai T, Fujishima I, Ryu H, Uemura K, Yokoyama T. Stereotactic interstitial laser-hyperthermia using Nd-YAG laser. Stereotact Funct Neurosurg. 1990;54–55:501–5.
13. Norred SE, Johnson JA. Magnetic resonance-guided laser induced thermal therapy for glioblastoma multiforme: a review. Biomed Res Int. 2014;2014:761312.
14. Missios S, Bekelis K, Barnett GH. Renaissance of laser interstitial thermal ablation. Neurosurg Focus. 2015;38(3):E13.
15. Chen Y, Ge M, Ali R, Jiang H, Huang X, Qiu B. Quantitative MR thermometry based on phase-drift

correction PRF shift method at 0.35 T. Biomed Eng Online. 2018;17(1):39.

16. Lewis MA, Staruch RM, Chopra R. Thermometry and ablation monitoring with ultrasound. Int J Hyperth. 2015;31(2):163–81.

17. Kolandaivelu A, Zviman MM, Castro V, Lardo AC, Berger RD, Halperin HR. Noninvasive assessment of tissue heating during cardiac radiofrequency ablation using MRI thermography. Circ Arrhythm Electrophysiol. 2010;3(5):521–9.

18. Eggert HR, Blazek V. Optical properties of human brain tissue, meninges, and brain tumors in the spectral range of 200 to 900 nm. Neurosurgery. 1987;21(4):459–64.

19. Fuentes D, Feng Y, Elliott A, Shetty A, McNichols RJ, Oden JT, et al. Adaptive real-time bioheat transfer models for computer-driven MR-guided laser induced thermal therapy. IEEE Trans Biomed Eng. 2010;57(5):1024–30.

20. Sloan AE, Ahluwalia MS, Valerio-Pascua J, Manjila S, Torchia MG, Jones SE, et al. Results of the NeuroBlate System first-in-humans Phase I clinical trial for recurrent glioblastoma: clinical article. J Neurosurg. 2013;118(6):1202–19.

21. Louis DN, Perry A, Reifenberger G, von Deimling A, Figarella-Branger D, Cavenee WK, et al. The 2016 World Health Organization classification of tumors of the central nervous system: a summary. Acta Neuropathol. 2016;131(6):803–20.

22. O'Beirn M, Benghiat H, Meade S, Heyes G, Sawlani V, Kong A, et al. The expanding role of radiosurgery for brain metastases. Medicines (Basel). 2018;5(3):pii: E90.

23. Wadhwa EL, Franc BL, Aboian M, Kim JY, Pampaloni M, Nicolaides T. Delayed fluorodeoxy-glucose positron emission tomography imaging in the differentiation of tumor recurrence and radiation necrosis in pediatric central nervous system tumors: case report and review of the literature. Cureus. 2018;10(9):e3364.

24. Muto M, Frauenfelder G, Senese R, Zeccolini F, Schena E, Giurazza F, et al. Dynamic susceptibility contrast (DSC) perfusion MRI in differential diagnosis between radionecrosis and neoangiogenesis in cerebral metastases using rCBV, rCBF and K2. Radiol Med. 2018;123(7):545–52.

25. Lamba N, Cagney DN, Brignell RH, Martin AM, Bessel LA, Catalano PR, et al. Neurosurgical resection and stereotactic radiation versus stereotactic radiation alone in patients with a single or solitary brain metastasis. World Neurosurgeon. 2019;122:e1557–61.

26. Ahluwalia M, Barnett GH, Deng D, Tatter SB, Laxton AW, Mohammadi AM, et al. Laser ablation after stereotactic radiosurgery: a multicenter prospective study in patients with metastatic brain tumors and radiation necrosis. J Neurosurg. 2018;130(3):804–11.

27. Ali MA, Carroll KT, Rennert RC, Hamelin T, Chang L, Lemkuil BP, et al. Stereotactic laser ablation as treatment for brain metastases that recur after stereo-tactic radiosurgery: a multiinstitutional experience. Neurosurg Focus. 2016;41(4):E11.

28. Tobler WD, Sawaya R, Tew JM Jr. Successful laser-assisted excision of a metastatic midbrain tumor. Neurosurgery. 1986;18(6):795–7.

29. Flickinger JC, Kondziolka D, Lunsford LD, Coffey RJ, Goodman ML, Shaw EG, et al. A multi-institutional experience with stereotactic radiosurgery for solitary brain metastasis. Int J Radiat Oncol Biol Phys. 1994;28(4):797–802.

30. Kim YH, Kim JW, Chung HT, Paek SH, Kim DG, Jung HW. Brain metastasis from renal cell carcinoma. Prog Neurol Surg. 2012;25:163–75.

31. Nozawa H, Ishihara S, Kawai K, Sasaki K, Murono K, Otani K, et al. Brain metastasis from colorectal cancer: predictors and treatment outcomes. Oncology. 2017;93(5):309–14.

32. Gallaher IS, Watanabe Y, DeFor TE, Dusenbery KE, Lee CK, Hunt MA, et al. BRAF mutation is associated with improved local control of melanoma brain metastases treated with gamma knife radiosurgery. Front Oncol. 2016;6:107.

33. Rostami R, Mittal S, Rostami P, Tavassoli F, Jabbari B. Brain metastasis in breast cancer: a comprehensive literature review. J Neuro-Oncol. 2016;127(3):407–14.

34. Eschrich SA, Pramana J, Zhang H, Zhao H, Boulware D, Lee JH, et al. A gene expression model of intrinsic tumor radiosensitivity: prediction of response and prognosis after chemoradiation. Int J Radiat Oncol Biol Phys. 2009;75(2):489–96.

35. Carpentier A, McNichols RJ, Stafford RJ, Itzcovitz J, Guichard JP, Reizine D, et al. Real-time magnetic resonance-guided laser thermal therapy for focal metastatic brain tumors. Neurosurgery. 2008;63(1 Suppl 1):ONS21–8; discussion ONS8–9.

36. Carpentier A, McNichols RJ, Stafford RJ, Guichard JP, Reizine D, Delaloge S, et al. Laser thermal therapy: real-time MRI-guided and computer-controlled procedures for metastatic brain tumors. Lasers Surg Med. 2011;43(10):943–50.

37. Hawasli AH, Bagade S, Shimony JS, Miller-Thomas M, Leuthardt EC. Magnetic resonance imaging-guided focused laser interstitial thermal therapy for intracranial lesions: single-institution series. Neurosurgery. 2013;73(6):1007–17.

38. Ewend MG, Morris DE, Carey LA, Ladha AM, Brem S. Guidelines for the initial management of metastatic brain tumors: role of surgery, radiosurgery, and radiation therapy. J Natl Compr Cancer Netw. 2008;6(5):505–13; quiz 14.

39. Levin VA, Bidaut L, Hou P, Kumar AJ, Wefel JS, Bekele BN, et al. Randomized double-blind placebo-controlled trial of bevacizumab therapy for radiation necrosis of the central nervous system. Int J Radiat Oncol Biol Phys. 2011;79(5):1487–95.

40. Rahmathulla G, Recinos PF, Valerio JE, Chao S, Barnett GH. Laser interstitial thermal therapy for focal cerebral radiation necrosis: a case report and literature review. Stereotact Funct Neurosurg. 2012;90(3):192–200.

41. Jolesz FA. Intraoperative imaging in neurosurgery: where will the future take us? Acta Neurochir Suppl. 2011;109:21–5.
42. Fabiano AJ, Alberico RA. Laser-interstitial thermal therapy for refractory cerebral edema from post-radiosurgery metastasis. World Neurosurg. 2014;81(3–4):652.e1–4.
43. Rao MS, Hargreaves EL, Khan AJ, Haffty BG, Danish SF. Magnetic resonance-guided laser ablation improves local control for postradiosurgery recurrence and/or radiation necrosis. Neurosurgery. 2014;74(6):658–67; discussion 67.
44. Rammo R, Asmaro K, Schultz L, Scarpace L, Siddiqui S, Walbert T, et al. The safety of magnetic resonance imaging-guided laser interstitial thermal therapy for cerebral radiation necrosis. J Neuro-Oncol. 2018;138(3):609–17.
45. Pruitt R, Gamble A, Black K, Schulder M, Mehta AD. Complication avoidance in laser interstitial thermal therapy: lessons learned. J Neurosurg. 2017;126(4):1238–45.
46. Willie JT, Laxpati NG, Drane DL, Gowda A, Appin C, Hao C, et al. Real-time magnetic resonance-guided stereotactic laser amygdalohippocampotomy for mesial temporal lobe epilepsy. Neurosurgery. 2014;74(6):569–85.
47. Jethwa PR, Barrese JC, Gowda A, Shetty A, Danish SF. Magnetic resonance thermometry-guided laser-induced thermal therapy for intracranial neoplasms: initial experience. Oper Neurosurg. 2012;71(suppl_1):ons133–ons45.
48. Wilfong AA, Curry DJ. Hypothalamic hamartomas: optimal approach to clinical evaluation and diagnosis. Epilepsia. 2013;54:109–14.
49. Sloan AE, Ahluwalia MS, Valerio-Pascua J, Manjila S, Torchia MG, Jones SE, et al. Results of the NeuroBlate System first-in-humans Phase I clinical trial for recurrent glioblastoma. J Neurosurg. 2013;118(6):1202–19.
50. Esquenazi Y, Kalamangalam GP, Slater JD, Knowlton RC, Friedman E, Morris S-A, et al. Stereotactic laser ablation of epileptogenic periventricular nodular heterotopia. Epilepsy Res. 2014;108(3):547–54.
51. Carpentier A, Chauvet D, Reina V, Beccaria K, Leclerq D, McNichols RJ, et al. MR-guided laser-induced thermal therapy (LITT) for recurrent glioblastomas. Lasers Surg Med. 2012;44(5):361–8.
52. Leonardi M, Lumenta C. Stereotactic guided laser-induced interstitial thermotherapy (SLITT) in gliomas with intraoperative morphologic monitoring in an open MR: clinical expierence. Minim Invasive Neurosurg. 2002;45(4):201–7.
53. Yin D, Thompson JA, Drees C, Ojemann SG, Nagae L, Pelak VS, et al. Optic radiation tractography and visual field deficits in laser interstitial thermal therapy for amygdalohippocampectomy in patients with mesial temporal lobe epilepsy. Stereotact Funct Neurosurg. 2017;95(2):107–13.

Integrating Systemic Therapy into the Management of Brain Metastases

8

John B. Fiveash, Anatoly Nikolaev, and Robert M. Conry

Introduction

The Food and Drug Administration oversees the approval of new drugs for human use in the United States. A drug that has not been previously approved for use in humans is termed a "new molecular entity." Each year there are 35–45 filings for new molecular entities and about 25 are approved. Although the numbers vary, each year about ten new oncology drugs are approved in the United States. This does not include expanded indications of existing drugs. Oncologists are faced with incomplete information on the safety and possible efficacy interactions of these new drugs when being combined with brain radiation therapy. The safety of these agents in combination brain radiation may be a function of the radiation volume, radiation dose schedule, drug mechanism of action, normal brain versus brain tumor penetrance, half-life, and timing of radiation vs drug exposure. This chapter will review the safety of various classes of systemic agents that are often prescribed in combination with brain radiation therapy for metastases. In some cases, there will be an opportunity to theoretically leverage potentially synergist efficacy of systemic agents and brain radiation safely. A proposed framework for treating patients with newer agents in the absence of clinical safety data is presented.

Evidence Base

Several factors will influence how brain radiation and systemic agents are integrated into the care of patients with metastases to the brain. Radiation volume (radiosurgery vs whole brain radiotherapy) and dose schedule significantly impact the risk of radiation necrosis and leukoencephalopathy, as well as skin dose. In considering how drugs may impact various toxicities of radiation, the timing and pharmacology of the agent are particularly relevant. Some agents require the drug to be present at the time of radiation, whereas others may simply have radiation recall or additive inflammatory potential. Many agents including large monoclonal antibodies may not penetrate non-enhancing regions of the brain but may reach areas of contrast enhancement where the blood–brain barrier is not fully intact. Other agents such as bevacizumab target blood vessel growth and may not need to cross blood–brain barrier.

J. B. Fiveash (✉)
Radiation Oncology, University of Alabama at Birmingham, Birmingham, AL, USA
e-mail: jfiveash@uab.edu

A. Nikolaev
Department of Radiation Oncology, University of Alabama at Birmingham, Birmingham, AL, USA

R. M. Conry
Division of Hematology & Oncology, University of Alabama at Birmingham, Birmingham, AL, USA

© Springer Nature Switzerland AG 2020
Y. Yamada et al. (eds.), *Radiotherapy in Managing Brain Metastases*,
https://doi.org/10.1007/978-3-030-43740-4_8

General Overview Studies

Historically, new drugs are studied in the metastatic setting with some washout period of typically 3–4 weeks separating the last treatment such as radiation. This results in clinical trials that do not meet the clinical needs to start systemic therapy and brain radiation without a long delay. In fact, the most often cited radiosurgical dose-finding study, RTOG 90-05, excluded patients that were planned to have systemic therapy within the next 3 months [1]. Finally, it is less common for patients with active CNS disease to be enrolled in prospective trials of new agents.

Two large retrospective studies have investigated the safety of brain RT with a variety of systemic agents. Investigators from Johns Hopkins reported on 193 patients receiving radiosurgery (SRS) and a variety of concurrent systemic therapy without any interruption. Concurrent therapy was judged to be safe across a variety of systemic therapies with no clear increase in the risk of myelosuppression or neurotoxicity [2]. Among 1650 patients treated with radiosurgery for brain metastases at the Cleveland Clinic, 445 received concurrent systemic therapy [3]. In this series, concurrent therapy was defined as treatment within five biologic half-lives. Overall, there was no increased risk of radiation necrosis for patients treated concurrently. However, subsets of patients who were at moderately high risk *of complications* included patients who received both whole-brain RT and SRS with concurrent systemic therapy and patients who were treated with VEGF or EGFR inhibitors. The toxicity events in this study included both symptomatic and asymptomatic radiation necrosis. A recent review attempted to evaluate the safety of systemic agents in combination with radiosurgery and identified gemcitabine, erlotinib, and vemurafenib as agents that had a higher rate of neurotoxicity in combination with brain radiation [4]. The evidence supporting these conclusions is explored further in the sections below.

Cytotoxic Agents

Conventional chemotherapeutic agents have historically been the mainstay of systemic treatment for a variety of cancers that spread secondarily to the central nervous system including non-small-cell lung cancer and breast cancer. In common tumor types, these drugs remain a standard salvage regimen after immunotherapy, or targeted agents are no longer efficacious. Many of these agents (e.g., cisplatin, taxanes, and gemcitabine) are radiation sensitizers and may impact non-CNS normal tissue such as skin or mucosa during whole-brain RT. In practice, cytotoxic chemotherapy is often given in cycles where the patient may not receive drug every week and radiosurgery can be delivered safely on an off-week. The use of whole-brain RT rather than radiosurgery may require a longer break, but there is some possibility to extrapolate safety from phase I trials in other tumor types such as glioblastoma. In highlighting several agents in this section, we will focus on endpoints where combinations of therapy may have more than additive toxicity or unique toxicity that may not be observed with sequential therapy.

Platinum Analogs

Cisplatin and carboplatin have a long history of use with concurrent radiation therapy at a variety of treatment sites. Prospective and retrospective studies in brain metastases and gliomas suggest these agents are generally safe during radiation therapy but large-scale randomized trials have not been conducted in all clinical settings. With the exception of high rates of ototoxicity with concurrent cisplatin and higher rates of myelosuppression, the use of concurrent platinum analogs and brain RT has been feasible [5]. Concurrent carboplatin is feasible with higher rates of hematologic toxicity in patients with medulloblastoma receiving craniospinal RT [6]. Oxaliplatin has mainly used clinically for colorectal cancer and has been studied less in patients receiving brain RT. In practice, it is generally feasible to delay concurrent brain RT to the off week(s) of chemotherapy cycles to minimize potential overlapping toxicity including fatigue. When one considers the potential risk of delaying brain RT when the cisplatin-based regimen is planned for systemic therapy, there is one randomized trial that attempt to study this question.

Robinet et al. randomized 176 patients to early vs delayed whole-brain RT with cisplatin and vinorelbine [7]. Specifically, the regimen included cisplatin 100 mg/m^2 on day 1 and vinorelbine 30 mg/m^2 on days 1, 8, 15, and 22. Cycles were repeated every 4 weeks. Patients were randomized to receive 30 Gy in ten fractions WBRT with cycle 1 versus evaluation after two cycles to receive brain RT if progressing. Patients randomized to delayed RT who were not progressing in the CNS could continue chemotherapy alone. There was no difference in overall survival between the early and delayed RT or toxicity suggesting that timing is less important. Cisplatin has also been combined safely with pemetrexed and whole-brain RT in a prospective phase II trial of patients with brain metastases from non-small-cell lung cancer [8]. Note that pemetrexed is related to folic acid, which is a class of chemotherapy drugs known as folate antimetabolites. The mechanism action is through inhibition of dihydrofolate reductase. Pemetrexed has been associated with higher rates of asymptomatic radiation necrosis (imaging changes) but not symptomatic necrosis in patients undergoing radiosurgery [9].

Taxanes

Paclitaxel and docetaxelare common cytotoxic agents administered with concurrent radiation therapy at a variety of tumor sites. There is limited penetration into normal CNS tissue [10]. Concurrent paclitaxel is feasible during wide field radiation treatment of gliomas [11, 12]. There is the potential for higher rates of skin and mucosal toxicity with concurrent whole-brain RT. No prospective trials have been completed with radiosurgery, but it is generally clinically feasible to treat with radiosurgery during an off week and limit interruptions in systemic therapy.

Antimetabolites

Antimetabolites are generally lower molecular weight compounds that interfere with DNA synthesis. Many of these agents including gem-

citabine and capecitabine are potent radiation sensitizers. Gemcitabine has limited penetration into the normal CNS but doses many-fold lower than the weekly systemic dose of 1000–1250 mg/m^2 can produce significant radiosensitization especially on skin and mucosa. Preclinical studies demonstrate that radiosensitization diminishes over 48–72 hours, suggesting that twice-weekly regimens may offer greater opportunity for radiosensitization. Twice weekly low-dose gemcitabine has been studied as a radiation sensitizer with doses up to 50 mg/m^2 thought to be feasible with whole-brain RT [13]. Dose escalation was limited by myelosuppression. Weekly gemcitabine has been studied with whole-brain RT and dose above 600 mg/m^2 were not feasible due to both neurotoxicity and myelosuppression [14]. It is easy to envision scenarios where poor coordination of care regarding start of RT and gemcitabine could result in a high risk of toxicity. Radiation recall reactions from gemcitabine have most often been described involving the skin and mucosa, but there is one report of CNS and optic nerve radiation recall [15].

Capecitabine and its metabolite 5-flurouracil (5-FU) are common agents utilized historically in the treatment of gastrointestinal and breast cancers. Capecitabine and lapatinib have been studied specifically as salvage regimen in patients with brain metastases from HER-2 positive breast cancer. Capecitabine has theoretical advantages compared to 5-FU including oral delivery, potentially higher CNS tumor concentrations as monotherapy, and the role of radiation therapy to increase CNS tumor concentrations. The final step of conversion of capecitabine ultimately to 5-FU inside tumor cells is controlled by thymidine phosphorylase (TP). TP activity inside tumor cells is increased by adding ionization radiation in an effect that lasts for weeks. In this case, 5-FU inside the cell acts as a radiation sensitizer and radiation further enhances 5-FU intratumoral concentrations for weeks after RT. Capecitabine is feasible with concurrent whole-brain RT for brain metastasis patients and in patients receiving 60 Gy partial brain RT for glioblastoma without excessive CNS toxicity [16–18]. The most likely clinical scenario to combine capecitabine and cranial RT is in patients with recurrent brain metastases from breast cancer where radiation dose might be limited due to prior treatment.

Methotrexate is an older agent historically employed in breast cancer but remains a standard agent in many lymphomas and leukemias. In addition to oncologic applications, it has a role as a lower dose oral anti-inflammatory agent. Large volume radiation concurrent or proceeding higher doses of methotrexate has been associated with higher rates of leukoencephalopathy [19]. Although methotrexate itself can cause this problem, it is possible that prior radiation could increase this risk changing CNS penetration. High-grade encephalopathy has been most frequently observed in older patients with CNS lymphomas, which received high-dose methotrexate after whole-brain RT. The risk seems to be lower if whole-brain RT is given after high-dose methotrexate. These experiences may be relevant to patients treated with methotrexate for leptomeningeal recurrences. Although some had advocated concurrent intrathecal methotrexate and brain RT for leptomeningeal tumors, a prospective trial found that 30 of 44 patients developed imaging findings suggestive of encephalopathy [20].

Other Cytotoxic Agents

Temozolomide is most commonly utilized with cranial RT for gliomas. It is clinically feasible but does increase the risk of pseudo-progression and myelosuppression. Because of the penetration into CNS tumors, it was commonly studied in brain metastasis patients prior to the immunotherapy era. A recent meta-analysis of six randomized trials of whole-brain RT with or without concurrent chemotherapy included three studies with concurrent temozolomide [21]. Although the regimens were clinically feasible, there was a higher rate of toxicity and no improvement in overall survival for patients receiving concurrent chemotherapy. A phase II trial from the University of Alabama at Birmingham found that adjuvant temozolomide starting immediately after radiosurgery for brain metastases was

feasible in patients not receiving other systemic agents [22].

Molecular Targeted Agents

Molecularly targeted agents include small molecule tyrosine kinase inhibitors and macromolecule monoclonal antibodies. Small molecule inhibitors are generally oral agents with shorter half-lives that can be stopped and restarted quickly to allow for safer brain radiation therapy. Monoclonal antibodies are often administered every 2 or 3 weeks. Stopping systemic therapy for several half-lives of monoclonal antibodies may not be clinically feasible. Although large macromolecules are not thought to easily cross the blood–brain barrier, MRI contrast-enhancing tumors have been imaged with PET labelled antibodies, suggesting a disrupted blood–brain barrier does allow antibodies to bind to brain metastases [23]. Furthermore, the anti-PD1 monoclonal antibody nivolumab thought to act primarily by activating exhausted tumor infiltrating lymphocytes has demonstrated an intracranial response rate of 20% in melanoma brain metastases [24].

EGFR targeted agents are particularly relevant in the treatment of selected patients with non-small-cell lung cancer. Erlotinib and gefitinib were the early agents approved in this class and are the most studied in combination with brain radiation therapy. Although several retrospective or single arm studies have demonstrated the safety of combining erlotinib with cranial radiation therapy, there is one randomized trial that should be highlighted. These small molecules have CNS actively and have been studied as radiation sensitizers at a variety of tumor sites. RTOG 0320 was three-arm trial randomizing patients to WBRT and radiosurgery (including standard of care chemotherapy as needed) vs adding erlotinib vs adding erlotinib and temozolomide. EGFR mutation was not required to enter this trial. The erlotinib arms trended to worse survival and had clearly worse overall toxicity apparently attributable to non-CNS events. A single patient developed high-grade brain necrosis. Although this trial is cited as evidence of higher-grade toxicity with erlotinib, it is not clear that the toxicity is more than additive or that patients to be maintained on erlotinib for systemic therapy should been managed differently in terms of cranial radiation or require a break. A second issue regarding these agents is whether RT should be added for selected patients with asymptomatic brain metastases. A large multi-institutional retrospective study of EGFR-naïve patients with newly diagnosed brain metastases patient found that patients who received erlotinib without radiation had inferior overall survival compared to patients who also received WBRT or radiosurgery [25]. Similar findings come from large meta-analyses of retrospective studies. Newer generation agents including osimertinib and afatinib have an overall response rate in the CNS of over 80–90% [25, 26]. The optimal combination and timing of EGFR agents and brain RT remain controversial in the absence of prospective clinical trials that include these newer agents in combination with radiosurgery.

Non-small-cell lung cancer with the ALK fusion occurs in about 3–5% of patients. An additional 1–2% will have a ROS mutation. Similar to EGFR-positive patients, ALK- or ROS-positive patients respond well to targeted agents and have a prolonged natural history. There are no prospective studies to define the safety of brain radiation with ALK-targeted agents. Therefore, a short break during cranial radiation may be indicated. For patients who are not candidates for radiosurgery and who would otherwise require WBRT, targeted therapy alone may be considered due to the high CNS response rates and long overall survival in these patients. The newest generation of ALK-targeted agents, such as alectinib, has superior CNS response and progression-free survival compared to crizotinib [27].

Case Vignette #1

Fifty-five-year-old female has a BRAF-positive melanoma and is receiving combination vemurafenib and trametinib with partial response in the lung and liver after 4 months of therapy. She presents with nausea and headache and is found to have ten brain metastases, the largest of which measures 2.3 cm in greatest diameter. Her body CT scans demonstrate continued response outside the CNS. In considering her radiation options, how will the radiation treatment volume necessitate changes to her systemic therapy schedule?

BRAF and MEK inhibitors are small molecule tyrosine kinase inhibitors that can penetrate the CNS although to a lesser degree than extracranial sites [28]. Mostly, these agents are utilized in the treatment of BRAF mutant melanoma. BRAF inhibitors including vemurafenib, dabrafenib, and encorafenib are potent radiation sensitizers and should be avoided during large volume radiation therapy including whole-brain RT due to high rates of skin and mucosal toxicity [29]. Pulmonary and hepatic hemorrhage has been described with concurrent RT [30]. It is controversial as to whether BRAF inhibitors increase the risk of radiosurgery toxicity, but high rates of necrosis and hemorrhage have been observed in some series. ECOG guidelines suggest a break of at least 3 days before and after WBRT and at least 1 day before and after radiosurgery [30]. Phase III trials combining BRAF and MEK inhibitors in advanced melanoma have reported hemorrhage events in 18% of patients with fatal intracranial hemorrhage in the setting of new or progressive brain metastases in approximately 2% [31, 32]. Thus, when managing patients with hemorrhagic melanoma brain metastases, holding BRAF and MEK inhibitors (e.g., trametinib, cobimetinib, binimetinib) should be considered in the acute setting.

Anti-HER2 therapies including monoclonal antibodies (e.g., trastuzumab) and small molecules (e.g., lapatinib, neratinib, tucatinib). Isolated CNS relapse is common for patients taking trastuzumab, suggesting inferior penetration of the antibody into the CNS. Lapatinib penetrates the CNS better as a small molecule and is often combined with capecitabine in the treatment of CNS metastases. A phase I trial of lapatinib and whole-brain radiation reported increased toxicity but attribution of some events was unclear [33]. This agent is currently being studied in NRG/RTOG 1119 with either whole-brain RT or radiosurgery. Trastuzumab has been reported to have a low rate of toxicity when combined with whole-brain radiation therapy [34]. A newer derivative of trastuzumab is T-DM1 or trastuzumab emtansine, an antibody drug conjugate. Despite being a macromolecule, this agent has CNS efficacy, and there are anecdotal reports of high-grade radiation necrosis in patients undergoing radiosurgery and systemic therapy with trastuzumab emtansine [35–38]. It is very unclear how to mitigate this potential risk since many of these patients did not have concurrent therapy.

VEGF Inhibitors

VEGF inhibitors include both monoclonal antibodies (e.g., bevacizumab) and oral tyrosine kinase inhibitors (e.g., sunitinib, sorafenib). Bevacizumab has been studied extensively with radiation in glioma and is generally safe to administer with cranial RT including with whole-brain RT [39]. Early in the development of bevacizumab, there was clinical concern regarding CNS bleeding. Large series including brain metastasis patients reveal a low risk of CNS hemorrhage [40, 41]. Bevacizumab reduces CNS edema and is one treatment option for patients with radiation necrosis [42]. All VEGF inhibitors have the potential to induce a clinical syndrome and imaging finding posterior reversible encephalopathy syndrome (PRES). PRES occurs in a variety of drugs and illnesses with vascular mediated hypertension including preeclampsia and is associated with bilateral symmetric FLAIR abnormalities on MRI generally starting in the posterior circulation and extending anteriorly [43].

In a large retrospective study from the Cleveland Clinic, oral VEGF inhibitors were associated with an increased risk of radiation necrosis (14.3% vs 6.6% without VEGF inhibitors) among a group of patients treated with radiosurgery either alone or in combination with whole-brain RT. The difference did not reach statistical significance in those who were treated with radiosurgery and no whole-brain RT. In a

prospective phase II trial, also at the Cleveland Clinic, sunitinib was studied as an adjuvant to radiosurgery with an acceptable safety profile [44]. In practice, most oral TKIs including VEGF inhibitors can be stopped for a brief period of time based upon half-life to avoid potential toxicity.

Case Vignette #2

Forty-five-year-old female has a history of T3bN0M0 melanoma of the right lower extremity treated with resection. The tumor was BRAF wild type, and she received no adjuvant therapy. She presents with a 1-month history of headaches and increasing left-sided motor weakness. CT reveals a single RLL nodule measuring 3 cm. MRI is shown in Fig. 8.1 and reveals a 2.4 cm right thalamic brain lesion. Biopsy of the chest nodule confirms metastatic melanoma. The neurosurgeon has seen the patient and is not recommending resection due to tumor location. Assuming the patient will receive immunotherapy,

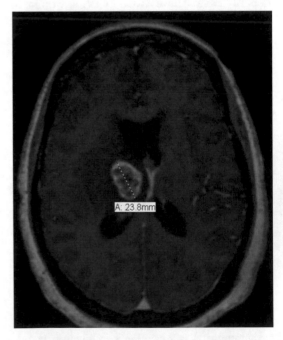

Fig. 8.1 Axial T1 post-contrast MRI image from Case Vignette #2 demonstrating a 2.4 cm right thalamic brain lesion

what radiation volume and dose schedule are recommended?

Immunotherapy

In 2018, the Nobel Prize in Physiology and Medicine was awarded to James Allison and Tasuku Honjo for their preclinical work on CTLA-4 and PD-1, respectively. Full translation of their basic science discoveries has taken nearly two decades, but checkpoint inhibitors are now the most common systemic anticancer treatments with clinical applications in a variety of tumor types including melanoma, non-small-cell lung cancer, head and neck cancer, bladder cancer, and others. In conjunction with additive or potentially synergistic effects on the treated tumor, it is hypothesized that treatment of the known CNS disease with radiosurgery may enhance the response to immunotherapy elsewhere. The clinical impact of the abscopal effect from brain treatment may be controversial, but it is present in preclinical models and small case series [45, 46]. Other immunotherapy regimens such as CAR-T cells are mainly utilized in hematologic malignancies and lymphomas but are under development in solid tumors that commonly metastasize to the brain.

Ipilimumab is a monoclonal antibody against CTLA-4 and was first approved in the treatment of melanoma in 2011. Early retrospective studies have found that ipilimumab in combination with radiosurgery is safe and improves CNS control and survival compared to historical controls, especially when given concurrently or in proximity [47, 48]. The safety of ipilimumab in combination with either whole-brain RT or radiosurgery has been explored in a phase I trial [49]. Ipilimumab 10 mg/kg currently only approved in the adjuvant setting was tolerable with radiosurgery, but the whole-brain RT arm did not complete accrual beyond 3 mg/kg, the approved dose for stage 4 melanoma. The currently available data do not support a break for ipilimumab when combined with radiosurgery. The potentially immunosuppressive effects of whole-brain radiation are discussed in the section below and serve

as one factor that may influence treatment decisions if immunotherapy is planned.

Anti-PD-1 agents including pembrolizumab and nivolumab were first approved to treat metastatic melanoma in 2014. As of 2019, anti-PD-1 and anti-PD-L1 agents are approved to treat nine different cancers. Similar to ipilimumab, the concurrent use of anti-PD-1 agents has been associated with improved response rates, CNS control, and overall survival, especially when administered concurrent with radiosurgery [50–52]. Multiple institutions are prospectively investigating the safety and optimal timing of these agents in the treatment of brain metastases. In addition, large randomized trials (CheckMate 548 and CheckMate 498) have completed accrual for glioblastoma treatment with 60 Gy fractionated therapy and anti-PD-1 agents, but no toxicity data has yet been reported. To date, there have been many retrospective studies suggesting relative safety, but results are mixed depending on endpoints [50, 51, 53–56]. Table 8.1 summarizes these data for studies that separate anti-PD-1 toxicity with an emphasis on concurrent therapy. Single-arm studies from Colorado and Alabama suggest there may be a higher rate of grade 3 radiosurgery toxicity than expected [52]. Larger studies from MGH and John Hopkins found no increased toxicity on multivariate analysis when radiosurgery is combined anti-PD-1 agents [50, 57]. The largest study to date is from Dana Farber with 115 patients treated with immunotherapy [53]. On multivariate analysis, patients receiving anti-PD-1 immunotherapy had over three times greater risk to develop symptomatic radiation necrosis compared to patients not receiving immunotherapy with radiosurgery. There is only one report of whole-brain RT in combination with anti-PD-1 where among 21 patients, one experienced grade 3 neurocognitive decline and one developed severe edema in the setting of tumor progression [55].

It is unknown whether dual checkpoint inhibition has greater CNS toxicity in combination with radiosurgery compared to anti-PD-1 agents. Dual checkpoint inhibition with ipilimumab and nivolumab for metastatic melanoma without brain involvement is associated with a threefold

Table 8.1 Retrospective studies of anti-PD-1 immunotherapy and cranial RT

	Number patients	Number tumors	Toxicity
Moffitt	26	73	1 (4%) grade 2 headache
MSKCC	21		1 (5%) grade 3 edema
Colorado	38 SRS	–	16% grade 2 or higher, 8% grade 3
UAB	43 SRS	126	11.6% of patients 4% of tumors Irreversible grade 3
Louisville	18 SRS	59	2 (3.4%) necrosis
Johns Hopkins	79 SRS	–	0–3% grade 3, no diff MVA
Brigham and Womens/Dana Faber	115 SRS	–	23/115 (21%) symptomatic necrosis
Sydney	6 SRS 21 WBRT	–	1/6 grade 3 necrosis 2/21 grade 3 neurocognitive and edema with progression
MGH	50 (various RT)	–	8–10% grade 3 No difference in grade 3 or greater compared to retrospective control.

greater incidence of serious immune-related adverse events (60%) than nivolumab alone. Many of the retrospective reports of dual checkpoint blockade with brain radiation lack details of the timing and doses of combination therapies. Further complicating interpretation of the literature is the variable use of steroids and assessment of immunotherapy associated imaging changes. These issues are discussed in a later section.

RT Factors

As one considers whether systemic therapy may increase the risk of brain RT, the traditional risk factors for radiation toxicity to the brain should not be overlooked. Randomized trials published since 2009 suggest that whole-brain RT has a higher risk of neurocognitive dysfunction beginning as early is 3–4 months after treatment [58, 59]. As systemic treatments for many malignancies advance, every effort should be made to avoid whole-brain radiation to preserve cognition in patients who survive for many years. For example, ipilimumab plus nivolumab in stage 4 melanoma provides 4-year overall survival of 53% [60]. For radiosurgery, treatment volume remains the dominant determinant of radiation toxicity. For example, in the dose escalation study RTOG 90-05, the hazard ratio for high-

grade toxicity for tumors 3.1–4 cm in greatest diameter was 16× greater than for tumors 2 cm or less. Dose-limiting toxicity was not identified for the smaller tumors with doses as high as 24 Gy evaluated. Others have found that the volumes of all dose levels from 8 to 18 Gy are predictive of radiation necrosis [61]. In practice, larger tumors treated with radiosurgery will have a high risk of toxicity, and very small tumors will have a low risk regardless of how systemic therapy is integrated. In a clinical scenario with a borderline radiosurgical target volume or new agent with inadequate data for safety, one potential tool to mitigate risk may be hypofractionation [62].

Areas of Uncertainty and Future Directions

Case Vignette #3

A 57-year-old male with metastatic melanoma developed headache and was diagnosed with a single brain metastasis. The radiosurgery plan is shown in Fig. 8.2 with the prescription isodose 20 Gy shown in yellow and 10 Gy in green. The patient starts anti-PD-1 therapy and returns 3 months later for follow-up. He is doing well clinically, and his systemic disease is responding.

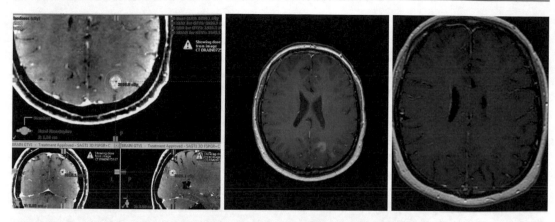

Fig. 8.2 Case Vignette #3 showing radiosurgery plan (left image)with the prescription isodose 20 Gy shown in yellow and 10 Gy in green. The patient starts anti-PD-1 therapy and returns 3 months later for follow-up (MRI middle pane). There is atypical imaging with irregular enhancement around the treated volume. Although this could be mistaken for tumor progression, in this case, the patient was observed, and the imaging change resolved at 6 months (right image). The imaging change at 3 months was inflammatory change related to immunotherapy and radiosurgery

How do you interpret his follow-up images? Is this tumor or possibly an effect of treatment? See the discussion on iRANO criteria below.

Immunotherapy Imaging Response

Immunotherapy can induce inflammatory changes in the brain parenchyma, pituitary, and pituitary stalk, in addition to the brain metastases themselves, referred to as "pseudoprogression." Parenchymal changes especially occur in brain exposed to a high dose of radiation. The iRANO criteria were devised to define imaging response in the setting of immunotherapy clinical trials for glioma, but these are also directly relevant in the clinical follow-up of brain metastasis patients receiving immunotherapy. The major lesson from these guidelines is that the MRI T1-enhancing abnormality can initially grow and then stabilize. If the patient is doing well clinically, and this is occurring early after starting immunotherapy, then observation should be strongly considered. Case #3 above shows enhancement surrounding the treated metastasis 3 months after radiosurgery and anti-PD-1. This patient was observed, and the image was normalized with associated complete response of the treated tumor.

Systemic Therapy Alone

Given the high CNS response rates of targeted agents (ERFR, ALK, BRAF) or immunotherapy checkpoint agents in selected patients, there is interest in delaying brain RT particularly in patients with asymptomatic brain metastases. For example, combined BRAF and MEK inhibition in 76 patients with asymptomatic melanoma brain metastases demonstrated as intracranial response rate of 58%, concordant with the extra-cranial response rate, and a 6.5-month median duration of response without radiotherapy (RT) [63, 64]. Phase II trials of checkpoint blockade without radiotherapy for asymptomatic melanoma brain metastases have shown intracranial responses in 20% of patients receiving single-agent nivolumab and 56% of patients following dual checkpoint blockade with ipilimumab plus nivolumab including 26% intracranial complete responses and 6-month progression-free survival in 67% of patients, which represents the most effective systemic therapy to date for melanoma brain metastases [32, 65]. The potential for higher rates of toxicity with checkpoint inhibitors in combination with radiosurgery complicates systemic treatment when steroids are required. To date, there are no randomized trials evaluating the optimal timing of these targeted agents or immunotherapy and radiation. Most brain metastases trials of systemic therapy alone have enrolled asymptomatic patients, so there is little information on patients with larger tumors, patients on steroids, or leptomeningeal tumors. A proposed trial in NRG Oncology will randomize patients with 1–15 melanoma brain metastases to dual immune checkpoint inhibitors alone vs checkpoint inhibitors plus radiosurgery. Most trials of immune checkpoint blockade in the absence of brain metastases have permitted a maximum steroid dose of 10 mg/day of prednisone (approximately 2 mg/day of dexamethasone) or equivalent for enrollment. A trial of ipilimumab for advanced melanoma with brain involvement allowed higher steroid doses but demonstrated a response rate approximately half that reported in trials limiting steroid use at enrollment to an adrenal replacement dose of 10 mg of daily prednisone. Thus, when treating melanoma brain metastases with checkpoint blockade, every effort should be made to limit dexamethasone to 2 mg daily or exceed that dose for as few days as possible. This issue is being prospectively studied in clinical trials (e.g., NCT03563729).

Lymphopenia – Role of Steroids and Radiation Volume

Preclinical studies from the University of Chicago suggest that high-dose radiation requires a functional immune system for optimal efficacy [66]. This has been demonstrated retrospectively in brain metastases patients undergoing treatment with immune checkpoint inhibitors and radiosurgery where an absolute lymphocyte count (ALC) below 1000 cells/μL was associated with inferior intracranial control [48]. Others have identified a beneficial effect of concurrent radiosurgery and immune checkpoint inhibitors that is partially dependent on having an ALC over 1000 [50]. Larger volume fractionated RT have been associated with lymphopenia at a variety of tumor sites [67]. Furthermore, a prolonged course of fractionated RT (# fractions >5) combined with PD-1 immune checkpoint blockade was found to be associated with an increased risk of severe lymphopenia (ANC < 500) [68]. In patients with metastatic non-small-cell lung cancer undergoing anti-PD-1 therapy, there is a strong association with use of prednisone over 10 mg/day and immunotherapy response, progression-free survival, and overall survival [69]. Taken together, there is strong rational to avoid excessive steroids in brain metastasis patients and to question any prophylactic steroids in patients receiving immune checkpoint inhibitors.

Conclusions and Recommendations

In an era of declining use of whole radiation therapy, focal radiation including radiosurgery offers additional advantages of minimizing the delay in administering systemic therapy and potentially less myelosuppression. High dose per fraction treatments may also offer theoretical advantages in combination with immunotherapy. Since the clinical evidence to define the optimal integration of systemic therapy and brain radiation therapy is lacking for most drugs, treating physicians are left to make pragmatic clinic decisions based upon extrapolations and preclinical studies and pharmacology. One practical strategy detailed in Fig. 8.3 is to limited breaks for most agents to a few days or a week for radiosurgery, and no breaks for some classes of drugs such as immunotherapy checkpoint inhibitors.

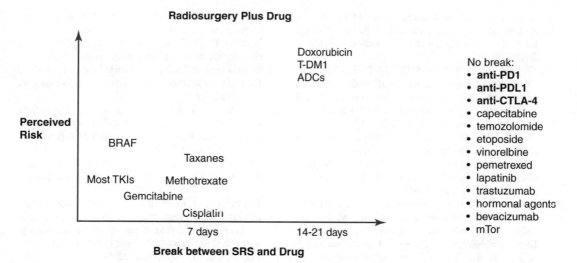

Fig. 8.3 Proposed schema to manage risk of combining CNS radiosurgery and systemic drugs as utilized at University of Alabama at Birmingham. Agents that have no break recommended are listed on the right. Other agents are plotted on the graph with the recommended break on the x-axis and the perceived risk to patient on the y-axis if no break was prescribed. Note that tumor volume may drive treatment decisions that deviate modestly from this schema, and that this schema only applies to radiosurgery patients and not those receiving whole-brain radiation therapy

Key Points
- Treatment volume is the largest predictor of brain radiosurgery toxicity such that very small tumors will have a very low risk of toxicity despite any concurrent systemic therapy, and larger tumors will have significant risk despite efforts to separate treatments temporally with a longer break.
- For brain metastases patients receiving most common cytotoxic agents, radiosurgery can be delivered safely during an off week, but whole-brain radiation therapy may necessitate longer delays.
- For patients receiving most molecular targeted therapies, brain radiation can be delivered safely with a short washout period depending on drug half-life.
- For patients receiving the most common immunotherapy agents, CNS control may be improved, but there are mixed studies on whether toxicity is worse. The use of steroids to manage symptoms may compromise the efficacy of immunotherapy, and larger volume whole-brain radiation therapy may further worsen myelosuppression.
- For borderline cases of treatment volume in patients receiving an agent with unknown risk, hypofractionation may be one option to potentially mitigate risk.

References

1. Shaw E, Scott C, Souhami L, et al. Radiosurgery for the treatment of previously irradiated recurrent primary brain tumors and brain metastases: initial report of radiation therapy oncology group protocol (90-05). Int J Radiat Oncol Biol Phys. 1996;34(3):647–54.
2. Shen CJ, Kummerlowe MN, Redmond KJ, Rigamonti D, Lim MK, Kleinberg LR. Stereotactic radiosurgery: treatment of brain metastasis without interruption of systemic therapy. Int J Radiat Oncol Biol Phys. 2016;95(2):735–42.
3. Kim JM, Miller JA, Kotecha R, et al. The risk of radiation necrosis following stereotactic radiosurgery with concurrent systemic therapies. J Neuro-Oncol. 2017;133(2):357–68.

4. Verduin M, Zindler JD, Martinussen HM, et al. Use of systemic therapy concurrent with cranial radiotherapy for cerebral metastases of solid tumors. Oncologist. 2017;22(2):222–35.

5. Quantin X, Bozonnat MC, Pujol JL. Recursive Partitioning Analysis Groups II–III brain metastases of non-small cell lung cancer: a phase II randomized study comparing two concurrent chemoradiotherapy regimens. J Thorac Oncol. 2010;5(6):846–51.

6. Jakacki RI, Burger PC, Zhou T, et al. Outcome of children with metastatic medulloblastoma treated with carboplatin during craniospinal radiotherapy: a Children's Oncology Group Phase I/II study. J Clin Oncol. 2012;30(21):2648–53.

7. Robinet G, Thomas P, Breton JL, et al. Results of a phase III study of early versus delayed whole brain radiotherapy with concurrent cisplatin and vinorelbine combination in inoperable brain metastasis of non-small-cell lung cancer: Groupe Francais de Pneumo-Cancerologie (GFPC) protocol 95-1. Ann Oncol. 2001;12(1):59–67.

8. Dinglin XX, Huang Y, Liu H, Zeng YD, Hou X, Chen LK. Pemetrexed and cisplatin combination with concurrent whole brain radiotherapy in patients with brain metastases of lung adenocarcinoma: a single-arm phase II clinical trial. J Neuro-Oncol. 2013;112(3):461–6.

9. Cagney DN, Martin AM, Catalano PJ, et al. Impact of pemetrexed on intracranial disease control and radiation necrosis in patients with brain metastases from non-small cell lung cancer receiving stereotactic radiation. Radiother Oncol. 2018;126(3):511–8.

10. Glantz MJ, Choy H, Kearns CM, et al. Paclitaxel disposition in plasma and central nervous systems of humans and rats with brain tumors. J Natl Cancer Inst. 1995;87(14):1077–81.

11. Glantz MJ, Chamberlain MC, Chang SM, Prados MD, Cole BF. The role of paclitaxel in the treatment of primary and metastatic brain tumors. Semin Radiat Oncol. 1999;9(2 Suppl 1):27–33.

12. Lederman G, Wronski M, Arbit E, et al. Treatment of recurrent glioblastoma multiforme using fractionated stereotactic radiosurgery and concurrent paclitaxel. Am J Clin Oncol. 2000;23(2):155–9.

13. Maraveyas A, Sgouros J, Upadhyay S, Abdel-Hamid AH, Holmes M, Lind M. Gemcitabine twice weekly as a radiosensitiser for the treatment of brain metastases in patients with carcinoma: a phase I study. Br J Cancer. 2005;92(5):815–9.

14. Huang YJ, Wu YL, Xie SX, Yang JJ, Huang YS, Liao RQ. Weekly gemcitabine as a radiosensitiser for the treatment of brain metastases in patients with non-small cell lung cancer: phase I trial. Chin Med J. 2007;120(6):458–62.

15. Jeter MD, Janne PA, Brooks S, et al. Gemcitabine-induced radiation recall. Int J Radiat Oncol Biol Phys. 2002;53(2):394–400.

16. Grunda JM, Fiveash J, Palmer CA, et al. Rationally designed pharmacogenomic treatment using concurrent capecitabine and radiotherapy for glioblastoma; gene expression profiles associated with outcome. Clin Cancer Res. 2010;16(10):2890–8.

17. Niravath P, Tham YL, Wang T, et al. A phase II trial of capecitabine concomitantly with whole-brain radiotherapy followed by capecitabine and sunitinib for brain metastases from breast cancer. Oncologist. 2015;20(1):13.

18. Chargari C, Kirova YM, Dieras V, et al. Concurrent capecitabine and whole-brain radiotherapy for treatment of brain metastases in breast cancer patients. J Neuro-Oncol. 2009;93(3):379–84.

19. Low S, Han CH, Batchelor TT. Primary central nervous system lymphoma. Ther Adv Neurol Disord. 2018;11:1756286418793562.

20. Pan Z, Yang G, He H, et al. Concurrent radiotherapy and intrathecal methotrexate for treating leptomeningeal metastasis from solid tumors with adverse prognostic factors: a prospective and single-arm study. Int J Cancer. 2016;139(8):1864–72.

21. Qin H, Pan F, Li J, Zhang X, Liang H, Ruan Z. Whole brain radiotherapy plus concurrent chemotherapy in non-small cell lung cancer patients with brain metastases: a meta-analysis. PLoS One. 2014;9(10):e111475.

22. Fiveash JB, Arafat WO, Naoum GE, et al. A phase 2 study of radiosurgery and temozolomide for patients with 1 to 4 brain metastases. Adv Radiat Oncol. 2016;1(2):83–8.

23. Dijkers EC, Oude Munnink TH, Kosterink JG, et al. Biodistribution of 89Zr-trastuzumab and PET imaging of HER2-positive lesions in patients with metastatic breast cancer. Clin Pharmacol Ther. 2010;87(5):586–92.

24. Long GV, Atkinson V, Lo S, et al. Combination nivolumab and ipilimumab or nivolumab alone in melanoma brain metastases: a multicentre randomised phase 2 study. Lancet Oncol. 2018;19(5):672–81.

25. Li SH, Liu CY, Hsu PC, et al. Response to afatinib in treatment-naive patients with advanced mutant epidermal growth factor receptor lung adenocarcinoma with brain metastases. Expert Rev Anticancer Ther. 2018;18(1):81–9.

26. Reungwetwattana T, Nakagawa K, Cho BC, et al. CNS response to osimertinib versus standard epidermal growth factor receptor tyrosine kinase inhibitors in patients with untreated EGFR-mutated advanced non-small-cell lung cancer. J Clin Oncol. 2018:JCO2018783118. https://doi.org/10.1200/JCO.2018.78.3118.

27. Gadgeel S, Peters S, Mok T, et al. Alectinib versus crizotinib in treatment-naive anaplastic lymphoma kinase-positive (ALK+) non-small-cell lung cancer: CNS efficacy results from the ALEX study. Ann Oncol. 2018;29(11):2214–22.

28. Mittapalli RK, Vaidhyanathan S, Dudek AZ, Elmquist WF. Mechanisms limiting distribution of the threonine-protein kinase B-RaF(V600E) inhibitor dabrafenib to the brain: implications for the treatment of melanoma brain metastases. J Pharmacol Exp Ther. 2013;344(3):655–64.

29. Pulvirenti T, Hong A, Clements A, et al. Acute radiation skin toxicity associated with BRAF inhibitors. J Clin Oncol. 2016;34(3):e17–20.

30. Anker CJ, Grossmann KF, Atkins MB, Suneja G, Tarhini AA, Kirkwood JM. Avoiding severe toxicity from combined BRAF inhibitor and radiation treatment: consensus guidelines from the Eastern Cooperative Oncology Group (ECOG). Int J Radiat Oncol Biol Phys. 2016;95(2):632–46.

31. Dummer R, Ascierto PA, Gogas HJ, et al. Encorafenib plus binimetinib versus vemurafenib or encorafenib in patients with BRAF-mutant melanoma (COLUMBUS): a multicentre, open-label, randomised phase 3 trial. Lancet Oncol. 2018;19(5):603–15.

32. Long GV, Stroyakovskiy D, Gogas H, et al. Combined BRAF and MEK inhibition versus BRAF inhibition alone in melanoma. N Engl J Med. 2014;371(20):1877–88.

33. Lin NU, Freedman RA, Ramakrishna N, et al. A phase I study of lapatinib with whole brain radiotherapy in patients with Human Epidermal Growth Factor Receptor 2 (HER2)-positive breast cancer brain metastases. Breast Cancer Res Treat. 2013;142(2):405–14.

34. Chargari C, Idrissi HR, Pierga JY, et al. Preliminary results of whole brain radiotherapy with concurrent trastuzumab for treatment of brain metastases in breast cancer patients. Int J Radiat Oncol Biol Phys. 2011;81(3):631–6.

35. Carlson JA, Nooruddin Z, Rusthoven C, et al. Trastuzumab emtansine and stereotactic radiosurgery: an unexpected increase in clinically significant brain edema. Neuro-Oncology. 2014;16(7):1006–9.

36. Geraud A, Xu HP, Beuzeboc P, Kirova YM. Preliminary experience of the concurrent use of radiosurgery and T-DM1 for brain metastases in HER2 positive metastatic breast cancer. J Neuro-Oncol. 2017;131(1):69–72.

37. Vilela MD, Longstreth WT Jr, Pedrosa HAS, Gil GOB, Duarte JM, Filho MAD. Progressively enlarging cerebellar hematoma concurrent with T-DM1 treatment. World Neurosurg. 2018;111:109–14.

38. Fabi A, Alesini D, Valle E, et al. T-DM1 and brain metastases: clinical outcome in HER2-positive metastatic breast cancer. Breast. 2018;41:137–43.

39. Levy C, Allouache D, Lacroix J, et al. REBECA: a phase I study of bevacizumab and whole-brain radiation therapy for the treatment of brain metastasis from solid tumours. Ann Oncol. 2014;25(12):2351–6.

40. Besse B, Lasserre SF, Compton P, Huang J, Augustus S, Rohr UP. Bevacizumab safety in patients with central nervous system metastases. Clin Cancer Res. 2010;16(1):269–78.

41. Socinski MA, Langer CJ, Huang JE, et al. Safety of bevacizumab in patients with non-small-cell lung cancer and brain metastases. J Clin Oncol. 2009;27(31):5255–61.

42. Levin VA, Bidaut L, Hou P, et al. Randomized double-blind placebo-controlled trial of bevacizumab therapy for radiation necrosis of the central nervous system. Int J Radiat Oncol Biol Phys. 2011;79(5):1487–95.

43. Abbas O, Shamseddin A, Temraz S, Haydar A. Posterior reversible encephalopathy syndrome after bevacizumab therapy in a normotensive patient. BMJ Case Rep. 2013;2013:1–4.

44. Ahluwalia MS, Chao ST, Parsons MW, et al. Phase II trial of sunitinib as adjuvant therapy after stereotactic radiosurgery in patients with 1–3 newly diagnosed brain metastases. J Neuro-Oncol. 2015;124(3):485–91.

45. Pfannenstiel LW, McNeilly C, Xiang C, et al. Combination PD-1 blockade and irradiation of brain metastasis induces an effective abscopal effect in melanoma. Onco Targets Ther. 2019;8(1):e1507669.

46. Grimaldi AM, Simeone E, Giannarelli D, et al. Abscopal effects of radiotherapy on advanced melanoma patients who progressed after ipilimumab immunotherapy. Onco Targets Ther. 2014;3:e28780.

47. Kiess AP, Wolchok JD, Barker CA, et al. Stereotactic radiosurgery for melanoma brain metastases in patients receiving ipilimumab: safety profile and efficacy of combined treatment. Int J Radiat Oncol Biol Phys. 2015;92(2):368–75.

48. An Y, Jiang W, Kim BYS, et al. Stereotactic radiosurgery of early melanoma brain metastases after initiation of anti-CTLA-4 treatment is associated with improved intracranial control. Radiother Oncol. 2017;125(1):80–8.

49. Williams NL, Wuthrick EJ, Kim H, et al. Phase 1 study of ipilimumab combined with whole brain radiation therapy or radiosurgery for melanoma patients with brain metastases. Int J Radiat Oncol Biol Phys. 2017;99(1):22–30.

50. Chen L, Douglass J, Kleinberg L, et al. Concurrent immune checkpoint inhibitors and stereotactic radiosurgery for brain metastases in non-small cell lung cancer, melanoma, and renal cell carcinoma. Int J Radiat Oncol Biol Phys. 2018;100(4):916–25.

51. Anderson ES, Postow MA, Wolchok JD, et al. Melanoma brain metastases treated with stereotactic radiosurgery and concurrent pembrolizumab display marked regression; efficacy and safety of combined treatment. J Immunother Cancer. 2017;5(1):76.

52. Stokes WA, Binder DC, Jones BL, et al. Impact of immunotherapy among patients with melanoma brain metastases managed with radiotherapy. J Neuroimmunol. 2017;313:118–22.

53. Martin AM, Cagney DN, Catalano PJ, et al. Immunotherapy and symptomatic radiation necrosis in patients with brain metastases treated with stereotactic radiation. JAMA Oncol. 2018;4(8):1123–4.

54. Yusuf MB, Amsbaugh MJ, Burton E, Chesney J, Woo S. Peri-SRS administration of immune checkpoint therapy for melanoma metastatic to the brain: investigating efficacy and the effects of relative treatment timing on lesion response. World Neurosurg. 2017;100:632–40.. e634

55. Liniker E, Menzies AM, Kong BY, et al. Activity and safety of radiotherapy with anti-PD-1 drug therapy in patients with metastatic melanoma. Onco Targets Ther. 2016;5(9):e1214788.

56. Ahmed KA, Stallworth DG, Kim Y, et al. Clinical out-
    comes of melanoma brain metastases treated with ste-
    reotactic radiation and anti-PD-1 therapy. Ann Oncol.
    2016;27(3):434–41.
57. Hubbeling HG, Schapira EF, Horick NK, et al. Safety
    of combined PD-1 pathway inhibition and intracra-
    nial radiation therapy in non-small cell lung cancer. J
    Thorac Oncol. 2018;13(4):550–8.
58. Chang EL, Wefel JS, Hess KR, et al. Neurocognition
    in patients with brain metastases treated with radio-
    surgery or radiosurgery plus whole-brain irradia-
    tion: a randomised controlled trial. Lancet Oncol.
    2009;10(11):1037–44.
59. Brown PD, Jaeckle K, Ballman KV, et al. Effect of
    radiosurgery alone vs radiosurgery with whole brain
    radiation therapy on cognitive function in patients
    with 1 to 3 brain metastases: a randomized clinical
    trial. JAMA. 2016;316(4):401–9.
60. Wolchok JD, Chiarion-Sileni V, Gonzalez R, et al.
    Overall survival with combined nivolumab and ipi-
    limumab in advanced melanoma. N Engl J Med.
    2017;377(14):1345–56.
61. Blonigen BJ, Steinmetz RD, Levin L, Lamba MA,
    Warnick RE, Breneman JC. Irradiated volume as a
    predictor of brain radionecrosis after linear accelera-
    tor stereotactic radiosurgery. Int J Radiat Oncol Biol
    Phys. 2010;77(4):996–1001.
62. Minniti G, Scaringi C, Paolini S, et al.
    Single-fraction versus multifraction (9 Gy x 3)
    stereotactic radiosurgery for large (>2 cm) brain
    metastases: a comparative analysis of local con-
    trol and risk of radiation-induced brain necro-
    sis. Int J Radiat Oncol Biol Phys. 2016;95(4):
    1142–8.
63. Davies MA, Saiag P, Robert C, et al. Dabrafenib plus
    trametinib in patients with BRAF(V600)-mutant mel-
    anoma brain metastases (COMBI-MB): a multicentre,
    multicohort, open-label, phase 2 trial. Lancet Oncol.
    2017;18(7):863–73.
64. Drago JZ, Lawrence D, Livingstone E, et al. Clinical
    experience with combination BRAF/MEK inhibitors
    for melanoma with brain metastases: a real-life multi-
    center study. Melanoma Res. 2019;29(1):65–9.
65. Tawbi HA, Forsyth PA, Algazi A, et al. Combined
    nivolumab and ipilimumab in melanoma metastatic to
    the brain. N Engl J Med. 2018;379(8):722–30.
66. Lee Y, Auh SL, Wang Y, et al. Therapeutic effects
    of ablative radiation on local tumor require CD8+ T
    cells: changing strategies for cancer treatment. Blood.
    2009;114(3):589–95.
67. Ellsworth SG. Field size effects on the risk and sever-
    ity of treatment-induced lymphopenia in patients
    undergoing radiation therapy for solid tumors. Adv
    Radiat Oncol. 2018;3(4):512–9.
68. Pike LRG, Bang A, Mahal BA, et al. The impact of
    radiation therapy on lymphocyte count and survival
    in metastatic cancer patients receiving PD-1 immune
    checkpoint inhibitors. Int J Radiat Oncol Biol Phys.
    2019;103(1):142–51.
69. Arbour KC, Mezquita L, Long N, et al. Impact of
    baseline steroids on efficacy of programmed cell
    death-1 and programmed death-ligand 1 blockade
    in patients with non-small-cell lung cancer. J Clin
    Oncol. 2018;36(28):2872–8.

Indications for Stereotactic Radiosurgery: Multiple Brain Metastases

9

Anurag Saraf and Tony J. C. Wang

Case Vignette

Case 1

A 63-year-old male with a past medical history of stage IIA (T2bN0M0) adenocarcinoma of the lung status post-stereotactic body radiotherapy (SBRT) (50 Gy in five fractions) 2 years ago, hypertension, and chronic obstructive pulmonary disease now presents with new onset seizure witnessed by wife and several bystanders on train. Patient had witnessed tonic-clonic seizure for 2 minutes and postictal state immediately afterwards. Patient is brought to the emergency department and found to be afebrile, vitals within normal limits, CBC and BMP within normal limits. CT of head with contrast shows three contrast-enhancing supratentorial lesions. CT of chest/abdomen/pelvis is unremarkable. MRI of brain with contrast demonstrates four supratentorial lesions (largest diameter 0.3 cm) and two infratentorial lesions (largest diameter 0.5 cm). Aggregate tumor volume is 2.7 cc.

A. Saraf
Department of Radiation Oncology, Massachusetts General Hospital, Boston, MA, USA

T. J. C. Wang (✉)
Department of Radiation Oncology, Columbia University Irving Medical Center, New York, NY, USA
e-mail: tjw2117@cumc.columbia.edu

Patient is managed with levetiracetam and reporting some chronic fatigue, otherwise he has no further seizures or focal symptoms. Patient is graded with a Karnofsky Performance Scale (KPS) score of 90. Prognostic indices score patient with Recursive Partitioning Analysis (RPA) Class I (KPS ≥ 70, age < 65, primary tumor controlled), Graded Prognostic Assessment (GPA) score of 2.0, and Lung-molGPA score of 2.0. Discussion including whole brain radiotherapy and SRS is made including the advantages and disadvantages of either options. Patient elects to receive SRS for all six lesions.

Patient is scheduled for routine surveillance follow-up with brain MRI every 3 months. At the 3- and 6-month follow-up appointment, the patient reports some fatigue without other symptoms with no evidence of new lesions or increase in size of previous lesions on brain MRI.

At the 9-month follow-up appointment, the patient reports being in good general health; however, brain MRI shows two new supratentorial lesions, with largest diameter of 0.3 cm and aggregate tumor volume of 1.2 cc. Patient is treated with SRS to each lesion and tolerates the procedure well. Patient is recommended to continue to follow up every 3 months with repeat imaging.

The 12-month follow-up patient reports some short-term memory loss and fatigue. Repeat brain MRI reveals seven new brain lesions with aggregate tumor volume of 5.1 cc. Patient is treated with whole brain radiation therapy (WBRT) with 30 Gy in ten fractions. Patient is discharged to start memantine extended-release daily. Patient presents to the 15-month follow-up with worsening short-term memory loss and gait abnormality. Patient is lost to follow-up after this appointment.

Key Points
- Indications for initial SRS treatment in the setting of multiple BM.
- Repeat SRS can serve as salvage therapy for limited number of BM recurrence.
- Salvage WBRT may be preferable over repeat SRS with high number of BM recurrence.

Introduction

Brain metastasis (BM) is the most common intracranial tumor, occurring in 10–30% of patients with cancer [1, 2]. One-third to one-half of patients present with more than one BM, and the proportion of patients presenting with more than three BM continues to increase [3–5]. Traditional treatment of multiple BM was with whole brain radiation therapy (WBRT) [6, 7]. However, numerous studies have found the cognitive toxicity and impaired quality of life (QoL) of WBRT to be excessive even in the context of multiple BM, and stereotactic radiosurgery (SRS) has become an ever-growing option [8–10].

In this chapter, multiple BM is defined as any case involving greater than one BM. Several studies have noted a difference in outcomes and treatment management in two distinct groups of patients with multiple BM: limited BM, defined as two to four BM, and extensive BM, defined as five or greater BM.

WBRT was recommended in the setting of multiple BM (particularly four or more metastases) for several perceptions: greater ability to treat micrometastatic disease burden, less concern for amount of total dose to normal brain tis-

sue compared to SRS, and less concern for total treatment time for multiple isocenters compared to SRS [1, 11, 12]. SRS is frequently given with WBRT to maximize disease control, since the omission of WBRT increases the risk of relapse [13]. Over the past several decades, randomized controlled trials and prospective data have addressed these perceptions and begun to swing treatment paradigms toward SRS over WBRT for multiple BM.

SRS brings several advantages for treatment of multiple BM over WBRT: better local control, greater sparing of normal tissue, less resource heavy in terms of possible fewer days of treatment, and more cost-effective. Prospective data have suggested that high-dose single-fraction radiation therapy has more durable local control than conventional radiation therapy for multiple BM with similar overall survival (OS). SRS also allows more localized treatment even for multiple, diffuse BM, leading to more sparing of normal brain tissue and better neurocognitive outcomes in the long term. With modern technology and delivery techniques, it is more feasible to treat multiple lesions with single isocenter setup, allowing for less treatment time and fewer resources needed for treatment. Finally, data have suggested that with the decrease in resources and decrease in adverse effects, SRS may be more cost-effective than WBRT even in the setting of extensive disease burden [14, 15].

Evidence Base

Limited Metastases

Traditionally, limited BM has been defined as up to 4 BM and has been the subject of the early studies looking at the safety and efficacy of SRS treatment for multiple BM.

The evidence of treating BM with SRS started with several studies comparing WBRT to SRS. First, several studies compared WBRT vs WBRT + SRS. RTOG 9508 was one of the first randomized controlled trials that compared WBRT to WBRT+ SRS in patients with 1–3 BM [6, 7]. It found a survival advantage in single brain metastasis patients with good prognosis (young age, good performance status, controlled primary tumor) with the addition of SRS (21.0 vs 10.3 months) compared to WBRT alone and found improved functional autonomy with preserved KPS over time. One caveat to this study is the lack of validated QoL outcomes, as there may be no benefit to patients who received salvage treatment after WBRT compared to WBRT with upfront SRS boost.

Next, several randomized studies studied SRS vs WBRT + SRS [10, 16–18]. These studies found that the addition of WBRT allowed for greater distant brain control (from 40–70% to 60–90%); however, there was no OS benefit; young patients aged less than 50 years may have better OS with SRS alone. On the other hand, neurocognition and QoL were greatly decreased with the addition of WBRT.

Finally, in the question of WBRT vs SRS, several studies have looked at toxicity and neurocognition. Brown et al. published a study involving patients with 1–3 BM comparing patients treated with SRS vs SRS + WBRT, with primary endpoint of neurocognitive function [10]. They found neurocognitive deterioration at 3 months was worse with the addition of WBRT (91% vs 63.5%, $p < 0.001$), and QoL was higher at 3 months with SRS alone ($p = 0.001$), with no difference in functional independence or median OS. Chang et al. reported a randomized control trial of patients with good prognosis with 1–3 BM randomized to SRS vs WBRT + SRS and found that the addition of WBRT increased neurocognitive decline (23% vs 49%, $p = 0.003$), as well as interestingly a survival benefit to delayed WBRT [16].

Except in the setting of large tumor diameter (greater than 3 cm), patients with limited BM should be managed with SRS and frequent surveillance monitoring.

Extensive Metastases

Extensive BM are traditionally defined as five or more BM. Patients with extensive BM were thought to be poor candidates for SRS and treated palliatively with WBRT. However, several recent studies have changed that mindset. Regarding the question of the number of BM treated with SRS, several studies have found good outcomes with fewer long-term side effects in limited BM versus more extensive disease. Table 9.1 demonstrates

Table 9.1 Prognostic indices in brain metastasis

Prognostic index	# Patients in study	Age	Performance status	ECM	Control of primary tumor	# BM	Vol. BM	Response to steroids	Classify by primary tumor	Primary tumor trait	Molecular trait
RPA [19]	1200	X	KPS	X	X						
SIR [20]	65	X	KPS	X	X	X	X				
BSBM [21]	110		KPS	X	X						
Rotterdam [22]	1292		ECOG	X				X			
GGS [23]	479	X	KPS	X							
GPA [24]	1960	X	KPS	X		X					
DS-GPA [25]	4259	X	KPS	X		X			X		
Updated DS-GPA [26]	3940								X	X	
Modified Breast-GPA [27]	1552	X	KPS			X			X	X	X
Lung-molGPA [28]	1833	X	KPS	X		X			X	X	X

RPA Recursive Partitional Analysis, *SIR* Score Index for Radiosurgery, *BSBM* Basic Score for Brain Metastases, *GGS* Golden Grading Score, *GPA* Graded Prognostic Assessment, *DS-GPA* Diagnostic Specific Graded Prognostic Assessment, *Lung-molGPA* Lung molecular Graded Prognostic Assessment, *KPA* Karnofsky Performance Score, *ECM* extracranial metastasis, *BM* brain metastasis, *Vol* volume outcomes of several studies that investigated SRS in the setting of extensive BM with at least 50 patients. In Case 1, the patient initially presented with six BM. Presented below is evidence for the benefit of using upfront SRS in the setting of extensive BM.

JLGK0901 was a Japanese study by Yamamoto et al. looking at survival and outcomes with SRS in 5–10 BM compared to 1 and 2–4 BM [8]. It was a non-inferiority prospective observational study of 1194 patients with 1–10 BM, with largest tumor volume < 10 cc and diameter < 3 cm, with total cumulative volume < 15 cc. It is one of the only non-retrospective studies looking at SRS for the treatment of greater than 5 BM, and several things were learned. Greater brain tumor burden was not associated with worse survival or neurologic death. With a median follow-up of 20.9 months, OS in patients with 1 tumor was 13.9 months compared to 2–4 tumors was 10.8 months and 5–10 tumors was 10.8 months, there was no difference in the two groups of multiple BM (HR 0.97, 95% CI 0.81–1.18, $p = 0.78$) (graphical representation in Fig. 9.1). Neurologic death was 10% in patients with 1 BM, 6% in patients with 2–4 BM, and 9% in patients with 5–10 BM ($p = 0.27$), suggesting systemic disease progression was the greatest factor in death for patients. Greater brain tumor burden did not affect intracranial relapse rates, as local failure was 16% in patients with 1 BM, 11% in patients with 2–4 BM, and 10% in patients with 5–10 BM, suggesting it is similar across all three cohorts. Grade 3–5 toxicity was also similar amongst all three cohorts, suggesting SRS for a greater tumor burden did not increase risk of adverse effects from treatment delivery.

Yamamoto did report that extensive BM treated with SRS was at higher risk of distant brain relapse compared to single brain metastasis. However, failure rate at 6 months was 40.0% for 2–4 BM and 45.9% for 5–10 BM ($p = 0.067$) suggesting no statistical difference for multiple BM with only SRS treatment. Leptomeningeal failure increased with greater metastatic burden, with 5–10 BM reporting the greater failure after 24 month at 21.9% vs 13.2% for 2–4 BM

($p = 0.035$). However, there is limited data to rule out the association with specific molecular subtypes, such as Her2-positive breast cancers or ALK-positive non-small-cell lung cancer (NSCLC).

One limited factor of current data is that multiple studies were inconsistent in whether patients with 5 BM were treated with or without WBRT and, therefore, if the SRS was salvage or upfront. There is no strong data currently in comparing salvage versus upfront SRS with respect to OS, local tumor control, or distant brain control.

Hughes et al. reported a multi-institution retrospective analysis of 2089 patients with up to 15 metastases treated with initial SRS [29]. Patients were stratified by number of BM, with 47% (989) with 1 BM, 42% (882) with 2–4 BM, and 10% (212) with 5–15 BM. Median overall survival of the cohort was 14.6 months for 1 BM, 9.5 months for 2–4 BM, and 7.5 months for 5–15 BM; multivariate analysis showed no difference in OS between 2–4 and 5–15 BM.

Several studies examining multiple metastases reported patients requiring frequent salvage rates. For example, Yamamoto et al. is one of the largest prospective trials examining patients with 5–10 BM showing no difference in OS, however, reported that 50% of patients developed new BM and 40% of patients required repeat and multiple courses of SRS [8]. Patients with multiple metastases require close monitoring with frequent serial MRI scans. Distant brain failure is known to increase with time, and surveillance MRI allows treatment of new lesions prior to symptoms or neurologic deterioration.

Chang et al. reported on 323 patients with BM treated by Gamma Knife stereotactic radiosurgery (GKRS) separated into patients with 1–5, 6–10, 11–15, and >15 BM [30]. While they found no difference in OS or local control between the groups, they reported that patients with >15 BM showed increased distant brain failure.

Other studies that have looked at treating up to 15+ BM have also found that the number of BM does not predict survival after SRS. Salvetti et al. published a single-institution retrospective study

Group	Median overall survival, months (95% CI)	HR (95% CI)	p value
1 tumour	13.9 (12.0–15.6)	0.76 (0.66–0.88)	0.0004
2–4 tumours	10.8 (9.4–12.4)	Reference	
5–10 tumours	10.8 (9.1–12.7)	0.97 (0.81–1.18)	0.78

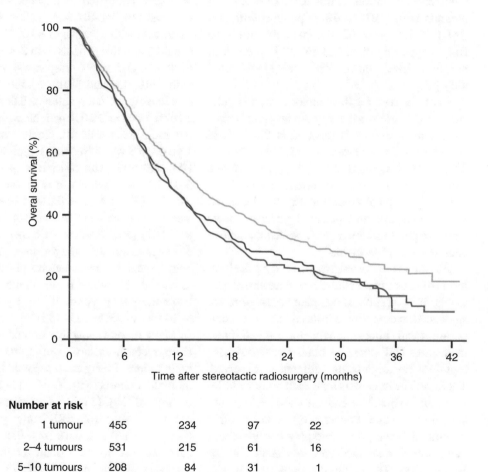

Number at risk

1 tumour	455	234	97	22
2–4 tumours	531	215	61	16
5–10 tumours	208	84	31	1

Fig. 9.1 Graphical representation of overall survival of 1 tumor vs 2–4 tumors vs 5+ tumors. Graphical representation of overall survival (OS) stratified by number of BM. In general, patients with 1 BM tend to have statistically significantly increased OS compared to patients with multiple BM; however, patients with 2–4 BM do not have statistically significant difference OS compared to patients with five or more BM. (From Yamamoto et al. [8]. Reproduced with permission from Elsevier)

of 96 patients with 5–15 BM that were treated with SRS with a median OS of 4.73 months [31]. They analyzed their results both using number of metastases as a continuous variable from 5 to 15, and as a dichotomous variable comparing 5–9 versus 10–15. In both instances, they found that number of metastases was not associated with a difference in OS.

Local Tumor Control

SRS local tumor control is impacted by multiple factors including diameter, volume, and dose prescribed. Local tumor control does not seem to be influenced by the number of metastases. Yamamoto et al. found that local recurrence at 6 months was 6.5% ($p = 0.45$) in patients with 1 BM, 3.0% in patients with 2–4 BM, and 4.3% ($p = 0.70$) in patients with 5–10 BM, suggesting that BM tumor burden does not affect local control when treated with SRS only [8].

Actuarial data for local tumor control is quite encouraging. Across multiple studies, local tumor control at 6 months is reported at 90–95%, at 12 months is reported at 75–90%, and at 24 months is reported at 60–75% [8, 16]. While patients may frequently experience distant brain failure, good local control allows for decreased repeat treatment and potential adverse effects from frequent treatment such as neurocognitive decline and radionecrosis.

As studies on extensive BM vary greatly in terms of tumor characteristics and treatment protocols, it is difficult to compare across different studies. However, single institution reports comparing local tumor control for limited brain metastases and extensive brain metastases have reported no significant difference observed. Therefore, most centers treat each brain metastasis as an independent entity not affected by considerations when concurrently treating other tumors. However, dose interplay considerations have been investigated and are detailed in the later section, "Dose Considerations."

Distant Brain Failure

Distant brain failure (DBF) is impacted by multiple factors including number of brain metastases, tumor histology and subtype, and prior treatments. Many reports of multiple BM outcomes include patients who have had prior WBRT, a known factor associated with decreased distant brain relapse. DBF is known to increase with time, with 40–60% of patients treated with

upfront SRS are likely to develop new brain lesions within 1 year of treatment [8, 32].

Patients with 1 BM have lower DBF than patients with more than 1 BM. However, patients with limited BM do not have lower DBF than patients with multiple BM. Yamamoto et al. found at 6 months patients with 1 BM had DBF of 23.9% compared to patients with 2–4 BM, who had DBF of 40.0%, which was statistically significant with a p value of <0.0001. However, at 6 and 12 months, patients with 2–4 BM had DBF of 40.0% and 54.5%, respectively, and patients with 5–10 BM had DBF of 45.9% and 63.8%, respectively, with a p value of 0.067, suggesting no difference in DBF in patients with greater than one brain metastasis [8]. Hughes et al. found at 1 year DBF was 30% with 1 BM, 41% with 2–4 BM, and 50% with 5–15 BM ($p < 0.01$). The 5–15 BM was associated with worse DBF than 2–4 BM (HR 1.43, $p < 0.01$); 1 BM was associated with favorable DBF than 2–4 BM (HR 0.70, $p < 0.01$) [29]. Predictors of DBF included age 65 years or greater, margin dose, and non-lung, breast, renal cell, or melanoma primary (reported as "other") histology. In separating the extensive BM cohort, they report DBF at 1 year of 42% in 5–10 BM vs 73% in 11–15 BM.

Many reports show that limited and extensive brain metastases have similar rates of distant brain failure. Chang et al. separated patients into multiple cohorts with 6–10, 11–15, and >15 metastases [30]. In this cohort, distant brain failure at 1 year for SRS only was 73% vs SRS + WBRT was 45% ($p = 0.02$). Therefore, data suggest worse distant brain failure for patients with more than 10 BM, although data are limited.

Salvage Therapy

In Case 1, we see the patient was initially treated with SRS for 6 BM but has distant brain failure 9 months after treatment with 2 new BM. Patients who progress after initial SRS for multiple BM have multiple salvage therapy options depending on clinical scenario: repeat SRS, salvage WBRT, or optimal supportive care.

Hughes et al. reported that crude rates of salvage SRS decreased and salvage WBRT increased with increasing number of BM [29]. Of patients with 1 BM, 27% had salvage SRS and 13% had WBRT; of patients with 2–4 BM, 24% had salvage SRS and 15% had WBRT; of patients with 5–15 BM, 21% had salvage SRS and 18% had WBRT. Patients with 5–15 BM were associated with lower risk of salvage SRS compared to patients with 2–4 BM. Time to WBRT was not statistically different between patients with 2–4 BM vs 5–15 BM. The authors suggest this may be related to institutional bias of non-radiotherapeutic salvage modalities or best supportive care at the time of progression in the 5–15 BM group.

Leptomeningeal Disease

Leptomeningeal disease (LMD) is a concern for SRS, where localized treatment spares the meninges compared to WBRT. Increasing tumor burden is associated with increased risk of LMD. Yamamoto et al. found that rate of LMD rates were highest in the patients with 5–10 BM cohort with a 2-year rate of 21.9%, versus 13.2% and 11% in the 2–4 cohort and single metastasis cohort, respectively [8]. It should be noted that their study did not report on difference in subgroups more likely to develop LMD, such as EGFR-positive or ALK-positive NSCLC, or HER2-positive or triple-negative breast cancer.

Toxicity

Toxicity related to SRS for the treatment of multiple BM is generally separated into acute and delayed effects. Acute effects tend to occur within the first weeks to months after treatment and are generally reversible, which may include fatigue, loss of appetite, dermatitis, alopecia, nausea, and vomiting, worsening neurologic symptoms. Delayed effects occur months after treatment and can be irreversible; the most severe may include radiation necrosis and neurocognitive impairment.

Modern NRG Protocols report toxicity based on the Common Terminology Criteria for Adverse Events (CTCAE) v5.0. Toxicity can be graded 1–5 as per CTCAE, with Grade 3 toxicity involving toxicity requiring significant toxicity not immediately life-threatening, hospitalization required, or limiting self-care ADL; Grade 4 with life-threatening consequences, or urgent intervention indicated; and Grade 5 involving death.

Grade 3–5 toxicity is not significantly worse in patients with multiple metastases compared to patients with single metastases. Yamamoto et al. reported in their cohort of 1194 patients treated with SRS, 8% developed any kind of adverse-event related to SRS only, and there was no difference in rates across cohorts of patients with 1, 2–4, and 5–10 BM. Grade 3–5 toxicity was less than 5% in each cohort [8]. Brown et al. published similar results in their study comparing SRS vs SRS + WBRT for 1–3 BM, with SRS only reporting 2.9% Grade 3–5 toxicity vs SRS + WBRT with 4.5% Grade 3–5 toxicity ($p = 0.72$) [10]. Concern for severe adverse effects for patients with SRS for multiple metastases should not be any more than treatment with WBRT or combined SRS + WBRT.

Neurocognition

A major concern of WBRT is the impact of neurocognition in patients and their resulting QoL. It is suggested that radiation therapy has adverse effect on the neurogenesis of the hippocampus, primarily affecting memory and recall. While the Mini-Mental Status Examination (MMSE) has been used to measure neurocognition in early studies, the test is not sensitive in detecting and correlating subtler neuro-psychological changes affected by radiation therapy. Hopkins Verbal Learning Test-Revised (HVLT-R) is one verbal neurocognitive test that tests a participant's total recall, delayed recall, and delayed recognition. It has been validated and incorporated into several randomized trials over time and corresponds better to cancer patients need for assistance in ADLs. In the question of multiple brain metastases, there is a correlation with total intracranial tumor volume is correlated with adverse neurocognitive performance at baseline. This question was directly addressed by several randomized controlled trials looking at cognitive deterioration, including learning and memory, over several months after treatment.

Chang et al. randomized 58 patients with 1–3 brain metastases to SRS plus WBRT versus SRS alone with a primary endpoint of deterioration on the HVLT-R 4 months after treatment [16]. The trial was stopped early on the basis that there was a 96% confidence that SRS plus WBRT resulted in inferior total recall than SRS alone at 4 months. Data suggested this decline in neurocognition persisted up to 6 months after treatment. Other neurocognitive tests showed executive function (as measured by COWA, Trail Making Test part B) also declined more severely in SRS plus WBRT compared to SRS alone. SRS only had greater median OS (15.2 vs 5.7 months) and 1 year OS (63% vs 21%, $p = 0.003$). SRS only had worse 1-year local control rate (67% vs 100%, $p = 0.012$) and 1-year distant brain tumor control rate (45% vs 73%, $p = 0.02$). Most patients in the SRS alone arm received salvage therapy, primarily with surgery or repeat SRS. Grade 3 and 4 toxicities were equivalent among both arms.

Brown et al. randomized 213 patients with 1–3 BM to SRS plus WBRT versus SRS alone with a primary endpoint of deterioration in multiple neurocognitive testing (including HVLT-R) 3 months after treatment, and a secondary endpoint for QoL [10]. Brown et al. found a significant decrease in neurocognition 3 months after treatment in patients treated with SRS plus WBRT in multiple different cognitive testing including immediate memory, delayed memory, and verbal fluency. They found these results persisted in patients beyond 6 months. They looked at 34 (16%) long-term survivors (defined as patients evaluated at 12 months) and found that neurocognitive decline was worse in SRS plus WBRT at 3 months (94.1% vs 45.5%, $p = 0.007$) and persisted at 12 months (94.4% vs 60%, $p = 0.04$), suggesting WBRT effects may not be temporary. Intracranial control was better in SRS plus WBRT, but OS was not significantly different (7.4 vs 10.4 months, $p = 0.92$). This suggests that while intracranial control is better with adjuvant WBRT, there is no different in OS with worsening neurocognition, and QoL that persists well after acute effects of WBRT.

Both trials found greater rates of cognitive deterioration in patients, with lower rates of intracranial relapse but no effect on OS. The lack of improvement in survival from WBRT is attributed to multiple factors in several trials, most prominent of which is the effectiveness of salvage therapies for intracranial progression with routine and frequent follow-up.

Quality of Life

Brown et al. utilized the Functional Assessment of Cancer Therapy-Brain tool to measure QoL, as well as the Barthel Index of Activities of Daily Living (ADL Index) to measure functional independence in patients after treatment [10]. There was better overall QoL at 3 months for patients treated with SRS alone compared to SRS plus WBRT (mean change from baseline −1.3 vs −10.9 points, $p = 0.002$), as well as functional well-being. Barthel ADL Index remained at high with no significant difference between the groups. They found in long-term survivors, who lived beyond 12 months, that the QoL measures at 3 months were significantly better in SRS alone, and some areas persisted beyond 9 months. Other studies have shown QoL decline with WBRT persist beyond 12 months, and the phenomenon is not partially reversible.

Kocher et al. reported the EORTC 22952-22601 Study of 359 patients with 1–3 BM randomized to SRS/surgery plus WBRT and SRS/surgery and observation [17]. The primary endpoint was time to functional independence as measured as change to World Health Organization (WHO) Performance Status (PS) score >2 (which correlates to individuals capable of limited self-care, completely disabled, or death). There was no difference between WBRT and observation (9.5 vs 10.0 months, $p = 0.71$). At 2 years, 22% were alive and functionally independent in both arms. Intracranial relapse and distant brain relapse were less in WBRT vs observation; however, overall survival was unchanged between WBRT and observation (10.9 vs 10.7 months, $p = 0.89$).

For greater than 5 BM, there is limited high-level evidence for neurocognitive function or quality of life between SRS alone and other treatment modalities. North American Gamma-knife Consortium is opening a randomized controlled trial (NAGKC 12–01) comparing radiosurgery to WBRT for patients with five or more metastases, with neurocognitive status and tumor control as the primary end points. These trials may also elucidate the concern of relapse after multiple brain metastases and patient QoL. Patients may have higher neurocognitive function and quality of life if they are monitored with serial MRI and salvaged as opposed to upfront WBRT without effect on overall survival.

Prognostic Index

Several prognostic indices have been formulated, tested, and validated over the past several years [19–28, 33, 34]. While older scores utilized clinical risk factors that tended to be more subjective, newer scores have found the number of brain metastases to be significantly associated with prognostic stratification, as well as disease subtype and molecular/genetic factors. Table 9.2 demonstrates several prognostic indices in the literature.

Recursive Partitioning Analysis (RPA) is the oldest and most commonly used prognostic index for patients with brain metastasis. Originally described in an analysis of outcomes of patients with brain metastases across several RTOG studies, RPA is a simple yet subjective metric that incorporates three metrics (age, KPS, primary tumor control) to group patients into three: Class I, Class II, Class III. Class I patients have the best prognosis consisting of patients with KPS ≥ 70, age < 65 years, and controlled primary tumor with no extracranial metastasis. Class III patients have the worst prognosis with KPS < 70. Class II consists of all other patients. Several studies analyzing SRS in multiple metastases have found that overall survival is associated with better RPA class and therefore can be used to pursue further treatment.

Table 9.3 demonstrates the median OS of the different stratified tiers within the prognostic indices that include number of BM as a risk factor. Graded Prognosis Assessment (GPA) and Diagnosis-Specific Graded Prognostic Assessment (dsGPA) are two newer prognostic indices that attempted to utilize more objective metrics in classification of patients with BM. The original GPA utilized age, KPS, the presence of extracranial metastases, number of brain metastases to group in a score 0–4, with 0 being the least favorable prognosis. While the GPA score was promising for several studies in brain metastases, data were more conflicting in the realm of SRS for multiple brain metastases. The newer dsGPA attempted to utilize primary cancer-specific factors into prognosis, such as breast cancer subtype and lung cancer molecular markers. This metric is newer and may be more validated in future studies.

Several prognostic indices can be used to evaluate the patient in the Introductory Case Vignette.

Table 9.2 Median overall survival by prognostic index tiers (in indices that include number of BM)

Prognostic index	Number of tiers	Median OS (mo)	Median OS in least favorable tier (mo)	Median OS in intermediate tiers (mo)	Median OS in most favorable tier (mo)
SIR [20]	3	6.8	2.9	7	31.4
GPA [24]	4	–	2.6	3.8–6.9	11
DS-GPA [25]	4	7.2	3.4	6.4–11.6	14.8
Updated ds-GPA [26]	4	7.2	3.1	5.4–8.7	16.7
Modified Breast-GPA [27]	4	8.5	2.6	9.2–19.9	28.8
Lung-molGPA (nonadenocarcinoma) [28]	3	9.2	5.3	9.8	12.8
Lung-molGPA (adenocarcinoma) [28]	4	15.2	6.9	13.7–26.5	46.8

SIR Score Index for Radiosurgery, *GPA* Graded Prognostic Assessment, *DS-GPA* Diagnostic Specific Graded Prognostic Assessment, *Lung-molGPA* Lung molecular Graded Prognostic Assessment

Table 9.3 Summary of studies reporting on SRS for patients with ≥5 brain metastases

Author (year)	Range of mets (number of patients)	Median follow up	Local recurrence	Distant brain failure	Overall survival
Hughes et al. (2019) [29]	5–15 BM (212)	48.7 mo	–	1 yr = 50% 2 yr = 54%	Median = 7.5 mo
Yamamoto et al. (2014) [8]	5–10 BM (208)	12 mo	1 yr = 6.5% 2 yr = 9.8%	1 yr = 63.8% 2 yr = 72%	Median = 10.8 mo
Salvetti (2013) [31]	5–15 BM (96)	4.1 mo	1 yr = 15.2% 2 yr = 25.1%	Total = 41%	5–9 BM = 4.8 mo 10–15 BM = 3.4 mo
Mohammadi et al. (2012) [35]	5–20 BM (178)	6.2 mo	3%	Total = 40% (median 2.1 mo)	Median = 6.7 mo
Chang (2010) [30]	6–10 BM (58) 11–15 BM (17) >15 BM (33)	10.7 mo 12.3 mo 8.0 mo	1 yr LC = 83% 1 yr LC = 92% 1 yr LC = 89%	1 yr = 47.2% 1 yr = 53.1% 1 yr = 80.3%	1 yr = 83% 1 yr = 92% 1 yr = 88%
Bhatnagar (2006) [36]	4–18 BM (205)	8 mo	1 yr = 29%	1 yr = 43%	Median = 8 mo

yr year, *mo* month, − not reported, *LC* local control

Based on RPA classification, the patient presents with KPS > 70, age < 65, and no extracranial metastases, grouping him into RPA Class I with a median OS of 7.1 months. Based on GPA classification, the patient presents with age > 60, KPS 90–100, number of BM > 3, and extracranial metastases absent groups him into GPA score 2.0 with a median OS of 6.5 months. Based on Lung-molGPA classification, the patient presents with age < 70, KPS 90–100, extracranial metastases absent, number of BM > 4, and EGFR/ALK status unknown, grouping him into Lung-mol GPA score of 2.0 with a median OS of 13.7 months.

Treatment Volume

The size of the largest BM can drive treatment decisions as well. Large brain metastasis measuring greater than 3 cm should be surgically removed rather than considered for SRS, resulting in greater overall survival, as well as functionally independent survival [37]. SRS for large tumors leads to risk of formation of edema, as well as delayed side effects. Two prospective controlled trials looked at the question of size of brain metastasis, randomizing to SRS versus surgery [38–40].

Several studies have suggested that aggregate tumor volume, rather than number of brain lesions, is more prognostic to clinical outcomes with SRS treatment. Bhatnagar et al. published a retrospective single institution report of 205 patients treated with four or more BM with SRS with median follow-up time of 8 months [36]. They found that total treatment volume was statistically associated with OS and local tumor control; however, number of brain metastasis is not statistically associated with clinical outcomes.

Smaller studies have further corroborated this finding. Grandhi et al. reported on a single institution retrospective analysis of 61 patients with 10 or more lesions treated with SRS only, with a median survival of 4 months [41]. In this study, they found that patients with 14 or more BM had significantly worse overall survival on multivariate analysis. However, they note that while other subgroups of number of BM were not associated with local control or survival, treatment volume was statistically significant and may be more predictive of outcome.

The argument that when comparing one patient with 2 BM with a total treatment volume of 5 cc versus another patient with 5 BM with a total treatment volume of 2 cc, the latter patient would have better chance at overall survival, and local tumor control is intuitive. Prospective and randomized studies are needed to further investigate this finding.

We can correlate these findings with the Case #1 Vignette. The patient initially presented with 6 BM with the largest individual tumor size of 0.5 cm and the tumor aggregate volume of 2.7 cc and was considered for upfront SRS treatment. The patient had DBF at 9 months with largest individual tumor size of 0.3 cm and aggregate tumor volume of 1.2 cc and was considered for salvage SRS. The patient then had DBF at 12 months with aggregate tumor volume of 5.1 cc, and WBRT was thought to be a better treatment option.

Dose Considerations

Recent studies have observed increased normal brain tissue dose spillage in treatment plans with greater than 3 BM [42–45]. In a multi-target treatment plan, radiation to the first target will invariably create background dose radiation to the subsequent targets and is incorporated into the treatment plan for subsequent targets. However, radiation of the subsequent targets will also affect the dose of the first target, creating a reciprocal dose effect [42, 43, 46]. Referred to as dose interplay effects, this is thought to be a major factor in increased normal tissue spillage in multi-target plans. This can lead to higher dose to normal brain tissue, which, as suggested earlier, can theoretically lead to toxicity including cognitive decline and radiation necrosis.

Different SRS platforms can also have variable effects depending on the number of beams, radiation source, and overall treatment plan approach. Ma et al. investigated treatment plans across different SRS platforms for multiple BM and found that dose conformality had greater variability in increasing number of targets across multiple SRS platforms [43]. Therefore, providers should be aware of the differences of treatment of the specific platform used for treatment and adjust treatment plans accordingly for increasing number of targets.

Ma et al. investigated treatment plans of increasing number of BM on different SRS platforms and found that increasing number of targets in an SRS platform can lead to decreasing conformity indices and variable isodose volumes [42]. The authors suggest up to a 20–30% reduction in prescription of dose to spare peripheral brain volume from dose non-conformality. Another study looked at optimizing Volumetric Modulated Arc Therapy (VMAT) linear accelerator plans by increasing the number of beams and optimizing for lowest normal tissue dose. The authors suggested that selecting higher number of optimized beams (such as the Broad-Range Optimization of Modulated Beam Approach, or BROOMBA) can decrease normal brain dose of multi-target treatment plans by as much as 65% [45].

Diagnosis

Patients who present with new brain lesions without a prior primary cancer diagnosis should have a full cancer workup. A comprehensive history and physical can help elucidate a primary cancer in 30% of patients with newly diagnosed brain metastasis. As lung cancer, breast cancer, and melanoma are the most common cancers that lead to multiple BM, a chest X-ray (CXR) should be the first imaging study performed, followed by a chest CT if the CXR is nondiagnostic. A CT of abdomen/pelvis and bone scan should be planned to determine extent of metastatic disease.

Patients presenting with a diagnosis of multiple BM should have history and physical and complete work up completed by a multidisciplinary team including Neurosurgery, Neuro-Oncology, and Radiation Oncology. Complete diagnostic workup of BM can include imaging and biopsy.

Imaging

Patients with suspected brain metastasis should have a contrast-enhanced magnetic resonance imaging of brain (MRI) for diagnosis. Contrast-enhanced MRI is more sensitive than non-enhanced MRI or CT with or without contrast and is important during surveillance to treat asymptomatic otherwise undetected lesions. Characteristic findings of brain metastases are contrast-enhancing lesions at the junction of the gray and white matter with circumscribed margins and surrounding edema.

Biopsy

Brain biopsy is performed when diagnosis via imaging is in doubt. Patients who present with multiple lesions are more characteristics of BM, and biopsy is usually deferred. About 80% of patients present with brain metastases after a primary tumor diagnosis, known as metachronous metastases. However, brain metastases that present at the same time as primary tumor diagnosis (synchronous metastases) and brain metastases that present before a primary tumor diagnosis (precocious metastases) may have a brain biopsy to help confirm primary tumor diagnosis through immunohistochemistry, as well as rule out other differential diagnoses of brain lesions such as primary brain tumor, infection, or inflammatory processes.

Management and Guidelines

Initial Management

Patients with newly diagnosed BM should first have symptoms managed if present. This may include corticosteroids for increased intracranial pressure, antiepileptics for control of seizures, management of thromboembolic disease, and/or surgical resection for decompression. Patients should have a complete staging workup to determine extent of metastatic disease and life expectancy.

Prognostic Index

No single prognostic index is recommended over any other. Commonly utilized indices include the Recursive Partitioning Analysis (RPA), the Graded Prognostic Assessment (GPA), and the more recent Diagnosis-Specific Graded Prognostic Assessment (dsGPA). Physicians should utilize tools to better categorize patients into survival time strata for management decisions, for predicting outcomes of interventions, and for comparing treatment results.

Setup

Patients can be treated on several different technologies that have stereotactic radiosurgery capabilities, including linear accelerators, Gamma Knife Radiosurgery (Fig. 9.2), or CyberKnife Radiosurgery. Patients can be treated in a single session that consists of positioning onto the machine, contouring dose deposition on computer software, and delivery of dose via machine. The treatment time is typically 45–90 minutes for a relatively simple case depending on number of BM, age of machine and radioactive material, and complexity of case. Patients can typically plan on spending half to a whole day in the clinic.

Radiation Dose

Several trials have looked at different efficacy and adverse effects associated with treatment dose and location. Two different treatment schemas are reproduced below. The first are treatment guidelines per RTOG 90-05, a frequently used treatment strategy by clinicians in the US and around the world. The second are treatment schemas of JLGK0901 (Yamamoto et al), a prospective observational trial; however, limitations of the study include a primarily Japanese population (with more favorable characteristics). Physicians should incorporate treatment strategies that are not only dependent on volume but also dependent on OAR constraints, prior radiation doses, and other clinical factors.

Treatment dose to 50–90% isodose line (measured in maximum diameter) per RTOG 90-05 [47]:

- Tumor diameter <2 cm = 20–24 Gy
- Tumor diameter 2–3 cm = 18 Gy
- Tumor diameter 3–4 cm = 15 Gy

Fig. 9.2 Gamma Knife Icon System. (**a**) and (**b**) Gamma Knife Icon radiosurgery system. The system uses daily Cone Beam CT comparison with planning CT co-registration and stereotactic imaging to monitor head positioning, as well as internal detectors to confirm accurate dose deposition. (This picture is provided by the Columbia University Department of Radiation Oncology)

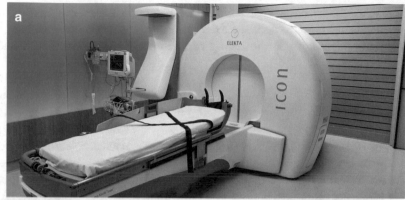

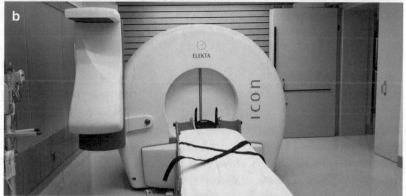

Treatment dose to lesion periphery (±2 Gy per clinical judgement) per JLGK0901 [8]:

- Tumor <4 cc = 22 Gy
- Tumor 4–10 cc = 20 Gy
- Brainstem tumor <1 cc = 20 Gy
- Brainstem tumor 1–4 cc = 18 Gy
- Brainstem tumor 4–10 cc = 16 Gy

Role for WBRT

Patients with multiple BM can be treated with WBRT in addition to SRS, keeping in mind WBRT is associated with increased tumor control but is also associated with decreased neuro-cognitive function and quality of life, with similar survival to SRS only. Hippocampal-sparing WBRT is currently under investigation (CC0001, see section "Future Directions" below for more details) and may be a suitable option for patients based on early reports.

Role for Surgery

Larger single tumors greater than 3 cm in diameter should be considered for surgery or fractionated radiosurgery. Other strategies include surgery and adjuvant SRS, neoadjuvant SRS followed by surgery.

Role for Palliative Care

For patients with poor life expectancy (less than 3 months), the use of WBRT may not significantly improve symptoms from WBRT treatment, and comfort measures is a reasonable option for patients. The QUARTZ trial was a phase 3 randomized controlled trial of 538 patients with NSCLC with BM unsuitable for surgery or SRS that compared optimal supportive care + WBRT vs optimal supportive care alone [48]. Overall survival was not statistically different between the two arms, and quality-adjusted life-years found a difference of 4.7 days. Poor performance status and active uncontrolled disease are risk factors for poor life expectancy in the setting of multiple brain metastases.

Timing of SRS

If new BM is seen on planning scan on the day of radiosurgery, it is reasonable to either treat all lesions visualized with SRS even if they exceed ten lesions or forgo SRS in favor of WBRT; there are insufficient high-quality data to suggest either would be more beneficial to the patient than the other.

Follow-Up

Patients should have close surveillance imaging with brain imaging (ideally Brain MRI) every 2–3 months for the first 6 months. If patients demonstrate new lesions, patients should be reevaluated by a multi-disciplinary team for salvage therapy or consideration of hospice care. Patients who do not demonstrate new lesions after the first 6 months may have been followed up with brain imaging every 3–4 months. Patients who are greater than 24 months away from initial treatment should be continued to be followed but be elected for more infrequent screening.

Areas of Uncertainty/Future Directions

Most studies reporting data on patients treated with greater than five brain metastases have several limitations. There is great range and variability with patient demographics and tumor characteristics, with brain metastases number ranging from 2 to 37 and volume ranging from 3.2 to 10.9 cc. Patient inclusion criteria vary greatly, from KPS to alternative treatment modality to primary histology. Most studies include some portion of patients that have had some treatment prior to SRS, including WBRT. There

is uncertainty in comparing outcomes of SRS as initial treatment versus SRS as salvage treatment with respect to local and distant brain control, as well as overall survival.

For greater than five brain metastases, no trial has looked directly at comparing WBRT to SRS. North American Gamma-Knife Consortium was a randomized controlled trial named: Neurocognitive Outcomes in Patients Treated With Radiotherapy for Five or More Brain Metastases (NAGKC 12–01; Clinical Trial Identifier: NCT01731704), with a study goal is to compare radiosurgery to WBRT for patients with five or more metastases, with neurocognitive status and tumor control as the primary end points. Unfortunately, the trial closed prior to enrollment due to insufficient staff. Whole Brain Radiotherapy (WBRT) Versus Stereotactic Radiosurgery (SRS) for 4 Upto 10 Brain Metastases (WBRT vs SRS) (Clinical Trial Identifier NCT02353000) is a Danish trial with a similar trial design and is currently active without patient recruitment [49]. Primary outcome is QoL, and secondary outcomes include OS, time to KPS >70, degree of independence, steroid use, and toxicity.

Pharmacological agents such as memantine during and after WBRT or donepezil after cranial radiotherapy have been tested for the prevention of cognitive dysfunction [50, 51]. However, although the effects of these agents in decreasing the cognitive effect of WBRT was statistically significant, the effect was minimal and did not affect decline in QoL associated with WBRT, nor affect other WBRT-related side effects (such as alopecia, fatigue, radiation necrosis).

The Canadian Cancer Trials Group (CCTG)/ Alliance groups have collaborated to open the study: Stereotactic Radiosurgery Compared with Whole Brain Radiotherapy (WBRT) for 5–15 brain metastases, which will randomize patients with 5–15 brain metastases to WBRT 30 Gy in 10 fractions + memantine daily versus SRS 18–20 or 22 Gy in single fraction (Clinical Trial Identifier: NCT03550391). The primary endpoint is to compare overall survival and neurocognitive progression-free survival between the two arms. Secondary endpoints include time to local/distant/leptomeningeal failure, difference in CNS failure patterns, number of salvage procedures, toxicity, and several QoL measures.

Hippocampal avoidance (HA) WBRT is a planning technique that avoids radiation dose to the hippocampal region during treatment for brain metastasis, with data showing infrequent presentation of brain metastasis in the hippocampal region. Retrospective and small prospective trials have shown delayed neurocognitive decline without worsened clinical outcome. Memantine Hydrochloride and Whole-Brain Radiotherapy With or Without Hippocampal Avoidance in Reducing Neurocognitive Decline in Patients With Brain Metastases (NRG CC001; Clinical Trial Identifier: NCT02360215) is a phase 2 trial assessing the effectiveness of hippocampal avoidance WBRT to delay neurocognitive failure. The primary endpoint is to assess neurocognitive function at 2, 4, 6, and 12 months after treatment utilized HVLT-R, COWA, and TMT testing. Early reports found that presented in abstract form to ASTRO 2018 found that memantine + HA WBRT reduced risk of cognitive failure and improved patient-reported symptoms. However, the logistics of the hippocampal avoidance WBRT should be noted, from high complexity and time of treatment plan creation compared to WBRT, as well as increased duration of time for treatment delivery.

Rapid advancements in immunotherapy have changed management for several patients with significant improvement in outcomes. Combining SRS with immunotherapy has been reported several times over the years with the benefit of enhanced antitumor immune response after radiation therapy. Also known as the abscopal effect, interest in combining these treatment modalities has spurred several prospective and randomized trials in the future. One example is the Phase I Clinical Study Combining L19-IL2 With SABR in Patients With Oligometastatic Solid Tumor (L19-IL2) (Clinical Trial Identifier: NCT02086721), which will look at dosing and toxicity of L19-IL2 (an immunocytokine) after SRS in patients with oligometastatic disease. While this trial will enroll several disease sites, BM is a common incidence among patients with oligometastatic disease (particularly in lung and breast) and may shed a light on future directions for SRS and immunotherapy in the setting of multiple BM.

Conclusions and Recommendations

- Treatment options for patients with multiple brain metastases include whole brain radiation treatment, surgery, stereotactic radiosurgery, as well as a combination of modalities as initial treatment and salvage treatment. Traditional management of multiple brain metastases is WBRT only.
- The advantages of SRS for brain metastases is that it avoids many of acute and late toxicities of WBRT, including alopecia, neurocognitive decline, with shorter overall treatment course.
- The disadvantages of SRS for brain metastases include localized treatment with increased risk of distant brain failure, and cost.
- Patients with multiple brain metastases are defined by two groups: limited brain metastases (1–4 BM) and multiple brain metastases (5+ BM).
- Several large randomized controlled trials demonstrated that patients with limited BM can be effectively treated with SRS only, with similar overall survival compared to WBRT only and better neurocognitive function and quality of life compared to WBRT.
- Data are limited but increasingly reassuring that patients with multiple brain metastases can effectively be treated with SRS only, with similar overall survival compared to WBRT, improved neurocognitive function and quality of life compared to WBRT.
- Patients treated with SRS have increased distant brain failure; however, salvage therapy with multiple courses of SRS is well tolerated and delays the need for WBRT as associated neurocognitive toxicity to last-line treatment.
- Data suggest that aggregate *volume* of tumor burden may be more representative of risk of clinical outcomes compared to *number* of brain metastases.

Future Directions

- WBRT vs SRS: WBRT vs SRS in 4–10 BM, primary endpoint: QoL
- CCTG Trial/Alliance: WBRT/Memantine vs SRS in 5–15 BM, primary endpoint: OS and neurocognitive function
- NRG CC001: WBRT/Memantine ± Hippocampal sparing, primary endpoint: neurocognitive function

References

1. Wen PY, Loeffler JS. Management of brain metastases. Oncology (Williston Park). 1999;13(7):941–54, 957–61; discussion 961–2, 9.
2. Johnson JD, Young B. Demographics of brain metastasis. Neurosurg Clin N Am. 1996;7(3):337–44.
3. Villa S, et al. Validation of the new graded prognostic assessment scale for brain metastases: a multicenter prospective study. Radiat Oncol. 2011;6:23.
4. Stelzer KJ. Epidemiology and prognosis of brain metastases. Surg Neurol Int. 2013;4(Suppl 4):S192–202.
5. Tabouret E, et al. Recent trends in epidemiology of brain metastases: an overview. Anticancer Res. 2012;32(11):4655–62.
6. Andrews DW, et al. Whole brain radiation therapy with or without stereotactic radiosurgery boost for patients with one to three brain metastases: phase III results of the RTOG 9508 randomised trial. Lancet. 2004;363(9422):1665–72.
7. Sperduto PW, et al. Secondary analysis of RTOG 9508, a phase 3 randomized trial of whole-brain radiation therapy versus WBRT plus stereotactic radiosurgery in patients with 1-3 brain metastases; poststratified by the graded prognostic assessment (GPA). Int J Radiat Oncol Biol Phys. 2014;90(3):526–31.
8. Yamamoto M, et al. Stereotactic radiosurgery for patients with multiple brain metastases (JLGK0901): a multi-institutional prospective observational study. Lancet Oncol. 2014;15(4):387–95.
9. Chang EL, et al. A pilot study of neurocognitive function in patients with one to three new brain metastases initially treated with stereotactic radiosurgery alone. Neurosurgery. 2007;60(2):277–83; discussion 283–4.
10. Brown PD, et al. Effect of radiosurgery alone vs radiosurgery with whole brain radiation therapy on cognitive function in patients with 1 to 3 brain metastases: a randomized clinical trial. JAMA. 2016;316(4):401–9.
11. Tsao MN, et al. Whole brain radiotherapy for the treatment of multiple brain metastases. Cochrane Database Syst Rev. 2006;(3):CD003869.
12. Borgelt B, et al. The palliation of brain metastases: final results of the first two studies by the Radiation Therapy Oncology Group. Int J Radiat Oncol Biol Phys. 1980;6(1):1–9.
13. Suzuki H, et al. Spontaneous haemorrhage into metastatic brain tumours after stereotactic radiosurgery using a linear accelerator. J Neurol Neurosurg Psychiatry. 2003;74(7):908–12.
14. Muller-Riemenschneider F, et al. Medical and health economic assessment of radiosurgery for the treatment of brain metastasis. GMS Health Technol Assess. 2009;5:Doc03.
15. Hall MD, et al. Cost-effectiveness of stereotactic radiosurgery with and without whole-brain radiotherapy for the treatment of newly diagnosed brain metastases. J Neurosurg. 2014;121(Suppl):84–90.
16. Chang EL, et al. Neurocognition in patients with brain metastases treated with radiosurgery or radiosurgery plus whole-brain irradiation: a randomised controlled trial. Lancet Oncol. 2009;10(11):1037–44.
17. Kocher M, et al. Adjuvant whole-brain radiotherapy versus observation after radiosurgery or surgical resection of one to three cerebral metastases: results of the EORTC 22952-26001 study. J Clin Oncol. 2011;29(2):134–41.
18. Aoyama H, et al. Neurocognitive function of patients with brain metastasis who received either whole brain radiotherapy plus stereotactic radiosurgery or radiosurgery alone. Int J Radiat Oncol Biol Phys. 2007;68(5):1388–95.
19. Gaspar L, et al. Recursive partitioning analysis (RPA) of prognostic factors in three Radiation Therapy Oncology Group (RTOG) brain metastases trials. Int J Radiat Oncol Biol Phys. 1997;37(4):745–51.
20. Weltman E, et al. Radiosurgery for brain metastases: a score index for predicting prognosis. Int J Radiat Oncol Biol Phys. 2000;46(5):1155–61.
21. Lorenzoni J, et al. Radiosurgery for treatment of brain metastases: estimation of patient eligibility using three stratification systems. Int J Radiat Oncol Biol Phys. 2004;60(1):218–24.
22. Lagerwaard FJ, et al. Identification of prognostic factors in patients with brain metastases: a review of 1292 patients. Int J Radiat Oncol Biol Phys. 1999;43(4):795–803.
23. Golden DW, et al. Prognostic factors and grading systems for overall survival in patients treated with radiosurgery for brain metastases: variation by primary site. J Neurosurg. 2008;109(Suppl):77–86.
24. Sperduto PW, et al. A new prognostic index and comparison to three other indices for patients with brain metastases: an analysis of 1,960 patients in the RTOG database. Int J Radiat Oncol Biol Phys. 2008;70(2):510–4.
25. Sperduto PW, et al. Diagnosis-specific prognostic factors, indexes, and treatment outcomes for patients with newly diagnosed brain metastases: a multi-institutional analysis of 4,259 patients. Int J Radiat Oncol Biol Phys. 2010;77(3):655–61.
26. Sperduto PW, et al. Summary report on the graded prognostic assessment: an accurate and facile diagnosis-specific tool to estimate survival

for patients with brain metastases. J Clin Oncol. 2012;30(4):419–25.

27. Subbiah IM, et al. Validation and development of a modified breast graded prognostic assessment as a tool for survival in patients with breast Cancer and brain metastases. J Clin Oncol. 2015;33(20):2239–45.

28. Sperduto PW, et al. Estimating survival in patients with lung cancer and brain metastases: an update of the graded prognostic assessment for lung cancer using molecular markers (lung-molGPA). JAMA Oncol. 2017;3(6):827–31.

29. Hughes RT, et al. Initial SRS for patients with 5 to 15 brain metastases: results of a multi-institutional experience. Int J Radiat Oncol Biol Phys. 2019;104:1091–8.

30. Chang WS, et al. Analysis of radiosurgical results in patients with brain metastases according to the number of brain lesions: is stereotactic radiosurgery effective for multiple brain metastases? J Neurosurg. 2010;113(Suppl):73–8.

31. Salvetti DJ, et al. Gamma Knife surgery for the treatment of 5 to 15 metastases to the brain: clinical article. J Neurosurg. 2013;118(6):1250–7.

32. Aoyama H, et al. Stereotactic radiosurgery with or without whole-brain radiotherapy for brain metastases: secondary analysis of the JROSG 99-1 randomized clinical trial. JAMA Oncol. 2015;1(4):457–64.

33. Saraf A, et al. Breast cancer subtype and stage are prognostic of time from breast cancer diagnosis to brain metastasis development. J Neuro-Oncol. 2017;134(2):453–63.

34. Tai CH, et al. Single institution validation of a modified graded prognostic assessment of patients with breast cancer brain metastases. CNS Oncol. 2018;7(1):25–34.

35. Mohammadi AM, et al. Role of Gamma Knife surgery in patients with 5 or more brain metastases. J Neurosurg. 2012;117(Suppl):5–12.

36. Bhatnagar AK, et al. Stereotactic radiosurgery for four or more intracranial metastases. Int J Radiat Oncol Biol Phys. 2006;64(3):898–903.

37. Tsao MN, et al. Radiotherapeutic and surgical management for newly diagnosed brain metastasis(es): an American Society for Radiation Oncology evidence-based guideline. Pract Radiat Oncol. 2012;2(3):210–25.

38. Lippitz B, et al. Stereotactic radiosurgery in the treatment of brain metastases: the current evidence. Cancer Treat Rev. 2014;40(1):48–59.

39. Vecht CJ, et al. Treatment of single brain metastasis: radiotherapy alone or combined with neurosurgery? Ann Neurol. 1993;33(6):583–90.

40. Patchell RA, et al. A randomized trial of surgery in the treatment of single metastases to the brain. N Engl J Med. 1990;322(8):494–500.

41. Grandhi R, et al. Stereotactic radiosurgery using the Leksell Gamma Knife Perfexion unit in the management of patients with 10 or more brain metastases. J Neurosurg. 2012;117(2):237–45.

42. Ma L, et al. Apparatus dependence of normal brain tissue dose in stereotactic radiosurgery for multiple brain metastases. J Neurosurg. 2011;114(6):1580–4.

43. Ma L, et al. Variable dose interplay effects across radiosurgical apparatus in treating multiple brain metastases. Int J Comput Assist Radiol Surg. 2014;9(6):1079–86.

44. McDonald D, et al. Comparison of radiation dose spillage from the Gamma Knife Perfexion with that from volumetric modulated arc radiosurgery during treatment of multiple brain metastases in a single fraction. J Neurosurg. 2014;121(Suppl):51–9.

45. Dong P, et al. Minimizing normal tissue dose spillage via broad-range optimization of hundreds of intensity modulated beams for treating multiple brain targets. J Radiosurg SBRT. 2016;4(2):107–15.

46. Sahgal A, et al. Prescription dose guideline based on physical criterion for multiple metastatic brain tumors treated with stereotactic radiosurgery. Int J Radiat Oncol Biol Phys. 2010;78(2):605–8.

47. Shaw E, et al. Single dose radiosurgical treatment of recurrent previously irradiated primary brain tumors and brain metastases: final report of RTOG protocol 90-05. Int J Radiat Oncol Biol Phys. 2000;47(2):291–8.

48. Mulvenna P, et al. Dexamethasone and supportive care with or without whole brain radiotherapy in treating patients with non-small cell lung cancer with brain metastases unsuitable for resection or stereotactic radiotherapy (QUARTZ): results from a phase 3, non-inferiority, randomised trial. Lancet. 2016;388(10055):2004–14.

49. Zindler JD, et al. Whole brain radiotherapy versus stereotactic radiosurgery for 4-10 brain metastases: a phase III randomised multicentre trial. BMC Cancer. 2017;17(1):500.

50. Brown PD, et al. Memantine for the prevention of cognitive dysfunction in patients receiving whole-brain radiotherapy: a randomized, double-blind, placebo-controlled trial. Neuro-Oncology. 2013;15(10):1429–37.

51. Rapp SR, et al. Donepezil for irradiated brain tumor survivors: a phase III randomized placebo-controlled clinical trial. J Clin Oncol. 2015;33(15):1653–9.

Hypofractionated Stereotactic Radiosurgery for Intact and Resected Brain Metastases

Erqi L. Pollom, Siyu Shi, and Scott G. Soltys

Introduction

Stereotactic radiosurgery (SRS), as defined by the neurosurgery and radiation oncology societies consensus statement [1], is a stereotactic irradiation in one to five fractions. Single-fraction SRS is an effective treatment option for many patients with both intact and resected brain metastases. For patients with large brain metastases who are not candidates for surgery, whole-brain radiotherapy has historically been considered the standard of care. Due to concern for poor local control and neurotoxicity associated with whole-brain radiotherapy, SRS has increasingly been explored for the treatment of these patients. However, clinicians have concern about increased toxicity with single-fraction SRS for larger targets or targets located near or within critical structures or eloquent brain, such as the brainstem, optic pathway, or motor cortex. Hypofractionated SRS over two to five fractions may be an alternative treatment that allows safe delivery of high cumulative doses to lesions suboptimally treated with single-fraction SRS due to size and/or location. There is accumulating clinical evidence showing that hypofractionated SRS can minimize risk to normal brain while maintaining acceptable local control, although the optimal dose and fractionation for this approach have yet to be determined. Other reviews have examined the outcomes of SRS versus hypofractionated SRS for benign and malignant brain tumors [2]; herein, we focus on the role and rationale of hypofractionation for brain metastases.

Limitations of Single-Fraction Radiosurgery

Single-fraction SRS dose is limited by risk of central nervous system toxicity. Adverse radiation effect (ARE), the imaging equivalent of histologically defined brain radiation necrosis, is the most common toxicity that occurs after SRS for tumors in or near the brain and can be associated with neurological deficits that can require management with steroids, bevacizumab, and, in some cases, surgical resection.

Factors that have been found to be correlated with the development of ARE include higher radiation dose, larger tumor volume, and volume of normal brain irradiated [3]. For recurrent, intact, previously irradiated primary brain tumors and brain metastases treated with escalating doses of single-fraction SRS, RTOG 90-05 found that normal brain tissue toxicity was significantly more likely to develop in patients with larger tumors. Compared to tumors smaller than 2 cm in maximum diameter, tumors with maximum diameters of 2–3 cm and 3–4 cm had, respectively,

E. L. Pollom (✉) · S. Shi · S. G. Soltys
Department of Radiation Oncology, Stanford University, Stanford, CA, USA
e-mail: erqiliu@stanford.edu

© Springer Nature Switzerland AG 2020
Y. Yamada et al. (eds.), *Radiotherapy in Managing Brain Metastases*,
https://doi.org/10.1007/978-3-030-43740-4_10

a 7.3 and 16.0 times higher risk of developing irreversible grade 3 or grade 4–5 central nervous system toxicity [3]. In addition to larger volume, increasing dose on this study was also associated with a greater risk of brain toxicity. Others have found that the risk of ARE correlates with the radio surgical volume encompassed by the 10-Gy or 12-Gy isodose line [4]. In a series of 206 patients with a total of 310 brain metastases treated with single-fraction SRS, the actuarial risk of ARE was up to 51% when the volume of receiving a dose of 12 Gy exceeded 10.9 cc [5]. Blonigen et al. similarly showed in a series of 63 patients with a total of 173 brain metastases that the risk of ARE is up to 69% when the volume of peritumoral normal brain receiving 10 and 12 Gy is greater than 14.5 and 10.8 cc, respectively [6].

For resected brain metastasis, the size of the preoperative lesion and volume of normal brain receiving 21 Gy have been found to be associated with incidence of radiation necrosis [7]. Although the addition of a margin around resection cavity improves local control [8], this also increases the volume of normal brain irradiated and, thus, can potentially increase risk of toxicity [9, 10].

In part due to the use of reduced doses to address these concerns for toxicity, larger lesions have been associated with lower control rates after single-fraction SRS. On the basis of the results of RTOG 90-05, the proposed single-fraction SRS doses for lesions with maximum diameter >2 cm, 2.1–3.0 cm, and 3.1–4.0 cm are 24 Gy, 18 Gy, and 15 Gy, respectively [3]. Using these doses, the 1-year local control rate has been reported to be only 49% and 45% for metastases 2.1–3.0 and 3.1–4.0 cm in diameter, respectively, compared with 85% for smaller lesions [11]. Similarly, Hasegawa et al. reported a 49% 1-year local control rate for tumors with a volume greater than 4 cc treated with single-fraction SRS [12]. In 153 brain metastases treated with single-fraction SRS using doses of 20 Gy or more, Chang et al. reported 1-year local control rates of 86% in tumors 1 cm or smaller in size and 56% in tumors greater than 1 cm [13]. A minimum prescribed isodose surface dose of 18 Gy and higher has been found to be associated with local control [14].

Radiobiology and Rationale of Hypofractionation

Hypofractionated SRS may allow the delivery of higher cumulative dose to larger targets while minimizing the risk of toxicity. Fractionation is a central tenet in radiotherapy that leverages the four Rs of classic radiation biology (repair, repopulation, reassortment, and reoxygenation) to expand the therapeutic window. Single-fraction SRS contradicts these conventional radiobiological principles but has been shown to be associated with excellent local control with acceptable toxicity for both metastatic and benign disease. A high level of precision and accuracy is required for delivering high doses of radiation to small targets. Previously, immobilization was achieved by invasively fixing the patient's head to a frame locked to the treatment couch. However, recent advances in image guidance and robotic-based systems have allowed the evolution of noninvasive, frameless radiosurgery which can facilitate the fractionated delivery of stereotactic radiotherapy with acceptable levels of accuracy [15–17]. Furthermore, recent preclinical and clinical studies on the radiobiology of single fraction, high-dose SRS have uncovered mechanisms of radiation different from that of conventionally fractionated radiotherapy. In addition to DNA double-strand breaks, single-fraction high-dose SRS may cause microvascular dysfunction and cell death through endothelial cell inflammation and apoptosis via the sphingomyelin pathway [18, 19]. There is still debate over whether there is a "new biology" beyond the classic radiobiologic paradigm of fractionation or simply higher biological effective dose (BED) that accounts for the efficacy of single-fraction SRS [20].

For malignant tumors, concern exists that single-fraction SRS results in a suboptimal therapeutic ratio between tumor control and late effects. As brain metastases comprise acutely responding neoplastic cells immediately surrounded by late responding normal brain tissue, Hall and Brenner argue that fractionated radiotherapy allows for normal tissue repair/recovery and offers the potential to exploit the different biologic responses and repair mechanisms between neoplastic and normal tissues to irradiation [21, 22]. Additionally, a radioresistant subpopulation of hypoxic cells may survive after single dose of radiation [23], leading to worse tumor control. Allowing for re-oxygenation over multiple fractions may improve tumor control outcomes. Expanding the therapeutic window may not be as important for smaller volumes treated with stereotactic techniques, as there is minimal dose spill outside the target volume. For larger volumes, hypofractionated SRS may offer an approach that leverages the radiobiologic advantages of both high doses per fraction and fractionation. Modeling studies suggest that treatment over 5–10 fractions provides the most gain in normal tissue sparing for fast growing tumor; the rate of improvement generally levels off at a large (i.e., >10 fractions) number of fractions [24].

Finally, there is emerging evidence that radiation treatment of tumors may have immune-stimulatory effects through immunogenic tumor cell death and enhanced recruitment of antitumor T cells and can be coupled with immunotherapy to improve cancer control outcomes [25, 26]. Diverse radiation regimens have been used in combination with immunotherapy, and recent data suggest that dose fractionation can determine the efficacy of combination treatment. Dewan et al. showed using breast and colon carcinoma models that while a single dose of 20 Gy was as effective as the fractionated regimens of 8 Gy × 3 and 6 Gy × 5 at controlling the growth of the irradiated tumor, only the two fractionated regimens were able to synergize with CTLA-4 blockade to induce antitumor T-cell immunity and inhibit a second palpable tumor outside the radiation field ("abscopal effect") [27]. It may be that single-fraction SRS damages the vasculature and may impair perfusion and transport of antigens and immune cells [28]. Molecular responses of cells irradiated with fractionated radiation have also been found to differ from single-dose radiation in vitro and in vivo, and they may contribute to the observed differences in effect of fractionated versus single-fraction radiation [29].

Clinical Experience with Hypofractionated SRS

Intact Metastases

Table 10.1 summarizes published studies of hypofractionated SRS for intact brain metastases and overall shows acceptable local control rates with hypofractionated regimens despite the large tumor volumes treated in many of these series. Also, the data suggest equivalent to improved toxicity rates compared to historical outcomes with single-fraction SRS.

A retrospective study by Minniti et al. of 289 patients with brain metastases with maximum diameters greater than 2 cm showed superior local control using a hypofractionated SRS regimen (9 Gy × 3 fractions) compared to single-fraction SRS, with 1-year local control rates of 90% versus 77%, respectively [45]. Furthermore, there was a lower risk of ARE (9% versus 18%) with hypofractionated SRS. In contrast, Wiggenraad et al. [52] found no difference in the local control rates or toxicity between hypofractionated SRS (8 Gy × 3) and single-fraction SRS (15 Gy) for large (volume >13 cc) brain metastases. Fokas et al. also found no difference in local control between hypofractionated SRS (using either 5 Gy × 7 or 4 Gy × 10) and single-fraction SRS; however, they found that grade 1–3 toxicity was significantly higher with single-fraction SRS (14%) compared with hypofractionated SRS (6% with 5 Gy × 7 and 2% with 4 Gy × 10) [34]. Another series found that 30 Gy in five fractions was associated with better local control than 24 Gy in five fractions (1-year local control 91% vs 75%) [41]. Some series have reported potentially worse local control with hypofractionated SRS for radioresistant histologies, although this may be due to lower BED of the hypofractionated regimens used [47]. These data suggest that hypofractionated regimens are safe but that clinicians should be vigilant to maintain a high BED, equivalent to single-fraction doses, for optimal local control.

While randomized studies comparing hypofractionated SRS over other techniques are lacking, the clinical experience so far suggests

Table 10.1 Selected hypofractionated SRS series for intact brain metastases

Author	Date	N (lesions)	Dose (Gy/fractions)	Lesion diameter or volume (median, range)	Histology	Margin (mm)	1-year LC (%)	Adverse radiation effect/necrosis[a] (%)
Aoki et al. [30]	2006	65	Median 24 (range 18–30)/3–5	>2 cm (n = 31); ≤ 2 cm (n = 34)	Lung, other	1	72	2
Aoyama et al. [31]	2003	159	35/4	3.3 cc, 0.006–48.3 cc	Lung, other	2	85	3
Ernst-stecken et al. [32]	2006	72	30–35/5	2.27 cm, 0.85–5.22 cm	Lung, melanoma, breast, colon, RCC, other	3	76	35
Fahrig et al. [33]	2007	228	30–35/5; 40/10; 35/7	PTV: 6.1 cc, 0.02–95.97 cc	Lung, melanoma, breast, rectal, RCC, other	3	72	1
Fokas et al. [34]	2012	122	35/7; 40/10	2.04 cc, 0.02–27.5 cc (35/7); 5.93 cc, 0.02–26.8 cc (40/10)	Lung, breast, melanoma, GI, GU, other	3	75 (35/7); 71 (40/10)	6 (35/7); 2 (40/10)
Higuchi et al. [35]	2009	46	30/3	17.6 cc (mean; SD 6.3 cc)	Lung, colon, breast, other	0	76	4
Kim et al. [36]	2011	49	36/6	PTV: 5.00 cc, 0.14–37.80 cc	Not reported	1	69	0
Kwon et al. [37]	2009	52	25/5; 20/5; 30/5; 36/6	1.16 cm, 1.7–31.2 cm	Lung, melanoma, other	1–2	68	6
Lindvall et al. [38]	2009	47	Median 38 (range 35–40)/5	6 cc, 0.6–26 cc	Lung, RCC, breast, melanoma, other	3	84 (at mean 3.7-month follow-up)	0
Lockney et al. [39]	2017	88	30/5	2.0 cm, 0.4–4.6 cm	Lung, breast, melanoma, other	2–5	81	4
Manning et al. [40]	2000	57	Median 27 (range 12–36)/3	2.16 cc	Lung, melanoma, breast, GI, RCC, thyroid	2	91 (at 6 months)	6
Marcrom et al. [41]	2017	182	25 or 30/5	1.68 cm, 0.31–5.50 cm	Lung, breast, melanoma, GI, GU, other	0–3	86	1

Märtens et al. [42]	2012	108	30/6; 30/5; 35/5; 28–40/7–10; 25/5	1.0 cc, 0.1–19.0 cc (upfront SRS); 2.0 cc, 0.1–29.2 cc (salvage SRS)	Lung, breast, melanoma, RCC, other	4	52	1
Matsuyama et al. [43]	2013	573	Peripheral BED10: Median 83.2 (range 19.1–89.6)/median 3 (range 2–10)	1.4 cc, 0.1–138.6 cc	Lung	1	95	2
Minniti et al. [44]	2014	171	27 (≥2 cm) or 36 (<2 cm)/3	10.1 cc, 1.6–48.4 cc	Lung, breast, melanoma, GI, RCC, other	1–3	88	6
Minniti et al. [45]	2016	138	27/3	17.9 cm, 5.6–54 cm	Lung, breast, colon, melanoma, RCC, other	1–2	91	3
Narayana et al. [46]	2007	20	30/5	3.5 cm, 2–5 cm	Lung, melanoma, RCC, breast, GI, ovary, sarcoma	3	70	5
Oermann et al. [47]	2013	74	20/2–5	2.5 cm (IQR 0.8–2.2 cm, radioresistant); 2.1 cm (IQR 1.4–2.8 cm, radiosensitive)	Melanoma, RCC, sarcoma, breast, lung	Not reported	Median 14.4 months (radioresistant); median 41.5 months (radiosensitive)	2
Ogura et al. [48]	2012	27	20–25 or 35/5	1.8 cm, 0.3–3.4 cm	Lung, breast, colon, other	2	87	5
Rajakesari et al. [49]	2014	70	25/5 (n = 61); 30/10; 32/8; 33/11; 24/8	1.7 cm, 0.4–6.4 cm	Lung, breast, melanoma, GI, RCC, other	Not reported	56	4
Saitoh et al. [50]	2010	78	39–42/3	1.2 cm, 0.4–3.8 cm	Lung	3	86	8
Tokuuye et al. [51]	1998	95	42/7; 48/8; 52/13 (for tumors >3 cm or close to critical structures)	Not reported	Lung, RCC, breast, other	2–3	91	8
Wiggenraad et al. [52]	2012	65	24/3	PTV > 13 cc or lesions in or close to brainstem (n = 47)	Lung, breast, melanoma, other	2	61	25%[b]

Abbreviations: *N* number, *LC* local control, *RCC* renal cell carcinoma, *PFS* progression-free survival, *cc* cubic centimeter, *GI* gastrointestinal, *WBRT* whole-brain radiation therapy, *GU* genitourethelial, *BED* biologically effective dose, *PTV* planning treatment volume, *SD* standard deviation, *IQR* interquartile range

[a]Clinically significant, requiring steroids

[b]Included pseudoprogression

that hypofractionated SRS may represent a better treatment option for larger metastatic brain tumors or those in close proximity to eloquent areas such as the brainstem or optic chiasm [44].

Resection Cavities

Surgery alone after resection of brain metastases is inadequate for local control [53–55]. Compared to postresection whole-brain radiotherapy, postresection SRS to the resection cavity results in improved cognition with no detriment to overall survival and has now become a standard of care treatment [56]. Numerous studies have reported outcomes of single-fraction SRS to small resection cavities with 1-year local control rates ranging from around 70% to 90% [8, 55, 57, 58]. As with intact lesions treated with SRS, cavities from large preoperative metastases (maximum diameter of 3 cm or greater) are more likely to recur locally after cavity SRS [59]. Increasing cavity volume is also associated with increased toxicity [7, 60]. Delaying SRS does not help reduce target volumes as there is minimal cavity shrinkage seen between the immediate postoperative scan to within a month following resection [61], and delay may be associated with inferior local control [62]. Hypofractionated SRS to the resection cavity has been shown to offer excellent local control rates, even for large brain metastases. Minniti et al. reported 1- and 2-year local control rates of 93% and 84%, respectively, and symptomatic radiation necrosis rate of only 5% with 9 Gy × 3 to the resection cavity [60]. Table 10.2 summarizes published studies of hypofractionated SRS for resected brain metastases.

Optimal Hypofractionated SRS Regimen

The optimal dose and fractionation schedule for hypofractionated SRS remain to be determined. Although the reliability of the linear–quadratic

(LQ) model has been questioned for SRS [75], BED based on the LQ model is most widely used clinically to compare the effects of various fractionation schedules. Local control has been associated with peripheral BED10 (using an alpha/beta ratio of 10 for tumor): one series found that the 1-year local control rate was 97% for BED10 greater than 80 Gy versus 90% for BED10 less than 80 Gy [43]. A recently published systematic review of SRS for brain metastases compared the BEDs of different SRS treatment schedules using an alpha/beta value of 12 Gy and found that a BED12 of at least 40 Gy (which corresponds to 25.5 Gy in three fractions or 20 Gy in single fraction) is necessary to obtain a 1-year local control >70% [52]. Similarly, in the postoperative setting, multisession SRS using BED10 ≥48 Gy to the resection cavity has been associated with improved local control. Surgical cavities treated with a BED10 ≥48 Gy (30 Gy in five fractions or 27 Gy in three fractions) had a 1-year local control of 100% compared to 33% for cavities treated with a lower BED10 [69].

Overall treatment time also needs to be explored in the setting of high doses per fraction. Studies in other organ sites have shown improved efficacy, toxicity, and quality of life with every other day dosing [76–78]. Radiobiologic studies suggest that the repair halftime for brain necrosis may be relatively long, with the potential of unrepaired damage still present after a 24-hour interval [79]. Reoxygenation may similarly require a longer time interval as hypoxia has been detected in lung tumors at 24–48 hours after a single fraction of radiation to the lung [80]. Increasing the interval of time between radiation fractions by delivering treatment on nonconsecutive days can allow for reassortment of remaining tumor cells into G2-M phase of the cell cycle and improved oxygenation and radiation sensitivity for subsequent fractions, thereby maximizing efficacy of the radiation. There is also time for repair and repopulation of normal cells in between the treatment sessions, thereby minimizing the risk of treatment. For patients with brain metastases not amenable to single-fraction

Table 10.2 Selected hypofractionated SRS series for resected brain metastases

Author	Date	N (cavities)	Dose (Gy/ fractions)	Cavity diameter or volume (median, range)	Histology	Margin (mm)	1-year LC (%)	Adverse radiation effect/ necrosis[a] (%)
Abuodeh et al. [63]	2016	77	25/5	8.92 cc, 0.17–54.2 cc	Lung, melanoma, RCC, breast, other	1–2	89	3
Ahmed et al. [64]	2014	65	20–30/5	8.06 cc, 0.13–54.25 cc	Lung, melanoma, RCC, breast, other	1–2	87	2
Ammirati et al. [65]	2014	36	30/5	10.25 cc, 1.04–67.52 cc	Lung, melanoma, breast, other	3	16% LF	8
Connolly et al. [66]	2013	33	40.05/15	3.3 cm, 1.7–5.7 cm	Lung, melanoma, breast, other	10	90	0
Do et al. [67]	2009	33	24–27.3/4–6	>3 cm (n = 16)	Lung, melanoma, breast, other	1–3	82	0
Doré et al. [7]	2017	103	23.1/3	>3 cm (n = 48)	Lung, RCC, breast, colon, melanoma, other	2	84	7
Keller et al. [68]	2017	189	33/3	7.6 cc, 0.2–48.81 cc	Lung, breast, GI, RCC, melanoma, other	2	88	19
Kumar et al. [69]	2018	43	28–30/3–5	3.1 cm (preoperative size)	Lung, breast, melanoma, other	2	23% LF	0
Ling et al. [70]	2015	100	Median 22 (range 10–28)/ median 3 (range 1–5)	PTV: 12.9 cc, 0.6–51.1 cc	Lung, melanoma, RCC, breast, other	0–1	72	6
Lockney et al. [39]	2017	143	30/5	3.2 cm, 0.7–6.3 cm	Lung, breast, melanoma, other	2–5	84	4
Pessina et al. [71]	2016	69	30/3	29 cc, 4.1–203.1 cc	Lung, melanoma, breast, other	3	100	9
Steinmann et al. [72]	2012	33	40/10, 35/7, 30/5	9.7 cc, 0.95–52.6 cc	Lung, melanoma, RCC, breast, other	4	71	0
Vogel et al. [73]	2015	33	Median 30 (range 16–35)/ median 5 (range 1–5)	3.8 cm, 2.8–6.7 cm	Lung, breast, melanoma, other	2–3	69	10
Wang et al. [74]	2011	37	24/3	>3 cm	Lung, melanoma, breast, kidney, colon	2–3	80	6

Abbreviations: *N* number, *LC* local control, *RCC* renal cell carcinoma, *GI* gastrointestinal, *cc* cubic centimeter, *cm* centimeter, *mm* millimeter, *LF* local failure
[a]Clinically significant, requiring steroids

SRS because of location or tumor size, Narayana et al. reported 1-year local control of 70% and steroid dependency in 15% of patients treated with 30 Gy in five fractions at two fractions per week [46]. However, other studies have found no benefit with every other day treatment compared to daily treatment [81].

A further extension of this concept is staged SRS treatment, in which fractions are separated by an even longer interval of at least few weeks. Staged SRS distributes high cumulative doses over time and allows for potentially smaller targets at subsequent treatment sessions. Higuchi et al. published the first report of staged SRS, in which patients with brain metastases of volume larger than 10 cc were treated with a total dose of 30 Gy over three staged fractions separated by 2-week interfraction intervals [35]. Overall tumor shrinkage was observed in 91% of the tumors, with tumor volumes decreasing by 19% and 40% at the second and third sessions. This approach resulted in 1-year local control rates of 76%, with only one patient developing grade 3 toxicity that required surgery. Other series have since been subsequently reported, showing similarly successful treatment of large brain metastases using staged SRS of 20–33 Gy over two sessions with minimal treatment-related morbidity [82–84]. Angelov et al. used a 30-day interfraction interval in order to allow for 10 half-lives for repair, assuming the repair half-time for late radiation effects in the brain is as long as 76 hours [79]. In their series of brain metastases greater than 2 cm treated with a median of 30 Gy in two sessions, they reported a 6-month local control rate of 88% and 6% of symptomatic radiation necrosis [83].

Indications for Surgery (Versus Radiosurgery) for Larger Lesions

For larger lesions, hypofractionated SRS has been shown as an effective primary treatment modality for large brain metastases that cannot be resected. While large brain metastases (those measuring greater than 2–3 cm in maximum diameter) are typically treated with resection followed by adjuvant radiation, surgical resection is sometimes not appropriate due to factors such as patients' performance status and comorbidities or extent of disease. In fact, a secondary analysis of EORTC 22952-26001 found that in patients with one to two brain metastases with a diameter of no greater than 4 cm, SRS was associated with improved early local control compared to surgical resection [85]. However, surgical resection is necessary in the following scenarios:

- Pathologic proof of metastatic disease is needed.
- Symptoms of edema/mass effect do not resolve with steroids.
- Symptoms that resolve with steroids but concern that the patient would be steroid dependent for weeks/months until the tumor shrinks (i.e., surgery would allow for more rapid resolution of edema/mass effect than with SRS alone).

Future Directions and Conclusions

Hypofractionated radiosurgery is a promising strategy for maximizing local control while minimizing toxicity, particularly for larger lesions or lesions in critical locations. While there is a wide range of acceptable fractionation regimens reported in the literature, maintaining a high BED (i.e., BED10 $\geq$48 Gy, equivalent to 27 Gy in three fractions) is important for optimal local control [52, 69]. Areas of uncertainty include how hypofractionated SRS compares with surgery for the treatment of larger brain metastases and how hypofractionated SRS compares with single-fraction SRS for the treatment of small brain metastases. Additional work is warranted in determining the optimal interfraction time interval and investigating novel approaches such as staged SRS.

Key Points
- For intact metastases and resection cavities greater than 2 cm in maximum diameter, data suggest improved tumor control and/or treatment-related toxicity with hypofractionated SRS over 2–5 days compared to single-fraction SRS.
- Maintain high BED equivalent to single-fraction doses for optimal local control with hypofractionation (i.e., BED10 ≥48 Gy, equivalent to 27 Gy in three fractions). Recommended radiosurgery doses for intact brain metastases and resection cavities are listed in Table 10.3.

Table 10.3 Recommended radiosurgery doses used at our institution for both intact metastases and resection cavities

Target maximum diameter (cm)	Dose (Gy/fractions)
<2 cm	20–24/1
2–3 cm	27–30/3 or 18/1
3–4	27/3
4–5	24/3
>5	25/5

Case Vignettes

Case 1: Postresection Cavity Hypofractionated SRS due to Size Along with Single-Fraction SRS for Small Intact Metastases

A 59-year-old woman with metastatic ovarian cancer presented with headaches, confusion, and visual disturbance due to a hemorrhagic brain metastasis measuring 4.8 × 4.9 cm in the left parieto-occipital lobe, with trace rim enhancement and surrounding vasogenic edema. She was started on antiseizure medication and steroids, which resulted in complete resolution of her symptoms. She underwent craniotomy for resection the hemorrhagic portion of her metastases followed by radiosur-

gery treatment 1 week later. On her radiosurgery planning MRI, the left parieto-occipital lesion measured 2.7 × 1.5 cm. Two additional lesions were seen in the left precentral gyrus (7 × 5 mm) and right frontal lobe (2 mm). The left parieto-occipital lesion was treated without margin to 27 Gy in three fractions with dose prescribed to the 72% isodose line (Fig. 10.1a). In a separate plan, the other two lesions were each treated together to 24 Gy in one fraction with dose prescribed to the 72% isodose line (Fig. 10.1b, c). She remains locally controlled at 1 year following radiosurgery, without neurological symptoms.

Case 2: Postresection Cavity Hypofractionated SRS over 5 Days due to Large Size

A 64-year-old woman with metastatic hormone-positive breast cancer presented with forgetfulness and abnormal behavior and was found to have a large cystic and solid right frontal mass measuring 5.5 cm with associated edema, subfalcine herniation, and midline shift. She underwent a gross total resection which revealed metastatic breast carcinoma. She was not able to undergo adjuvant radiosurgery until 2 months after her resection. At the time of her treatment planning, there was a thick rim of enhancement of the resection cavity margins, concerning for recurrent tumor. She underwent radiosurgery to the resection cavity with 2-mm margin to 25 Gy in five fractions. She developed nodular leptomeningeal progression 3 months following radiosurgery for which she completed whole-brain radiotherapy (Fig. 10.2).

Case 3: Hypofractionated SRS over 3 Days due to Large Size and Location

A 65-year-old woman with metastatic ovarian carcinoma, previously treated with SRS 6 months ago for four brain metastases, pre-

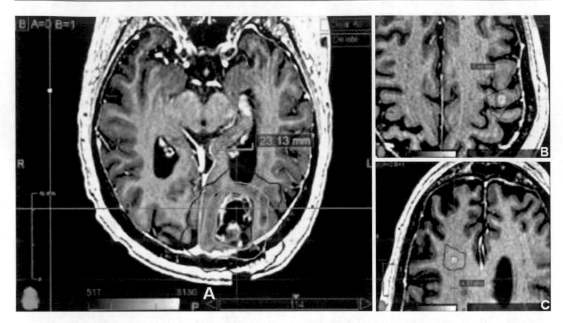

Fig. 10.1 Postresection cavity hypofractionated SRS due to size along with single-fraction SRS for small intact metastases. (**a**) Left parieto-occipital lesion (2.7 × 1.5 cm), status postresection of hemorrhagic portion, treated to 27 Gy in three fractions prescribed to the 72% isodose line (green 27 Gy, light blue 13.5 Gy, dark blue 6.75 Gy). (**b** and **c**) Left precentral gyrus lesion (7 × 5 mm) and right frontal lobe lesion (2 mm) treated in a separate plan to 24 Gy in one fraction prescribed to the 72% isodose line (green 24 Gy, light blue 12 Gy, dark blue 6 Gy)

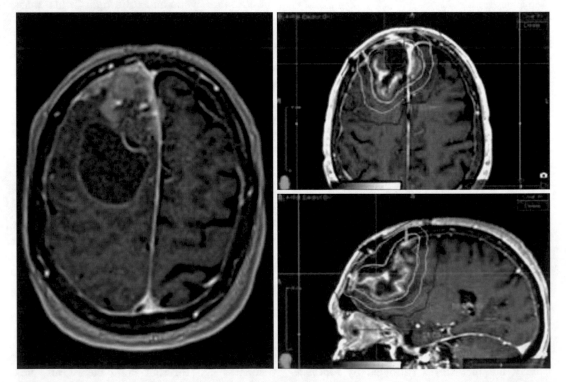

Fig. 10.2 Axial and sagittal views of right frontal resection cavity with 2-mm margin treated with 25 Gy in five fractions prescribed to the 72% isodose line. The preoperative MRI was fused with the postoperative images to aid in contouring the target volume. The preoperative extent rather than entire surgical tract was covered

sented with mild diplopia on far lateral gaze. MRI revealed a 2.7 × 2.7 cm metastasis in the pons. She received 24 Gy in three consecutive daily fractions to the 72% isodose line. Follow-up

MRI 9 months later revealed continued shrinkage of the tumor with no adverse radiation effect (Fig. 10.3).

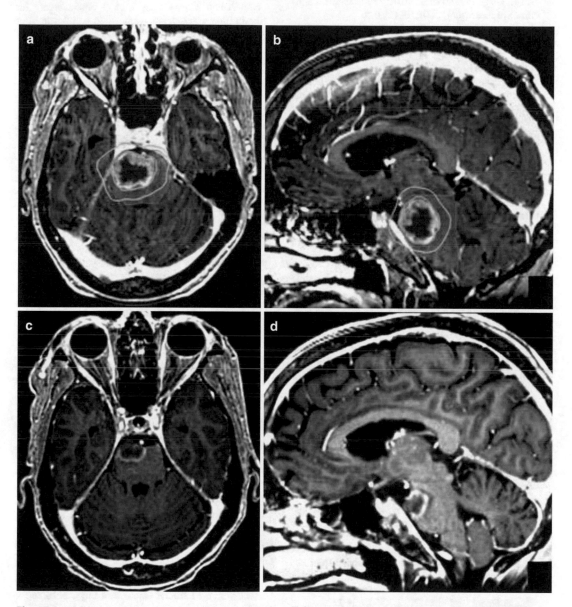

Fig. 10.3 Axial and sagittal views of pontine metastasis treated with 24 Gy (green isodose line) in three consecutive daily fractions to the 72% isodose line (**a** and **b**). Also shown is the 50% dose line in cyan (12 Gy isodose line). Follow-up MRI 9 months later (**c** and **d**) revealed continued shrinkage of the tumor with no adverse radiation effect

References

1. Barnett GH, Linskey ME, Adler JR, Cozzens JW, Friedman WA, Heilbrun MP, et al. Stereotactic radiosurgery—an organized neurosurgery-sanctioned definition. J Neurosurg. 2007;106(1):1–5.
2. Kirkpatrick JP, Soltys SG, Lo SS, Beal K, Shrieve DC, Brown PD. The radiosurgery fractionation quandary: single fraction or hypofractionation? Neuro Oncol. 2017;19(suppl_2):ii38–49.
3. Shaw E, Scott C, Souhami L, Dinapoli R, Kline R, Loeffler J, et al. Single dose radiosurgical treatment of recurrent previously irradiated primary brain tumors and brain metastases: final report of RTOG protocol 90-05. Int J Radiat Oncol Biol Phys. 2000;47(2):291–8.
4. Korytko T, Radivoyevitch T, Colussi V, Wessels BW, Pillai K, Maciunas RJ, et al. 12 Gy gamma knife radiosurgical volume is a predictor for radiation necrosis in non-AVM intracranial tumors. Int J Radiat Oncol Biol Phys. 2006;64(2):419–24.
5. Minniti G, Clarke E, Lanzetta G, Osti MF, Trasimeni G, Bozzao A, et al. Stereotactic radiosurgery for brain metastases: analysis of outcome and risk of brain radionecrosis. Radiat Oncol Lond Engl. 2011;6:48.
6. Blonigen BJ, Steinmetz RD, Levin L, Lamba MA, Warnick RE, Breneman JC. Irradiated volume as a predictor of brain radionecrosis after linear accelerator stereotactic radiosurgery. Int J Radiat Oncol Biol Phys. 2010;77(4):996–1001.
7. Doré M, Martin S, Delpon G, Clément K, Campion L, Thillays F. Stereotactic radiotherapy following surgery for brain metastasis: predictive factors for local control and radionecrosis. Cancer Radiother. 2017;21(1):4–9.
8. Choi CYH, Chang SD, Gibbs IC, Adler JR, Harsh GR, Lieberson RE, et al. Stereotactic radiosurgery of the postoperative resection cavity for brain metastases: prospective evaluation of target margin on tumor control. Int J Radiat Oncol Biol Phys. 2012;84(2):336–42.
9. Kirkpatrick JP, Wang Z, Sampson JH, McSherry F, Herndon JE, Allen KJ, et al. Defining the optimal planning target volume in image-guided stereotactic radiosurgery of brain metastases: results of a randomized trial. Int J Radiat Oncol Biol Phys. 2015;91(1):100–8.
10. Nataf F, Schlienger M, Liu Z, Foulquier JN, Grès B, Orthuon A, et al. Radiosurgery with or without a 2-mm margin for 93 single brain metastases. Int J Radiat Oncol Biol Phys. 2008;70(3):766–72.
11. Vogelbaum MA, Angelov L, Lee S-Y, Li L, Barnett GH, Suh JH. Local control of brain metastases by stereotactic radiosurgery in relation to dose to the tumor margin. J Neurosurg. 2006;104(6):907–12.
12. Hasegawa T, Kondziolka D, Flickinger JC, Germanwala A, Lunsford LD. Brain metastases treated with radiosurgery alone: an alternative to whole brain radiotherapy? Neurosurgery. 2003;52(6):1318–26.
13. Chang EL, Hassenbusch SJ, Shiu AS, Lang FF, Allen PK, Sawaya R, et al. The role of tumor size in the radiosurgical management of patients with ambiguous brain metastases. Neurosurgery. 2003;53(2):272–81.
14. Shiau C-Y, Sneed PK, Shu H-KG, Lamborn KR, McDermott MW, Chang S, et al. Radiosurgery for brain metastases: relationship of dose and pattern of enhancement to local control. Int J Radiat Oncol Biol Phys. 1997;37(2):375–83.
15. Adler JR Jr, Chang SD, Murphy MJ, Doty J, Geis P, Hancock SL. The Cyberknife: a frameless robotic system for radiosurgery. Stereotact Funct Neurosurg. 1997;69(1–4):124–8.
16. Fuss M, Salter BJ, Cheek D, Sadeghi A, Hevezi JM, Herman TS. Repositioning accuracy of a commercially available thermoplastic mask system. Radiother Oncol. 2004;71(3):339–45.
17. Li G, Ballangrud A, Chan M, Ma R, Beal K, Yamada Y, et al. Clinical experience with two frameless stereotactic radiosurgery (fSRS) systems using optical surface imaging for motion monitoring. J Appl Clin Med Phys. 2015;16(4):149–62.
18. Paris F, Fuks Z, Kang A, Capodieci P, Juan G, Ehleiter D, et al. Endothelial apoptosis as the primary lesion initiating intestinal radiation damage in mice. Science. 2001;293(5528):293–7.
19. Ch'ang H-J, Maj JG, Paris F, Xing HR, Zhang J, Truman J-P, et al. ATM regulates target switching to escalating doses of radiation in the intestines. Nat Med. 2005;11(5):484–90.
20. Brown JM, Koong AC. High-dose single-fraction radiotherapy: exploiting a new biology? Int J Radiat Oncol Biol Phys. 2008;71(2):324–5.
21. Brenner DJ, Martel MK, Hall EJ. Fractionated regimens for stereotactic radiotherapy of recurrent tumors in the brain. Int J Radiat Oncol Biol Phys. 1991;21(3):819–24.
22. Hall EJ, Brenner DJ. The radiobiology of radiosurgery: rationale for different treatment regimes for AVMs and malignancies. Int J Radiat Oncol Biol Phys. 1993;25(2):381–5.
23. Brown JM, Diehn M, Loo BW. Stereotactic ablative radiotherapy should be combined with a hypoxic cell radiosensitizer. Int J Radiat Oncol Biol Phys. 2010;78(2):323–7.
24. Ma L, Sahgal A, Descovich M, Cho Y-B, Chuang C, Huang K, et al. Equivalence in dose fall-off for isocentric and nonisocentric intracranial treatment modalities and its impact on dose fractionation schemes. Int J Radiat Oncol Biol Phys. 2010;76(3):943–8.
25. Demaria S, Golden EB, Formenti SC. Role of local radiation therapy in cancer immunotherapy. JAMA Oncol. 2015;1(9):1325.
26. Demaria S, Bhardwaj N, McBride WH, Formenti SC. Combining radiotherapy and immunotherapy: a revived partnership. Int J Radiat Oncol Biol Phys. 2005;63(3):655–66.
27. Dewan MZ, Galloway AE, Kawashima N, Dewyngaert JK, Babb JS, Formenti SC, et al.

Fractionated but not single-dose radiotherapy induces an immune-mediated abscopal effect when combined with anti-CTLA-4 antibody. Clin Cancer Res. 2009;15(17):5379–88.

28. Park HJ, Griffin RJ, Hui S, Levitt SH, Song CW. Radiation-induced vascular damage in tumors: implications of vascular damage in ablative hypofractionated radiotherapy (SBRT and SRS). Radiat Res. 2012;177(3):311–27.

29. Tsai M-H, Cook JA, Chandramouli GVR, DeGraff W, Yan H, Zhao S, et al. Gene expression profiling of breast, prostate, and glioma cells following single versus fractionated doses of radiation. Cancer Res. 2007;67(8):3845–52.

30. Aoki M, Abe Y, Hatayama Y, Kondo H, Basaki K. Clinical outcome of hypofractionated conventional conformation radiotherapy for patients with single and no more than three metastatic brain tumors, with noninvasive fixation of the skull without whole brain irradiation. Int J Radiat Oncol Biol Phys. 2006;64(2):414–8.

31. Aoyama H, Shirato H, Onimaru R, Kagei K, Ikeda J, Ishii N, et al. Hypofractionated stereotactic radiotherapy alone without whole-brain irradiation for patients with solitary and oligo brain metastasis using noninvasive fixation of the skull. Int J Radiat Oncol Biol Phys. 2003;56(3):793–800.

32. Ernst-Stecken A, Ganslandt O, Lambrecht U, Sauer R, Grabenbauer G. Phase II trial of hypofractionated stereotactic radiotherapy for brain metastases: results and toxicity. Radiother Oncol. 2006;81(1):18–24.

33. Fahrig A, Ganslandt O, Lambrecht U, Grabenbauer G, Kleinert G, Sauer R, et al. Hypofractionated stereotactic radiotherapy for brain metastases: results from three different dose concepts. Strahlenther Onkol. 2007;183(11):625–30.

34. Fokas E, Henzel M, Surber G, Kleinert G, Hamm K, Engenhart-Cabillic R. Stereotactic radiosurgery and fractionated stereotactic radiotherapy: comparison of efficacy and toxicity in 260 patients with brain metastases. J Neuro-Oncol. 2012;109(1):91–8.

35. Higuchi Y, Serizawa T, Nagano O, Matsuda S, Ono J, Sato M, et al. Three-staged stereotactic radiotherapy without whole brain irradiation for large metastatic brain tumors. Int J Radiat Oncol Biol Phys. 2009;74(5):1543–8.

36. Kim Y-J, Cho KH, Kim J-Y, Lim YK, Min HS, Lee SH, et al. Single-dose versus fractionated stereotactic radiotherapy for brain metastases. Int J Radiat Oncol Biol Phys. 2011;81(2):483–9.

37. Kwon AK, DiBiase SJ, Wang B, Hughes SL, Milcarek B, Zhu Y. Hypofractionated stereotactic radiotherapy for the treatment of brain metastases. Cancer. 2009;115(4):890–8.

38. Lindvall P, Bergström P, Löfroth P-O, Tommy Bergenheim A. A comparison between surgical resection in combination with WBRT or hypofractionated stereotactic irradiation in the treatment of solitary brain metastases. Acta Neurochir. 2009;151(9):1053–9.

39. Lockney NA, Wang DG, Gutin PH, Brennan C, Tabar V, Ballangrud A, et al. Clinical outcomes of patients with limited brain metastases treated with hypofractionated (5 × 6 Gy) conformal radiotherapy. Radiother Oncol. 2017;123(2):203–8.

40. Manning MA, Cardinale RM, Benedict SH, Kavanagh BD, Zwicker RD, Amir C, et al. Hypofractionated stereotactic radiotherapy as an alternative to radiosurgery for the treatment of patients with brain metastases. Int J Radiat Oncol Biol Phys. 2000;47(3):603–8.

41. Marcrom SR, McDonald AM, Thompson JW, Popple RA, Riley KO, Markert JM, et al. Fractionated stereotactic radiation therapy for intact brain metastases. Adv Radiat Oncol. 2017;2(4):564–71.

42. Märtens B, Janssen S, Werner M, Frühauf J, Christiansen H, Bremer M, et al. Hypofractionated stereotactic radiotherapy of limited brain metastases: a single-centre individualized treatment approach. BMC Cancer. 2012;12:497.

43. Matsuyama T, Kogo K, Oya N. Clinical outcomes of biological effective dose-based fractionated stereotactic radiation therapy for metastatic brain tumors from non-small cell lung cancer. Int J Radiat Oncol Biol Phys. 2013;85(4):984–90.

44. Minniti G, D'Angelillo RM, Scaringi C, Trodella LE, Clarke E, Matteucci P, et al. Fractionated stereotactic radiosurgery for patients with brain metastases. J Neuro-Oncol. 2014;117(2):295–301.

45. Minniti G, Scaringi C, Paolini S, Lanzetta G, Romano A, Cicone F, et al. Single-fraction versus multifraction (3 × 9 Gy) stereotactic radiosurgery for large (>2 cm) brain metastases: a comparative analysis of local control and risk of radiation-induced brain necrosis. Int J Radiat Oncol Biol Phys. 2016;95(4):1142–8.

46. Narayana A, Chang J, Yenice K, Chan K, Lymberis S, Brennan C, et al. Hypofractionated stereotactic radiotherapy using intensity-modulated radiotherapy in patients with one or two brain metastases. Stereotact Funct Neurosurg. 2007;85(2–3):82–7.

47. Oermann EK, Kress M-AS, Todd JV, Collins BT, Hoffman R, Chaudhry H, et al. The impact of radiosurgery fractionation and tumor radiobiology on the local control of brain metastases: clinical article. J Neurosurg. 2013;119(5):1131–8.

48. Ogura K, Mizowaki T, Ogura M, Sakanaka K, Arakawa Y, Miyamoto S, et al. Outcomes of hypofractionated stereotactic radiotherapy for metastatic brain tumors with high risk factors. J Neuro-Oncol. 2012;109(2):425–32.

49. Rajakesari S, Arvold ND, Jimenez RB, Christianson LW, Horvath MC, Claus EB, et al. Local control after fractionated stereotactic radiation therapy for brain metastases. J Neuro-Oncol. 2014;120(2):339–46.

50. Saitoh J, Saito Y, Kazumoto T, Kudo S, Ichikawa A, Hayase N, et al. Therapeutic effect of Linac-based stereotactic radiotherapy with a micro-multileaf collimator for the treatment of patients with brain metastases from lung cancer. Jpn J Clin Oncol. 2010;40(2):119–24.

51. Tokuuye K, Akine Y, Sumi M, Kagami Y, Murayama S, Nakayama H, et al. Fractionated stereotactic radiotherapy of small intracranial malignancies. Int J Radiat Oncol Biol Phys. 1998;42(5):989–94.

52. Wiggenraad R, Kanter AV, Kal HB, Taphoorn M, Vissers T, Struikmans H. Dose-effect relation in stereotactic radiotherapy for brain metastases. A systematic review. Radiother Oncol. 2011;98(3):292–7.

53. Patchell RA, Tibbs PA, Regine WF, Dempsey RJ, Mohiuddin M, Kryscio RJ, et al. Postoperative radiotherapy in the treatment of single metastases to the brain: a randomized trial. JAMA. 1998;280(17):1485–9.

54. Kocher M, Soffietti R, Abacioglu U, Villà S, Fauchon F, Baumert BG, et al. Adjuvant whole-brain radiotherapy versus observation after radiosurgery or surgical resection of one to three cerebral metastases: results of the EORTC 22952-26001 study. J Clin Oncol. 2011;29(2):134–41.

55. Mahajan A, Ahmed S, McAleer MF, Weinberg JS, Li J, Brown P, et al. Post-operative stereotactic radiosurgery versus observation for completely resected brain metastases: a single-centre, randomised, controlled, phase 3 trial. Lancet Oncol. 2017;18(8):1040–8.

56. Brown PD, Ballman KV, Cerhan JH, Anderson SK, Carrero XW, Whitton AC, et al. Postoperative stereotactic radiosurgery compared with whole brain radiotherapy for resected metastatic brain disease (NCCTG N107C/CEC·3): a multicentre, randomised, controlled, phase 3 trial. Lancet Oncol. 2017;18(8):1049–60.

57. Soltys SG, Adler JR, Lipani JD, Jackson PS, Choi CYH, Puataweepong P, et al. Stereotactic radiosurgery of the postoperative resection cavity for brain metastases. Int J Radiat Oncol Biol Phys. 2008;70(1):187–93.

58. Brennan C, Yang TJ, Hilden P, Zhang Z, Chan K, Yamada Y, et al. A phase 2 trial of stereotactic radiosurgery boost after surgical resection for brain metastases. Int J Radiat Oncol Biol Phys. 2014;88(1):130–6.

59. Ojerholm E, Miller D, Geiger GA, Lustig RA. Stereotactic radiosurgery to the resection bed for intracranial metastases and risk of leptomeningeal carcinomatosis. J Neurosurg. 2014;121:9.

60. Minniti G, Esposito V, Clarke E, Scaringi C, Lanzetta G, Salvati M, et al. Multidose stereotactic radiosurgery (9 Gy × 3) of the postoperative resection cavity for treatment of large brain metastases. Int J Radiat Oncol Biol Phys. 2013;86(4):623–9.

61. Atalar B, Choi CYH, Harsh GR, Chang SD, Gibbs IC, Adler JR, et al. Cavity volume dynamics after resection of brain metastases and timing of postresection cavity stereotactic radiosurgery. Neurosurgery. 2013;72(2):180–5.

62. Iorio-Morin C, Ezahr Y. Early Gamma Knife stereotactic radiosurgery to the tumor bed of resected brain metastasis for improved local control. J Neurosurg. 2014;121:6.

63. Abuodeh Y, Ahmed KA, Naghavi AO, Venkat PS, Sarangkasiri S, Johnstone PAS, et al. Postoperative stereotactic radiosurgery using 5-Gy × 5 sessions in the management of brain metastases. World Neurosurg. 2016;90:58–65.

64. Ahmed KA, Freilich JM, Abuodeh Y, Figura N, Patel N, Sarangkasiri S, et al. Fractionated stereotactic radiotherapy to the post-operative cavity for radioresistant and radiosensitive brain metastases. J Neuro-Oncol. 2014;118(1):179–86.

65. Ammirati M, Kshettry VR, Lamki T, Wei L, Grecula JC. A prospective phase II trial of fractionated stereotactic intensity modulated radiotherapy with or without surgery in the treatment of patients with 1 to 3 newly diagnosed symptomatic brain metastases. Neurosurgery. 2014;74(6):586–94.

66. Connolly EP, Mathew M, Tam M, King JV, Kunnakkat SD, Parker EC, et al. Involved field radiation therapy after surgical resection of solitary brain metastases—mature results. Neuro Oncol. 2013;15(5):589–94.

67. Do L, Pezner R, Radany E, Liu A, Staud C, Badie B. Resection followed by stereotactic radiosurgery to resection cavity for intracranial metastases. Int J Radiat Oncol Biol Phys. 2009;73(2):486–91.

68. Keller A, Doré M, Cebula H, Thillays F, Proust F, Darié I, et al. Hypofractionated stereotactic radiation therapy to the resection bed for intracranial metastases. Int J Radiat Oncol Biol Phys. 2017;99(5):1179–89.

69. Kumar AMS, Miller J, Hoffer SA, Mansur DB, Coffey M, Lo SS, et al. Postoperative hypofractionated stereotactic brain radiation (HSRT) for resected brain metastases: improved local control with higher BED10. J Neuro-Oncol. 2018;139(2):449–54.

70. Ling DC, Vargo JA, Wegner RE, Flickinger JC, Burton SA, Engh J, et al. Postoperative stereotactic radiosurgery to the resection cavity for large brain metastases: clinical outcomes, predictors of intracranial failure, and implications for optimal patient selection. Neurosurgery. 2015;76(2):150–7.

71. Pessina F, Navarria P, Cozzi L, Ascolese AM, Maggi G, Riva M, et al. Outcome evaluation of oligometastatic patients treated with surgical resection followed by hypofractionated stereotactic radiosurgery (HSRS) on the tumor bed, for single, large brain metastases. Sherman JH, editor. PLoS One. 2016;11(6): e0157869.

72. Steinmann D, Maertens B, Janssen S, Werner M, Frühauf J, Nakamura M, et al. Hypofractionated stereotactic radiotherapy (hfSRT) after tumour resection of a single brain metastasis: report of a single-centre individualized treatment approach. J Cancer Res Clin Oncol. 2012;138(9):1523–9.

73. Vogel J, Ojerholm E, Hollander A, Briola C, Mooij R, Bieda M, et al. Intracranial control after Cyberknife radiosurgery to the resection bed for large brain metastases. Radiat Oncol. 2015;10(1):221. Available from: http://www.ro-journal.com/content/10/1/221.

74. Wang C-C, Floyd SR, Chang C-H, Warnke PC, Chio C-C, Kasper EM, et al. Cyberknife hypofractionated stereotactic radiosurgery (HSRS) of resection cavity after excision of large cerebral metastasis: efficacy and safety of an 800 cGy × 3 daily fractions regimen. J Neurooncol. 2012;106(3):601–10.

75. Park C, Papiez L, Zhang S, Story M, Timmerman RD. Universal survival curve and single fraction equivalent dose: useful tools in understanding potency of ablative radiotherapy. Int J Radiat Oncol Biol Phys. 2008;70(3):847–52.

76. Quon HC, Ong A, Cheung P, Chu W, Chung HT, Vesprini D, et al. Once-weekly versus every-other-day stereotactic body radiotherapy in patients with prostate cancer (PATRIOT): a phase 2 randomized trial. Radiother Oncol. 2018;127(2):206–12.

77. Alite F, Stang K, Balasubramanian N, Adams W, Shaikh MP, Small C, et al. Local control dependence on consecutive vs. nonconsecutive fractionation in lung stereotactic body radiation therapy. Radiother Oncol. 2016;121(1):9–14.

78. Jain S, Poon I, Soliman H, Keller B, Kim A, Lochray F, et al. Lung stereotactic body radiation therapy (SBRT) delivered over 4 or 11 days: a comparison of acute toxicity and quality of life. Radiother Oncol. 2013;108(2):320–5.

79. Bender ET. Brain necrosis after fractionated radiation therapy: is the halftime for repair longer than we thought? Med Phys. 2012;39(11):7055–61.

80. Kclada OJ, Decker RH, Nath SK, Johung KL, Zheng M-Q, Huang Y, et al. High single doses of radiation may induce elevated levels of hypoxia in early-stage non-small cell lung cancer tumors.

Int J Radiat Oncol Biol Phys. 2018;102(1):174–83.

81. Samson P, Rehman S, Juloori A, DeWees T, Roach M, Bradley J, et al. Local control for clinical stage I non-small cell lung cancer treated with 5-fraction stereotactic body radiation therapy is not associated with treatment schedule. Pract Radiat Oncol. 2018;8(6):404–13.

82. Yomo S, Hayashi M, Nicholson C. A prospective pilot study of two-session Gamma Knife surgery for large metastatic brain tumors. J Neuro-Oncol. 2012;109(1):159–65.

83. Angelov L, Mohammadi AM, Bennett EE, Abbassy M, Elson P, Chao ST, et al. Impact of 2-staged stereotactic radiosurgery for treatment of brain metastases ≥ 2 cm. J Neurosurg. 2018;129:366–82.

84. Yomo S, Hayashi M. A minimally invasive treatment option for large metastatic brain tumors: long-term results of two-session Gamma Knife stereotactic radiosurgery. Radiat Oncol Lond Engl. 2014;9:132.

85. Churilla TM, Chowdhury IH, Handorf E, Collette L, Collette S, Dong Y, et al. Comparison of local control of brain metastases with stereotactic radiosurgery vs surgical resection: a secondary analysis of a randomized clinical trial. JAMA Oncol. 2019;5(2):243–7. Available from: https://jamanetwork.com/journals/jamaoncology/fullarticle/2713842.

Target Delineation for Radiosurgery (Including Postoperative Cavity Radiosurgery) in Brain Metastases

11

Balamurugan A. Vellayappan, Mei Chin Lim, Clement Yong, Kejia Teo, Shawn Malone, and Simon Lo

Case Vignettes

Case 1

A 76-year-old woman presented with a known history of metastatic breast cancer (ER/PR negative, Her 2 positive). She had been previously treated with stereotactic radiosurgery (SRS) for two brain lesions located in the frontal lobe and left cerebellum 2 years prior. She now presents with gait unsteadiness. T1-contrast-enhanced MRI shows two large cerebellar metastases (cer-

ebellar vermis 1.9 cm × 1.6 cm, right cerebellar hemisphere 1.8 cm × 2.3 cm), with mass effect and effacement of the fourth ventricle causing early hydrocephalus. She underwent resection of the larger superficial lesion in the right cerebellar hemisphere. Systemic staging scans showed the extracranial disease to be controlled. She was then treated with hypofractionated stereotactic radiotherapy (HSRT) to the cavity and residual metastasis (25 Gy in five fractions, prescribed to the 80% isodose line). Her imaging and target volumes are presented in Fig. 11.1.

Case 2

A 70-year-old woman presented with headache and left hemiparesis. T1-contrast-enhanced MRI showed a predominantly cystic metastasis in the right frontal lobe, measuring 5 cm × 4 cm. Five other small subcentimeter BMs were noted. Biopsy of the lung lesion showed a non-small-cell lung adenocarcinoma, with molecular subtype exhibiting EGFR mutation in exon 20 (denoting resistance to tyrosine-kinase inhibitors), ALK/ROS1 negative, and PDL1 score of 11%. She underwent Ommaya reservoir insertion to drain the large cystic metastases, with a view to perform single-fraction SRS thereafter. Unfortunately, there was relatively quick cyst fluid reaccumu-

B. A. Vellayappan (✉)
Department of Radiation Oncology, National University Cancer Institute Singapore, National University Health System, Singapore, Singapore
e-mail: bala_vellayappan@nuhs.edu.sg

M. C. Lim · C. Yong
Department of Diagnostic Imaging, National University Hospital, National University Health System, Singapore, Singapore

K. Teo
Department of Neurosurgery, National University Hospital, National University Health System, Singapore, Singapore

S. Malone
The Ottawa Hospital Regional Cancer Center, Ottawa, ON, Canada

S. Lo
Department of Radiation Oncology, University of Washington School of Medicine, Seattle, WA, USA

© Springer Nature Switzerland AG 2020
Y. Yamada et al. (eds.), *Radiotherapy in Managing Brain Metastases*,
https://doi.org/10.1007/978-3-030-43740-4_11

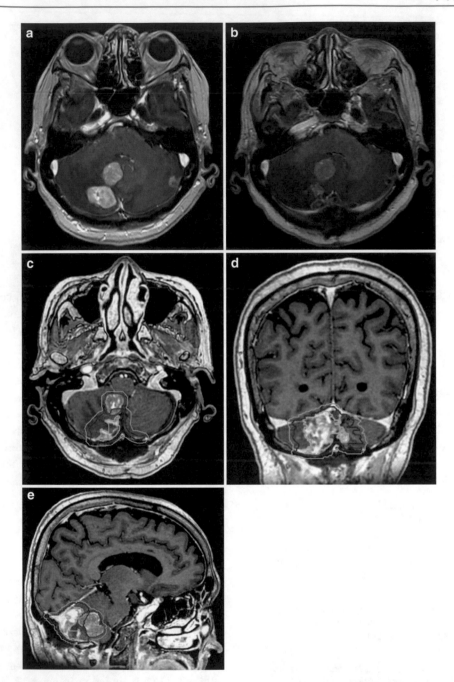

Fig. 11.1 (**a**) Preoperative axial T1-contrast imaging showing two cerebellar metastases causing effacement of the 4th ventricle. (**b**) Postoperative axial T1-contrast imaging demonstrating resection of the larger superficial lesion. (**c–e**) Target volume definition: postoperative cavity (lime green), cavity clinical target volume (blue), gross tumor volume for intact metastasis (red), and planning target volume (olive green)

lation and therefore the patient had to undergo resection of the dominant right frontal BM. She was treated with HSRT to the right frontal resection cavity (30 Gy in five fractions prescribed to 80% isodose line) and SRS to the remaining lesions. The relevant imaging and target volumes for the right frontal cavity are shown in Fig. 11.2.

Introduction

Brain metastases (BMs) occur in up to 60% of patients with cancer and cause morbidity and mortality in these patients [1]. This number is expected to increase due to more effective systemic therapy, which is able to provide extracranial tumor control, and due to more sensitive brain imaging, which is able to detect small volume metastases.

Approximately one-half of patients with BM present with a single metastatic lesion [2]. Since the brain is devoid of lymphatic vessels, cancer cells can enter the brain only via a hematogenous route [3]. Certain cancer primaries have a predilection to seed the brain and account for up to 80% of BM – these include primary lung, melanoma, breast, and renal cell cancers [4]. BMs are commonly situated in the cerebral hemispheres (80%) at the gray–white matter junction where tumor cells lodge at the final capillary arborization [5]. The cerebellar hemispheres (15%) and basal ganglia (3%) are less frequently involved [6].

In this chapter, we will briefly review the imaging features and treatment approach of BM. In particular, we will provide a practical approach for the use of SRS for BM, including the postoperative scenario.

Imaging Features of BM on CT and MRI

Computed tomography (CT) is often used as an initial screening tool for symptomatic patients, as it allows early recognition of time-critical events, such as intracranial mass effect, hydro-cephalus, and hemorrhagic events [7]. Iodinated intravenous contrast helps diagnosis when metastases may not be large enough to cause mass effect or have significant peritumoral edema, but unfortunately, contrast-enhanced CT alone can have a false negative rate of up to 19%, especially in locations with significant volume of bone causing beam hardening, such as in the low frontotemporal region and posterior fossa [8].

MRI is clearly the imaging modality of choice for the evaluation and delineation of BM. Multiple studies have unequivocally confirmed its superiority over CT for the detection of subcentimeter lesions and leptomeningeal carcinomatosis [8–11]. On T1-weighted imaging (T1WI), BMs are typically isointense to hypointense in appearance. Hemorrhagic BMs, which are commonly seen with lung and renal cell cancers, are hyperintense on T1WI (Fig. 11.3). BMs from melanoma are also hyperintense on T1WI due to the T1 hyperintensity of melanin. On T2-weighted imaging (T2WI), BM are typically hyperintense, unless there has been an underlying hemorrhage. The presence of vasogenic edema, which occurs due to blood–brain barrier disruption, is best assessed on T2WI and will show hyperintense white matter changes surrounding the BM. Frequently, BM tends to demonstrate facilitated diffusion (elevated values on apparent diffusion coefficient [ADC] maps with high value on diffusion-weighted imaging [DWI]) as opposed to restricted diffusion seen in cerebral abscesses (low ADC values) [12].

Intravenous infusion of gadolinium during image acquisition increases metastasis detection. The postcontrast sequences are generally T1WI with or without fat-suppression techniques. Angiogenesis stimulated by the metastasis lacks the blood–brain barrier and facilitates leakage of gadolinium into the interstitial tissues, causing avid parenchymal enhancement (Fig. 11.4) by altering the local proton magnetic environment. In larger BM, especially those with hemorrhage or cystic changes, the tumoral enhancement tends to be heterogeneous (due to central necrosis). Delaying

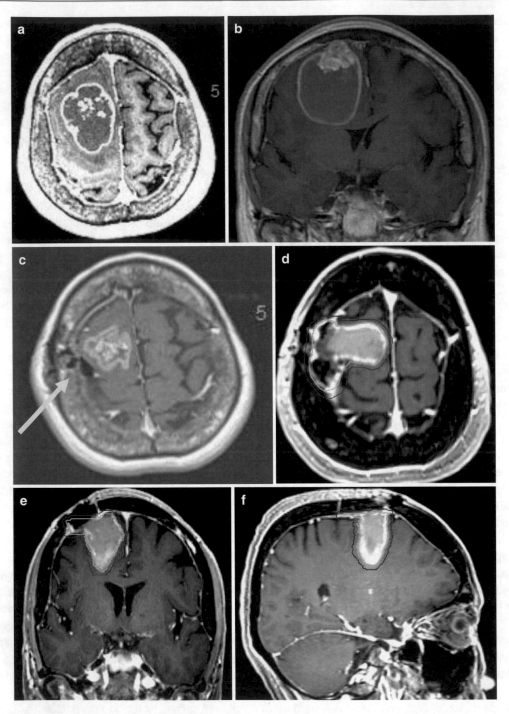

Fig. 11.2 (**a**, **b**) Axial and coronal T1-contrast MRI showing a large cystic metastasis in the R frontal lobe. Rim enhancement is demonstrated and nodularities are seen superiorly. Dural contact is seen on image (**b**). (**c**) Collapse of the cystic lesion after insertion of Ommaya reservoir (yellow arrow). (**d–f**) Images showing the target volume for stereotactic treatment. Note that the resection tract and overlying dura are included and the overlying. CTV (green outline), PTV (red outline)

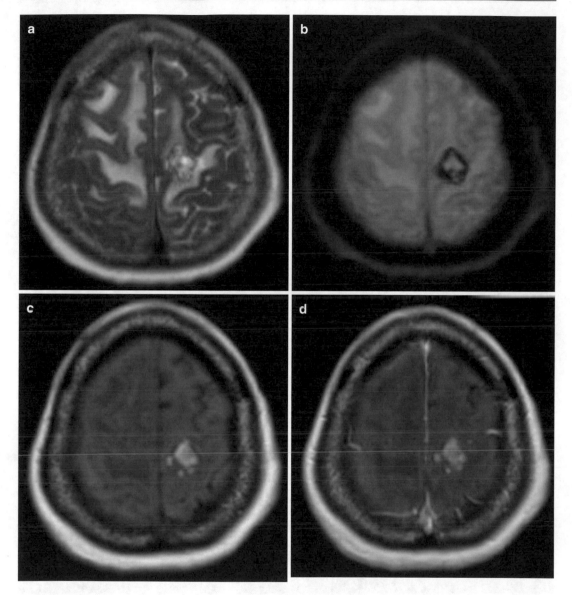

Fig. 11.3 Cystic hemorrhagic BM in a 56-year-old man with known metastatic lung cancer. (**a**) Axial T2WI sequence demonstrates a lobulated T2W hyperintense mass in the left frontal lobe with prominent surrounding vasogenic edema. Note the presence of vasogenic edema also in the right frontal lobe. (**b**) Axial T2* gradient echo sequence shows that the mass has peripheral hemosiderin rim from chronic blood products. (**c**) Precontrast T1WI VIBE sequence shows that that mass is inherently bright, suggestive of the presence of methemoglobin which is seen in subacute blood products. (**d**) Postcontrast T1WI VIBE sequence again shows T1W hyperintensity of the left frontal lobe mass. True enhancement cannot be accurately ascertained in the presence of hemorrhage

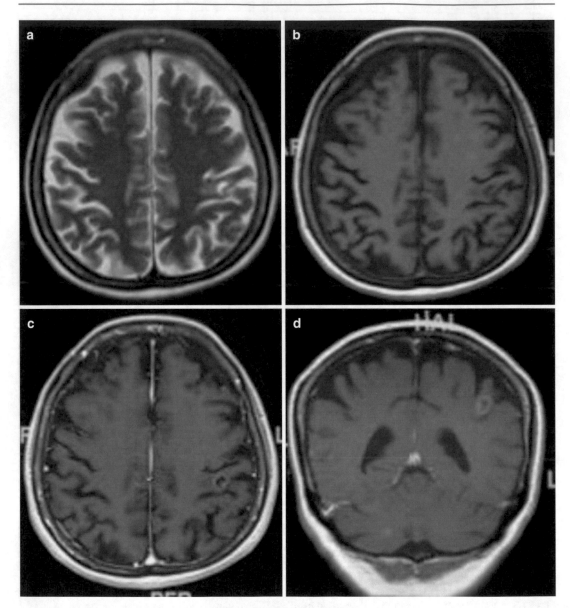

Fig. 11.4 Ring-enhancing BM in a 73-year-old man with known metastatic lung cancer. (**a**) Axial T2WI sequence reveals a small T2W hyperintense lesion in the left frontal lobe with mild surrounding edema. (**b**) Precontrast axial T1WI VIBE sequence shows that the lesion is slightly hypointense, which demonstrates ring enhancement on (**c**) postcontrast axial T1WI VIBE sequence and (**d**) postcontrast coronal T1WI sequence. Another small ring-enhancing BM is seen in the right cerebellar hemisphere (**d**)

imaging by 10–15 min after gadolinium administration increases the conspicuity and detection of small metastases, perhaps by permitting more gadolinium to diffuse out through the relatively small surface area of the small metastasis' neovasculature [13].

Evolution of BM Management

BMs, unfortunately, are associated with a high mortality rate with the median survival typically being measured in months. As such, many have assumed a fatalistic approach upon the diagnosis of BM and withhold aggressive cancer treatment. Whole-brain radiotherapy (WBRT) came into the foray when an early study showed that it improved survival, compared to historical controls who were treated with corticosteroids alone [14]. Due to its wide availability, ease of administration, and relatively low cost, it was considered to be the standard treatment until recently. In more recent years, advances in neuroimaging, neurosurgery, and systemic therapeutics have afforded longer survival in patients, and consequently, the long-term effects of WBRT have caused heightened concerns [15]. Moreover, WBRT alone has not produced sustained local intracranial control, and more efficacious modalities were favored [16, 17].

Stereotactic Radiosurgery (SRS)

SRS refers to the delivery of radiation, in one session, using multiple focused beams to deposit an ablative dose to the tumor in a highly conformal manner (while avoiding high doses to surrounding brain tissue). Notably, the inherent characteristics of BM, such as spherical shape, well-demarcated border, and absence of normal brain parenchyma inside the tumor volume, make them suitable for the delivery of SRS.

Although there are no published randomized controlled trials (RCT) comparing SRS to WBRT, many prospective studies have shown SRS alone to have superior local control rates [18–22]. In addition, the detriment in quality of life (QoL) and neurocognition seen with WBRT have prompted many to defer the routine use of adjuvant WBRT [23]. There are now a multitude of platforms available to perform intracranial SRS, and these include Gamma Knife, CyberKnife, or linear-accelerator-based technologies [24]. A full review of these technologies is beyond the scope of this chapter, but readers are encouraged to know the intricate differences between these machines [25].

Surgery

With the rise and efficacy of SRS, the indications of surgical resection are generally reserved for patients with large tumors exhibiting mass effect, surgically accessible lesions causing neurological deficits or when the diagnosis is uncertain (for confirmation of tumor histology). The goal is to achieve gross-total resection of the tumor. Most metastatic tumors have a pseudocapsule that facilitates en bloc removal. For larger tumors, only an intralesional resection may be possible (i.e., tumor debulking). If resections are performed in a piecemeal fashion, the risk of local recurrence remains exceedingly high without adjuvant treatment. For example, a recent single-center RCT reported the risk of local recurrence after resection to be 56% at 12 months [26].

Adjuvant WBRT had been demonstrated, nearly 20 years earlier, in an RCT to reduce the risk of intracranial recurrence postresection; however, this increased locoregional control comes at a cost of QoL and neurocognitive impairment with no survival benefit [27]. This trade-off prompted investigators to explore the use of "limited" brain radiotherapy, in lieu of WBRT. Initial results showed that the local control rates were comparable to historical WBRT series and superior to observation alone [28]. Surprisingly, the group with the least conformal plan had the best control rates, suggesting that marginal misses through suboptimal target delineation or local tumor infiltration may be contributory.

A follow-on study demonstrated that using a 2-mm margin around the resection cavity decreased local failure rates without causing more toxicity [29]. Brown et al. recently reported the NCCTG N107C/RTOG 12-70 trial which compared resection cavity SRS to WBRT [21]. Although the overall survival was not different between arms, the SRS-only arm had improved cognitive-deterioration-free survival. However, one has to note that the WBRT arm did demonstrate improved intracranial control. Possible explanations for this include overconservative target delineation and/or interobserver variation in target delineation, and inadequate radiosurgery dose prescription for large cavities.

Patient Selection for SRS

In general, patients should be well selected for SRS. Factors to consider for patient selection include age, performance status, extracranial tumor control, number, and volume of brain metastases. Median life expectancy can be estimated using prognostic algorithms, such as the disease-specific graded prognostic assessment (ds-GPA) [30]. With regard to maximal lesion size, various trials have allowed patients with a maximal lesion diameter of 5 cm to be enrolled [31]. Large lesions may not be suitable for single-fraction SRS, as the risk of complications (in particular symptomatic radionecrosis) increases. Strategies for the management of large BM are discussed elsewhere in this book.

Patient Immobilization

Patient immobilization is a critical step in the delivery of SRS, as errors in localization have been shown to contribute most to treatment failure [32, 33].

Frame-based SRS has traditionally been used for SRS. This involves rigid fixation of a MRI-compatible stereotactic metallic frame, using pins, into the outer table of the skull. Frame-based techniques provide submillimeter accuracy. Fiducial coordinates, which are built into the metallic frame system, are subsequently used for locating the isocenter during treatment delivery. It is usually well tolerated; however, there remains a small risk of infection and bleeding at the site of pin placement.

In recent years, frameless SRS is increasingly being used as it allows for patient comfort and reproducible setup while maintaining a high level of precision. A custom-made near-rigid thermoplastic face mask is utilized, together with bite blocks and vacuum-cushioned neck rests or customized thermoplastic headrests. Image-guidance systems such as on-board cone-beam CT (CBCT) are used for pretreatment image verification or stereoscopic x-rays for monitoring the skull position during treatment. To improve patient immobilization, both interfractional and intrafractional motions need to be reduced. Interfractional motion can be reduced significantly by utilizing online imaging, together with a 6 degree-of-freedom robotic couch. Guckenberger et al. reported that the setup error (while using a frame-less system) can be reduced from 3.9 ± 1.7 mm to 0.9 ± 0.6 mm by adding CBCT image guidance [34]. However, the residual error (caused by intrafractional motion) of 0.9 mm remained. Additional stereoscopic imaging to monitor and correct intrafraction motion is possible with specially equipped linear accelerators and CyberKnife platforms. Interfractional motion has been shown to be reduced by the use of bite blocks [35].

In single-fraction SRS with online correction, only intrafractional motion needs to be considered. Both frame-based and frameless systems have been shown to have low levels of intrafraction motion (mean intrafractional shift 0.4 ± 0.3 mm vs 0.7 ± 0.5 mm) [36]. However, 3% of frame-based patients in that same study showed an intrafraction shift of 1 mm or more, whereas 22% of frameless patients showed an intrafraction shift of 1 mm or more. Overall treatment time prolongation has been reported to increase intrafractional motion, and we try to keep treatment times for frameless SRS within 20 min [34].

Simulation and Required Pretreatment Imaging

For most treatment platforms, other than Gamma Knife, a simulation CT is required. Having CT imaging is useful for electron density calculations, especially in skull base locations where air cavities can cause dose inhomogeneity by altering electronic equilibrium. In addition, compared to MRI, CT has superior spatial accuracy, as it is not subject to distortion. As such, if enough landmarks can be identified on both CT and MRI, the spatial accuracy of the MRI (which is used for target delineation) can be verified.

For simulation, the patient must be comfortable and pain-free throughout the procedure. Patients with claustrophobia may not be suitable candidates for SRS. Excessive use of sedatives or anxiolytics increases risk, as monitoring patients with impaired levels of consciousness during simulation and treatment can be challenging. We typically position patients straight and supine with arms by their side. A knee pillow is provided for comfort. As mentioned earlier, there are multiple options for immobilization, and these include both frame-based and frameless systems (thermoplastic mask with or without bite block). We typically use CT settings of 120 kV and 350 mA and scan the patient from vertex to the bottom of C3 vertebrae using a helical scanning approach. This allows reformatting the data into any slice thickness. We recommend axial slices of 1-mm thickness. A CT localizer box is placed over the patient's head prior to the scan. This is used for referencing 2D fiducial coordinates, which are then used to calculate treatment isocenter. Adhesive metallic point markers can also be used to establish the isocenter at the time of simulation (which can then be used to establish treatment isocenters). The use of iodinated contrast during CT simulation is optional and is not routinely recommended for patients undergoing MRI for target delineation.

Pretreatment Imaging

A contrast-enhanced MRI is critical for BM SRS. Each department should protocolize the MRI settings for SRS planning. A minimum field strength of 1.5 Tesla and slice thickness of 2 mm or less is recommended [37]. We recommend that all patients undergoing SRS have a recent high-resolution volumetric MRI (as close to, or at least within 1–2 weeks of the treatment date). Garcia and colleagues have shown that BMs grow at an average of 0.02 ml/day, with a projected increase in volume by 1.35-fold at 2 weeks [38]. Similarly, Salkeld and colleagues showed that changes in management were more frequently needed if there was more than 1-week

interval between cavity SRS planning MRI and the actual delivery of SRS [39].

The current standard stereotactic MR imaging protocol used at NCIS is performed on a 3-Tesla (3 T) Siemens MAGNETOM Skyra MRI system (Siemens Medical Solutions, Erlangen, Germany) with a Siemens Head/Neck 20-channel coil. The SRS protocol is used in complement of a full diagnostic MRI study, and only the SRS postcontrast isotropic T1W gradient echo sequence (GRE) is described below. The MRI contrast used is gadoterate meglumine (Dotarem®, Guerbet, Roissy CDG, France), a macrocyclic gadolinium-based contrast agent. This is administered intravenously at a standard 0.01 mmol/kg dose at a rate of 2 cc/second, followed by a 10-cc saline flush. The postcontrast sequence is performed approximately 10 min after injection [13]. The isotropic T1W GRE imaging used is a volumetric interpolated brain examination (VIBE) T1W sequence, which is a radiofrequency spoiled 3D GRE sequence (TR/ TE = 6.36/2.46 ms, 15° flip angle), with gapless 1.0-mm slice thickness, matrix of 256 × 256, and a field of view (FOV) of 256 mm. Slice oversampling of 15% is performed to prevent aliasing artifact of the slices. It is recommended that the images are acquired without angulation (to facilitate CT-MR co-registration).

Higher doses of gadolinium have proven advantages over standard doses in detecting small metastases [40, 41]. A report that found triple dose contrast-enhanced MRI superior for metastasis detection to delayed imaging with standard dose [42] was performed using 5- to 10-mm-thick slices, and thus may not be applicable for modern SRS applications. Double doses of gadolinium were shown to provide a more precise delineation of the gross tumor volume for radiosurgery [43]. Notwithstanding the improved detection, the use of higher contrast doses has been associated with increased false positives (such as mistaking normal vascular enhancement for small BM) [44].

Special mention is needed to highlight the inherent spatial and geometric distortion present in MRI images. Although these are typically subtle, such distortions can significantly impact the accuracy of SRS. These arise due to factors including static-field inhomogeneity, eddy currents, and gradient nonlinearity [45, 46]. Distortions are more pronounced with lesions at the radial margin of the magnetic field (i.e., periphery of the brain), with reported errors of up to 2 mm. Neumann and colleagues showed that distortion is more marked with the higher strength gradient coils such as a 7-Tesla scanner, as opposed to the 1.5- and 3-Tesla machines commonly used in current practice [47]. Thankfully, most modern MRI scanners come with distortion correction algorithms, which can reduce this error by up to 60% [47]. Without the use of distortion correction, Seibert et al. reported up to 4-mm medial displacement of GTV (on MRI compared to CT), where 28% of patients would have a geometric miss [48].

The above issues can lead to errors with co-registration (with simulation CT). Although these MRI scanners usually come under the purview of diagnostic radiology, where tissue contrast for diagnosis is the primary objective, they should be checked for millimeter-level spatial resolution periodically. The AAPM have set up Task Group 117 to provide guidance and propose quality checks that are recommended in MR scanners which are used for SRS imaging data [49].

Automatic co-registration tools, which usually come in-built with contouring software, are now common and can be used for image fusion [50]. Any registration should be manually checked prior to target delineation. Structures which are easily visible on CT and MRI can be used to verify the fusion, including dural surfaces (falx, tentorium), ventricular system (particularly the choroid plexus which is often calcified on CT), and bony anatomy (cochlea, internal acoustic meatus, optic canal, clivus, sella). The fusion is particularly important at the site of the disease (i.e., region of interest). An example of image co-registration verification is shown in Fig. 11.5. The spatial accuracy of the overall process of image acquisition, co-registration, and target delineation can be assessed by comparing the contours of a tumor such as a vestibular schwannoma, where the intracanalicular portion (outlined on gadolinium-enhanced MRI) should fit perfectly into the internal auditory canal in the petrous bone (visualized on CT).

Situations with MRI Contraindications

Although high-resolution MRI is much preferred for target delineation, situations exist where MRI is contraindicated (such as presence of pacemaker or severe renal impairment). In such situations, we recommend a high-resolution CT with iodinated contrast (slice thickness 1 mm) in place of MRI. At our center, we perform CT imaging

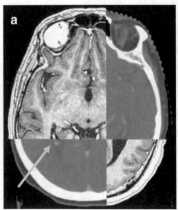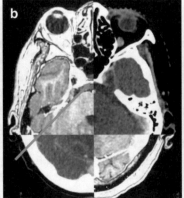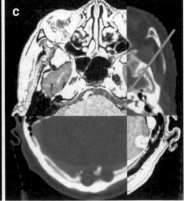

Fig. 11.5 (**a**) CT/MR fusion verification using checker box. Lateral ventricle aligning perfectly, with the calcified choroid plexus visible on both MRI and CT (yellow arrow). (**b**) Clivus aligning on both CT and MRI (green arrow), with left-right fusion being verified using basilar artery. (**c**) Internal acoustic meatus and cochlea are aligned (blue arrow)

on a GE Healthcare Revolution scanner (120 kV; 300 mA; helical rotation; primary iterative reconstruction at 0.625-mm slice thickness) with injection of 50 ml of iodinated contrast (Omnipaque 350 mg I/ml) at 0.7 ml/s. The scan is performed 2 min after injection. Previous studies have recommended protocols using injections of 200 ml of iodinated contrast (Angiovist-370) with up to a 1-h delay in order to improve detection [51, 52]. This is weighed against the fact that the area of enhancement often became larger and its margin became less well defined with time [53]. This is not routinely practiced, as current helical CT with submillimeter slice thickness often reduces the effect of partial voluming seen in older scanners. For patients on renal dialysis, gadolinium contrast administration for MRI is relatively contraindicated; such patients can still receive iodinated contrast for CT, as it will be removed during dialysis. A gross tumor volume (GTV) to clinical target volume (CTV) margin of 1–2 mm is advisable when MRI is contraindicated.

Target Delineation of BM (GTV, CTV)

Once image fusion has been verified, delineation of the target and OAR should be performed. For cases with uncertainty (such as postoperative), we recommend involving the neuroradiologist and/or neurosurgeon in target delineation. The window levels on the MRI should be adjusted so that the borders of the lesion can be clearly identified. Unlike CT, there are no presets for MRI window levels. The window levels for MRI are known to be affected by tissue-specific parameters and operator-specific parameters (such as receiver bandwidth, flip angle, and matrix size) As such, we recommend that window levels are adjusted manually using visual feedback.

Situation

De Novo BM

Target delineation for de novo BM is relatively straightforward. The GTV (gross tumor vol-

ume) should be easily visible on the T1-contrast-enhanced MRI. Image magnification is advised for small lesions. The delineated GTV should be verified and adjusted on the sagittal and coronal planes. Often enlarged feeder vessels can be seen beside the well-demarcated BM. It is controversial if these should be included in the GTV. In our practice at NCIS and UW, we do not routinely include the feeder vessels in the GTV.

Generally, a clinical target volume (to account for microscopic extension) is not required in SRS. Baumert and colleagues conducted an autopsy-based assessment on the infiltration of BM [54]. In their study, they evaluated 76 specimens and showed that 63% showed tumor infiltration beyond the grossly visible boundary. Histological subtypes such as small cell and melanoma showed a depth of infiltration >1 mm and other subtypes <1 mm.

Noel et al. showed that an addition of 1-mm CTV margin (on 1.5-Tesla MRI) improved 2-year local control rates [55]. However, this study was performed before 2000 – it is possible that the resolution of the MRI used in that era was suboptimal. Nataf et al. compared using a 0- vs 2-mm margin (GTV–PTV) and did not show improved local control, additionally there were more complications in the 2-mm margin group [56]. Likewise, findings from a randomized controlled trial from Duke University (discussed below) also suggest a higher complication rate with a larger PTV margin [57].

BM Involving Dura or Dural-Based BM
A distinction has to be made between leptomeningeal metastases (LM) and BM involving the dural layer of the meninges (i.e., pachymeninges). LM is generally considered a contraindication for SRS, and often WBRT or intrathecal therapy is recommended. However, for BM involving the dura, or skull vault metastases with dural involvement, SRS can be performed safely. The GTV is best delineated on T1-contrast-enhanced MRI sequence. We recommend a 5-mm CTV margin along the dura to include microscopic disease. The CTV margin need not include brain parenchyma.

Based on a prior interobserver comparison study, which has been presented only in abstract form, the greatest amount of variability occurred in two scenarios – meningeal involvement and hemorrhagic lesions [58]. As such, it may be prudent to seek the opinion of neuroradiologists and neurosurgeons in such situations.

BM with Cystic or Hemorrhagic Component

Certain primary histological subtypes, in particular non-small-cell lung carcinoma, are prone to cystic BM. The cyst content is better visualized on the T2 sequence. However, the cyst wall may be nodular and always enhances on the T1 contrast sequence. Historically, it has been thought the cystic BMs have a poorer prognosis overall and do not respond as well as solid BM [59, 60]. At times, the large volume associated with cystic BM precludes single-fraction SRS. Strategies have been attempted to drain the cyst (using an Ommaya reservoir) followed by SRS to the lesion on the same day (like in Case 2 vignette). It is unclear how this compares to fractionated SRT. In any case, the entire cyst wall should be included in the GTV.

Hemorrhagic BM are seen more commonly with melanoma, RCC, and NSCLC, but are often seen in choriocarcinoma or papillary thyroid cancer metastases. The intratumoral bleed is expected to reduce in extent as clot resorption takes place. However, the lesion may progress or rebleed during the convalescent period. It is expected that the entire lesion is contaminated with cancer cells, and therefore should be included in the GTV.

Resection Cavity

Resection of BM is often done in a piecemeal fashion, and multiple studies have demonstrated a local recurrence rate of 50–85%, which can potentially translate to inferior survival if routine surveillance and salvage strategies are not in place [20, 26, 27, 61, 62]. Where surgery is done through en-bloc technique, lower local recurrence rates (14% at 1 year) have been reported [63], but this is an outlier in the literature.

Controversy exists if the resection corridor should be included in the target volume for cav-

ity SRS [64]. For example, the randomized trial reported by Kepka et al., and the N107C trial, excludes the surgical tract and postoperative edema from their CTV [21, 65]. Notably, early reports showed a higher incidence of leptomeningeal dissemination postcavity SRS of about 10% [66], with breast cancer identified as a risk factor for leptomeningeal dissemination. It is also postulated that leptomeningeal dissemination may occur due to a geographical miss during cavity SRS, rather than the procedure itself [67]. As such, expert consensus guidelines have been formulated for the use of cavity SRS, and these are summarized in Table 11.1, with case examples shown in Fig. 11.6 [68]. It is clear that the clinical target volume should account for changes seen on the postoperative scan and include potential adjacent areas harboring microscopic disease.

Especially in cavity SRS, postoperative changes may obscure the borders of the tumor bed and may resemble residual tumor. It is pertinent to review surgical operative notes to determine what type of surgery has been performed and seek opinion from the surgeon and neuroradiologist if in doubt. Based on the consensus guideline, the largest variability was seen in cases where the

Table 11.1 Recommendations for CTV delineation in the postoperative setting

	Recommendation
All cases	Fusion of preoperative MRI (T1-weighted, gadolinium-enhanced) imaging to aid volume definition CTV should include entire surgical tract (seen on postoperative CT and axial T1-weight gadolinium-enhanced MRI) and exclude postoperative edema
Situation:	
Preoperative dural contact	Extension of CTV by 5–10 mm along the dura (next to bone flap) to account for microscopic disease extension
Without dural contact	Extension of CTV by 1–5 mm along the bone flap
Preoperative venous sinus contact	Extension of CTV by 1–5 mm into the adjacent sinus

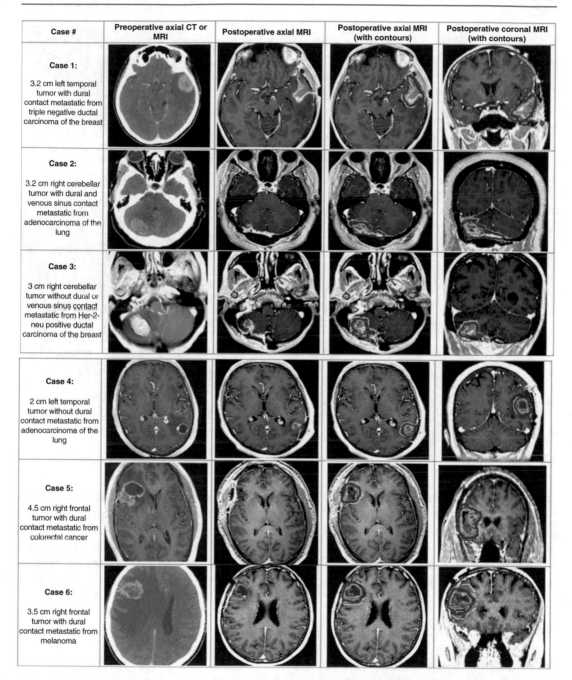

Fig. 11.6 Individual and consensus clinical target volume contours in resected brain metastases. Consensus contours shown in thick red and individual contours in other colors. Abbreviations: CT computed tomography, MRI magnetic resonance imaging. (From Soliman et al. [68]. Reprinted with permission from Elsevier)

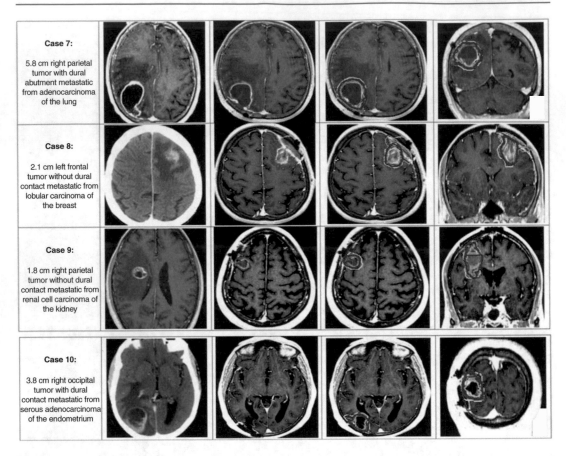

Case 7:				
5.8 cm right parietal tumor with dural abutment metastatic from adenocarcinoma of the lung				

| Case 8: | | | | |
| 2.1 cm left frontal tumor without dural contact metastatic from lobular carcinoma of the breast | | | | |

| Case 9: | | | | |
| 1.8 cm right parietal tumor without dural contact metastatic from renal cell carcinoma of the kidney | | | | |

| Case 10: | | | | |
| 3.8 cm right occipital tumor with dural contact metastatic from serous adenocarcinoma of the endometrium | | | | |

Fig. 11.6 (continued)

BM was located infratentorially, or close to a venous sinus and/or dura. In all cases, CTV definition should be done with the aid of T1-weighted gadolinium-enhanced postoperative MRI scan, obtained 1–3 weeks post-resection, and as close to the proposed radiosurgery date as feasible.

PTV Margin

PTV margin is highly reliant on the platform used to treat BM. It is institution specific, and rigorous in-house quality assurance should be performed to determine the adequate PTV. For example, when rigid fixation is used, a PTV margin of 0–1 mm is usually adequate [69, 70]. In contrast, a 2- to 3-mm margin may be required with a thermoplastic mask. The availability of a 6 degree-of-freedom couch is particularly useful to correct for rotational errors [71]. Undoubtedly,

the risk of geographical miss decreases with a larger PTV margin. However, a bigger volume of normal brain tissue will be included in the PTV and consequently treated to a high dose. A randomized controlled trial has shown that the risk of radionecrosis increases when a 3-mm PTV (vs 1-mm) margin is used (12.5% vs 2.5%) [57].

Dose Selection

Dose selection is primarily determined by the volume or diameter of the PTV. Somewhat counterintuitively, the prescription dose is lowered for larger volumes, in order to reduce the risk of treatment complications. This practice is based on data borne out of the RTOG 90-05 Phase 1 trial [72]. Lesions below ≤20 mm were safely treated with 24 Gy, 21–30 mm with 18 Gy, and 31–40 mm with 15 Gy. However, these data are

Table 11.2 Volume-based recommendation for single-session SRS dose selection used in N107c trial [21]

Volume-based recommendation for single-session SRS dose selection used in N107c trial [21]		Alternative dosing using 5 fraction stereotactic radiation
<4.2 cc	20 Gy	N/A
4.2–8 cc	18 Gy	30–35Gy in 5 fractions
8–14.4 cc	17 Gy	25–30 Gy in 5 fractions
14.4–20 cc	15 Gy	
20–30 cc	14 Gy	25 Gy in 5 fractions
30-cc to 5-cm maximum transverse diameter	12 Gy	

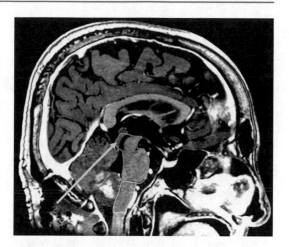

Fig. 11.7 Sagittal T1 MRI showing the midbrain and pons (green outline) and medulla (yellow outline). Yellow arrow showing the tectal plate at the posterior midbrain

based on a mixture of recurrent primary and secondary brain tumors, and all patients had prior radiation.

Postoperative cavities tend to be irregularly shaped, and using lesion diameter to select dose can be challenging. The N107C trial, which included resection cavities, used a volume-based method for dose selection [21] (Table 11.2).

In our practice, for lesions above 3-cm diameter (14.1 cc), we prefer to use a 3 or 5 HSRT approach [73]. Regardless of fraction number, the target delineation methodology for gross tumor volume is similar.

Delineation of OAR

We recommend readers refer to an organs-at-risk delineation guide published by Scoccianti et al. in 2015 [74].

1. Brainstem: The brainstem is a critical organ and is regarded with high priority during SRS planning. Exceeding the dose limits of the brainstem may result in radionecrosis and consequent effects such as cranial neuropathy, motor weakness, or in worst case, death from respiratory depression. The brain stem consists of three substructures (mid-brain, pons, and medulla) and spans from the posterior clinoid process to the foramen magnum.

   While contouring the brainstem, it is useful to note that the brainstem is surrounded by cerebrospinal fluid. We find that visualizing

the brainstem on the sagittal plane is helpful for organ delineation (Fig. 11.7). The pons is the thickest part of the brainstem, and typically, it measures about 3 cm in length. Errors in delineation, such as excluding the quadrigeminal plate (also known as tectal plate) located at the posterior part of the midbrain, are common.

The periphery of the brainstem has been reported to be more tolerant to radiation; however, this is not supported by strong evidence. Dose constraints for the medulla are lower than that of the midbrain and pons [75]. Depending on the type of immobilization used, we recommend a 1- to 2-mm PRV (planning organ-at-risk volume).

2. Optic apparatus

   (a) Optic apparatus consists of left and right optic nerves and the optic chiasm. They exist in continuity and have similar dose constraints, but they are labeled individually. Injury to these structures presents with visual deficits (such as blurred vision, color impairment, or visual field defects).

   (b) Optic nerves are easily identified on both CT and MRI. They originate at the posterior part of the globe and are surrounded by intraorbital fat. The intracanalicular portion of the optic nerve lies within the optic canal. Optic canals are best identified on bone window settings using the coronal plane.

(c) Optic chiasm lies above the tuberculum sella (where the pituitary gland is located) and in between the clinoid segment of the internal carotid arteries. It is surrounded by CSF (chiasmatic cistern). The pituitary stalk is an important landmark to identify as the optic chiasm lies anterior to it. The chiasm can be visualized easily on high-resolution CT and MRI images. It is important to note that the chiasm is usually sloping upwards, and this is best visualized on the sagittal plane (Fig. 11.8).

(d) Care must be taken that the optic nerves and chiasm are contoured in continuity. Leaving gaps in the contouring may lead to the treatment planning system inadvertently dumping hot spots in those areas which will not be reported on dose–volume histograms.

3. Cochlea

The cochlea is a small spiral-shaped fluid-filled organ which is involved in hearing. The cochlea is located in the petrous part of the temporal bone, anterior to the labyrinth and lateral to the internal auditory canal. Impairment of cochlear function may result in hearing loss and/or tinnitus. The cochlea is best identified on T2 sequence or CT bone window (Fig. 11.9) [76].

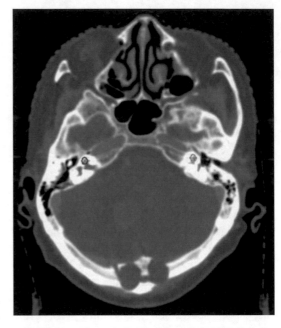

Fig. 11.9 Axial CT bone window with right (pink) and left (orange) cochlea outlined

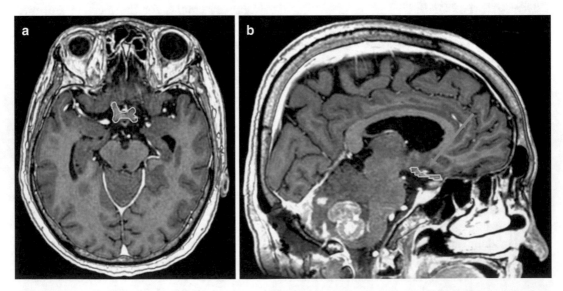

Fig. 11.8 (**a**) Axial T1 MRI showing the optic chiasm. (**b**) Axial T1 MRI demonstrating the upslope of the optic chiasm (blue arrow)

Complication and Mitigation Strategies

Dose limits for the organs-at-risk are suggested in Table 11.3.

Use of Corticosteroids

The routine use of corticosteroids during SRS is controversial. Patients with large amounts of perilesional edema may benefit from a short course of steroids during and after SRS. Duration and dose of corticosteroids should be determined based on symptoms, but typically last between 1 and 2 weeks [84].

Use of Anticonvulsants

Although seizures have been reported to occur post-SRS, we do not routinely use anticonvulsants prophylactically. For patients with a prior history of seizures, anticonvulsants should be continued [84].

Posterior Fossa Location

Lesions in the posterior fossa may result in obstructive hydrocephalus from compression of the fourth ventricle. SRS-induced perilesional edema may cause exacerbation of this effect, and covering the patient with dexamethasone periprocedure may be useful. However, there is no evidence for the use of prophylactic ventriculo-peritoneal shunts.

Area Postrema Location

SRS of BM close to the area postrema can induce severe nausea and vomiting. Prophylactic administration of medications such as 5-HT3 antagonists to prevent nausea and vomiting for patients being treated to this area will greatly minimize the risk of this unpleasant complication.

Follow-Up

With SRS-alone strategy, there remains a relatively high distant intracranial failure rate of 50% at 1 year. As such, regular surveillance imaging is needed. We typically perform post-SRS MR imaging at 4–6 weeks, and every 2–3 months thereafter.

Areas of Uncertainty

Timing of Postoperative Cavity SRS

The balance of allowing for surgical wound healing and not delaying local and systemic therapy has to be considered when selecting the optimal

Table 11.3 Recommended dose limits for organs-at-risk

OAR	1 fraction	3 fractions	5 fractions	References	Endpoint
Brainstem	Dmax: 15Gy	Dmax: 23.1 Gy	Dmax: 31Gy	[77, 78]	G3+ cranial neuropathy
	D(0.5 cc) <10Gy	D(0.5 cc) <18Gy	D(0.5 cc) <23Gy		
	Dmax: 12.5 Gy	–	–	[78]	
Optic pathway	Dmax: 10Gy	Dmax: 17.4 Gy	Dmax: 25Gy	[79]	G3+ optic neuritis
	D(0.2 cc): <8Gy	D(0.2 cc): <15.3 Gy	D(0.2 cc): <23Gy		
	Dmax: 12 Gy	Dmax: 19.5 Gy	Dmax: 25 Gy	[80]	
Cochlea	Dmax: 12 Gy	Dmax: 20 Gy	Dmax: 27.5Gy	[77]	G3+ hearing loss
	Dmax:4 Gy			[81]	High chance of hearing preservation if <4 Gy
Brain (brain parenchyma – GTV)	V10 <10.5 cc,V12<7.9 cc	N/A	V20<20cc	[82, 83]	Symptomatic radionecrosis

time for the administration of SRS. Prior studies have found that the risk of local recurrence increases if there was a delay of more than 3 weeks from surgery to SRS [85]. Atalar and colleagues have shown that the majority of changes occur immediately after surgery (0–3 days), after which there was no significant reduction in cavity volume [86]. In contrast, Patel et al. have shown that the cavity size increased by a median of 28% (immediate postoperative cavity compared to cavity size at 3 weeks later) [87]. As such, most studies recommend performing SRS between 1 and 3 weeks.

Preoperative Versus Postoperative SRS

Preoperative SRS is a novel concept, where the tumor is sterilized prior to resection. Compared to resection cavity SRS, preoperative SRS has been shown to have less interindividual contouring variability [88]. Atalar et al. have reported that the average size of the target volume to be smaller postoperatively; however, there is a wide variation in their result (−29%, range −82% to 1258%) [86]. Moreover, the possible need to include the surgical tract, together with a 2-mm-PTV margin, makes the overall treatment volume of cavity SRS large.

Investigators from North Carolina have studied this prospectively, where surgery is performed a median of 1 day following SRS (range 0–17 days), and have shown it be effective and safe with no cases developing radionecrosis [89]. However, there is no level 1 evidence supporting the use of preoperative SRS. It remains to be seen if preoperative SRS can lead to decreased rates of radiation necrosis and LMD. This topic is further detailed in Chap. 6.

Existing Guidelines

Society guidelines are available to guide the overall management of BM [23, 90]. The German Society for Radiation Oncology has published its guidelines on the implementation of SRS for BM [91]. Consensus guidelines have been published on the contouring of completely resected BM [68].

Key Points

- Each department performing SRS should protocolize the MRI sequence being used for target delineation.
- Distortion correction algorithms should be utilized, and quality assurance procedures should be periodically performed for MRI scanners used in SRS treatment planning.
- Image fusion must be manually verified by the radiation oncologist prior to target delineation.
- Time between MRI acquisition and treatment delivery should be minimized.
- A multidisciplinary approach for target delineation, involving neuroradiologists and/or neurosurgeons, is recommended for cases with uncertainty (such as postoperative cavity SRS).
- Both OAR and target delineation should be performed on MRI and cross-verified on CT images.
- CTV margin is recommended in postoperative cavity SRS where there is contact with the meningeal surfaces. PTV margin will vary depending on type of immobilization and image verification performed.

References

1. Lassman AB, DeAngelis LM. Brain metastases. Neurol Clin. 2003;21(1):1–23. vii.
2. Lohr F, Pirzkall A, Hof H, Fleckenstein K, Debus J. Adjuvant treatment of brain metastases. Semin Surg Oncol. 2001;20(1):50–6.
3. Armulik A, Genove G, Mae M, Nisancioglu MH, Wallgard E, Niaudet C, et al. Pericytes regulate the blood-brain barrier. Nature. 2010;468(7323):557–61.
4. Barnholtz-Sloan JS, Sloan AE, Davis FG, Vigneau FD, Lai P, Sawaya RE. Incidence proportions of brain metastases in patients diagnosed (1973–2001) in the Metropolitan Detroit Cancer Surveillance System. J Clin Oncol. 2004;22(14):2865–72.
5. Hwang TL, Close TP, Grego JM, Brannon WL, Gonzales F. Predilection of brain metastasis in gray

and white matter junction and vascular border zones. Cancer. 1996;77(8):1551–5.

6. Fink KR, Fink JR. Imaging of brain metastases. Surg Neurol Int. 2013;4(Suppl 4):S209–19.

7. Barajas RF Jr, Cha S. Imaging diagnosis of brain metastasis. Prog Neurol Surg. 2012;25:55–73.

8. Schellinger PD, Meinck HM, Thron A. Diagnostic accuracy of MRI compared to CCT in patients with brain metastases. J Neuro-Oncol. 1999;44(3):275–81.

9. Sze G, Milano E, Johnson C, Heier L. Detection of brain metastases: comparison of contrast-enhanced MR with unenhanced MR and enhanced CT. AJNR Am J Neuroradiol. 1990;11(4):785–91.

10. Watanabe M, Tanaka R, Takeda N. Correlation of MRI and clinical features in meningeal carcinomatosis. Neuroradiology. 1993;35(7):512–5.

11. Iaconetta G, Lamaida E, Rossi A, Signorelli F, Manto A, Giamundo A. Leptomeningeal carcinomatosis: review of the literature. Acta Neurol (Napoli). 1994;16(4):214–20.

12. Al-Okaili RN, Krejza J, Wang S, Woo JH, Melhem ER. Advanced MR imaging techniques in the diagnosis of intraaxial brain tumors in adults. Radiographics. 2006;26(Suppl 1):S173–89.

13. Kushnirsky M, Nguyen V, Katz JS, Steinklein J, Rosen L, Warshall C, et al. Time-delayed contrast-enhanced MRI improves detection of brain metastases and apparent treatment volumes. J Neurosurg. 2016;124(2):489–95.

14. Chao JH, Phillips R, Nickson JJ. Roentgen-ray therapy of cerebral metastases. Cancer. 1954;7(4):682–9.

15. Nieder C, Spanne O, Mehta MP, Grosu AL, Geinitz H. Presentation, patterns of care, and survival in patients with brain metastases: what has changed in the last 20 years? Cancer. 2011;117(11):2505–12.

16. Patchell RA, Tibbs PA, Walsh JW, Dempsey RJ, Maruyama Y, Kryscio RJ, et al. A randomized trial of surgery in the treatment of single metastases to the brain. N Engl J Med. 1990;322(8):494–500.

17. Kondziolka D, Patel A, Lunsford LD, Kassam A, Flickinger JC. Stereotactic radiosurgery plus whole brain radiotherapy versus radiotherapy alone for patients with multiple brain metastases. Int J Radiat Oncol Biol Phys. 1999;45(2):427–34.

18. Aoyama H, Shirato H, Tago M, Nakagawa K, Toyoda T, Hatano K, et al. Stereotactic radiosurgery plus whole-brain radiation therapy vs stereotactic radiosurgery alone for treatment of brain metastases: a randomized controlled trial. JAMA. 2006;295(21):2483–91.

19. Chang EL, Wefel JS, Hess KR, Allen PK, Lang FF, Kornguth DG, et al. Neurocognition in patients with brain metastases treated with radiosurgery or radiosurgery plus whole-brain irradiation: a randomised controlled trial. Lancet Oncol. 2009;10(11):1037–44.

20. Kocher M, Soffietti R, Abacioglu U, Villa S, Fauchon F, Baumert BG, et al. Adjuvant whole-brain radiotherapy versus observation after radiosurgery or surgical resection of one to three cerebral metastases: results of the EORTC 22952-26001 study. J Clin Oncol. 2011;29(2):134–41.

21. Brown PD, Ballman KV, Cerhan JH, Anderson SK, Carrero XW, Whitton AC, et al. Postoperative stereotactic radiosurgery compared with whole brain radiotherapy for resected metastatic brain disease (NCCTG N107C/CEC.3): a multicentre, randomised, controlled, phase 3 trial. Lancet Oncol. 2017;18(8):1049–60.

22. Yamamoto M, Kawabe T, Sato Y, Higuchi Y, Nariai T, Watanabe S, et al. Stereotactic radiosurgery for patients with multiple brain metastases: a case-matched study comparing treatment results for patients with 2–9 versus 10 or more tumors. J Neurosurg. 2014;121(Suppl):16–25.

23. Available from: https://www.astro.org/Patient-Care-and-Research/Clinical-Practice-Statements/ASTRO-39;s-guideline-on-brain-metasteses.

24. Andrews DW, Bednarz G, Evans JJ, Downes B. A review of 3 current radiosurgery systems. Surg Neurol. 2006;66(6):559–64.

25. Sahgal A, Ruschin M, Ma L, Verbakel W, Larson D, Brown PD. Stereotactic radiosurgery alone for multiple brain metastases? A review of clinical and technical issues. Neuro-Oncology. 2017;19(suppl 2):ii2–ii15.

26. Mahajan A, Ahmed S, McAleer MF, Weinberg JS, Li J, Brown P, et al. Post-operative stereotactic radiosurgery versus observation for completely resected brain metastases: a single-centre, randomised, controlled, phase 3 trial. Lancet Oncol. 2017;18(8):1040–8.

27. Patchell RA, Tibbs PA, Regine WF, Dempsey RJ, Mohiuddin M, Kryscio RJ, et al. Postoperative radiotherapy in the treatment of single metastases to the brain: a randomized trial. JAMA. 1998;280(17):1485–9.

28. Soltys SG, Adler JR, Lipani JD, Jackson PS, Choi CY, Puataweepong P, et al. Stereotactic radiosurgery of the postoperative resection cavity for brain metastases. Int J Radiat Oncol Biol Phys. 2008;70(1):187–93.

29. Choi CY, Chang SD, Gibbs IC, Adler JR, Harsh GR, Lieberson RE, et al. Stereotactic radiosurgery of the postoperative resection cavity for brain metastases: prospective evaluation of target margin on tumor control. Int J Radiat Oncol Biol Phys. 2012;84(2):336–42.

30. Sperduto PW, Kased N, Roberge D, Xu Z, Shanley R, Luo X, et al. Summary report on the graded prognostic assessment: an accurate and facile diagnosis-specific tool to estimate survival for patients with brain metastases. J Clin Oncol. 2012;30(4):419–25.

31. Andrews DW, Scott CB, Sperduto PW, Flanders AE, Gaspar LE, Schell MC, et al. Whole brain radiation therapy with or without stereotactic radiosurgery boost for patients with one to three brain metastases: phase III results of the RTOG 9508 randomised trial. Lancet. 2004;363(9422):1665–72.

32. Lutz W, Winston KR, Maleki N. A system for stereotactic radiosurgery with a linear accelerator. Int J Radiat Oncol Biol Phys. 1988;14(2):373–81.

33. Klein EE, Hanley J, Bayouth J, Yin FF, Simon W, Dresser S, et al. Task Group 142 report: quality assurance of medical accelerators. Med Phys. 2009;36(9):4197–212.

34. Guckenberger M, Roesch J, Baier K, Sweeney RA, Flentje M. Dosimetric consequences of translational and rotational errors in frame-less image-guided radiosurgery. Radiat Oncol. 2012;7:63.

35. Theelen A, Martens J, Bosmans G, Houben R, Jager JJ, Rutten I, et al. Relocatable fixation systems in intracranial stereotactic radiotherapy. Accuracy of serial CT scans and patient acceptance in a randomized design. Strahlenther Onkol. 2012;188(1):84–90.

36. Ramakrishna N, Rosca F, Friesen S, Tezcanli E, Zygmanszki P, Hacker F. A clinical comparison of patient setup and intra-fraction motion using frame-based radiosurgery versus a frameless image-guided radiosurgery system for intracranial lesions. Radiother Oncol. 2010;95(1):109–15.

37. Anzalone N, Essig M, Lee SK, Dorfler A, Ganslandt O, Combs SE, et al. Optimizing contrast-enhanced magnetic resonance imaging characterization of brain metastases: relevance to stereotactic radiosurgery. Neurosurgery. 2013;72(5):691–701.

38. Garcia MA, Anwar M, Yu Y, Duriseti S, Merritt B, Nakamura J, et al. Brain metastasis growth on preradiosurgical magnetic resonance imaging. Pract Radiat Oncol. 2018;8(6):e369–e76.

39. Salkeld AL, Hau EKC, Nahar N, Sykes JR, Wang W, Thwaites DI. Changes in brain metastasis during radiosurgical planning. Int J Radiat Oncol Biol Phys. 2018;102(4):727–33.

40. Yuh WT, Engelken JD, Muhonen MG, Mayr NA, Fisher DJ, Ehrhardt JC. Experience with high-dose gadolinium MR imaging in the evaluation of brain metastases. AJNR Am J Neuroradiol. 1992;13(1):335–45.

41. Sze G, Johnson C, Kawamura Y, Goldberg SN, Lange R, Friedland RJ, et al. Comparison of single- and triple-dose contrast material in the MR screening of brain metastases. AJNR Am J Neuroradiol. 1998;19(5):821–8.

42. Yuh WT, Tali ET, Nguyen HD, Simonson TM, Mayr NA, Fisher DJ. The effect of contrast dose, imaging time, and lesion size in the MR detection of intracerebral metastasis. AJNR Am J Neuroradiol. 1995;16(2):373–80.

43. Subedi KS, Takahashi T, Yamano T, Saitoh J, Nishimura K, Suzuki Y, et al. Usefulness of double dose contrast-enhanced magnetic resonance imaging for clear delineation of gross tumor volume in stereotactic radiotherapy treatment planning of metastatic brain tumors: a dose comparison study. J Radiat Res. 2013;54(1):135–9.

44. Togao O, Hiwatashi A, Yamashita K, Kikuchi K, Yoshiura T, Honda H. Additional MR contrast dosage for radiologists' diagnostic performance in detecting brain metastases: a systematic observer study at 3 T. Jpn J Radiol. 2014;32(9):537–44.

45. Sumanaweera TS, Glover GH, Binford TO, Adler JR. MR susceptibility misregistration correction. IEEE Trans Med Imaging. 1993;12(2):251–9.

46. Baldwin LN, Wachowicz K, Fallone BG. A two-step scheme for distortion rectification of magnetic resonance images. Med Phys. 2009;36(9):3917–26.

47. Neumann JO, Giese H, Biller A, Nagel AM, Kiening K. Spatial distortion in MRI-guided stereotactic procedures: evaluation in 1.5-, 3- and 7-Tesla MRI scanners. Stereotact Funct Neurosurg. 2015;93(6):380–6.

48. Seibert TM, White NS, Kim GY, Moiseenko V, McDonald CR, Farid N, et al. Distortion inherent to magnetic resonance imaging can lead to geometric miss in radiosurgery planning. Pract Radiat Oncol. 2016;6(6):e319–e28.

49. Available from: https://www.aapm.org/org/structure/?committee_code=TG117.

50. Knisely JP, Bond JE, Yue NJ, Studholme C, de Lotbinière AC. Image registration and calculation of a biologically effective dose for multisession radiosurgical treatments. Technical note. J Neurosurg. 2000 Dec;93 Suppl 3:208-18.

51. Sighvatsson V, Ericson K, Tomasson H. Optimising contrast-enhanced cranial CT for detection of brain metastases. Acta Radiol. 1998;39(6):718–22.

52. Davis PC, Hudgins PA, Peterman SB, Hoffman JC Jr. Diagnosis of cerebral metastases: double-dose delayed CT vs contrast-enhanced MR imaging. AJNR Am J Neuroradiol. 1991;12(2):293–300.

53. Blatt DR, Friedman WA, Agee OF. Delayed computed tomography contrast enhancement patterns in biopsy proven cases. Neurosurgery. 1993;32(4):560–9.

54. Baumert BG, Rutten I, Dehing-Oberije C, Twijnstra A, Dirx MJ, Debougnoux-Huppertz RM, et al. A pathology-based substrate for target definition in radiosurgery of brain metastases. Int J Radiat Oncol Biol Phys. 2006;66(1):187–94.

55. Noel G, Simon JM, Valery CA, Cornu P, Boisserie G, Hasboun D, et al. Radiosurgery for brain metastasis: impact of CTV on local control. Radiother Oncol. 2003;68(1):15–21.

56. Nataf F, Schlienger M, Liu Z, Foulquier JN, Gres B, Orthuon A, et al. Radiosurgery with or without A 2-mm margin for 93 single brain metastases. Int J Radiat Oncol Biol Phys. 2008;70(3):766–72.

57. Kirkpatrick JP, Wang Z, Sampson JH, McSherry F, Herndon JE 2nd, Allen KJ, et al. Defining the optimal planning target volume in image-guided stereotactic radiosurgery of brain metastases: results of a randomized trial. Int J Radiat Oncol Biol Phys. 2015;91(1):100–8.

58. Clavier J, Antoni D, Bauer N, Guillerme F, Truntzer P, Atlani D, et al. Delineation of brain metastases for stereotactic radiation therapy: an interobserver contour comparison. Int J Radiat Oncol Biol Phys. 2014;90(1):S311.

59. Sun B, Huang Z, Wu S, Ding L, Shen G, Cha L, et al. Cystic brain metastasis is associated with poor prognosis in patients with advanced breast cancer. Oncotarget. 2016;7(45):74006–14.

60. Goodman KA, Sneed PK, McDermott MW, Shiau CY, Lamborn KR, Chang S, et al. Relationship between pattern of enhancement and local control of brain metastases after radiosurgery. Int J Radiat Oncol Biol Phys. 2001;50:139-46.

61. DeAngelis LM, Mandell LR, Thaler HT, Kimmel DW, Galicich JH, Fuks Z, et al. The role of postoperative radiotherapy after resection of single brain metastases. Neurosurgery. 1989;24(6):798–805.

62. Smalley SR, Schray MF, Laws ER Jr, O'Fallon JR. Adjuvant radiation therapy after surgical resection of solitary brain metastasis: association with pattern of failure and survival. Int J Radiat Oncol Biol Phys. 1987;13(11):1611–6.

63. Patel AJ, Suki D, Hatiboglu MA, Abouassi H, Shi W, Wildrick DM, et al. Factors influencing the risk of local recurrence after resection of a single brain metastasis. J Neurosurg. 2010;113(2):181–9.

64. Brennan C, Yang TJ, Hilden P, Zhang Z, Chan K, Yamada Y, et al. A phase 2 trial of stereotactic radiosurgery boost after surgical resection for brain metastases. Int J Radiat Oncol Biol Phys. 2014;88(1):130–6.

65. Kepka L, Tyc-Szczepaniak D, Bujko K, Olszyna-Serementa M, Michalski W, Sprawka A, et al. Stereotactic radiotherapy of the tumor bed compared to whole brain radiotherapy after surgery of single brain metastasis: results from a randomized trial. Radiother Oncol. 2016;121(2):217–24.

66. Atalar B, Modlin LA, Choi CY, Adler JR, Gibbs IC, Chang SD, et al. Risk of leptomeningeal disease in patients treated with stereotactic radiosurgery targeting the postoperative resection cavity for brain metastases. Int J Radiat Oncol Biol Phys. 2013;87(4):713–8.

67. Johnson MD, Avkshtol V, Baschnagel AM, Meyer K, Ye H, Grills IS, et al. Surgical resection of brain metastases and the risk of leptomeningeal recurrence in patients treated with stereotactic radiosurgery. Int J Radiat Oncol Biol Phys. 2016;94(3):537–43.

68. Soliman H, Ruschin M, Angelov L, Brown PD, Chiang VLS, Kirkpatrick JP, et al. Consensus contouring guidelines for postoperative completely resected cavity stereotactic radiosurgery for brain metastases. Int J Radiat Oncol Biol Phys. 2018;100(2):436–42.

69. Prabhu RS, Dhabaan A, Hall WA, Ogunleye T, Crocker I, Curran WJ, et al. Clinical outcomes for a novel 6 degrees of freedom image guided localization method for frameless radiosurgery for intracranial brain metastases. J Neuro-Oncol. 2013;113(1):93–9.

70. Dhabaan A, Schreibmann E, Siddiqi A, Elder E, Fox T, Ogunleye T, et al. Six degrees of freedom CBCT-based positioning for intracranial targets treated with frameless stereotactic radiosurgery. J Appl Clin Med Phys. 2012;13(6):3916.

71. Mancosu P, Reggiori G, Gaudino A, Lobefalo F, Paganini L, Palumbo V, et al. Are pitch and roll compensations required in all pathologies? A data analysis of 2945 fractions. Br J Radiol. 2015;88(1055):20150468.

72. Shaw E, Scott C, Souhami L, Dinapoli R, Kline R, Loeffler J, et al. Single dose radiosurgical treatment of recurrent previously irradiated primary brain tumors and brain metastases: final report of RTOG protocol 90-05. Int J Radiat Oncol Biol Phys. 2000;47(2):291–8.

73. Brenner DJ, Martel MK, Hall EJ. Fractionated regimens for stereotactic radiotherapy of recurrent tumors in the brain. Int J Radiat Oncol Biol Phys. 1991;21(3):819–24.

74. Scoccianti S, Detti B, Gadda D, Greto D, Furfaro I, Meacci F, et al. Organs at risk in the brain and their dose-constraints in adults and in children: a radiation oncologist's guide for delineation in everyday practice. Radiother Oncol. 2015;114(2):230–8.

75. Benedict SH, Yenice KM, Followill D, Galvin JM, Hinson W, Kavanagh B, et al. Stereotactic body radiation therapy: the report of AAPM Task Group 101. Med Phys. 2010;37(8):4078–101.

76. Pacholke HD, Amdur RJ, Schmalfuss IM, Louis D, Mendenhall WM. Contouring the middle and inner ear on radiotherapy planning scans. Am J Clin Oncol. 2005;28(2):143–7.

77. Timmerman RD. An overview of hypofractionation and introduction to this issue of seminars in radiation oncology. Semin Radiat Oncol. 2008;18(4):215–22.

78. Mayo C, Yorke E, Merchant TE. Radiation associated brainstem injury. Int J Radiat Oncol Biol Phys. 2010;76(3 Suppl):S36–41.

79. Mayo C, Martel MK, Marks LB, Flickinger J, Nam J, Kirkpatrick J. Radiation dose-volume effects of optic nerves and chiasm. Int J Radiat Oncol Biol Phys. 2010;76(3 Suppl):S28–35.

80. Grimm J, LaCouture T, Croce R, Yeo I, Zhu Y, Xue J. Dose tolerance limits and dose volume histogram evaluation for stereotactic body radiotherapy. J Appl Clin Med Phys. 2011;12(2):3368.

81. Tamura M, Carron R, Yomo S, Arkha Y, Muraciolle X, Porcheron D, et al. Hearing preservation after Gamma Knife radiosurgery for vestibular schwannomas presenting with high-level hearing. Neurosurgery. 2009;64(2):289–96. Discussion 96.

82. Ernst-Stecken A, Ganslandt O, Lambrecht U, Sauer R, Grabenbauer G. Phase II trial of hypofractionated stereotactic radiotherapy for brain metastases: results and toxicity. Radiother Oncol. 2006;81(1):18–24.

83. Blonigen BJ, Steinmetz RD, Levin L, Lamba MA, Warnick RE, Breneman JC. Irradiated volume as a predictor of brain radionecrosis after linear accelerator stereotactic radiosurgery. Int J Radiat Oncol Biol Phys. 2010;77(4):996–1001.

84. Soffietti R, Abacioglu U, Baumert B, Combs SE, Kinhult S, Kros JM, et al. Diagnosis and treatment of brain metastases from solid tumors: guidelines from the European Association of Neuro-Oncology (EANO). Neuro-Oncology. 2017;19(2):162–74.

85. Iorio-Morin C, Masson-Cote L, Ezahr Y, Blanchard J, Ebacher A, Mathieu D. Early Gamma Knife stereotactic radiosurgery to the tumor bed of resected brain metastasis for improved local control. J Neurosurg. 2014;121(Suppl):69–74.

86. Atalar B, Choi CY, Harsh GR, Chang SD, Gibbs IC, Adler JR, et al. Cavity volume dynamics after resection of brain metastases and timing of postresection cavity stereotactic radiosurgery. Neurosurgery. 2013;72(2):180–5. Discussion 5.

87. Patel RA, Lock D, Helenowski IB, Chandler JP, Sachdev S, Tate MC, et al. Postsurgical cavity evolution after brain metastasis resection: how soon should postoperative radiosurgery follow? World Neurosurg. 2018;110:e310–e4.

88. Vellayappan BA, Doody J, Vandervoort E, Szanto J, Sinclair J, Caudrelier JM, et al. Pre-operative versus post-operative radiosurgery for brain metastasis: effects on treatment volume and inter-observer variability. J Radiosurg SBRT. 2018;5(2):89–97.

89. Asher AL, Burri SH, Wiggins WF, Kelly RP, Boltes MO, Mehrlich M, et al. A new treatment paradigm: neoadjuvant radiosurgery before surgical resection of brain metastases with analysis of local tumor recurrence. Int J Radiat Oncol Biol Phys. 2014;88(4):899–906.

90. Soffietti R, Cornu P, Delattre JY, Grant R, Graus F, Grisold W, et al. EFNS Guidelines on diagnosis and treatment of brain metastases: report of an EFNS Task Force. Eur J Neurol. 2006;13(7):674–81.

91. Kocher M, Wittig A, Piroth MD, Treuer H, Seegenschmiedt H, Ruge M, et al. Stereotactic radiosurgery for treatment of brain metastases. A report of the DEGRO Working Group on Stereotactic Radiotherapy. Strahlenther Onkol. 2014;190(6):521–32.

Indications for Whole-Brain Radiation Therapy

12

Michael Huo, Fabio Ynoe de Moraes,
Matthew Foote, Mark B. Pinkham,
Gustavo N. Marta, and John H. Suh

Case Vignette

A 52-year-old Caucasian man presents with increasing fatigue, cough, weight loss, headaches, nausea, ataxia, and right arm weakness. His comorbidities include chronic obstructive pulmonary disease, hypertension, and hypercholesterolemia. He is a current smoker with a

M. Huo (✉)
Radiation Medicine Program, Princess Margaret Cancer Centre, Toronto, ON, Canada

Department of Radiation Oncology, University of Toronto, Toronto, ON, Canada

School of Medicine, The University of Queensland, Brisbane, QLD, Australia

F. Y. de Moraes
Department of Oncology, Division of Radiation Oncology, Kingston General Hospital, Queens University, Kingston, ON, Canada

M. Foote · M. B. Pinkham
School of Medicine, The University of Queensland, Brisbane, QLD, Australia

Department of Radiation Oncology, Princess Alexandra Hospital, Brisbane, Australia

G. N. Marta
Department of Radiation Oncology, Hospital Sírio-Libanês and Instituto do Câncer de Estado de São Paulo (ICESP) – Faculdade de Medicina da Universidade de São Paulo (FMUSP), São Paulo, Brazil

J. H. Suh
Department of Radiation Oncology, Taussig Cancer Institute, Cleveland Clinic, Cleveland, OH, USA

60 pack-year history. CT of the chest/abdomen/pelvis reveals a 5 cm left upper lobe mass, enlarged mediastinal adenopathy, and a 3 cm left adrenal mass. CT of the head reveals 16 enhancing brain lesions ranging in size from 4 mm to 18 mm with no hydrocephalus and minimal midline shift, with mild-to-moderate associated vasogenic edema. MRI brain (Fig. 12.1) reveals the aforementioned intracranial disease on CT, plus an additional nine lesions measuring up to 4 mm.

He is admitted to hospital and commenced on dexamethasone 8 mg daily with symptomatic improvement. A subsequent CT-guided biopsy of the lung mass reveals lung adenocarcinoma, TTF-1 positive. No ALK or EGFR mutations are detected, and PDL1 expression is less than 1%. He is referred to radiation oncology for further management of his brain metastases.

Given the number and size of brain metastases, he is deemed unsuitable for neurosurgical resection and radiosurgery. His performance status improves to ECOG 1 (ECOG 3 at presentation) after 24 hours of dexamethasone, with resolution of his weakness, headaches, and ataxia. He is evaluated by radiation oncology, and whole-brain radiation therapy is commenced – 30 Gy in 10 fractions. He tolerates this treatment well, though with nausea requiring ondansetron and fatigue. He is gradually weaned off dexamethasone over 2 weeks and proceeds on to systemic therapy over the next 6 months, with a surveillance MRI brain at 3 months revealing a

© Springer Nature Switzerland AG 2020
Y. Yamada et al. (eds.), *Radiotherapy in Managing Brain Metastases*,
https://doi.org/10.1007/978-3-030-43740-4_12

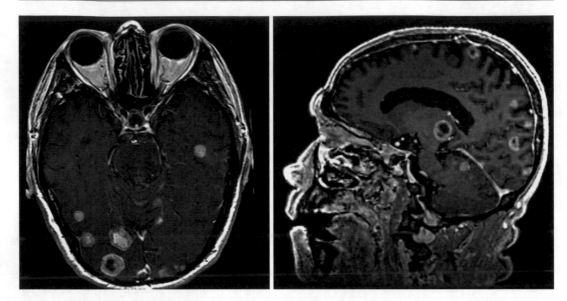

Fig. 12.1 MRI Brain demonstrating widespread brain metastases from NSCLC

stability or partial regression of all of his treated lesions, with no new lesions developing.

Introduction

Whole-brain radiation therapy (WBRT) is a historically established treatment for patients with brain metastases, with an improvement in overall survival in many patients [1]. A 2005 systematic review including eight randomized controlled trials found a median survival of 3.2–5.8 months following WBRT, compared to 2–3 months in patients managed with steroids and best supportive care [2]. Furthermore, WBRT is typically delivered via relatively simple techniques, such as opposed lateral fields with appropriate shielding for lenses (Fig. 12.2), making this treatment approach globally available. A typical WBRT dosimetry is shown in Fig. 12.3.

However, the landscape of brain metastasis management has dramatically changed with the advent of stereotactic radiosurgery (SRS) and systemic therapies with intracranial efficacy such as targeted therapy and immunotherapy [3]. The role of WBRT has gradually reduced over time due to high-quality evidence demonstrating that it can be safely omitted in lieu of the aforemen-

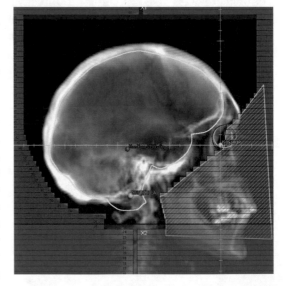

Fig. 12.2 Traditional WBRT fields

tioned treatments in selected cases. Furthermore, newer randomized evidence has emerged suggesting a reduced role in some patients of poorer performance status, which comprise a proportion of those with brain metastases [4].

Nonetheless, local treatments such as surgical resection and radiosurgery are not always feasible for a variety of reasons, including high intracranial disease volume, advanced age, poor

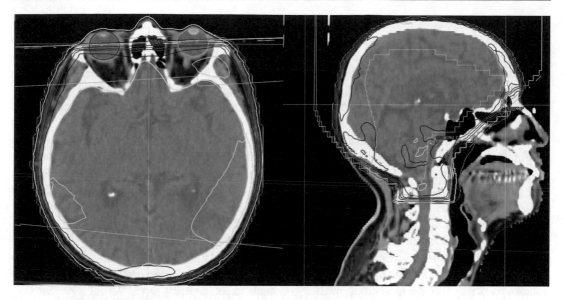

Fig. 12.3 Typical WBRT dosimetry

performance status, and high systemic disease burden. Early studies suggest that a high proportion of brain metastases patients present with multiple lesions, and high-quality randomized evidence is still awaited regarding the utility of more focal therapies where more than four brain metastases are present [5].

WBRT has the ability to treat both gross and microscopic disease, preventing the development of new gross metastatic disease and its associated symptoms. The duration of response is highly variable, with a previous systematic review suggesting between 1 and 8 months [2]. A relatively high rate of symptom improvement has been demonstrated, with 64–83% of patients benefiting in early studies [6]. It also may have utility in the setting of leptomeningeal disease, and for reirradiation of select patients following both SRS and WBRT– though definitive high-quality data are lacking. Of note, most randomized data were prior to the availability of more effective systemic therapies such as targeted therapy and immunotherapy, with a large proportion of patients having non-small cell lung cancer – for which systemic treatment has improved dramatically. Thus, patients may both live longer following WBRT, and be at increased risk of developing late toxicity due to improved survival.

While intracranial disease is often the limiting factor for prognosis and quality-of-life in patients with brain metastases, patients nonetheless have multiple competing risks for survival, quality of life, and neurocognitive function. Not all patients may be appropriate for upfront treatment to their brain metastases, depending on multiple patient, tumor, and treatment factors. There may not always be a clear, ideal treatment approach. As such, a degree of individual judgment must be applied when recommending treatment for brain metastases.

The aim of this chapter is to review the current status and future direction of WBRT for patients with brain metastases.

Patient Selection

In patients of poor performance status, supportive care alone could be considered, in favor of WBRT. A 2005 systematic review by Pease et al. found that median survival following WBRT correlated with RPA class, a prognostic measure initially established by Gaspar et al. [2, 7]. Specifically, median survival among five observational studies where RPA was measured was as follows: 8.3 months for RPA class I, 4.4 months for class II, and 2.4 months for class III [7]. More recently, a UK and Australian phase 3 noninferiority trial evaluating quality of life in NSCLC patients treated with WBRT versus supportive care alone (with dexamethasone) suggested no significant difference between the two arms [4]. Quality-adjusted life years were 46.4 and 41.7 days, respectively, while median overall survival was only 51 vs 49 days – perhaps reflective of the patient population eligible for the study, i.e., patients were required to be unsuitable for surgery or SRS. Of note, this is significantly higher than historical means found in early WBRT trials (which did not all have cross-sectional imaging) in the order of 1 month. The QUARTZ trial, however, did suggest that certain subgroups may still benefit from WBRT – patients under the age of 60 had improved survival with WBRT. Additionally, there were nonstatistically significant correlations between overall survival and RPA score, GPA score, performance status, and controlled primary tumor.

Caution should be applied when generalizing these results to all patients of limited performance status, as there are some caveats. These relate to the lack of use of other anti-cancer treatments, unreported potential selection bias with patient recruitment, no clear measure of intracranial disease burden, and an unreported rate of neurological death. Additionally, the quality-of-life tool was not brain-specific, and was potentially affected by many factors outside of intracranial disease. Nonetheless, this was an important study confirming that best supportive care alone is a reasonable approach for patients of poor performance status, though individual judgment should still be applied.

Gaspar et al. and Sperduto et al. found that grouping by recursive partitioning analysis (RPA) and graded prognostic assessment (GPA) were prognostic, and developed prognostic scoring systems to assist with patient selection [7, 8]. In 2017, Sperduto et al. further updated GPA grouping with respect to lung and melanoma molecular markers [9, 10]. Specifically for melanoma, BRAF-mutant disease was found to be a positive prognostic factor, along with number of brain metastases, extracranial disease burden, and the previously known variables of age and performance status. In the setting of lung adenocarcinoma, EGFR and ALK mutation status were significant prognostic variables. Of note, patients with the best prognosis with respect to age, performance status, extracranial disease burden, number of brain metastases, and mutation status had a median survival of up to 46.8 months. While many of these factors would suggest that such patients are more suitable for focal therapy such as SRS or surgery, BRAF status and EGFR/ALK status should be factored into when considering the appropriateness of WBRT in patients unsuitable for focal therapy.

The 2018 National Cancer Comprehensive Network (NCCN) recommendations for brain metastases describe both WBRT and SRS as appropriate options for patients with newly diagnosed or stable systemic disease and limited brain metastases – though SRS is the preferred approach [11]. Of note, "limited brain metastases" is an evolving definition, typically reflective of a relatively low number and volume of intracranial disease though variable depending upon the clinical situation. For those with widespread systemic disease and limited systemic treatment options, but limited brain metastases, WBRT or supportive care is suggested. For patients with extensive brain metastases, deemed to be all cases which are not limited in terms of number or size of metastases, WBRT and SRS are both options though SRS should especially be considered in patients of good performance status. While not explicitly outlined in NCCN Guidelines, systemic therapy such as immunotherapy or targeted therapy may also be options in the setting of extensive brain metastases, particularly in the setting of low-volume asymptomatic disease. WBRT remains the standard of care for certain histologies such as small-cell lung cancer.

Fractionation Schedules for WBRT

The most common and established fractionation schedules are 30 Gy in 10 fractions or 20 Gy in 5 fractions [2, 12]. Differences in dose, timing, and fractionation do not appear to significantly impact survival following WBRT, based on consensus from a number of randomized studies [13]. This was reinforced by a 2018 Cochrane review which found no benefit to higher biologically equivalent dose regimens [12]. However, there appeared to be worse overall survival compared to 30 Gy in 10 fractions, when results of three trials comparing 20 Gy in five fractions, 10 Gy in one fraction and 12 Gy in two fractions were pooled, with a hazard ratio of 1.21 ($p = 0.01$.) When 20 Gy in 5 fractions and 30 Gy in 10 fractions were compared in two randomized trials, there was similar overall survival and neurological function. Additionally, neurological function improvement appeared to worsen with lower-dose WBRT (HR 1.74).

Postoperative Setting

Prior to the advent of stereotactic radiosurgery, postoperative WBRT had been the treatment of choice following surgical resection of a solitary brain metastasis.

Influencing this practice was a randomized controlled trial in 1990 by Patchell et al. which found that surgical resection has a survival benefit for solitary lesions compared with biopsy and WBRT [14]. Specifically, median survival was 40 weeks with surgery and WBRT, compared to 15 weeks with biopsy and WBRT, while local recurrence was 20% versus 50%, respectively. Subsequent to this, Patchell et al. compared postoperative WBRT following surgery versus surgery alone in another RCT in 1998 [15]. Local recurrence was significantly reduced with WBRT, with a rate of 10% versus 46% though median survival was limited at 43 and 48 weeks. Overall intracranial recurrence was 18% with adjuvant WBRT versus 70% without. Neurological death was also reduced: 14% versus 44%, though no differences were seen in overall survival or duration of functional independence.

Further supporting this, a 1994 randomized trial by Noordijk et al. found that in the setting of solitary brain metastasis, surgery plus WBRT led to improved overall survival (10 months vs

6 months median), compared with WBRT alone [16]. Age and extracranial disease burden were also strong prognostic factors.

More recently, EORTC 22952–26001 randomized 359 patients to either WBRT or observation after local treatment (surgical resection or radiosurgery) in the setting of 1–3 brain metastases [17]. Of note, overall survival was similar between WBRT and observation at 10.9 months versus 10.7 months. WBRT reduced the 2-year local relapse rate from 59% to 27% following surgery, and 31% to 19% following radiosurgery respectively. WBRT reduced distant intracranial progression from 42% to 23% after surgery, and from 48% to 33% after SRS. Salvage therapies were used far more frequently in the observation arm, at 51% compared with 16%. Importantly, none of these findings translated to a significant difference in duration of functional independence, which was the primary endpoint, likely due to adequate surveillance, leading to detection and treatment of asymptomatic recurrences, as well as extracranial disease progression causing greater disability in comparison.

SRS alone is an alternative postoperative treatment, which has been demonstrated to have significant local control benefits via multiple retrospective studies and two recent randomized trials. In 2017, Mahajan et al. found that surgical bed recurrence was significantly reduced following adjuvant SRS to the surgical cavity (to a median dose of 16 Gy, range 12–18 Gy) in the setting of complete resection of 1–3 metastases, compared with observation alone [18]. Surgical bed control was 72% with SRS versus 43% for observation at 12 months. Of note, local control of the cohort as a whole worsened with increasing tumor size: greater than 90% for <2.5 cm maximal diameter; 46% for 2.5–3.5 cm, and 43% for >3.5 cm. Adjuvant SRS had a significant local control benefit in all settings. In a second randomized trial, Brown et al. found higher rates of tumor bed control with adjuvant WBRT compared with SRS, but also significantly increased cognitive deterioration at 6 months (85% vs 52%), despite improved intracranial control – that is, WBRT had a greater negative effect on neurocognitive function than disease progression

[19]. Again, no overall survival benefit to WBRT was found. A trial published in June 2018 by Kayama et al. randomized patients who had surgical resection of four or fewer lesions to postoperative WBRT, or either SRS to non-resected lesions or MRI surveillance and salvage SRS [20]. The SRS/observation arm was found to be noninferior in terms of overall survival (15.6 months for both), though intracranial progression-free survival was lower without WBRT (4 months versus 10.4 months). Of note, 16.4% of patients receiving WBRT experienced grade 2–4 cognitive dysfunction 3 months posttreatment, compared to 7.7% of those on the SRS/observation arm.

There is one randomized phase III trial which suggested comparable surgical bed control and no difference in neurological death between adjuvant SRS and WBRT. Kepka et al. found via phase III RCT that surgical bed control was comparable between adjuvant stereotactic radiotherapy to the cavity and WBRT (74% vs 75%), with no difference in neurologic death [21]. However, this trial was underpowered and should be interpreted with caution.

Overall, the published literature to date suggest that WBRT may not be the ideal postoperative treatment in the setting of 1–3 brain metastases due to no difference in overall survival and higher toxicity compared with SRS to the cavity alone. Based on current data, radiosurgery to the operative bed should be considered the standard of care.

Reirradiation Following WBRT

Progression of intracranial disease is a common scenario following WBRT. Typically, patients of reasonable performance status with limited disease may be suitable for surgery or salvage stereotactic radiosurgery – with similar indications and contraindications to the upfront setting. However, patients who are not suitable for salvage local treatments may derive benefit from repeat WBRT though the dose to disease is reduced, and control is typically less durable.

Early observational data published in 1996 suggest that reirradiation with WBRT confers symptomatic benefit in up to 71% of patients, with a subsequent median survival of 4 months [22]. In this retrospective study, 86 patients received a median reirradiation dose of 20 Gy after a median first course of 30 Gy. The median age was 58 and most patients were ECOG 2 or 3. Of note, levels of significant toxicity were low, though this should be considered in the context of a short median survival – i.e., patients may not have lived long enough to develop severe neurocognitive toxicity. In concordance with this, the median duration of response was 2.75 months.

A 2010 paper by Ammrati et al. reviewed the evidence to date for WBRT reirradiation following initial WBRT [23]. Three retrospective studies of 52, 72, and 86 patients were found, with median survival following WBRT ranging from 4 to 5.6 months [22, 24, 25]. The average reirradiation dose was 20–25 Gy, with the rate of neurological function improvement ranging from 31% to 70%. In terms of long-term toxicity, two series reported a single patient each developing symptoms of dementia attributed to repeat WBRT.

Since then, further retrospective reviews of 10, 134, 28, and 49 patients have been published by Son et al., Scharp et al., Ozgen et al., and Guo et al., respectively [26–29]. These reviews found median survival to range from 2.8 to 5.2 months following reirradiation, without reports of severe toxicity. Three studies reported partially improved or stable neurological symptoms in 51–83%, while one study reported symptom improvement in 39% without reporting how many were stable. A summary of more recent reirradiation series is presented in Table 12.1.

Logie et al. performed a pooled multi-institutional retrospective analysis of 205 patients [30]. Patients of RPA class I had a median survival of 7.5 months following reirradiation; for class II, MS was 5.2 months, and for class III, 2.9 months. Karnofsky Performance Status <80, extracranial disease burden, time interval between courses <9 months, small cell histology, and uncontrolled primary site correlated with shorter MS.

Importantly, the rate of significant complications following reirradiation appears low, though

Table 12.1 Summary of whole brain reirradiation after upfront WBRT

Paper	Year	Patients	Age	Median first dose (Gy)	Median second dose (Gy)	Outcome measure	Median OS (months)
Wong et al.	1996	86	58 median	30	20	Symptom resolution or clinical improvement – 70%	4
Cooper et al.	1990	52	57.3 mean	30	25	Stable or clinical improvement at 2–4 weeks – 94%	5
Sadikov et al.	2007	72	56.5 median	20	25	Stable or clinical improvement – 73%	4.1
Son et al.	2012	10	59 mean	35	21.6	Symptom resolution or clinical improvement – 80%	5.2
Scharp et al.	2014	134	57 median	30	20	Stable or clinical improvement – 83%	2.8
Ozgen et al.	2013	28	52 median	30	25	Symptom resolution or clinical improvement – 39%	3
Guo et al.	2016	49	56 median	30	20	Stable or improved neurologic symptoms – 51%	3
Logie et al.	2017	205	55 median	20	20	–	3.6

this may be in part due to the limited survival of such patients [31]. It is unclear if this remains the case due to newer systemic therapies affording patients longer overall survival, given the potentially longer timeframe to develop late neurocognitive toxicity.

WBRT Salvage Following SRS

Patients who develop intracranial progression following SRS may also be treated with WBRT if they are no longer suitable for further local treatments. Typically, no alteration of WBRT dose/fractionation is required following SRS, unless critical structures such as the brain stem or optic chiasm were taken close to tolerance in the initial course of treatment.

Leptomeningeal Disease

Patients who develop leptomeningeal disease (Fig. 12.4) typically have a dismal prognosis, with a high proportion concurrently experiencing progressive disease at a systemic level [32]. Thus, symptom palliation and preservation of quality of life is the key goal in this setting, particularly as

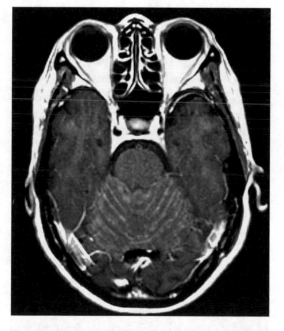

Fig. 12.4 Example of leptomeningeal disease of posterior fossa from NSCLC

symptoms often include highly morbid cranial nerve deficits. Often, steroids alone are insufficient for managing complications of leptomeningeal disease. As such, WBRT may have a role in the palliative management of these patients, with the potential to reduce tumor bulk and restore CSF flow [31].

Unfortunately, outcome data to conclusively show symptomatic benefit from WBRT are lacking. A retrospective review of 27 breast or lung cancer patients treated with WBRT alone for leptomeningeal carcinomatosis found a median OS of 8.1 weeks [33]. Perhaps highlighting the poor prognosis of this scenario, only four patients had follow-up MRI studies – of whom three had improvement in radiological appearances. No quality of life results were reported.

Another review of 125 patients with NSCLC showed no improvement in overall survival with WBRT [34]. Of note, 34% of patients had symptoms of raised intracranial pressure; median overall survival was 3 months; WBRT doses ranged from 30 Gy in 10 fractions to 37.5 Gy in 15 fractions. Again, no data regarding quality of life and symptom resolution were reported.

In summary, WBRT may have a role to play in the symptom management of leptomeningeal disease – though definitive data to demonstrate quality of life benefits are lacking.

Prophylactic Cranial Irradiation

WBRT is also used in the prophylactic setting, and remains a standard consideration in the management of small cell lung cancer (SCLC). This has been demonstrated by randomized trials and a systematic review, summarized in Table 12.2.

In the limited-stage setting, a meta-analysis by Auperin et al. found that prophylactic cranial irradiation (PCI) improved 3 year overall survival from 15.3% to 20.7%, while also improving the rate of disease-free survival and lowering the risk of brain metastasis development from 59% to 33% [35]. Of note, this was in the setting of complete remission following thoracic treatment, in an era where MRI was not routinely performed. Furthermore, CTs were not routinely performed prior to treatment.

In the extensive stage setting, an EORTC trial published in 2007 found benefits to both overall survival (27% vs 13% at 1 year) and incidence of

Table 12.2 Summary of PCI Data

Stage	Data	Outcome	Result (%)
Limited	Meta-analysis	3-year OS with PCI	20
	Auperin et al.	3-year OS without PCI	15
		Risk of BM with PCI	33
		Risk of BM without PCI	59
Extensive	Randomized trial	1-year OS with PCI	27
	EORTC 2007	1-year OS without PCI	13
		Symptomatic BM at 1 year with PCI	15
		Symptomatic BM at 1 year without PCI	40
	Randomized trial	1-year OS with PCI	48
	Takahashi et al.	1-year OS without PCI	54
	MRI staging	Incidence of BM with	48
		Incidence of BM without	69

symptomatic brain metastases (15% vs 40% at 1 year) for PCI [36]. As such, PCI is the standard of care in patients who are responding to systemic therapy with ES-SCLC. This is now complicated by the recent publication of a randomized trial where 3-monthly MRI brain imaging was utilized, with the subsequent findings of no overall survival benefit in those without MRI-apparent disease, compared with observation (OS 48% vs 54% at 1 year) [37]. The incidence of brain metastases was still reduced from 69% to 48% with PCI. Of note, 58% received delayed brain radiotherapy after being initially observed. A notable limitation of this study is that participating centers accrued approximately one patient per year. As such, the observation may be considered as an alternative to PCI in the extensive-stage setting, but is not currently the standard of practice.

To guide dose/fractionation decisions, a randomized trial comparing 25 Gy in 10 fractions with higher doses (36 Gy in 18 fractions and a hyperfractionated schedule of 36 Gy in 24 fractions twice-daily) found no benefit to higher doses [38]. As such, PCI of 25 Gy remains the standard of care. A 2012 analysis of RTOG 0212, a component of the aforementioned trial, found that patients treated with 36 Gy experienced significantly more chronic neurotoxicity compared with 25 Gy [39].

PCI has been investigated for non-small cell lung cancer, but no overall survival or disease-free survival benefits were demonstrated in a randomized RTOG trial of 356 patients [40]. As such, it is not routinely recommended. Of note, the incidence of brain metastases at 7.7% following PCI versus 18% on observation was comparatively lower compared with trials involving SCLC.

1–3 Brain Metastases – WBRT ± SRS

The role of WBRT has gradually diminished over time – this is most apparent in the setting of limited brain metastases, due to the advent of stereotactic radiosurgery and emerging data to show significant delayed neurocognitive toxicity from WBRT.

RTOG 9508 randomized patients with 1–3 newly diagnosed brain metastases to either WBRT or WBRT followed by SRS boost [41]. A survival advantage was shown for patients with a single unresectable brain metastasis for the addition of SRS to WBRT over WBRT alone. Additionally, improvement in Karnofsky performance status was found for patients receiving both treatments, compared to those receiving WBRT alone. The rate of neurologic death did not differ between the two groups. A secondary analysis of RTOG 9508 published in 2014 found that the overall survival advantage also extended to patients of Graded Prognostic Assessment (GPA) score 3.5–4.0, whether they had one, two, or three brain metastases [42]. This did not extend to patients of lower GPA scores.

A Cochrane review by Patil et al. on the topic of WBRT alone versus WBRT plus SRS corroborated this [43]. In the setting of a single brain metastasis less than 3 cm in diameter with controlled primary disease, WBRT plus SRS conferred not only a local control benefit compared with WBRT alone, but also a benefit in overall survival, as well as improvements in steroid requirements and performance status (KPS unchanged in 43% at 6 months versus 28%). Of note, when all patients are included (i.e., those with more than one metastasis), there was no survival benefit.

1–4 Brain Metastases – SRS ± WBRT

The above trials have suggested that SRS when added to WBRT has significant benefits for 1–3 brain metastases. In this section, we will examine the evidence for omission of WBRT outright on the basis of non-inferior survival and avoidance of delayed neurocognitive toxicity.

Randomized trials from NCCTG N0574 (a phase III RCT of SRS with or without WBRT for 1–3 brain metastases) and the MD Anderson Cancer Center found that the addition of WBRT to SRS resulted in inferior cognitive function following treatment [44, 45]. There was an improvement in intracranial disease control with the addition of WBRT, but not overall survival. The 1 year CNS progression rates were higher in the SRS alone arms – 73% and 35% versus 27% and 12%, respectively. N0574 in particular found deficits in terms of immediate recall, memory, and verbal fluency (92% vs 64%), while the MD Anderson trial found deterioration in learning and memory function. As such, potential advantages to omitting WBRT include avoidance of neurocognitive toxicity, minimal recovery time, and minimal delay for reinitiation of systemic therapy.

Churilla et al. performed a subset analysis of NCCTG N0574 of NSCLC patients with favorable prognoses. They found no significant differences in overall survival for patients receiving WBRT + SRS compared to SRS alone, despite improved intracranial control [46]. This is in contrast to the JROSG-99 trial which suggested an OS benefit to WBRT when added to SRS in favorable-prognosis NSCLC patients [47]. However, a significantly higher proportion of patients were likely to have EGFR mutation positivity in a

Japanese study population, resulting in improved survival. The interpretation of these trials is that in a Western population, it is likely that the addition of WBRT to SRS does not result in an overall survival benefit – despite higher rates of intracranial failure, for which salvage options exist.

A Japanese trial of 132 patients with 1–4 brain metastases treated with radiosurgery alone or WBRT plus radiosurgery found an increased local control rate of 89% with WBRT and SRS, versus 73% for SRS alone [48]. Distant intracranial failure was reduced from 64% to 42%. Concordant with other similar trials, there was no significant reduction in overall survival with the omission of WBRT, while rates of neurological death were unchanged. Functional independence is another measure which has been found to be similar between SRS and SRS + WBRT. The EORTC 22952–26001 trial specifically assessed duration of functional independence, with no difference found between WBRT + SRS versus SRS alone [17]. Overall survival was also similar.

A meta-analysis of phase three trials of SRS with or without WBRT for 1–4 brain metastases (pooled results of 364 patients from three RCTs) confirmed better OS and lower rates of distant brain failure for patients with a single brain metastasis [49]. Age was found to correlate with treatment outcome – specifically, if under 50, the addition of WBRT to SRS was actually detrimental to OS despite greater intracranial control. Reasons for this may include the effectiveness of salvage therapy and delay of systemic therapy. Of note, the risk of neurological death was reduced with adjuvant WBRT compared with WBRT upon progression. This was most pronounced in those under 50 years of age, from 39% to 22% though not statistically significant. As such, adjuvant WBRT may still have a role in select high-risk individuals, though this is yet to be clearly defined.

The time factor involved with WBRT following SRS probably has an impact. Of note, Chang et al. found that patients in the SRS alone arm received systemic therapy over 1 month earlier than patients in the SRS plus WBRT arm [45]. This also translated to a median of two more cycles of systemic therapy.

A specific paper outlining quality of life results from EORTC 22952–26001 revealed that quality of life was improved in patients receiving local therapy (surgery or radiosurgery) alone versus local therapy plus WBRT, in the setting of 1–3 brain metastases [50]. This was particularly significant for global health status at 9 months, physical functioning at 2 months, cognitive functioning at 12 months, and fatigue at 2 months – suggesting impacts of WBRT at more than just an early or late time point. Adverse impacts for WBRT were found on hair loss, appetite, nausea, drowsiness, and social functioning.

These trials have thus established SRS alone as the standard of care in patients of suitable performance status with limited brain metastases. It can be seen that the addition of WBRT does not improve overall survival, while having adverse effects on quality of life. Reasons for SRS alone may include the early detection of asymptomatic brain metastases via MRI observation, and the efficacy of salvage treatments implemented before significant clinical deterioration.

Future Directions – 4+ Brain Metastases

The role of WBRT may continue to change in the future, on the basis of early observational data suggesting suitability for SRS for greater than four metastases – leading to ongoing randomized trials investigating this hypothesis.

In 2014, Yamamoto et al. published a multi-institutional prospective observational study of SRS alone for patients with 1–10 brain metastases (JLGK0901) [51, 52]. For patients with a limited volume of intracranial disease, they found that the number of brain metastases did not correlate with outcome, thus identifying SRS as a potentially suitable treatment for patients of good performance status (KPS 80 or higher) with cumulative disease volume of less than or equal to 15 cc. Overall survival for 5–10 metastases was similar to 2–4 brain metastases (10.8 vs 10.8 months), as was the risk of neurological death (4.3% vs 1.7%) and the risk of distant intracranial progression (63.8% vs 54.5%) – while only 9% of patients received salvage WBRT. Of note, mini-mental state examination (MMSE) scores were maintained similar to baseline in greater than 90% of patients at 12 months, and greater than 86% of patients at 48 months. Additionally, the rate of complications (approximately 12% for any complications; 2–3% for grade 3 or higher) was no different between single, 2–4 and 5–10 treated lesions.

There are currently no published randomized data investigating SRS +/− WBRT in patients with four or more brain metastases. A current MD Anderson study is randomizing patients with 4–15 brain metastases to SRS or WBRT (NCT01592968), while a Netherlands trial of WBRT versus SRS for patients with 4–10 brain metastases is underway with a primary endpoint of quality of life at 3 months compared with baseline (NCT02353000) [53]. If these trials are positive, the role of WBRT in the setting of multiple brain metastases may continue to diminish.

Impact of Systemic Therapies with CNS Activity

The role of targeted therapies and immunotherapics has impacted the role of WBRT in select patients, primarily due to enhanced blood-brain barrier penetration of these agents [54]. These therapies have expanding roles for histologies which comprise a significant proportion of patients with brain metastases, such as non-small cell lung cancer and melanoma [5, 55]. Typically, suitable patients will have low-volume, asymptomatic disease. For illustrative purposes, an MRI scan of a patient treated upfront with systemic therapy is shown in Fig. 12.5.

Melanoma represents an area where immunotherapy and targeted therapy have altered the systemic treatment armamentarium, including for intracranial disease. For BRAF-mutant disease, dabrafenib, vemurafenib, and trametinib have been proven to have some degree of effectiveness for brain metastases. Earlier studies found response rates ranging from 6.7% to 39% for dabrafenib and vemurafenib alone, though progression-free survival was relatively short at 4 months or fewer [56, 57]. More promising results have been found for combination therapy consisting of dabrafenib and trametinib, an oral MEK inhibitor [58]. Intracranial response rates range from 44% to 60%, though intracranial progression free survival remains modest at 5–7 months at best.

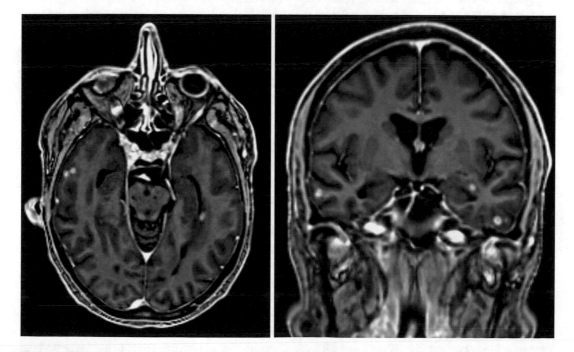

Fig. 12.5 MRI Brain of patient with low-volume intracranial disease, treated with targeted therapy

Ipilimumab, an anti-CTLA-4 monoclonal antibody, has demonstrated a response rate of 24% for asymptomatic melanoma brain metastases [59]. However, efficacy considerably decreases if steroids are required for symptom management (a common scenario), with a drop in response rates to only 10%. Furthermore, median intracranial PFS remains low at only 6 weeks. The most promising immunotherapy thus far appears to be anti-PD-1 antibodies such as pembrolizumab. In 2016, Goldberg et al. found pembrolizumab has an intracranial response rate of 22% in melanoma patients and 33% for NSCLC for a group of patients with a lesion size of 1.9 cm or less [60]. A recently published randomized phase 2 trial found that nivolumab in combination with ipilimumab resulted in a response rate of 46% with combination therapy, compared with 20% for nivolumab alone and 6% for ipilimumab alone [61]. Grade 3 or higher toxicity occurred in 54% of patients on combination therapy. In BRAF-mutant patients who progress despite targeted therapy, the response rate for combined immunotherapy was only 16%, highlighting a worse overall biology. Response rates were less than 10% in the setting of leptomeningeal disease or ongoing steroid requirements. Further consolidating these findings, a single-arm, phase II trial involving the same systemic therapy in 94 asymptomatic patients found 58% of patients had either stable disease (2%), partial response (30%), or a complete response (26%) [62]. Maximal lesional size was 3 cm, while 76% of patients had one or two lesions only. Consistent with other trials, grade 3 or higher toxicity occurred in 55% of patients.

As such, the role of upfront immunotherapy and targeted therapy for metastatic melanoma is for carefully selected patients with asymptomatic disease in non-eloquent locations, where progression would not result in rapid and severe morbidity. The importance of adequate MRI surveillance should not be underestimated particularly due to the PFS seen in published data to date, with salvage SRS or WBRT remaining an option.

Standard chemotherapy for lung cancer has limited CNS penetrance [63]. Sperduto et al. investigated the role of the addition of either temozolomide or erlotinib to WBRT and SRS for NSCLC in a phase III RTOG trial [64]. Accrual was relatively limited, and no overall survival benefit was found; there was a non-statistically significant deleterious effect (13.4 months versus 6.3 and 6.1 months), suggested to be due to increased toxicity.

Targeted therapies for EGFR-mutant and ALK-rearranged NSCLC have demonstrated intracranial efficacy, resulting in a dramatic change in treatment options for low volume asymptomatic brain metastases [54, 65, 66]. It should be recognized however that such subsets of NSCLC represent a minority of patients, particularly in Western populations. In the setting of EGFR-mutant NSCLC, relatively high intracranial response rates are seen with erlotinib, gefitinib, and osimertinib – in the order of 50–80%, with PFS ranging from 6 to 12 months. For ALK-rearranged NSCLC, intracranial response rates for crizotinib are around 20%, while newer agents such as alectinib, brigatinib, and ceritinib have improved response rates of 50–70% [67–70]. Brigatinib, in particular, demonstrated very promising intracranial progression-free survival of up to 18 months. Thus, for EGFR-mutant and ALK-rearranged NSCLC, WBRT or SRS can potentially be delayed for asymptomatic patients with low volume disease, who are managed with systemic therapy and adequate intracranial surveillance. It is unknown whether salvage SRS or WBRT are as effective when deferred upfront. Immunotherapy is also being investigated for non-mutant NSCLC, though definitive data in this setting are awaited.

Despite the aforementioned studies, caution should be adopted when considering omission of brain radiotherapy. Retrospective data published in 2016 suggest that deferral of radiotherapy in patients with EGFR-mutant NSCLC was associated with inferior overall survival [71]. The duration of response of many agents is relatively short, while most trials were phase II single-arm studies. A 2017 update from the same authors corroborated this, with median OS for patients treated with upfront SRS, WBRT, and EGFR-TKIs being 46 months, 30 months, and 25 months, respectively [72]. This highlights the need for prospective randomized data to guide the optimal sequencing of therapy, given the suggestion for a survival detriment with deferral of radiotherapy. Furthermore, the optimal timing and sequencing of therapy is not yet established. When choosing a management strategy, the overall clinical context should be considered – including factors such as lesion size, location, intracranial and extracranial disease burden, expected effectiveness of systemic therapy, and the overall pace of disease progression.

Her-2 positive breast cancer is another histology where targeted therapy has shown some promise. The phase II LANDSCAPE trial found an intracranial response rate of 65.9% in 45 patients with HER-2 positive breast cancer to lapatinib and capecitabine [73]. Median intracranial progression-free survival was 5.5 months, though 49% of patients experienced grade 3 or 4 toxicity. Prior to this, options were disappointing – Freedman et al. conducted a prospective trial of neratinib for 40 patients with Her-2 positive metastatic breast cancer brain metastases; the CNS objective response rate was 8%, with median progression-free survival of 1.9 months (patients were imaged every 2 months routinely) and a grade 3 toxicity rate of over 20% [74].

The optimal sequencing of systemic therapy and radiotherapy is unclear. A 2016 review paper by Kroeze et al. suggested that concurrent targeted therapy or immunotherapy with stereotactic radiotherapy appears to be well tolerated, with low rates of increased toxicity – apart from BRAF inhibitors, where high rates of severe toxicity are observed [75]. However, only limited data were found for more modern immunotherapies such as pembrolizumab and nivolumab; thus, clinicians should proceed with caution and maintain close contact with medical oncologists prior to and during treatment.

Neurotoxicity and HA-WBRT

Delayed neurocognitive toxicity is a recognized side effect of WBRT. However, it must be considered that intracranial disease progression can have significant effects on neurocognition as well – in many cases more so than the effect of treatment. Most patients with brain metastases in initial trials investigating the neurocognitive sequelae of WBRT did not live beyond 6 months [76]. Nonetheless, debilitating dementia associated with WBRT is rare – but patients treated with high doses per fraction (>3.5 Gy) and high total doses may be particularly susceptible [77]. This should be considered when counselling patients.

Radiotherapy-induced damage to neural stem cells may contribute to cognitive decline following RT, with clinical data suggesting a dose-response correlation specific to the hippocampus [78, 79]. The advent of IMRT has enabled conformal avoidance of the hippocampal neural stem cell compartment, and hippocampal-avoidance WBRT (HA-WBRT) [80, 81]. Technical requirements for HA-WBRT are summarized in Table 12.3 [82, 83], with an example of contours shown in Fig. 12.6, and dosimetry shown in Fig. 12.7.

To demonstrate the utility of hippocampal dose-avoidance, RTOG 0933 was a phase 2 single-arm trial which found a mean relative decline in Hopkins Verbal Learning Test-Revised Delayed Recall of 7% from baseline following HA-WBRT – substantially lower than a historical control of 30% for traditional WBRT [82]. Additionally, there was no decline in quality of life scores. Based on this trial, a median hippocampal dose of <9 Gy and Dmax of <16 Gy were suggested. These constraints are listed in Table 12.3.

Table 12.3 Requirements and dose constraints for HA-WBRT

Aspect	Requirements
Imaging	3D axial thin-slice MRI (<1.5 mm slices)
Simulation	Fusion with radiotherapy planning CT (slice thickness 2.5 mm or less)
Technique	Intensity modulated radiation therapy, volumetric modulated arc therapy, or helical tomotherapy
Contours	Hippocampus contours
	Hippocampal avoidance volume (5 mm expansion on hippocampi)
Dose constraints	Hippocampus: Maximum 16 Gy
	Hippocampus: <9 Gy to 100%
	Hippocampal avoidance volume: Maximum 30 Gy

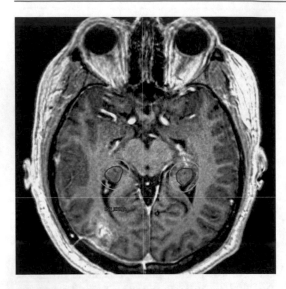

Fig. 12.6 Hippocampal contours on MRI

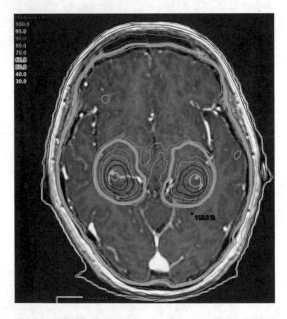

Fig. 12.7 Hippocampal avoidance (HA)-WBRT dosimetry

Further guidance in relation to hippocampal dose constraints comes from a Gondi et al. study which prospectively evaluated the relationship between hippocampal dose and long-term neurocognitive function for benign or low-grade adult brain tumors treated with fractionated stereotactic radiotherapy [84]. A dose of 7.3 Gy (equivalent dose in 2 Gy-fractions) to 40% or more of

bilateral hippocampi correlated with impairment in delayed recall at 18 months.

Radioprotective agents such as memantine have been investigated. RTOG 0614 was a multi-institutional RCT which found that the use of memantine, an N-methyl-D-aspartate (NMDA) receptor antagonist, did not significantly reduce the rate of decline in delayed recall at 24 weeks when used during WBRT [85]. However, there was significantly longer time to cognitive decline in the memantine arm (at 24 weeks, 54% compared to 65%), as well as higher executive function, processing speed and delayed recognition while the medication exhibited minimal toxicity. However, there remains some uncertainty regarding interpretation of the results, given a majority of patients had died or progressed at 24 weeks, resulting in only 149 analyzable patients.

Preliminary results of NCT02360215 were recently presented [86]. This was a phase III trial of WBRT with memantine, with or without hippocampal avoidance with a primary endpoint of time to neurocognitive failure. Results to date, presented in October 2018, revealed a reduction in neurocognitive failure rate at 6 months from 69.1% to 58% for conventional WBRT versus HA-WBRT, respectively, while achieving similar intracranial control and overall survival. The full results are eagerly awaited.

NCT02635009 will investigate the role of HA-WBRT for prophylactic cranial irradiation in SCLC, with time to deterioration in episodic memory being one of the primary outcomes.

Overall, there are early data to suggest neurocognitive protective effects of measures such as hippocampal avoidance and memantine, though trials are ongoing. It is unclear what effect such measures will have on the use of WBRT, particularly as SRS alone is under investigation for 4–15 metastases.

> **Key Points**
> • The role of WBRT has diminished over time due to advances in radiosurgery and systemic therapy, with a growing body of literature demonstrating com-

parably favorable efficacy and toxicity. Particularly in the setting of limited brain metastases, SRS is now considered the standard of care in place of WBRT.

- WBRT nonetheless continues to have a role in patients unsuitable for SRS who are of reasonable performance status – particularly those with leptomeningeal disease and for prophylactic cranial irradiation in the setting of SCLC. It also continues to have a role in the reirradiation setting, either after SRS or repeated after a first course of WBRT, though the prognosis of these patients is typically poor.

- In patients of poor performance status, best supportive care can be considered in place of WBRT, though this should be considered in the context of individual patient factors. In asymptomatic patients with low-volume intracranial disease and effective upfront targeted therapy or immunotherapy options, both SRS and WBRT can be reserved for future progression in select cases. Caution should be applied when withholding upfront radiotherapy and individual judgement should always be utilized, as well as multidisciplinary discussion with medical oncologists and neurosurgeons.

- Delayed neurotoxicity from WBRT can be mediated by hippocampal-avoidance WBRT, with recent randomized data showing significant benefits. Randomized trials are underway to evaluate the role of SRS compared with WBRT in the setting of 4–15 brain metastases and limited overall intracranial disease volume. These trials are eagerly awaited, as they will likely continue to shape the modern management of brain metastases, and, in particular, the role of WBRT.

References

1. Borgelt B, Gelber R, Kramer S, Brady LW, Chang CH, Davis LW, Perez CA, Hendrickson FR. The palliation of brain metastases: final results of the first two studies by the Radiation Therapy Oncology Group. Int J Radiat Oncol Biol Phys. 1980;6(1):1–9.
2. Pease NJ, Edwards A, Moss LJ. Effectiveness of whole brain radiotherapy in the treatment of brain metastases: a systematic review. Palliat Med. 2005;19(4):288–99.
3. Moraes FY, Taunk NK, Marta GN, Suh JH, Yamada Y. The rationale for targeted therapies and stereotactic radiosurgery in the treatment of brain metastases. Oncologist. 2016;21(2):244–51.
4. Mulvenna P, Nankivell M, Barton R, Faivre-Finn C, Wilson P, McColl E, Moore B, Brisbane I, Ardron D, Holt T, Morgan S, Lee C, Waite K, Bayman N, Pugh C, Sydes B, Stephens R, Parmar MK, Langley RE. Dexamethasone and supportive care with or without whole brain radiotherapy in treating patients with non-small cell lung cancer with brain metastases unsuitable for resection or stereotactic radiotherapy (QUARTZ): results from a phase 3, non-inferiority, randomised trial. Lancet. 2016;388(10055):2004–14.
5. Delattre JY, Krol G, Thaler HT, Posner JB. Distribution of brain metastases. Arch Neurol. 1988;45(7):741–4.
6. McTyre E, Scott J, Chinnaiyan P. Whole brain radiotherapy for brain metastasis. Surg Neurol Int. 2013;4(Suppl 4):S236–44.
7. Gaspar L, Scott C, Rotman M, Asbell S, Phillips T, Wasserman T, McKenna WG, Byhardt R. Recursive partitioning analysis (RPA) of prognostic factors in three Radiation Therapy Oncology Group (RTOG) brain metastases trials. Int J Radiat Oncol Biol Phys. 1997;37(4):745–51.
8. Sperduto PW, Kased N, Roberge D, Xu Z, Shanley R, Luo X, Sneed PK, Chao ST, Weil RJ, Suh J, Bhatt A, Jensen AW, Brown PD, Shih HA, Kirkpatrick J, Gaspar LE, Fiveash JB, Chiang V, Knisely JP, Sperduto CM, Lin N, Mehta M. Summary report on the graded prognostic assessment: an accurate and facile diagnosis-specific tool to estimate survival for patients with brain metastases. J Clin Oncol. 2012;30(4):419–25.
9. Sperduto PW, Jiang W, Brown PD, Braunstein S, Sneed P, Wattson DA, Shih HA, Bangdiwala A, Shanley R, Lockney NA, Beal K, Lou E, Amatruda T, Sperduto WA, Kirkpatrick JP, Yeh N, Gaspar LE, Molitoris JK, Masucci L, Roberge D, Yu J, Chiang V, Mehta M. Estimating survival in melanoma patients with brain metastases: an update of the graded prognostic assessment for melanoma using molecular markers (melanoma-molGPA). Int J Radiat Oncol Biol Phys. 2017;99(4):812–6.

10. Sperduto PW, Yang TJ, Beal K, Pan H, Brown PD, Bangdiwala A, Shanley R, Yeh N, Gaspar LE, Braunstein S, Sneed P, Boyle J, Kirkpatrick JP, Mak KS, Shih HA, Engelman A, Roberge D, Arvold ND, Alexander B, Awad MM, Contessa J, Chiang V, Hardie J, Ma D, Lou E, Sperduto W, Mehta MP. Estimating survival in patients with lung cancer and brain metastases: an update of the graded prognostic assessment for lung cancer using molecular markers (lung-molGPA). JAMA Oncol. 2017;3(6):827–31.

11. National Comprehensive Cancer Network. Central nervous system cancers (version 1. 2018). https://www.nccn.org/professionals/physician_gls/pdf/cns.pdf. Accessed 22 Oct 2018.

12. Tsao MN, Xu W, Wong RK, Lloyd N, Laperriere N, Sahgal A, Rakovitch E, Chow E. Whole brain radiotherapy for the treatment of newly diagnosed multiple brain metastases. Cochrane Database Syst Rev. 2018;1:CD003869.

13. Khuntia D, Brown P, Li J, Mehta MP. Whole-brain radiotherapy in the management of brain metastasis. J Clin Oncol. 2006;24(8):1295–304.

14. Patchell RA, Tibbs PA, Walsh JW, Dempsey RJ, Maruyama Y, Kryscio RJ, Markesbery WR, Macdonald JS, Young B. A randomized trial of surgery in the treatment of single metastases to the brain. N Engl J Med. 1990;322(8):494–500.

15. Patchell RA, Tibbs PA, Regine WF, Dempsey RJ, Mohiuddin M, Kryscio RJ, Markesbery WR, Foon KA, Young B. Postoperative radiotherapy in the treatment of single metastases to the brain: a randomized trial. JAMA. 1998;280(17):1485–9.

16. Noordijk EM, Vecht CJ, Haaxma-Reiche H, Padberg GW, Voormolen JH, Hoekstra FH, Tans JT, Lambooij N, Metsaars JA, Wattendorff AR, et al. The choice of treatment of single brain metastasis should be based on extracranial tumor activity and age. Int J Radiat Oncol Biol Phys. 1994;29(4):711–7.

17. Kocher M, Soffietti R, Abacioglu U, Villà S, Fauchon F, Baumert BG, Fariselli L, Tzuk-Shina T, Kortmann RD, Carrie C, Ben Hassel M, Kouri M, Valeinis E, van den Berge D, Collette S, Collette L, Mueller RP. Adjuvant whole-brain radiotherapy versus observation after radiosurgery or surgical resection of one to three cerebral metastases: results of the EORTC 22952–26001 study. J Clin Oncol. 2011;29(2):134–41.

18. Mahajan A, Ahmed S, McAleer MF, Weinberg JS, Li J, Brown P, Settle S, Prabhu SS, Lang FF, Levine N, McGovern S, Sulman E, McCutcheon IE, Azeem S, Cahill D, Tatsui C, Heimberger AB, Ferguson S, Ghia A, Demonte F, Raza S, Guha-Thakurta N, Yang J, Sawaya R, Hess KR, Rao G. Post-operative stereotactic radiosurgery versus observation for completely resected brain metastases: a single-centre, randomised, controlled, phase 3 trial. Lancet Oncol. 2017;18(8):1040–8.

19. Brown PD, Ballman KV, Cerhan JH, Anderson SK, Carrero XW, Whitton AC, Greenspoon J, Parney IF, Laack NNI, Ashman JB, Bahary JP, Hadjipanayis CG, Urbanic JJ, Barker FG 2nd, Farace E, Khuntia D, Giannini C, Buckner JC, Galanis E, Roberge D. Postoperative stereotactic radiosurgery compared with whole brain radiotherapy for resected metastatic brain disease (NCCTG N107C/CEC·3): a multicentre, randomised, controlled, phase 3 trial. Lancet Oncol. 2017;18(8):1049–60.

20. Kayama T, Sato S, Sakurada K, Mizusawa J, Nishikawa R, Narita Y, Sumi M, Miyakita Y, Kumabe T, Sonoda Y, Arakawa Y, Miyamoto S, Beppu T, Sugiyama K, Nakamura H, Nagane M, Nakasu Y, Hashimoto N, Terasaki M, Matsumura A, Ishikawa E, Wakabayashi T, Iwadate Y, Ohue S, Kobayashi H, Kinoshita M, Asano K, Mukasa A, Tanaka K, Asai A, Nakamura H, Abe T, Muragaki Y, Iwasaki K, Aoki T, Watanabe T, Sasaki H, Izumoto S, Mizoguchi M, Matsuo T, Takeshima H, Hayashi M, Jokura H, Mizowaki T, Shimizu E, Shirato H, Tago M, Katayama H, Fukuda H, Shibui S, Japan Clinical Oncology Group. Effects of surgery with salvage stereotactic radiosurgery versus surgery with whole-brain radiation therapy in patients with one to four brain metastases (JCOG0504): a phase III, noninferiority, randomized controlled trial. J Clin Oncol. 2018:JCO2018786186.

21. Kępka L, Tyc-Szczepaniak D, Bujko K, Olszyna-Serementa M, Michalski W, Sprawka A, Trąbska-Kluch B, Komosińska K, Wasilewska-Teśluk E, Czeremszyńska B. Stereotactic radiotherapy of the tumor bed compared to whole brain radiotherapy after surgery of single brain metastasis: results from a randomized trial. Radiother Oncol. 2016;121(2):217–24.

22. Wong WW, Schild SE, Sawyer TE, Shaw EG. Analysis of outcome in patients reirradiated for brain metastases. Int J Radiat Oncol Biol Phys. 1996;34(3):585–90.

23. Ammirati M, Cobbs CS, Linskey ME, Paleologos NA, Ryken TC, Burri SH, Asher AL, Loeffler JS, Robinson PD, Andrews DW, Gaspar LE, Kondziolka D, McDermott M, Mehta MP, Mikkelsen T, Olson JJ, Patchell RA, Kalkanis SN. The role of retreatment in the management of recurrent/progressive brain metastases: a systematic review and evidence-based clinical practice guideline. J Neuro-Oncol. 2010;96(1):85–96.

24. Cooper JS, Steinfeld AD, Lerch IA. Cerebral metastases: value of reirradiation in selected patients. Radiology. 1990;174(3 Pt 1):883–5.

25. Sadikov E, Bezjak A, Yi QL, Wells W, Dawson L, Millar BA, Laperriere N. Value of whole brain re-irradiation for brain metastases–single centre experience. Clin Oncol (R Coll Radiol). 2007;19(7):532–8.

26. Son CH, Jimenez R, Niemierko A, Loeffler JS, Oh KS, Shih HA. Outcomes after whole brain reirradiation in patients with brain metastases. Int J Radiat Oncol Biol Phys. 2012;82(2):e167–72.

27. Scharp M, Hauswald H, Bischof M, Debus J, Combs SE. Re-irradiation in the treatment of patients with cerebral metastases of solid tumors: retrospective analysis. Radiat Oncol. 2014;9:4.

28. Ozgen Z, Atasoy BM, Kefeli AU, Seker A, Dane F, Abacioglu U. The benefit of whole brain reirradia-

tion in patients with multiple brain metastases. Radiat Oncol. 2013;8:186.

29. Guo S, Balagamwala EH, Reddy C, Elson P, Suh JH, Chao ST. Clinical and radiographic outcomes from repeat whole-brain radiation therapy for brain metastases in the age of stereotactic radiosurgery. Am J Clin Oncol. 2016;39(3):288–93.

30. Logie N, Jimenez RB, Pulenzas N, Linden K, Ciafone D, Ghosh S, Xu Y, Lefresne S, Wong E, Son CH, Shih HA, Wong WW, Tyldesley S, Dennis K, Chow E, Fairchild AM. Estimating prognosis at the time of repeat whole brain radiation therapy for multiple brain metastases: the reirradiation score. Adv Radiat Oncol. 2017;2(3):381–90.

31. Nguyen TD, DeAngelis LM. Brain metastases. Neurol Clin. 2007;25(4):1173–92.

32. Wang N, Bertalan MS, Brastianos PK. Leptomeningeal metastasis from systemic cancer: review and update on management. Cancer. 2018;124(1):21–35.

33. Gani C, Müller AC, Eckert F, Schroeder C, Bender B, Pantazis G, Bamberg M, Berger B. Outcome after whole brain radiotherapy alone in intracranial leptomeningeal carcinomatosis from solid tumors. Strahlenther Onkol. 2012;188(2):148–53.

34. Morris PG, Reiner AS, Szenberg OR, Clarke JL, Panageas KS, Perez HR, Kris MG, Chan TA, DeAngelis LM, Omuro AM. Leptomeningeal metastasis from non-small cell lung cancer: survival and the impact of whole brain radiotherapy. J Thorac Oncol. 2012;7(2):382–5.

35. Aupérin A, Arriagada R, Pignon JP, Le Péchoux C, Gregor A, Stephens RJ, Kristjansen PE, Johnson BE, Ueoka H, Wagner H, Aisner J. Prophylactic cranial irradiation for patients with small-cell lung cancer in complete remission. Prophylactic Cranial Irradiation Overview Collaborative Group. N Engl J Med. 1999;341(7):476–84.

36. Slotman B, Faivre-Finn C, Kramer G, Rankin E, Snee M, Hatton M, Postmus P, Collette L, Musat E, Senan S, EORTC Radiation Oncology Group and Lung Cancer Group. Prophylactic cranial irradiation in extensive small-cell lung cancer. N Engl J Med. 2007;357(7):664–72.

37. Takahashi T, Yamanaka T, Seto T, Harada H, Nokihara H, Saka H, Nishio M, Kaneda H, Takayama K, Ishimoto O, Takeda K, Yoshioka H, Tachihara M, Sakai H, Goto K, Yamamoto N. Prophylactic cranial irradiation versus observation in patients with extensive-disease small-cell lung cancer: a multicentre, randomised, open-label, phase 3 trial. Lancet Oncol. 2017;18(5):663–71.

38. Le Péchoux C, Dunant A, Senan S, Wolfson A, Quoix E, Faivre-Finn C, Ciuleanu T, Arriagada R, Jones R, Wanders R, Lerouge D, Laplanche A, Prophylactic Cranial Irradiation (PCI) Collaborative Group. Standard-dose versus higher-dose prophylactic cranial irradiation (PCI) in patients with limited-stage small-cell lung cancer in complete remission after chemotherapy and thoracic radiotherapy (PCI 99–01, EORTC 22003–08004, RTOG 0212, and IFCT

99–01): a randomised clinical trial. Lancet Oncol. 2009;10(5):467–74.

39. Wolfson AH, Bae K, Komaki R, Meyers C, Movsas B, Le Pechoux C, Werner-Wasik M, Videtic GM, Garces YI, Choy H. Primary analysis of a phase II randomized trial Radiation Therapy Oncology Group (RTOG) 0212: impact of different total doses and schedules of prophylactic cranial irradiation on chronic neurotoxicity and quality of life for patients with limited-disease small-cell lung cancer. Int J Radiat Oncol Biol Phys. 2011;81(1):77–84.

40. Gore EM, Bae K, Wong SJ, Sun A, Bonner JA, Schild SE, Gaspar LE, Bogart JA, Werner-Wasik M, Choy H. Phase III comparison of prophylactic cranial irradiation versus observation in patients with locally advanced non-small-cell lung cancer: primary analysis of radiation therapy oncology group study RTOG 0214. J Clin Oncol. 2011;29(3):272–8.

41. Andrews DW, Scott CB, Sperduto PW, Flanders AE, Gaspar LE, Schell MC, Werner-Wasik M, Demas W, Ryu J, Bahary JP, Souhami L, Rotman M, Mehta MP, Curran WJ Jr. Whole brain radiation therapy with or without stereotactic radiosurgery boost for patients with one to three brain metastases: phase III results of the RTOG 9508 randomised trial. Lancet. 2004;363(9422):1665–72.

42. Sperduto PW, Shanley R, Luo X, Andrews D, Werner-Wasik M, Valicenti R, Bahary JP, Souhami L, Won M, Mehta M. Secondary analysis of RTOG 9508, a phase 3 randomized trial of whole-brain radiation therapy versus WBRT plus stereotactic radiosurgery in patients with 1–3 brain metastases; poststratified by the graded prognostic assessment (GPA). Int J Radiat Oncol Biol Phys. 2014;90(3):526–31.

43. Patil CG, Pricola K, Sarmiento JM, Garg SK, Bryant A, Black KL. Whole brain radiation therapy (WBRT) alone versus WBRT and radiosurgery for the treatment of brain metastases. Cochrane Database Syst Rev. 2017;9:CD006121.

44. Brown PD, Jaeckle K, Ballman KV, Farace E, Cerhan JH, Anderson SK, Carrero XW, Barker FG 2nd, Deming R, Burri SH, Ménard C, Chung C, Stieber VW, Pollock BE, Galanis E, Buckner JC, Asher AL. Effect of radiosurgery alone vs radiosurgery with whole brain radiation therapy on cognitive function in patients with 1 to 3 brain metastases: a randomized clinical trial. JAMA. 2016;316(4):401–9.

45. Chang EL, Wefel JS, Hess KR, Allen PK, Lang FF, Kornguth DG, Arbuckle RB, Swint JM, Shiu AS, Maor MH, Meyers CA. Neurocognition in patients with brain metastases treated with radiosurgery or radiosurgery plus whole-brain irradiation: a randomised controlled trial. Lancet Oncol. 2009;10(11):1037–44.

46. Churilla TM, Ballman KV, Brown PD, Twohy EL, Jaeckle K, Farace E, Cerhan JH, Anderson SK, Carrero XW, Garces YI, Barker FG 2nd, Deming R, Dixon JG, Burri SH, Chung C, Ménard C, Stieber VW, Pollock BE, Galanis E, Buckner JC, Asher AL. Stereotactic radiosurgery with or without whole-brain radiation therapy for limited brain metastases: a secondary

analysis of the North Central Cancer Treatment Group N0574 (Alliance) randomized controlled trial. Int J Radiat Oncol Biol Phys. 2017;99(5):1173–8.

47. Aoyama H, Tago M, Shirato H, Japanese Radiation Oncology Study Group 99–1 (JROSG 99–1) Investigators. Stereotactic radiosurgery with or without whole-brain radiotherapy for brain metastases: secondary analysis of the JROSG 99–1 randomized clinical trial. JAMA Oncol. 2015 Jul;1(4):457–64.

48. Aoyama H, Shirato H, Tago M, Nakagawa K, Toyoda T, Hatano K, Kenjyo M, Oya N, Hirota S, Shioura H, Kunieda E, Inomata T, Hayakawa K, Katoh N, Kobashi G. Stereotactic radiosurgery plus whole-brain radiation therapy vs stereotactic radiosurgery alone for treatment of brain metastases: a randomized controlled trial. JAMA. 2006;295(21):2483–91.

49. Sahgal A, Aoyama H, Kocher M, Neupane B, Collette S, Tago M, Shaw P, Beyene J, Chang EL. Phase 3 trials of stereotactic radiosurgery with or without whole-brain radiation therapy for 1 to 4 brain metastases: individual patient data meta-analysis. Int J Radiat Oncol Biol Phys. 2015;91(4):710–7.

50. Soffietti R, Kocher M, Abacioglu UM, Villa S, Fauchon F, Baumert BG, Fariselli L, Tzuk-Shina T, Kortmann RD, Carrie C, Ben Hassel M, Kouri M, Valeinis E, van den Berge D, Mueller RP, Tridello G, Collette L, Bottomley A. A European Organisation for Research and Treatment of Cancer phase III trial of adjuvant whole-brain radiotherapy versus observation in patients with one to three brain metastases from solid tumors after surgical resection or radiosurgery: quality-of-life results. J Clin Oncol. 2013;31(1):65–72.

51. Yamamoto M, Serizawa T, Shuto T, Akabane A, Higuchi Y, Kawagishi J, Yamanaka K, Sato Y, Jokura H, Yomo S, Nagano O, Kenai H, Moriki A, Suzuki S, Kida Y, Iwai Y, Hayashi M, Onishi H, Gondo M, Sato M, Akimitsu T, Kubo K, Kikuchi Y, Shibasaki T, Goto T, Takanashi M, Mori Y, Takakura K, Saeki N, Kunieda E, Aoyama H, Momoshima S, Tsuchiya K. Stereotactic radiosurgery for patients with multiple brain metastases (JLGK0901): a multi-institutional prospective observational study. Lancet Oncol. 2014;15(4):387–95.

52. Yamamoto M, Serizawa T, Higuchi Y, Sato Y, Kawagishi J, Yamanaka K, Shuto T, Akabane A, Jokura H, Yomo S, Nagano O, Aoyama H. A multi-institutional prospective observational study of stereotactic radiosurgery for patients with multiple brain metastases (JLGK0901 study update): irradiation-related complications and long-term maintenance of mini-mental state examination scores. Int J Radiat Oncol Biol Phys. 2017;99(1):31–40.

53. Zindler JD, Bruynzeel AME, Eekers DBP, Hurkmans CW, Swinnen A, Lambin P. Whole brain radiotherapy versus stereotactic radiosurgery for 4–10 brain metastases: a phase III randomised multicentre trial. BMC Cancer. 2017;17(1):500.

54. Venur VA, Ahluwalia MS. Targeted therapy in brain metastases: ready for primetime? Am Soc Clin Oncol Educ Book. 2016;35:e123–30.

55. Yawn BP, Wollan PC, Schroeder C, Gazzuola L, Mehta M. Temporal and gender-related trends in brain metastases from lung and breast cancer. Minn Med. 2003;86(12):32–7.

56. Long GV, Trefzer U, Davies MA, Kefford RF, Ascierto PA, Chapman PB, Puzanov I, Hauschild A, Robert C, Algazi A, Mortier L, Tawbi H, Wilhelm T, Zimmer L, Switzky J, Swann S, Martin AM, Guckert M, Goodman V, Streit M, Kirkwood JM, Schadendorf D. Dabrafenib in patients with Val600Glu or Val600Lys BRAF-mutant melanoma metastatic to the brain (BREAK-MB): a multicentre, open-label, phase 2 trial. Lancet Oncol. 2012;13(11):1087–95.

57. McArthur GA, Maio M, Arance A, Nathan P, Blank C, Avril MF, Garbe C, Hauschild A, Schadendorf D, Hamid O, Fluck M, Thebeau M, Schachter J, Kefford R, Chamberlain M, Makrutzki M, Robson S, Gonzalez R, Margolin K. Vemurafenib in metastatic melanoma patients with brain metastases: an open-label, single-arm, phase 2, multicentre study. Ann Oncol. 2017;28(3):634–41.

58. Davies MA, Saiag P, Robert C, Grob JJ, Flaherty KT, Arance A, Chiarion-Sileni V, Thomas L, Lesimple T, Mortier L, Moschos SJ, Hogg D, Márquez-Rodas I, Del Vecchio M, Lebbé C, Meyer N, Zhang Y, Huang Y, Mookerjee B, Long GV. Dabrafenib plus trametinib in patients with BRAF(V600)-mutant melanoma brain metastases (COMBI-MB): a multicentre, multicohort, open-label, phase 2 trial. Lancet Oncol. 2017;18(7):863–73.

59. Margolin K, Ernstoff MS, Hamid O, Lawrence D, McDermott D, Puzanov I, Wolchok JD, Clark JI, Sznol M, Logan TF, Richards J, Michener T, Balogh A, Heller KN, Hodi FS. Ipilimumab in patients with melanoma and brain metastases: an open-label, phase 2 trial. Lancet Oncol. 2012;13(5):459–65.

60. Goldberg SB, Gettinger SN, Mahajan A, Chiang AC, Herbst RS, Sznol M, Tsiouris AJ, Cohen J, Vortmeyer A, Jilaveanu L, Yu J, Hegde U, Speaker S, Madura M, Ralabate A, Rivera A, Rowen E, Gerrish H, Yao X, Chiang V, Kluger HM. Pembrolizumab for patients with melanoma or non-small-cell lung cancer and untreated brain metastases: early analysis of a non-randomised, open-label, phase 2 trial. Lancet Oncol. 2016;17(7):976–83.

61. Long GV, Atkinson V, Lo S, Sandhu S, Guminski AD, Brown MP, Wilmott JS, Edwards J, Gonzalez M, Scolyer RA, Menzies AM, McArthur GA. Combination nivolumab and ipilimumab or nivolumab alone in melanoma brain metastases: a multicenter randomised phase 2 study. Lancet Oncol. 2018;19(5):672–81.

62. Tawbi HA, Forsyth PA, Algazi A, Hamid O, Hodi FS, Moschos SJ, Khushalani NI, Lewis K, Lao CD, Postow MA, Atkins MB, Ernstoff MS, Reardon DA, Puzanov I, Kudchadkar RR, Thomas RP, Tarhini A, Pavlick AC, Jiang J, Avila A, Demelo S,

Margolin K. Combined nivolumab and ipilimumab in melanoma metastatic to the brain. N Engl J Med. 2018;379(8):722–30.

63. Postmus PE, Smit EF. Chemotherapy for brain metastases of lung cancer: a review. Ann Oncol. 1999;10(7):753–9.

64. Sperduto PW, Wang M, Robins HI, Schell MC, Werner-Wasik M, Komaki R, Souhami L, Buyyounouski MK, Khuntia D, Demas W, Shah SA, Nedzi LA, Perry G, Suh JH, Mehta MP. A phase 3 trial of whole brain radiation therapy and stereotactic radiosurgery alone versus WBRT and SRS with temozolomide or erlotinib for non-small cell lung cancer and 1 to 3 brain metastases: Radiation Therapy Oncology Group 0320. Int J Radiat Oncol Biol Phys. 2013;85(5):1312–8.

65. Welsh JW, Komaki R, Amini A, Munsell MF, Unger W, Allen PK, Chang JY, Wefel JS, McGovern SL, Garland LL, Chen SS, Holt J, Liao Z, Brown P, Sulman E, Heymach JV, Kim ES, Stea B. Phase II trial of erlotinib plus concurrent whole-brain radiation therapy for patients with brain metastases from non-small-cell lung cancer. J Clin Oncol. 2013;31(7):895–902.

66. Mok TS, Wu Y-L, Ahn M-J, Garassino MC, Kim HR, Ramalingam SS, Shepherd FA, He Y, Akamatsu H, Theelen WS, Lee CK, Sebastian M, Templeton A, Mann H, Marotti M, Ghiorghiu S, Papadimitrakopoulou VA, AURA3 Investigators. Osimertinib or platinum-pemetrexed in EGFR T790M-positive lung cancer. N Engl J Med. 2017;376(7):629–40.

67. Costa DB, Shaw AT, Ou SH, Solomon BJ, Riely GJ, Ahn MJ, Zhou C, Shreeve SM, Selaru P, Polli A, Schnell P, Wilner KD, Wiltshire R, Camidge DR, Crinò L. Clinical experience with crizotinib in patients with advanced ALK-rearranged non-small-cell lung cancer and brain metastases. J Clin Oncol. 2015;33(17):1881–8.

68. Gadgeel SM, Gandhi L, Riely GJ, Chiappori AA, West HL, Azada MC, Morcos PN, Lee RM, Garcia L, Yu L, Boisserie F, Di Laurenzio L, Golding S, Sato J, Yokoyama S, Tanaka T, Ou SH. Safety and activity of alectinib against systemic disease and brain metastases in patients with crizotinib-resistant ALK-rearranged non-small-cell lung cancer (AF-002JG): results from the dose-finding portion of a phase 1/2 study. Lancet Oncol. 2014;15(10):1119–28.

69. Crinò L, Ahn MJ, De Marinis F, Groen HJ, Wakelee H, Hida T, Mok T, Spigel D, Felip E, Nishio M, Scagliotti G, Branle F, Emeremni C, Quadrigli M, Zhang J, Shaw AT. Multicenter phase II study of whole-body and intracranial activity with ceritinib in patients with ALK-rearranged non-small-cell lung cancer previously treated with chemotherapy and crizotinib: results from ASCEND-2. J Clin Oncol. 2016;34(24):2866–73.

70. Kim DW, Tiseo M, Ahn MJ, Reckamp KL, Hansen KH, Kim SW, Huber RM, West HL, Groen HJM, Hochmair MJ, Leighl NB, Gettinger SN, Langer CJ, Paz-Ares Rodríguez LG, Smit EF, Kim ES, Reichmann W, Haluska FG, Kerstein D, Camidge DR. Brigatinib in patients with crizotinib-refractory anaplastic lymphoma kinase-positive non-small-cell lung cancer: a randomized, multicenter phase II trial. J Clin Oncol. 2017;35(22):2490–8.

71. Magnuson WJ, Yeung JT, Guillod PD, Gettinger SN, Yu JB, Chiang VL. Impact of deferring radiation therapy in patients with epidermal growth factor receptor-mutant non-small cell lung cancer who develop brain metastases. Int J Radiat Oncol Biol Phys. 2016;95(2):673–9.

72. Magnuson WJ, Lester-Coll NH, Wu AJ, Yang TJ, Lockney NA, Gerber NK, Beal K, Amini A, Patil T, Kavanagh BD, Camidge DR, Braunstein SE, Boreta LC, Balasubramanian SK, Ahluwalia MS, Rana NG, Attia A, Gettinger SN, Contessa JN, Yu JB, Chiang VL. Management of brain metastases in tyrosine kinase inhibitor-naïve epidermal growth factor receptor-mutant non-small-cell lung cancer: a retrospective multi-institutional analysis. J Clin Oncol. 2017;35(10):1070–7.

73. Bachelot T, Romieu G, Campone M, Diéras V, Cropet C, Dalenc F, Jimenez M, Le Rhun E, Pierga JY, Gonçalves A, Leheurteur M, Domont J, Gutierrez M, Curé H, Ferrero JM, Labbe-Devilliers C. Lapatinib plus capecitabine in patients with previously untreated brain metastases from HER2-positive metastatic breast cancer (LANDSCAPE): a single-group phase 2 study. Lancet Oncol. 2013;14(1):64–71.

74. Freedman RA, Gelman RS, Wefel JS, Melisko ME, Hess KR, Connolly RM, Van Poznak CH, Niravath PA, Puhalla SL, Ibrahim N, Blackwell KL, Moy B, Herold C, Liu MC, Lowe A, Agar NY, Ryabin N, Farooq S, Lawler E, Rimawi MF, Krop IE, Wolff AC, Winer EP, Lin NU. Translational breast cancer research consortium (TBCRC) 022: a phase II trial of neratinib for patients with human epidermal growth factor receptor 2-positive breast cancer and brain metastases. J Clin Oncol. 2016;34(9):945–52.

75. Kroeze SG, Fritz C, Hoyer M, Lo SS, Ricardi U, Sahgal A, Stahel R, Stupp R, Guckenberger M. Toxicity of concurrent stereotactic radiotherapy and targeted therapy or immunotherapy: a systematic review. Cancer Treat Rev. 2017;53:25–37.

76. Brown PD, Ahluwalia MS, Khan OH, Asher AL, Wefel JS, Gondi V. Whole-brain radiotherapy for brain metastases: evolution or revolution? J Clin Oncol. 2018;36(5):483–91.

77. DeAngelis LM, Delattre JY, Posner JB. Radiation-induced dementia in patients cured of brain metastases. Neurology. 1989;39(6):789–96.

78. Monje ML, Mizumatsu S, Fike JR, Palmer TD. Irradiation induces neural precursor-cell dysfunction. Nat Med. 2002;8(9):955–62.

79. Monje ML, Vogel H, Masek M, Ligon KL, Fisher PG, Palmer TD. Impaired human hippocampal neurogenesis after treatment for central nervous system malignancies. Ann Neurol. 2007;62(5):515–20.

80. Gondi V, Tomé WA, Mehta MP. Why avoid the hippocampus? A comprehensive review. Radiother Oncol. 2010;97(3):370–6.

81. Kazda T, Jancalek R, Pospisil P, Sevela O, Prochazka T, Vrzal M, Burkon P, Slavik M, Hynkova L, Slampa P, Laack NN. Why and how to spare the hippocampus during brain radiotherapy: the developing role of hippocampal avoidance in cranial radiotherapy. Radiat Oncol. 2014;9:139.

82. Gondi V, Pugh SL, Tome WA, Caine C, Corn B, Kanner A, Rowley H, Kundapur V, DeNittis A, Greenspoon JN, Konski AA, Bauman GS, Shah S, Shi W, Wendland M, Kachnic L, Mehta MP. Preservation of memory with conformal avoidance of the hippocampal neural stem-cell compartment during whole-brain radiotherapy for brain metastases (RTOG 0933): a phase II multi-institutional trial. J Clin Oncol. 2014;32(34):3810–6.

83. Gondi V, Tolakanahalli R, Mehta MP, Tewatia D, Rowley H, Kuo JS, Khuntia D, Tomé WA. Hippocampal-sparing whole-brain radiotherapy: a "how-to" technique using helical tomotherapy and linear accelerator-based intensity-modulated radiotherapy. Int J Radiat Oncol Biol Phys. 2010;78(4):1244–52.

84. Gondi V, Hermann BP, Mehta MP, Tomé WA. Hippocampal dosimetry predicts neurocognitive function impairment after fractionated stereotactic radiotherapy for benign or low-grade adult brain tumors. Int J Radiat Oncol Biol Phys. 2013;85(2):348–54.

85. Brown PD, Pugh S, Laack NN, Wefel JS, Khuntia D, Meyers C, Choucair A, Fox S, Suh JH, Roberge D, Kavadi V, Bentzen SM, Mehta MP, Watkins-Bruner D, Radiation Therapy Oncology Group (RTOG). Memantine for the prevention of cognitive dysfunction in patients receiving whole-brain radiotherapy: a randomized, double-blind, placebo-controlled trial. Neuro-Oncology. 2013;15(10):1429–37.

86. Gondi V, Deshmukh S, Brown P, Wefel J, Tome W, Brune D, Bovi J, Robinson C, Khuntia D, Grosshans DR, Konski AA, Roberge D, Kundapur V, Devisetty K, Shah SA, Usuki KY, Anderson BM, Mehta MP, Kachnic LA. Preservation of neurocognitive function (NCF) with conformal avoidance of the hippocampus during whole brain radiotherapy (HA-WBRT) for brain metastases: preliminary results of phase III trial NRG oncology CC001. Int J Radiat Oncol Biol Phys. 2018;102(3):s5.

Particle Therapy for the Treatment of Brain Metastases

13

Jeremy Brownstein, Hooney D. Min, Marc Bussiere, and Helen A. Shih

Abbreviations

ASL	Acute Severe Lymphopenia
CIT	Carbon Ion Therapy
IMPT	Intensity Modulated Proton Therapy
IMRT	Intensity Modulated Radiation Therapy
LET	Linear Energy Transfer
MGH	Massachusetts General Hospital
PBS	Pencil Beam Scanning
PBT	Proton Beam Therapy
PSP	Passively Scattered Protons
RBE	Relative Biological Effectiveness
SOBP	Spread-Out Bragg Peak
SRS	Stereotactic Radiosurgery
VMAT	Volumetric Modulated Arc Therapy

J. Brownstein (✉)
Department of Radiation Oncology, Massachusetts General Hospital, Boston, MA, USA

Department of Radiation Oncology, Comprehensive Cancer Center, The Ohio State University, Columbus, Ohio, USA
e-mail: jeremy.brownstein@osumc.edu

H. D. Min
College of Medicine, Seoul National University, Seoul, South Korea

M. Bussiere
Stereotactic Physics, Department of Radiation Oncology, Massachusetts General Hospital, Boston, MA, USA

H. A. Shih
Proton Therapy Centers, Department of Radiation Oncology, Massachusetts General Hospital, Boston, MA, USA

Case Vignettes

Case 1

A fifty-five-year-old gentleman and nonsmoker with metastatic non-small-cell lung cancer initially presented 3 years ago with a persistent cough of 3 months even after asthma medication adjustments and steroids. Workup revealed a right upper lobe lung mass with mediastinal adenopathy, biopsy confirming moderately differentiated adenocarcinoma. Staging revealed several sites of osseous and multiple brain metastases. He received whole-brain radiation therapy 30 Gy in 10 fractions and had no further CNS disease for 3 years while on systemic therapy. On routine staging, he was then found to have developed two new asymptomatic left frontal metastases. He was treated with proton SRS, 18 Gy (RBE) to each lesion, well tolerated and with high conformality, minimizing unaffected brain reirradiation (Fig. 13.1a, b).

Case 2

A forty-six-year-old female presented with BRAF mutant metastatic melanoma, who was initially diagnosed 4 years prior with a pruritic pigmented scalp lesion that was resected. She underwent wide local excision, which was found to be of 5 mm depth and with 2/5 sentinel lymph nodes positive.

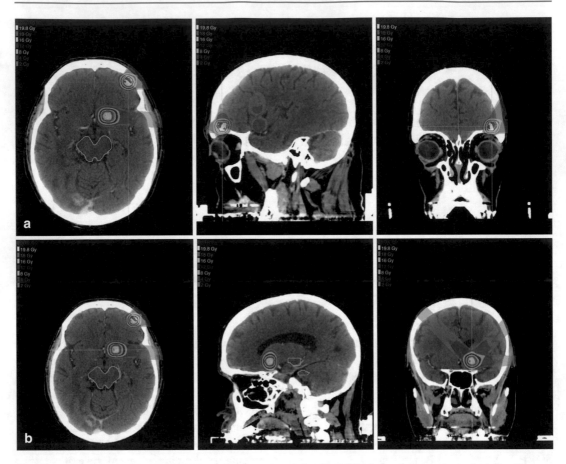

Fig. 13.1 Proton SRS plans of two left frontal non-small-cell lung cancer brain metastases along the anterior skull base treated on the same day: (**a**) lesion just superior to the left orbit and (**b**) lesion just superior to the left optic nerve and anterior to the chiasm. Maximum sparing to the surrounding normal tissues is achieved with proton therapy

Despite more comprehensive local and nodal excision that was negative for additional disease, she recurred with pulmonary metastases 14 months from initial diagnosis, underwent BRAF-directed therapy for 5 months followed by immunotherapy at the time of progression. Four months later, she developed her first intracranial metastases in the right occipital lobe and left thalamus. These were irradiated without incident. One year later, she developed further asymptomatic intracranial disease of a right temporal and left anterior frontal brain metastases. Given the peripheral locations and moderate size of the left frontal lesion, she was treated with proton SRS to minimize collateral brain radiation exposure (Fig. 13.2a, b).

Proton Basics

Dose Distribution

In Proton Beam Therapy (PBT), a beam of protons is accelerated to high energies using either a *cyclotron* or a *synchrotron*, and is then modulated, focused and shaped to target the desired treatment volume. Protons in PBT interact with matter primarily via *proton–electron reactions* and thus deposit dose differently than do photons used in external beam radiation therapy (i.e., megavoltage X-rays and high energy Gamma Rays), which primarily interact via *Compton scattering* [1]. Photons are deeply penetrating.

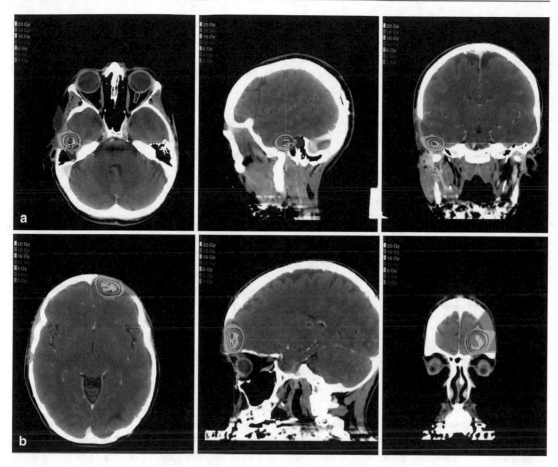

Fig. 13.2 Proton SRS plans of two melanoma brain metastases treated on the same day: (**a**) a lesion of the right temporal skull base and anterior to the cochlea and (**b**) an intermediate size lesion along the left anterior frontal convexity. Each plan achieves maximal sparing of the surrounding brain

Following an initial buildup, the dose they deposit gradually decreases throughout the full length of the beam path [2]. On the other hand, protons slow down as they traverse tissues and eventually halt. Contrary to the gentle slope of photon dose distributions, the dose deposited by protons increases dramatically as the proton beam slows, peaking in a narrow burst (known as the Bragg peak) before plummeting to zero as the protons abruptly stop (Fig. 13.3). Since the range of protons in tissues is finite with minimal dose deposited beyond the Bragg peak, protons can be used to treat a target while sparing normal tissues just beyond the target, yielding a potential advantage as compared to photons.

Scattering and Modulation

The water-equivalent depth of the Bragg peak is energy-dependent and roughly proportional to the initial energy squared [D_{WET} [3] $= 0.0022 \times E$ $(MeV)^{1.77}$] [4]. Monoenergetic protons exit the accelerator in the form of a "pencil beam," which is only a few millimeters in diameter. Unaltered, this beam would create a very narrow field with a Bragg peak depositing dose in tissue spanning only a few millimeters in depth. As most clinically relevant targets span 1–20 cm in the traverse and longitudinal axes, a monoenergetic pencil beam will not suffice for most treatments. Therefore, a polyenergetic beam must be

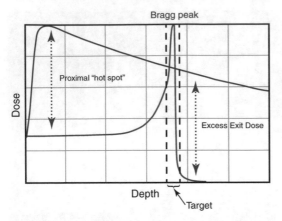

Fig. 13.3 Dose distribution of therapeutic photon and proton beams. Dose as a function of depth is demonstrated for photons (red) and protons (blue). For photons, the maximum dose occurs proximal to the target. Within the beam path, this "hot spot" will receive a higher dose than the target. Photons also continue to deposit dose distal to the target, resulting in unnecessary exit dose. Within a proton beam, dose increases with increasing depth, reaching a maximum in the Bragg peak. The choice of beam energy is chosen such that the Bragg peak falls within the target. Distal to the Bragg peak, dose decreases precipitously, resulting in minimal exit dose

employed with energies chosen to create overlapping Bragg peaks throughout the depth of the target, and the beam must be altered to cover the width of the treatment volume. This can be achieved using scattering and scanning technology.

Scattering, also referred to as *passive scattering*, was the mainstream therapeutic technology for the first several decades of clinical application. A homogeneous dose distribution in depth can be created by superimposing monoenergetic beams of differing energies. This can be achieved by introducing one of a number of modulation devices. One common method passes the pencil beam through a *spinning compensator wheel* that contains spokes of varying thickness. As the pencil beam encounters progressively thicker spokes, the resultant protons will have incrementally lower energy and will produce ever-shallower Bragg peaks. The arc-length of each spoke reflects the relative weight of the corresponding peak. Alternatively, a pencil beam can be passed through a *ridge filter* – a static block with an echinate surface of repeating finely spaced ridged

spikes. Protons that have encountered the tip of a spike will have lower energy than protons encountering a valley. In both methods, a number of Bragg peaks are produced which combine to form a so-called "spread-out Bragg peak" (SOBP). Modulators devices are specifically designed such that the SOBP produces a uniform physical dose throughout the breadth of the target volume (Fig. 13.4). For a detailed description of passive scatter techniques, please refer to Refs. [5–7]. With passive scattering, the narrow polyenergetic beam is broadened by passing through one or more scattering devices which helps spread the dose profile laterally (i.e., *double scattering*). Patient and field-specific *apertures* made of brass, Cerrobend, or created with a multileaf collimator conform the beam to the lateral contours of the target and around critical structures. Patient- and field-specific *range compensators* fabricated from plastics or wax are also used to further conform the SOBP to the distal edge of the target [7].

In contrast, *scanning* systems (i.e., Pencil Beam Scanning or PBS) utilize bending magnets to sweep the monoenergetic pencil beam laterally across the treatment field (much like the electron beam is swept across a phosphorescent screen in an old-fashioned cathode-ray television), allowing the dose to be "painted" onto tissue at a given depth. The deep surface of the target is treated first with the highest energy protons. The primary beam energy is then decreased incrementally and successive shallower layers are similarly painted with the dose. As one can modulate the intensity of the pencil beam as it sweeps across the field and/or modulates the time the beam spends at each location, this technique is often referred to as *intensity modulated proton therapy* (IMPT). Like X-ray-based intensity modulated radiation therapy (IMRT), IMPT also employs inverse planning and optimization; however, due to the ability of protons to form Bragg peaks, IMPT can utilize fewer fields and inherently eliminates exit dose, significantly decreasing integral dose as compared to IMRT [8]. While there are advantages and disadvantages to both passive scattering and scanning systems, most newer systems employ scanning technology (i.e., IMPT), as this

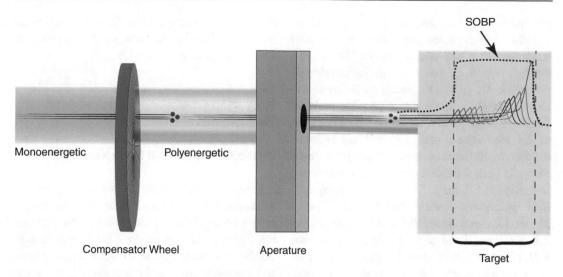

Fig. 13.4 Schematic of a passively modulated proton beam. A monoenergetic proton beam leaving a cyclotron or synchrotron interacts with a spinning modulation wheel (variable depth of modulator wheel not depicted). The resultant polyenergetic beam is collimated through an aperture before encountering the target. The configuration of the modulation wheel is specifically chosen to yield of a spectrum of energies that deposit Bragg peaks throughout the breadth of the target, called a "spread-out Bragg peak" (SOBP). (Image modified with permission from the following Brownstein et al. [12])

technique allows for far greater conformation of both the distal AND the proximal edge of target. Because most passively scattered beams have *uniform range modulation* (i.e., the "thickness" of the SOBP is approximately constant), using a range compensator to conform the distal SOBP to the deep contour of a target will, by necessity, impact proximal SOBP as well – potentially resulting in hot spots superficial to the target. Conversely, a scanning platform affords more freedom in the placement of pencil beam segments, allowing for *variable range modulation*. Furthermore, IMPT enables variable dose intensity to be delivered to a target within a given treatment (i.e., simultaneous integrated boost) [9], and allows for additional optimization to account for range uncertainties [10] and/or incorporate biological factors [11] (discussed below).

Biological Factors

There are many forms of ionizing radiation, ranging from massless photons to heavy atomic nuclei traveling at relativistic speeds. The biological impacts of radiation depend not only on the quantity of dose delivered but also on how it interacts with matter. Photons deposit energy sparsely, imparting DNA damage that can frequently be repaired (i.e., single strand breaks). Heavy ions are more potent than photons because, within their Bragg peak, they deposit radiation in dense ionization tracks that can impart highly clustered, irreparable DNA damage (i.e., double strand breaks, dicentric rings, etc.). For example, the damage imparted by carbon and heavier ions can be equivalent to the damage caused by a threefold higher dose of X-rays [12]. Heavy ions are thus termed as high Linear Energy Transfer (LET) radiation in that a large amount of energy is deposited over a shorter distance compared to low LET radiation photons [13]. To compare doses between modalities, the Relative Biological Effectiveness (RBE) is defined as the dose ratio of X-rays to the particle of interest required to cause the same biological effect (i.e., in the above example, the RBE of carbon ions is 3 because a threefold higher dose of X-rays is required to induce the same damage) [14].

Protons are considered "low LET" radiation but are nonetheless more potent than X-rays. In most clinical applications, protons are generally assumed to have a constant RBE of 1.1, imply-ing that a given proton treatment is biologically equivalent to a 10% higher dose of X-rays [15]. For this reason, proton doses are frequently ref-erenced in Gy (RBE) to specify the X-ray equiv-alent dose [14]. However, a growing body of literature suggests that assuming a uniform RBE of 1.1 may ignore clinically relevant nuances. Similar to the carbon ions, as a proton slows along its path it deposits energy with increasing intensity and density. Thus, slow-moving pro-tons approaching their end-of-range have a higher LET and their RBE can be greater than 1.1. Since the distal edge of a target volume has a greater fraction of slow-moving protons than the proximal edge, the RBE tends to increase with increasing depth assuming the target vol-ume has uniform physical dose. Paganetti et al. (2014) described the increase in proton RBE over the course of a uniform SOBP: the RBE is ~1.1 in the entrance region, ~1.15 in the center, ~1.35 in the distal edge, and ~1.7 in the distal fall off [16]. Thus, placing the distal edge of a target volume in a radiosensitive organ under the assumption of a uniform RBE of 1.1 may result in a biologically effective overdose of 20%. Peeler et al. (2016) reviewed a series of pediatric patients treated with PBT for ependymoma and retrospectively calculated LET using Monte Carlo simulations. They noted a significant asso-ciation on univariate analysis between treatment-related changes on T2 MRI and higher LET_{max} within their CTV [17].

RBE is complex and is dependent on many variables. In addition to LET and dose-per-fraction, RBE is also influenced by biological factors such as histology, the tissue's intrinsic radiosensitivity/capacity for repair, and tumor oxygenation [18]. Recently, several groups have noted that cytogenetics may also impact RBE. Mutations in the DNA Homologous Repair and Fanconi Anemia pathways result in increased susceptibility to proton-mediated cell kill and thus a higher RBE [3, 19]. While many RBE modeling techniques are currently under investi-gation that include both physical and biological factors, there remains no clear consensus as to how to incorporate a variable RBE into proton treatment planning and most centers continue to assume a uniform RBE of 1.1 [20].

Proton Stereotactic Radiosurgery Techniques

Immobilization and Image Guidance

Effective immobilization is of critical importance to ensure accurate target localization. Compared with photon SRS, errors in setup can have an even greater impact on the dose distribution as the depth of the Bragg peak is extremely sensitive to changes in depth and density of tissues proxi-mal to the target. The immobilization devices used for proton SRS are specially designed to limit particle scattering. An example of an immo-bilization frame that has been developed for pro-ton therapy of brain tumors is the Massachusetts General Hospital (MGH) modified Gill-Thomas-Cosman frame, comprising a rounded carbon fiber occipital support, low-density cushion, and a dental mold fixed to a stereotactic cranial ring (Fig 13.5a). This device is used in the treatment of intracranial targets that do not extend to the base of the skull but requires that the patient has good dentition to create excellent and reproduc-ible immobilization. Alternative fixation devices, which do not use dental fixation, make use of thermoplastic masks and custom occipital cush-ions for a comfortable yet reproducible immobi-lization while being designed with consideration for the sensitivities associated with proton ther-apy [21].

Cone Beam CT and automated localization systems are now being integrated into many newer proton therapy platforms [22]. However, these developments are recent and some estab-lished proton centers continue to employ calvar-ial fiducial markers to rigorously triangulate patient position and ensure accurate treatment delivery (Fig 13.5b). Fiducial marker placement can be performed as an outpatient procedure by a neurosurgeon in 15–20 minutes with minimal risk of complications.

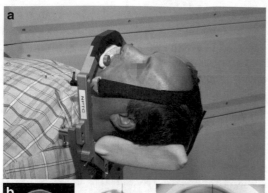

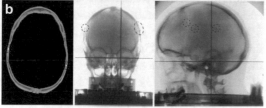

Fig. 13.5 Proton treatment immobilization and localization. (**a**) The modified Gill-Thomas-Cosman mask achieves reproducible noninvasive immobilization with a Velcro strap that secures the patient's forehead and a custom dental tray that rigidly associates with his/her dentition. (**b**) Fiducials are placed via a minimally invasive procedure deep to the outer table of the calvarium. CT (left panel) demonstrates well-placed fiducials (red circles). Pretreatment onboard kV imaging (middle and right panel) sets the isocenter by aligning to fiducials (red circles) with ± 0.5 mm accuracy

Dosimetric Considerations

As intracranial tumors often reside in close proximity to important avoidance structures, the best-achievable radiation plans may necessitate either incomplete target coverage or exceeding normal tissue constraints. To this end, many groups have evaluated which modality – photons or protons – can best maximize intracranial target coverage while minimizing normal tissue toxicities. Bolsi et al. simultaneously planned 12 cases (5 meningiomas, 5 acoustic neuromas, and 2 pituitary adenomas) with 3D conformal photon radiotherapy, IMRT, stereotactic arc photon therapy, spot-scanning protons, and passively scattered protons. All modalities had excellent target coverage but those planned with protons demonstrated significantly lower mean radiation dose to the brain-

stem, eyes, and uninvolved brain [23]. Freund et al. compared 13 cases of pediatric CNS tumors planned for fractionated radiotherapy with contemporary Volumetric Modulated Arc Therapy (VMAT), passively scattered protons (PSP), and IMPT. Compared to VMAT, both PSP and IMPT had significantly higher maximum brain dose, lower brain volume receiving low dose radiation, and a lower predicted risk of brain necrosis [24].

Proton Beam Dosimetry

While PBS systems are adept at treating irregular volumes, brain metastases are frequently small and spherical, and can thus be approached with simpler modulation techniques. *Single scattering systems* are well suited for irradiating small targets that do not require the lateral beam spreading needed for larger lesions. Here a pencil beam is passed through low-Z material to achieve the desired Bragg peak pull-back. While the resultant field has a nonuniform dose distribution, the central portion is sufficiently flat and can be collimated to treat small targets with excellent dose homogeneity. Compared to more complicated scanning techniques, single scattering systems can be designed with smaller effective source diameters and larger source-to isocenter distances to produce a narrower lateral penumbra at shallow depth compared to double scattering systems. Safai et al. also noted that for targets <14 cm depth in water (i.e., most intracranial targets), the lateral penumbra of a collimated passively scattered beam is sharper compared to that of a pencil beam, even for a smaller PBS beam spot of 3 mm. For example, they found that for a target at 4 cm depth in water, the lateral 80% – 20% penumbra of PBS (3 mm spot size) was 1 cm compared to ~3 mm for a collimated beam [25]. Others have found that adding a collimator to a PBS platform significantly improves lateral penumbra at depths <11 cm in water [26]. The authors note that these observations cannot be broadly applied, as proton beam profiles are highly dependent on the specifics of the individual system.

Clinical Applications

Benign Intracranial Lesions

Owing to their favorable dose distribution, proton therapy platforms are of interest in stereotactic radiosurgery. Protons are a particularly appealing option for the treatment of benign intracranial lesions as patients often have an excellent prognosis and limiting dose to uninvolved brain becomes a greater priority. MGH has published several series detailing their experience with proton-SRS in the treatment of vestibular schwannomas [27], pituitary adenomas [28, 29], and arteriovenous malformations [30, 31]. For a detailed and comprehensive clinical discussion regarding the proton-SRS, please refer to the following [32].

Proton SRS for Brain Metastases

There are limited data regarding the use of proton stereotactic radiosurgery for the treatment of brain metastases. MGH has published the only series to date, reporting their experience treating 815 brain metastases in 370 patients between 1991 and 2016 [33]. Median age of patients included was 61 and most had an excellent performance status with 2/3 having Karnofsky Performance Status ≥ 80%. A variety of tumor histologies were represented with a non-small-cell lung cancer implicated in a plurality of patients (34%) followed by melanoma (28%) and breast cancer (17%). Approximately half of patients had no extracranial disease and approximately one half only had a single metastasis.

Patients were treated at the Harvard Cyclotron Laboratory until construction of Francis H. Burr Proton Center at MGH main campus was completed in 2001. Patients included in this series were immobilized with different techniques depending upon the clinical context (described above). All patients underwent placement of calvarial fiducial markers to ensure accurate setup with orthogonal X-rays. Target volumes ranged 0.02–23.3 cm^3 (mean 1.6 cm^3; median 0.6 cm^3) and delivered dose ranged 8–28 Gy (mean 17.3; median 18 Gy (RBE)).

With a median follow up of 9.2 months, oncologic outcomes were comparable to those reported in photon SRS series. Local failure at 6 and 12 months was 4.3% and 8.5%, respectively; distant CNS failure rates at 6 and 12 months was 39% and 48%, respectively; and median overall survival was 12.4 months. Treatments were well tolerated with only 11% incidence of Grade 2+ acute toxicity, and pathologically confirmed radionecrosis occurring in 3.6% at 1 year. The authors conducted retrospective analysis of 10 patients with 3–4 brain metastases, comparing the achieved proton dose distribution with the distribution achievable using photon-SRS techniques. They noted a significantly lower volume of brain receiving 4 Gy with protons compared to photons. Figure 13.6 demonstrates a similar comparison of one such patient who was initially treated with proton SRS and was subsequently re-planned post hoc with contemporary high-density MLC VMAT.

Heavy Charged Particle SRS for Brain Metastases

There is growing interest in the use of heavier charged particles to treat certain tumors due to their improved dosimetric and radiobiological properties. There are 11 treatment centers in Europe and Asia that utilize Heavy Ion Therapy such as carbon ions, with several more currently under construction [34]. Compared to protons, carbon ions have sharper lateral penumbrae, and have a significantly higher RBE within their Bragg peaks. These advantages make carbon ion therapy (CIT) suitable for treating radio-resistant tumors adjacent critical structures [35]. A retrospective study of patients with low/intermediate grade skull base chondrosarcoma treated with CIT at Heidelberg Ion Beam Therapy Center demonstrated local control rates of 96% and 90% at 3 and 4 years, respectively [36], comparing favorably to patients treated with protons [37, 38]. However, to our knowledge, there are no large published series of patients with brain metastases treated with CIT or other heavy ions. While doing so would be technically feasible, it may not be practical, as availability of CIT is scarce, and this

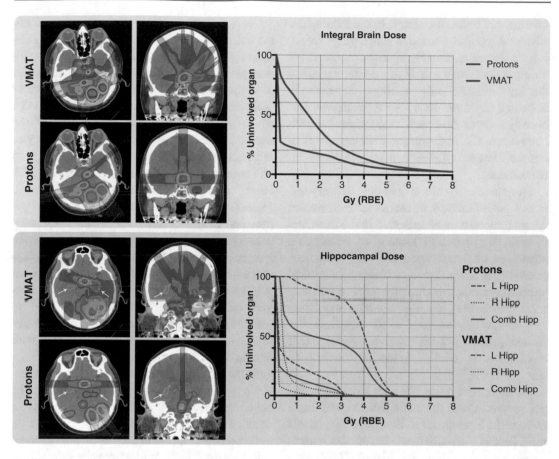

Fig. 13.6 Comparison of Proton-SRS vs. VMAT-SRS in a patient with multiple brain metastases. Blue box: Representative slices showing the dose distribution of VMAT plan (upper panels) and protons (lower panels). DVH (right) demonstrates that the proton plan yields a lower volume of uninvolved brain receiving low doses compared with photons (mean dose 0.96 vs 2.03 Gy). Purple panel: Representative slices showing the dose distribution of VMAT plan (upper panels) and protons (lower panels) with the hippocampi labeled with white arrows. DVH (right) demonstrates that the proton plan yields a lower dose to left hippocampus (mean dose 0.68 vs. 3.75 Gy, respectively), right hippocampus (mean dose 0.07 vs. 0.54 Gy, respectively), and bilateral hippocampi (mean dose 0.39 vs. 2.22 Gy, respectively). Of note, neither proton nor VMAT plans were specifically optimized to avoid the hippocampi

modality is unlikely to offer a significant advantage over other radiosurgery platforms.

Discussion

Some physicians have raised concerns vis-a-vis routinely employing proton-SRS in the treatment of brain metastases. In response to the Harvard experience presented above, Kirkpatrick et al. reiterate that local control and intracranial progression with protons are not improved compared to historical series treating brain metastases with photon-SRS – an expected finding given that proton patients were treated with similar, if not more modest doses [39]. They further point out that data are lacking as to whether the decreased integral dose seen with protons translates into improved neurocognition, especially given the poor prognosis associated with brain metastases. They hypothesize that the cost for proton centers to deliver proton-SRS may be much higher than photon-SRS while yielding similar outcomes.

The authors of this chapter agree that there are currently insufficient data to justify routinely recommending proton-SRS over photon-SRS in the treatment of brain metastases. In most instances, advanced photon platforms employing VMAT can easily and efficiently simultaneously target multiple metastases with highly conformal radiotherapy utilizing only a single or multiple isocenter(s). Since many such platforms frequently include on-board image guidance with cone-beam CT and surface tracking, invasive immobilization and/or fiducial markers are unnecessary.

Despite improvements in photon delivery and image-guided therapy, there are specific instances where protons may be indicated in the treatment of brain metastases. PBT can offer a dosimetric advantage, particularly with large or irregular targets [40] and can facilitate sparing of critical structures within a modest proximity of the treatment volume [41]. Thus, proton-SRS may facilitate ablative treatment of brain metastases for certain patients with a disadvantageous tumor distribution in whom photon-SRS cannot be safely delivered.

Advances in systemic therapy have led to longer survival times for many patients with brain metastases. Sperduto et al. have recently updated the Disease Specific – Grade Prognostic Assessment (DS-GPA) for non-small-cell lung cancer. Those in the highest prognostic group from *Alk*-mutated or *EGFR*-mutated adenocarcinoma (DS-GPA 3.5–4) have a median survival of 47 months, including some afflicted with >4 brain metastases [42]. Similarly, those in the favorable prognostic group with metastatic Her2+ cancer have a median survival of 27 months [43]. With new successes in targeted systemic therapies, there is an ever-growing population of patients with "favorable risk" metastatic disease who may live with their cancer for many years, even after developing brain metastases. For such patients, it will be important to explore whether employing proton-SRS to decrease integral brain dose will lead to tangible improvements in neurocognitive outcomes.

Excess integral dose can have deleterious effects that extend beyond uninvolved brain. Under physiological conditions, the brain receives approximately 16% of cardiac output with a heart–heart transit time of approximately 30 seconds [44]. Yovino et al. sought to quantify the unintentional radiation dose imparted to circulating lymphocytes during a course of radiotherapy for malignant glioma. Through careful modeling, they calculated that the mean dose of radiation to circulating lymphocytes was ~2 Gy, which would be expected to kill half of the exposed lymphocytes; and 99% of lymphocytes received >0.5 Gy, which would be expected to kill at least 10% of exposed lymphocytes [45]. Huang et al. observed and employed a logistic regression of 183 patients with high-grade glioma and demonstrated a significant association between V25 Gy and development of acute severe lymphopenia (ASL) [46, 47]. This study and others [48] have also described a correlation between ASL and worse overall survival. Of note, the integral radiation doses of uninvolved brain in patients receiving fractionated treatment for glioma are far higher than those anticipated with photon SRS for brain metastases. Nonetheless, with the growing role immunotherapy in metastatic patients, it is increasingly important to be cognoscente of how radiotherapy impacts the immune system.

In conclusion, proton SRS is an effective and safe treatment for brain metastases. While there are currently no indications for its routine use over photon SRS, protons may better facilitate safe treatment of large volume disease and may yield a lower integral dose for patients with several small volume metastases. Further investigation is needed to determine if this lower integral dose translates into superior neurocognitive outcomes or better protects anti-cancer immunity.

Key Points

- PBT has a dosimetric advantage compared to photon radiotherapy. Unlike deeply penetrating photons that deposit dose throughout the entirety of their beam path, protons halt at a specific depth depositing most of their dose at the end of range within a narrow Bragg peak. This results in minimal exit dose deposited distal to the target.

- Proton-SRS is a safe and effective treatment for brain metastases, resulting in better low-dose sparing and similar oncologic outcomes compared to photon-SRS.
- Given that advanced photon-SRS platforms are widely available and can deliver highly conformal treatments that frequently meet all desired constraints, the authors of this chapter do not recommend routinely employing proton-SRS in the treatment of brain metastases.
- Off protocol Proton-SRS should only be considered in cases where ablative treatment is indicated, but photon-SRS cannot achieve desired constraints.
- Future studies are needed to determine if the decreased exit dose afforded by proton-SRS can better protect antitumor immunity or can better spare long-term neurocognition in patients with a favorable prognosis.

References

1. Newhauser WD, Zhang R. The physics of proton therapy. Phys Med Biol. 2015;60(8):R155–209.
2. Almond PR, Biggs PJ, Coursey BM, Hanson WF, Huq MS, Nath R, et al. AAPM's TG-51 protocol for clinical reference dosimetry of high-energy photon and electron beams. Med Phys. 1999;26(9):1847–70.
3. Willers H, Allen A, Grosshans D, McMahon SJ, von Neubeck C, Wiese C, et al. Toward A variable RBE for proton beam therapy. Radiother Oncol. 2018;128(1):68–75.
4. Bortfeld T. An analytical approximation of the Bragg curve for therapeutic proton beams. Med Phys. 1997;24(12):2024–33.
5. Wilson RR. Radiological use of fast protons. Radiology. 1946;47(5):487–91.
6. Larsson B. Pre-therapeutic physical experiments with high energy protons. Br J Radiol. 1961;34:143–51.
7. Paganetti H. Proton therapy physics. Boca Raton: CRC Press; 2016.
8. Trofimov A, Bortfeld T. Optimization of beam parameters and treatment planning for intensity modulated proton therapy. Technol Cancer Res Treat. 2003;2(5):437–44.
9. Madani I, Lomax AJ, Albertini F, Trnkova P, Weber DC. Dose-painting intensity-modulated proton ther-

apy for intermediate- and high-risk meningioma. Radiat Oncol. 2015;10:72.
10. Paganetti H. Range uncertainties in proton therapy and the role of Monte Carlo simulations. Phys Med Biol. 2012;57(11):R99–117.
11. Giantsoudi D, Grassberger C, Craft D, Niemierko A, Trofimov A, Paganetti H. Linear energy transfer-guided optimization in intensity modulated proton therapy: feasibility study and clinical potential. Int J Radiat Oncol Biol Phys. 2013;87(1):216–22.
12. Brownstein JM, Wisdom AJ, Castle KD, Mowery YM, Guida P, Lee CL, et al. Characterizing the potency and impact of carbon ion therapy in a primary mouse model of soft tissue sarcoma. Mol Cancer Ther. 2018;17(4):858–68.
13. Durante M, Loeffler JS. Charged particles in radiation oncology. Nat Rev Clin Oncol. 2009;7(1):37–43.
14. International Atomic Energy Agency. Dose reporting in ion beam therapy. Vienna: International Atomic Energy Agency; 2007.
15. Paganetti H, Niemierko A, Ancukiewicz M, Gerweck LE, Goitein M, Loeffler JS, et al. Relative biological effectiveness (RBE) values for proton beam therapy. Int J Radiat Oncol Biol Phys. 2002;53(2):407–21.
16. Paganetti H. Relative biological effectiveness (RBE) values for proton beam therapy. Variations as a function of biological endpoint, dose, and linear energy transfer. Phys Med Biol. 2014;59(22):R419–72.
17. Peeler CR, Mirkovic D, Titt U, Blanchard P, Gunther JR, Mahajan A, et al. Clinical evidence of variable proton biological effectiveness in pediatric patients treated for ependymoma. Radiother Oncol. 2016;121(3):395–401.
18. Hall EJ, Giaccia AJ. Radiobiology for the radiologist. Philadelphia: Wolters Kluwer Health/Lippincott Williams & Wilkins; 2012.
19. Fontana AO, Augsburger MA, Grosse N, Guckenberger M, Lomax AJ, Sartori AA, et al. Differential DNA repair pathway choice in cancer cells after proton- and photon-irradiation. Radiother Oncol. 2015;116(3):374–80.
20. McMahon SJ, Paganetti H, Prise KM. LET-weighted doses effectively reduce biological variability in proton radiotherapy planning. Phys Med Biol. 2018;63(22):225009.
21. Yerramilli D, Bussière MR, Loeffler JS, Shih HA. Proton beam therapy (for CNS tumors). In: Chang EL, Brown PD, Lo SS, Sahgal A, Suh JH, editors. Adult CNS radiation oncology: principles and practice. Cham: Springer International Publishing; 2018. p. 709–22.
22. Hua C, Yao W, Kidani T, Tomida K, Ozawa S, Nishimura T, et al. A robotic C-arm cone beam CT system for image-guided proton therapy: design and performance. Br J Radiol. 2017;90(1079):20170266.
23. Bolsi A, Fogliata A, Cozzi L. Radiotherapy of small intracranial tumours with different advanced techniques using photon and proton beams: a treatment planning study. Radiother Oncol. 2003;68(1):1–14.

24. Freund D, Zhang R, Sanders M, Newhauser W. Predictive risk of radiation induced cerebral necrosis in pediatric brain cancer patients after VMAT versus proton therapy. Cancers. 2015;7(2):617–30.

25. Safai S, Bortfeld T, Engelsman M. Comparison between the lateral penumbra of a collimated double-scattered beam and uncollimated scanning beam in proton radiotherapy. Phys Med Biol. 2008;53(6):1729–50.

26. Winterhalter C, Lomax A, Oxley D, Weber DC, Safai S. A study of lateral fall-off (penumbra) optimisation for pencil beam scanning (PBS) proton therapy. Phys Med Biol. 2018;63(2):025022.

27. Weber DC, Chan AW, Bussiere MR, Harsh IVGR, Ancukiewicz M, Barker IIFG, et al. Proton beam radiosurgery for vestibular schwannoma: tumor control and cranial nerve toxicity. Neurosurgery. 2003;53(3):577–88.

28. Wattson DA, Tanguturi SK, Spiegel DY, Niemierko A, Biller BMK, Nachtigall LB, et al. Outcomes of proton therapy for patients with functional pituitary adenomas. Int J Radiat Oncol Biol Phys. 2014;90(3):532–9.

29. Petit JH, Biller BM, Yock TI, Swearingen B, Coen JJ, Chapman P, et al. Proton stereotactic radiotherapy for persistent adrenocorticotropin-producing adenomas. J Clin Endocrinol Metab. 2008;93(2):393–9.

30. Hattangadi-Gluth JA, Chapman PH, Kim D, Niemierko A, Bussière MR, Stringham A, et al. Single-fraction proton beam stereotactic radiosurgery for cerebral arteriovenous malformations. Int J Radiat Oncol Biol Phys. 2014;89(2):338–46.

31. Hattangadi JA, Chapman PH, Bussière MR, Niemierko A, Ogilvy CS, Rowell A, et al. Planned two-fraction proton beam stereotactic radiosurgery for high-risk inoperable cerebral arteriovenous malformations. Int J Radiat Oncol Biol Phys. 2012;83(2):533–41.

32. Shih HA, Chapman PH, Loeffler JS. Proton beam radiosurgery: clinical experience. In: Lozano AM, Gildenberg PL, Tasker RR, editors. Textbook of stereotactic and functional neurosurgery. Berlin, Heidelberg: Springer Berlin Heidelberg; 2009. p. 1131–7.

33. Atkins KM, Pashtan IM, Bussiere MR, Kang KH, Niemierko A, Daly JE, et al. Proton stereotactic radiosurgery for brain metastases: a single-institution analysis of 370 patients. Int J Radiat Oncol Biol Phys. 2018;101(4):820–9.

34. Particle Therapy Co-operative Group. Particle therapy facilities in clinical operation. 2018. Available from: https://www.ptcog.ch/index.php/facilities-in-operation.

35. Durante M, Loeffler JS. Charged particles in radiation oncology. Nat Rev Clin Oncol. 2010;7(1):37–43.

36. Schulz-Ertner D, Nikoghosyan A, Hof H, Didinger B, Combs SE, Jakel O, et al. Carbon ion radiotherapy of skull base chondrosarcomas. Int J Radiat Oncol Biol Phys. 2007;67(1):171–7.

37. Ares C, Hug EB, Lomax AJ, Bolsi A, Timmermann B, Rutz HP, et al. Effectiveness and safety of spot scanning proton radiation therapy for chordomas and chondrosarcomas of the skull base: first long-term report. Int J Radiat Oncol Biol Phys. 2009;75(4):1111–8.

38. Mizoe JE. Review of carbon ion radiotherapy for skull base tumors (especially chordomas). Rep Pract Oncol Radiother. 2016;21(4):356–60.

39. Kirkpatrick JP, Laack NN, Halasz LM, Minniti G, Chan MD. Proton therapy for brain metastases: a question of value. Int J Radiat Oncol Biol Phys. 2018;101(4):830–2.

40. Fossati P, Vavassori A, Deantonio L, Ferrara E, Krengli M, Orecchia R. Review of photon and proton radiotherapy for skull base tumours. Rep Pract Oncol Radiother. 2016;21(4):336–55.

41. Adeberg S, Harrabi S, Bougatf N, Verma V, Windisch P, Bernhardt D, et al. Dosimetric comparison of proton radiation therapy, volumetric modulated arc therapy, and three-dimensional conformal radiotherapy based on intracranial tumor location. Cancers. 2018;10(11):401.

42. Sperduto PW, Yang TJ, Beal K, Pan H, Brown PD, Bangdiwala A, et al. Estimating survival in patients with lung cancer and brain metastases: an update of the graded prognostic assessment for lung cancer using molecular markers (Lung-molGPA). JAMA Oncol. 2017;3(6):827–31.

43. Sperduto PW, Kased N, Roberge D, Xu Z, Shanley R, Luo X, et al. Effect of tumor subtype on survival and the graded prognostic assessment for patients with breast cancer and brain metastases. Int J Radiat Oncol Biol Phys. 2012;82(5):2111–7.

44. Ganong WF. Review of medical physiology. 21st ed. Boston: McGraw-Hill; 2003.

45. Yovino S, Kleinberg L, Grossman SA, Narayanan M, Ford E. The etiology of treatment-related lymphopenia in patients with malignant gliomas: modeling radiation dose to circulating lymphocytes explains clinical observations and suggests methods of modifying the impact of radiation on immune cells. Cancer Investig. 2013;31(2):140–4.

46. Petr J, Platzek I, Hofheinz F, Mutsaerts H, Asllani I, van Osch MJP, et al. Photon vs. proton radiochemotherapy: effects on brain tissue volume and perfusion. Radiother Oncol. 2018;128(1):121–7.

47. Huang J, DeWees TA, Badiyan SN, Speirs CK, Mullen DF, Fergus S, et al. Clinical and dosimetric predictors of acute severe lymphopenia during radiation therapy and concurrent temozolomide for high-grade glioma. Int J Radiat Oncol Biol Phys. 2015;92(5):1000–7.

48. Vaios EJ, Nahed BV, Muzikansky A, Fathi AT, Dietrich J. Bone marrow response as a potential biomarker of outcomes in glioblastoma patients. J Neurosurg. 2017;127(1):132–8.

Special Topics in Brain Metastases Management

14

James Byrne, Kevin S. Oh, and Nancy Wang

Osseous Skull Base Metastases

Case Vignette

Case 1

A 71-year-old female with stage IV rectal cancer presents with progressively worsening diplopia, right-sided ptosis, right eye blurriness, and disconjugate gaze. Head CT demonstrates a lytic component involving the right anterior clinoid process. MRI brain confirms a lobulated mass causing compression of the optic nerve within the optic canal and third nerve within the superior orbital fissure.

Introduction

Skull base metastases are rare and have been found in approximately 4% of cancer patients [1]. These metastases may be clinically silent but can become symptomatic when their growth produces pain or compression of cranial nerves or vasculature. As to be expected, cancers that have a tropism for bone are the most common histologies that lead to skull base metastases, including prostate, breast, lymphoma, renal cell carcinoma, and lung cancer [2].

Evidence Base

Diagnosis

While most skull base metastases are asymptomatic, the most common symptomatic clinical presentation is a cranial neuropathy in approximately 21% of patients [3]. Compression or damage to extraocular motor nerves, trigeminal, or hypoglossal nerves is among the most common neuropathies. Distinct syndromes can arise from cranial nerve dysfunction and vascular compression adjacent to the associated basal foramina and sinuses that comprise the skull base. These include orbital syndrome, parasellar/sellar syndrome, middle fossa syndrome, jugular foramen syndrome, and occipital condyle syndrome [4]. Table 14.1 summarizes the signs and symptoms of each syndrome.

The diagnosis of skull base metastases involves dedicated imaging of adequate resolution, including noncontrast CT head, which covers the mastoids, temporal bone, and entire skull base, and MRI brain, specifically non-Gadolinium

J. Byrne
Department of Radiation Oncology, Harvard Radiation Oncology Program, Boston, MA, USA

K. S. Oh (✉)
Department of Radiation Oncology, Massachusetts General Hospital, Boston, MA, USA
e-mail: koh2@mgh.harvard.edu

N. Wang
Division of Neuro-Oncology, Department of Neurology, Massachusetts General Hospital, Boston, MA, USA

© Springer Nature Switzerland AG 2020
Y. Yamada et al. (eds.), *Radiotherapy in Managing Brain Metastases*,
https://doi.org/10.1007/978-3-030-43740-4_14

(Gd) contrast-enhanced T1-weighted images. The CT may demonstrate a space-occupying lesion with bone destruction (Fig. 14.1), and MRI may demonstrate a contrast-enhancing mass (Fig. 14.2) and involvement of the adjacent cranial nerves, dura, or brain parenchyma or exten-

Table 14.1 Syndromes in skull base metastases

Location	Symptoms	Signs
Orbit	Supraorbital headache Diplopia	Proptosis Ophthalmoplegia +/− Facial numbness +/− Decreased vision +/− Periorbital swelling
Parasellar (sella turcica, petrous apex)	Frontal headache Diplopia	Ophthalmoplegia Facial numbness (V1) Periorbital swelling
Middle fossa (petrous ridge)	Facial numbness Paresthesias Atypical facial pain	Facial numbness (V2, V3) Abducens palsy (anterior ridge) Facial palsy (posterior ridge)
Jugular foramen	Occipital pain Hoarseness Dysphagia	Cranial nerve palsies (IX, X, XI)
Occipital condyle	Occipital pain Dysarthria	Cranial nerve palsy (XII)

From Laigle-Donadey et al. [1]. With permission from Springer Nature

sion through skull base foramina into the masticator space or paranasal sinuses, for example [5]. Imaging is critical for determining next steps in management and delineating key structures for radiation or surgical intervention. In cases where pathological confirmation of metastatic disease is needed, endoscopic biopsy or other minimally invasive techniques are used when possible.

Management

Treatment of skull base metastases may require a combination of radiation therapy, surgery, and systemic therapy. Radiation therapy is the mainstay of treatment for patients requiring palliation of pain or neurologic dysfunction [6, 7]. The rate of neurological improvement after radiation therapy is closely related to the speed of the treatment after the onset of the symptoms. Surgery is a viable option in select patients; however, neurovascular structure involvement complicates surgical attempts to avoid significant morbidity and obtain clear margins. For certain histologies that are historically radioresistant, surgery may provide a significant therapeutic benefit compared to radiation alone. For those with asymptomatic and nonthreatening disease who are not in need of urgent local therapy, systemic therapy alone or surveillance may be the appropriate choice.

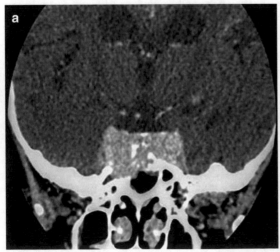 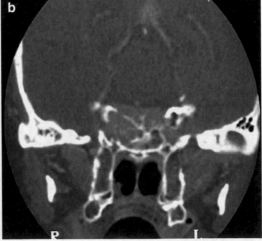

Fig. 14.1 Contrast coronal CT-scan reconstructions with soft-tissue windows (**a**) and bone windows (**b**) showing a strongly enhancing, well-delineated mass invading the sphenoid body with marked bone erosion. (From Laigle-Donadey et al. [1]; with permission from Springer Nature)

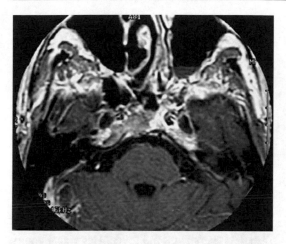

Fig. 14.2 Axial T1-weighted MRI after gadolinium administration shows an enhancing lesion invading the clivus and the posterior part of the sphenoid sinus close to the noninvaded Meckel's cavum. (From Laigle-Donadey et al. [1]; with permission from Springer Nature)

Radiation Therapy for Skull Base Metastases

Radiotherapy was used in ~70% of patients with prostate cancer skull base metastases in a report from Svare et al. [8]. Radiation provides excellent relief of pain and improvement in neurologic function [6, 7]. There are a variety of factors that govern the radiation dose and fractionation scheme, including the size of the lesion and proximity to critical structures.

Conventionally Fractionated Photon Radiation Therapy

The primary radiation modality for skull base metastases is conventionally fractionated photon radiation. Conventionally fractionated radiation provides significant symptom relief in the majority of patients. A retrospective analysis from Memorial-Sloan Kettering Cancer Center demonstrated that 37 of 43 patients with skull base metastases achieved symptomatic relief with conventionally fractionated radiation. Of these patients, seven had complete resolution of their cranial nerve deficits [9]. Another retrospective series evaluated the radiation management of skull base metastases from castrate-resistant prostate cancer. The majority of patients experienced a complete or partial

clinical response to radiation therapy. Unfortunately, two thirds of patients died within 3 months from treatment from their burden of metastatic disease. It was emphasized that patients should undergo radiation treatment as soon as possible after diagnosis to improve the likelihood of symptom resolution [10, 11]. Historically, opposed lateral beam and three-field arrangements were predominantly used for skull base metastases [11]. However, because modern imaging is able to better delineate bony disease, intensity-modulated radiation therapy (IMRT) is now heavily used to minimize dose to nontarget structures, such as the optic apparatus, pituitary, and neurocognitive centers [12].

Stereotactic Radiosurgery

Stereotactic radiosurgery (SRS) has shown promise in the treatment of skull base metastases. Small retrospective case series have shown high local control rates between 67% and 95% [13, 14] and low complication rates (6%) [13]. SRS also has been shown to provide excellent symptom relief. Furthermore, another series involving stereotactic radiotherapy (SRT) (regimen of 44 Gy in five fractions) has shown low rates of toxicity (15% grade 3 and 0% grade 4+) in patients with previously irradiated locally advanced or recurrent head and neck malignancies involving the skull base [15]. A series of patients treated with Gamma Knife (GK) radiosurgery for treatment of skull base metastases causing trigeminal neuralgia showed that 60% of patients were pain free at 6 months and 40% of patients discontinued analgesic use due to lack of pain [16]. With appropriate immobilization and on-board imaging, the use of SRS may be an alternative for management.

Areas of Uncertainty

The choice of radiation dose for conventional fractionation remains controversial. There are multiple randomized trials that demonstrated similar short-term pain relief when comparing single-fraction (e.g., 8 Gy × 1) vs. multifraction regimens (e.g., 4 Gy × 6) [17, 18]. However, the data regarding selection of dose for skull base metastases, in particular, are limited to retrospective studies. There are reports of improved rates of neurologic recovery with the use of higher doses of radiation (36 Gy) compared to standard doses (30 Gy in 10 fractions), and this benefit may be a function of histology and differences in radiosensitivity [19, 20]. Prospective studies evaluating the efficacy and safety of methods such as SRS, as well as combination radiation and systemic therapy (i.e., immunotherapy), are warranted.

Conclusions and Recommendations

A high index of suspicion based on new-onset cranial nerve deficit or craniofacial pain in patients with cancer is important to facilitate early diagnosis. In general, early treatment is crucial if one wishes to improve potentially disabling symptoms. The primary treatment for palliation is radiotherapy in most cases. When administered soon after the appearance of symptoms, radiation can provide significant symptomatic relief of pain and neurologic dysfunction. SRS is another effective form of treatment but is limited by the size of the lesion and proximity of critical structures, such as the optic apparatus. A minority of patients are selected for surgical resection.

Key Points

- The most common clinical presentation of a skull base metastasis is a cranial neuropathy.
- Radiation therapy is the primary treatment modality for skull base metastases.
- Early treatment is crucial to improve potentially disabling symptoms and maximize palliation.
- No class 1 evidence exists to guide decisions on how radiation should be delivered for skull base metastases.

Choroidal Metastases

Case Vignette

Case 2

A 69-year-old female with a history of stage IV ER+/PR+/HER2− breast cancer who initially reports blurriness of vision and then flashes in her left eye presents. Her last exam 2 years ago was within normal limits. She is seen by an ophthalmologist, who diagnoses a metastasis in the left choroid, estimated to measure 16 mm × 15 mm, located 0 disc diameters from the optic disc and 0 disc diameters from the fovea. Her visual acuity is measured as 20/20 in the right eye and 20/70 in the left eye. She is deemed to be a good candidate for eye-conserving therapy.

Introduction

Choroidal metastases, although rare, are the most common intraocular malignancy. Patients often present with blurred vision, floaters, phosphenes, or pain [21, 22]. In approximately 15–20% of breast cancer patients who are diagnosed with choroidal metastases, they are detected during routine staging procedures or eye exams [23]. Their incidence has steadily increased likely due to methods for early detection and improvements in survival for patients with hematogenous metastases. In one series from the Liverpool Ocular Oncology Centre, choroidal metastases were noted to be the first sign of metastatic disease in up to a third of patients with cancer [21]. The most common primary sites for choroidal metastases are breast and lung [22, 23]. Metastases originating from breast cancer are often bilateral or multifocal, whereas those originating from lung cancer are typically unilateral and unifocal [22, 23].

Evidence Base

Diagnosis

Early detection of choroidal metastases is critical for preservation or reversal of visual decline. The diagnosis of choroidal metastases requires a mul-

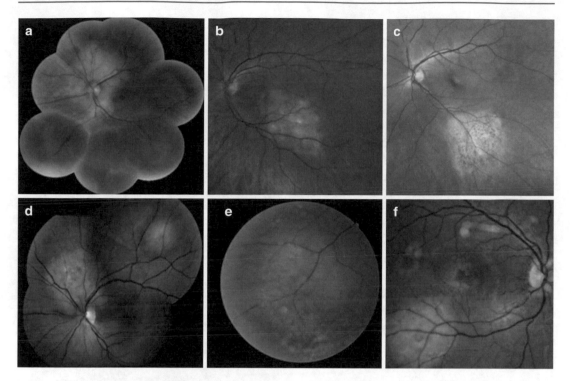

Fig. 14.3 Fundus photography: (**a**) lung carcinoma: pale yellow color; (**b**) breast carcinoma: lobular creamy white color; (**c**) prostate carcinoma: amelanotic mass; (**d**) renal carcinoma: temporal orange-color mass associated to another pale yellow juxtapapillary mass; (**e**) lung carci- noid tumor: orange color; (**f**) thyroid tumor: subfoveal orange-color mass associated to another inferior white mass. (From Mathis et al. [24]; with permission from Elsevier)

timodality approach to determine the extent of disease and management approach. Diagnostic methods have greatly improved and now include indocyanine green angiography, optical coher- ence tomography (OCT), spectral domain-OCT, fundoscopy (Fig. 14.3), and ultrasonography. Pathological confirmation by choroidal tumor biopsy may be needed to confirm the histology [24]. Furthermore, a significant portion of patients with choroidal metastases will have extra-ocular metastases as well [25]. MRI brain is recommended in cases of choroidal metastases because of the high risk of concomitant brain metastases, particularly in those with lung and breast cancer (32% and 62%, respectively, in some series) [26, 27].

Management

Choroidal metastases may result in loss of vision and, ultimately, loss of autonomy. The primary goal of treatment involves preventing or revers- ing the impairment of visual function. Avoiding enucleation is a primary concern, as there are associated functional and psychological conse- quences. In general, swift action may stop irre- versible blindness. Therefore, because of the speed and reliability of response, radiation ther- apy is the mainstay of treatment [24]. In many cases, a combination of systemic and local treat- ments is used to recover clinical decline and pro- vide local control.

Radiation Therapy for Choroidal Metastases

Options for radiation therapy vary widely with respect to method, dose and fractionation, and tar- get. The major techniques used in the treatment of choroidal metastases include photon radiation therapy, proton radiation therapy, and plaque brachytherapy. Within photon radiation therapy, fractionated 3D conformal conventional, frac- tionated intensity-modulated radiation therapy

(IMRT), and stereotactic radiosurgery/radiation therapy (SRS/SRT) are the major categories of modalities [24]. These choices are governed by the local extent of disease, proximity to the macula, number of lesions, prognosis, and goals of care. Each radiation modality has unique technical considerations including dose and fractionation, conformality, treatment time, and access to the technique. Table 14.2 shows the tolerance doses for standard fractionation. All these considerations must be accounted for in a risk–benefit analysis, acknowledging the fact that normal tissue can better tolerate smaller doses per fraction, but there is a continuum of responses depending on dose per fraction and total dose. Many cases of choroidal metastases are adequately treated with standard palliative fractionation, such as 3 Gy × 10. However, historically radioresistant tumors (e.g., melanoma and renal cell carcinoma) may benefit from higher dose per fraction, which may affect the macula [28].

Radiation Planning

The setup and immobilization for treatment planning are entirely dependent on the modality of radiation therapy. In most cases, the patient's head is immobilized using custom immobilization with a thermoplastic or rigid mask. For reproducibility, the patient is asked to close their eyes and maintain a downward or straight gaze. For target delineation, high-resolution MRI and, when available, planar fundus images (Fig. 14.4) are fused to the planning CT scan. In the case of unilateral involvement, one can employ a 3D conformal technique such as a wedged-pair or noncoplanar beams. In cases of bilateral involvement or high suspicion for contralateral micrometastasis (such as in the presence of concurrent multiple brain metastases), parallel-opposed lateral fields may be used. A CTV expansion from the GTV is generally 5 mm. Depending on the type of immobilization, an additional expansion of 0–5 mm is applied for the PTV [29]. The treatment planning process of determining beam number and arrangement will be a function of the radiation modality.

Table 14.2 Organs at risk in orbital radiation

Tissue	Dose objection for standard fractionation	Comments
Lens	Mean lens dose <0.5 Gy avoids lens opacities Mean lens dose <5–8 Gy avoids symptomatic cataracts	Radiation-induced cataract occurs generally 1–3 years after irradiation
Cornea	Maximal dose to cornea <40–60 Gy avoids risk of keratitis, ulcer, or edema Perforation is rare and seen only above 60 Gy	
Lacrimal gland	Volume of lacrimal gland receiving 30 Gy < 50%	
Retina	Volume of retina receiving 45 Gy < 50%	Significant retinopathy occurred typically 3 months to 3 years after radiotherapy, depending on the dose and other medical conditions
Optic nerve	Maximal dose to optic nerve <55 Gy	Radiation-induced optic neuropathy occurs between 3 months and 8 years after treatment with a peak at 18 months
Chiasm	Maximal dose to the chiasm <55 Gy	Chiasm is posterior and generally preserved in the treatment of choroidal metastases

From Mathis et al. [24]. With permission from Elsevier
Standard fractionation = 1.8–2.0 Gy per fraction

Stereotactic Radiosurgery

The data for SRS in the management of choroidal metastases appear promising, but they are limited to case series. In a case series of 10 patients, SRS (12–20 Gy) resulted in long-term tumor control in all patients [29]. Tumor regression was noted in 5 of 10 patients, but only 4 of 10 patients had stability or improved of their vision; no chronic radiation-induced toxicities were noted [29]. Others have found that there were no acute com-

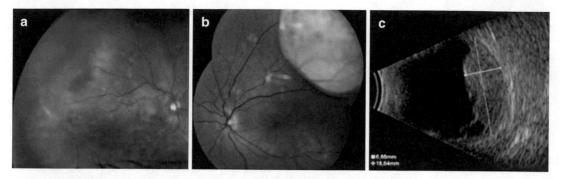

Fig. 14.4 Voluminous choroidal metastases. (**a**) Retinophotography of choroidal metastasis from a nasopharyngeal cancer; (**b, c**) retinophotography of choroidal metastasis from a neuroendocrine tumor and corresponding ultrasonography. Yellow marker: thickness (height); green marker: diameter (base). (From Mathis et al. [24]; with permission from Elsevier)

plications using GK radiosurgery (range 15–25 Gy), except the sample size was quite limited (i.e., seven patients). Limitations of this approach include long treatment times, eye tracking, and complete immobilization of the eye. To overcome these limitations, anesthetic ocular blocks and bridle suture were used to limit eye movement [30].

Proton Radiation

Proton radiation for choroidal metastases is performed at a limited number of centers worldwide. At Massachusetts General Hospital, a retrospective analysis of 77 patients with choroidal metastases treated with 20 Gy in two fractions demonstrated 94% local control over a median follow-up of 7.7 months. Approximately 31% of patients experienced an adverse event, and visual acuity was improved or stable in 38% of treated eyes [31]. Most published studies involve passive scattering proton therapy, and there are very little data on pencil beam scanning proton therapy. A drawback of proton therapy is the limited potential sparing of the macula in tumors located in the posterior pole. For tumors in proximity to the macula, a smaller dose per fraction is preferred to spare normal tissues. To assist with target delineation and tracking, fiducials are placed around the tumor and tracked prior to treatment. Additionally, infrared cameras may enable immediate interruption of the proton beam if a patient changes their gaze [24].

Plaque Brachytherapy

Plaque brachytherapy involves the placement of a radioactive isotope for a prescribed timeframe. The plaque is typically sutured onto the sclera near the tumor and remains in place until the therapeutic dose has been delivered (typically 2–4 days). The most commonly used isotope is iodine-125 due to the low dose rate. In one of the largest series of 36 patients, plaque brachytherapy enabled tumor regression in all patients and a complete response rate of 94% of cases who received a dose range 45–70 Gy. They noted that the complicated rate was low, and the most common complications were retinopathy, optic neuropathy, and cataracts [32]. Overall, plaque brachytherapy is a good treatment option, albeit more invasive than external beam radiation therapy. It is only offered at specialized centers.

Sequelae of Radiation Therapy

The early complications of radiation therapy involve radiodermatitis, focal alopecia, conjunctivitis, and xerophthalmia. The late complications, which may occur months to years after treatment, can include continued conjunctivitis, xerophthalmia, cataracts, hormonal imbalance, reduced visual acuity, and damage to normal brain tissue. Depending on prognosis, disease control must be balanced by the complications, especially in long-term survivors. Radiation-induced macular damage reaches its peak at 2 years, and adverse effects should be considered in context of overall prognosis. Sparing of the macula and optic disc are important to preserve vision with external beam radiotherapy as well as brachytherapy [33], and the ability to achieve sparing is more dependent on proximity to the gross disease.

Areas of Uncertainty

It remains unclear what the best radiation treatment modality is for treating choroidal metastases. There are no prospective randomized trials comparing the effectiveness and side effect profiles of the different modalities. These efforts are made challenging by the rarity of choroidal metastases and limited access to treatment modalities across centers.

Conclusions and Recommendations

Radiation therapy is a primary treatment for choroidal metastases. Radiation therapy can be used alone or in combination with systemic therapy especially in the context of diffuse metastatic disease. Various radiation treatment modalities can be used to manage choroidal metastases, including conventionally fractionated radiation therapy, stereotactic radiation therapy/SRS, proton therapy, and plaque brachytherapy.

> **Key Points**
> - Choroidal metastases are typically diagnosed as blurred vision, floaters, phosphenes, or pain.
> - Radiation therapy is a primary treatment modality for choroidal metastases.
> - Major radiation modalities include conventionally fractionated radiation, stereotactic radiation therapy, proton radiation therapy, and plaque brachytherapy.
> - It remains unclear what the most optimal radiation treatment modality is for choroidal metastases.

Brainstem Metastases

Case Vignette

Case 3

A 60-year-old woman with a history of clinical stage II (T2 N0 M0) ER/PR-negative and HER2-positive invasive ductal carcinoma of the right breast receives neoadjuvant T-DM1 and pertuzumab on a clinical trial. She then undergoes a right mastectomy with sentinel lymph node biopsy. Pathology reveals a pathologic complete response with 0/3 sentinel nodes involved. She then receives adjuvant Taxol, Herceptin, and Pertuzumab for four cycles followed by Herceptin every 3 weeks for 1 year. One year later, she presents with a headache and right > left leg weakness. MRI brain is ordered and demonstrates a cystic rim-enhancing pontine mass as demonstrated in Fig. 14.5.

Introduction

Metastases within the brainstem comprise only 5% of all cases, which reflects the distribution of relative blood flow to each region of the brain. The management of brainstem metastases has several unique challenges. Although there is a wealth of randomized data regarding the risks and benefits of SRS for brain metastases, patients with brainstem metastases are excluded from these trials due to the concern that commonly used SRS doses exceed brainstem tolerance [34–36]. With respect to radiation therapy, the dose limitations of the surrounding brainstem make the delivery of a safe ablative dose unachievable whether treatment is single fraction, hypofractionated, or fractionated. The clinician is inevitably challenged to find the lowest dose felt to be both efficacious and safe. Brainstem metastases are not considered surgically accessible for upfront management nor as a salvage option. Progression of metastases with the brainstem often leads to rapid and unsalvageable neurologic death.

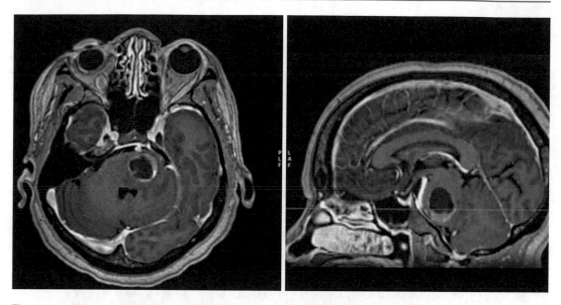

Fig. 14.5 Axial and sagittal T1 postgadolinium sequences demonstrating a cystic brainstem lesion with nodular enhancement along the inferior and left lateral aspects

Evidence Base

Single-Fraction Stereotactic Radiosurgery

Outcomes of brainstem metastases treated with radiation therapy are reported in several small single-institution studies using single-fraction SRS [37–47]. As reflected in Table 14.3, most of the series used GK-based radiosurgery and included fewer than 50 patients. Local control ranged from 75% to 95% with a median dose generally ranging from 13 to 16 Gy in a single fraction. Radiosurgery-related complications were generally less than 10%, although methodology for reporting was inconsistent across studies. Several studies reported poorer local control with larger tumor volumes [37, 40, 42, 43] or historically radioresistant histologies such as melanoma or renal cell carcinoma [37, 39]. Trifiletti et al. published the largest pooled dataset through the International Gamma Knife Research Foundation, which included 547 patients treated with GK for brainstem metastases. The median margin dose was 16 Gy (prescribed to 50% isodose level). Local control and overall survival at 12 months were 81.8% and 32.7%, respectively.

Severe radiosurgery-induced toxicity (≥ grade 3) resulted in 7.4% of cases [48].

Safety is the primary consideration when selecting the dose and fractionation for radiation therapy to a brainstem metastasis. The Quantitative Analyses of Normal Tissue Effects in the Clinic (QUANTEC) guidelines compiled the available data regarding various neural elements including the brainstem. As part of this effort, Mayo et al. compiled available safety data for irradiation of the brainstem using various fractionation schedules [49]. Based on available data, this effort concluded that the entire brainstem may be treated to 54 Gy using conventional fractionation with minimal risk, and smaller volumes (up to 10 mL) may be irradiated to a maximum of 59 Gy in fraction sizes of 2 Gy or less. In this context, the risk of neuropathy or necrosis is believed to be less than 5%. The available safety data for single-fraction radiosurgery are limited to only five studies with a range of doses and prescription points. For single-fraction SRS treatments, the risk of toxicity to the brainstem increases for doses >12 Gy. However, experience is accumulating on single-fraction SRS to the brainstem for metastatic disease, which is unique

Table 14.3 Single-institution series of radiosurgery for brainstem metastases

Author	Year	N	SRS modality	Median dose (range)	Local control	OS (month, median)	Toxicity
Hatiboglu et al.	2011	60	LINAC	15 Gy (8–18)	76% crude	4	20% SRS-related complications
Hussain et al.	2007	22	GK	16 Gy (14–23)	100% crude	8.5	5% hemiparesis after SRS
Kased et al.	2008	42	GK	16 Gy (10–19.8)	77% at 1 year	9	9.5% SRS-related complications
Kawabe et al.	2012	200	GK	18 Gy (12–25)	82% at 2 years	6	One death and six asymptomatic radiographic peritumor changes
Kilburn et al.	2014	44	GK	18 Gy (10–22)	74% at 1 year	6	9% SRS-related complications
Koyfman et al.	2010	43	GK	15 Gy (9.6–24)	85% at 1 year	5.8	No grade 3–4 toxicities observed
Lin et al.	2012	45	LINAC	14 Gy (10–17)	88% at 1 year	11.6	4.7% complication rate at 2 years
Lorenzoni et al.	2009	25	GK	20 Gy (15–24)	95% crude	11.1	No SRS-induced complications documented
Peterson et al.	2014	41	GK	17 Gy	91% crude	22% at 12 months	One patient died of hemorrhage after treatment
Sengoz et al.	2013	44	GK	16 Gy (10–20)	96% crude	8	4% asymptomatic radiographic peritumoral changes
Shuto et al.	2003	25	GK	13 Gy mean (8–18)	77% crude	4.9	8% radiation-induced injury

SRS stereotactic radiosurgery, *LINAC* linear accelerator-based radiosurgery, *GK* Gamma Knife radiosurgery, *OS* overall survival

in that the target displaces as opposed to infiltrates brainstem parenchyma, thereby affording the possibility of a higher dose as long as it is located within gross disease. Foote et al. reported the largest study including 149 patients with vestibular schwannoma treated with LINAC-based SRS between 10 and 22.5 Gy [50]. Based on univariate analysis, significant risk factors for facial neuropathy and any cranial neuropathy were Dmax ≥17.5 Gy and 12.5 Gy, respectively. Therefore, it was concluded that there was a significant increase in nerve complication for peripheral doses ≥15 Gy.

Hypofractionated Stereotactic Regimens

Many institutions, especially those employing linear accelerator-based systems, choose to use hypofractionated strategies for the treatment of brainstem metastases. Hypofractionated radiation refers to treatment using daily doses ≥4 Gy/day, which is often used in conjunction with techniques for stereotactic body radiation therapy

(SBRT). Common regimens include 8 Gy × 3 and 6 Gy × 5. These dose and fractionation schedules are based on modeled safety profiles using the linear quadratic (LQ) equation to calculate the "nBED2/2," which is the biologic effective dose in 2-Gy equivalent fractions assuming an alpha/beta ratio of 2. It should be noted that the reliability of this model is controversial in the setting of high dose per fraction. Clark et al. reviewed 77 patients with both benign and malignant brain tumors treated to a dose of 7 Gy × 6 (to 90% iso-dose surface) and reported brainstem complications in 4 of 20 patients treated for meningioma [51]. Using the linear quadratic model, complications correlated with a mean BED >70 Gy assuming alpha/beta of 2.5 Gy.

Future Directions

The emergence of more effective and durable systemic therapy for brain metastases may obviate the need for radiation therapy, especially in high-risk locations such as the brainstem. For example, in melanoma, the intracranial response rates to single-agent ipilimumab, single-agent PD-1 blockade, or combination of ipilimumab and nivolumab are as high as 10–25%, 25–35%, and 55%, respectively, and these responses are often durable [52–54]. In patients with known driver mutations, there are now widely available targeted agents with CNS penetration and intracranial response rates generally <60–70%. These include erlotinib and osimertinib for EGFR-mutant non–small-cell lung cancer (NSCLC), alectinib for ALK-mutant NSCLC, and various BRAF/MEK inhibitors for BRAF-mutant melanoma. However, the durability of response to targeted agents is limited by the development of resistance pathways. Therefore, the roles of radiation therapy in the upfront or salvage settings of brainstem metastases will need to be redefined. Moreover, immunotherapy and targeted agents may increase the risks of high-dose radiation by either potentiating the risk of radionecrosis or by lengthening the natural history of disease.

Conclusions and Recommendations

The brainstem is a rare location for metastatic disease. Given its inaccessible surgical location, radiation remains the mainstay of therapy. The published literature for single-fraction radiosurgery for brainstem metastases is limited to small single-institution series and a pooled data set. Overall, with doses of 13–24 Gy in a single fraction, the local control is felt to be 75–95% with treatment-related complications generally reported as <10%. Hypofractionated regimens are commonly used in order to increase the safety profile, but there is no consensus regarding the optimal fractionation schedule. Lastly, the growing number of systemic options and concern for increased risk of radionecrosis may lead clinicians to become increasingly conservative with radiation therapy in the context of immunotherapy and targeted agents.

Key Points
- The brainstem is a clinically high-risk location for metastatic disease that requires a more conservative approach.
- The mainstay of therapy is radiation, which can be delivered with SRS, hypofractionation, or conventionally fractionated treatments. Most of the available data are in the context of SRS.
- Emerging systemic therapy with intracranial activity, such as immunotherapy and targeted agents, may obviate the need for radiation therapy for brainstem metastases.

Dural-Based Metastases

Case Vignette

Case 4

A 58-year-old man with metastatic salivary duct adenocarcinoma of the right parotid involving bone, liver, and lung presents with several weeks of right arm weakness. Since his diagnosis 4 years ago, he has received multiple lines of systemic therapy, currently on cyclophosphamide/doxorubicin. He presents with several weeks of increasing confusion. An MRI brain is obtained, which reveals multiple hemorrhagic brain metastases, including a dominant right temporal dural-based metastasis with extension into the calvarium, associated edema, and mass effect (Fig. 14.6).

Introduction

In addition to metastasizing to the brain parenchyma or cerebrospinal fluid, tumor cells may also metastasize to the dura mater. This may be associated with extension into the epidural or subdural space, and direct intraparenchymal invasion may be seen in up to a third of patients

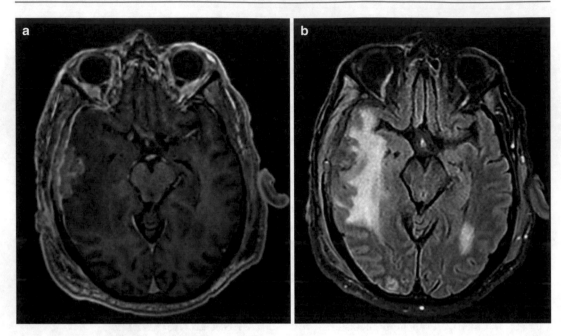

Fig. 14.6 Gadolinium-enhanced brain MRI shows a dural-based lesion in the right temporal region demonstrating irregular, heterogeneous enhancement. There is associated right frontotemporal pachymeningeal thickening and extension into the adjacent calvarium. There is significant surrounding edema and local mass effect resulting in leftward midline shift (**b**). Additional regions of T2/FLAIR hyperintensity in the left temporo-occipital lobe and right occipital lobe correspond to intraparenchymal lesions that are not well visualized in (**a**)

[55]. Frequently, dural-based metastases are seen concurrently with intraparenchymal or calvarial metastases. Dural-based metastases are relatively rare, with an incidence of 9–14% based on autopsy series [4]. Dural-based metastases are more frequent in breast, prostate, lung, and hematologic malignancies (i.e., chloromas) and are often seen in advanced stage disease with associated poor prognosis. Metastasis is thought to occur by direct invasion (particularly in the setting of calvarial metastasis) or hematogenous spread.

Prognosis is similar to that of intraparenchymal brain metastases with a median overall survival of approximately 6 months and death largely due to systemic progression [55, 56]. A retrospective study of 122 patients with dural-based metastases found that lower KPS and lung cancer were poor prognostic factors [55]. Hematologic malignancies, breast and prostate cancer, and isolated or solitary dural-based metastases are favorable prognostic factors [56]. Despite multiple available treatment modalities including surgery, radiation, and systemic therapy, dural-based metastases frequently cause significant neurologic dysfunction and morbidity.

Evidence Base

Diagnosis

Gadolinium-enhanced magnetic resonance imaging (MRI) is the imaging modality of choice and may provide clues regarding the extraparenchymal origin, including the presence of a dural tail, CSF cleft, displaced subarachnoid vessels, and overlying reactive calvarial changes. Dural-based metastases are usually avidly enhancing and biconvex or lenticular in shape, in contrast to primary epidural or subdural metastases which tend to be more crescentic in appearance [55]. Adjacent vasogenic edema or mass effect may be seen. Compromise of vascular structures may lead to infarct or intraparenchymal hemorrhage. Dural-based metastases may also be associated with subdural hematomas. The differential diagnosis for a dural-based enhancing mass includes both neoplastic (e.g., meningioma, schwannoma, hemangiopericytoma, and lymphoma) and non-neoplastic causes (e.g., sarcoidosis, empyema, and osteomyelitis when bone lesions are associated).

Presenting symptoms depend on location and are often nonspecific. Dural-based metastases are often diagnosed incidentally on screening or surveillance imaging. Deficits may result from direct mass effect on underlying brain parenchyma or edema, which may lead to headache and other signs of increased intracranial pressure. Lesions in the skull base often present as cranial neuropathies. Seizures and focal neurologic deficits such as weakness may occur.

Management

Treatment modalities include surgery, radiation, and chemotherapy, although data are mostly based on retrospective studies. For dural-based metastases with symptoms limited to pain and not requiring urgent decompression, radiation therapy plays an important role in providing local control and symptom relief. Radiation therapy is usually fractionated, such as 30 Gy in 10 fractions [57], but a higher equivalent BED may be considered for historically radioresistant histologies. Highly conformal fractionated radiation techniques should be used to spare uninvolved tissue, and stereotactic or image-guided therapy should be considered when adjacent to critical structures, such as in skull base lesions. SRS may be used for smaller lesions away from critical tissues, with one retrospective study showing up to 85% local tumor control rate in prostate cancer dural-based metastases [58]. Prescription doses of 15–24 Gy are commonly used. Hypofractionated stereotactic radiation therapy (e.g., 9 Gy × 3 or 6 Gy × 5) may be considered for lesions exceeding 3 cm in maximum diameter. Surgical resection remains the standard for pathologic diagnosis and often leads to rapid relief of symptoms due to mass effect or edema. Postoperative adjuvant radiation may be administered if there is incomplete resection or evidence of brain invasion.

As dural-based metastases are outside the blood–brain barrier, systemic therapy may be effective, and choice of agent should depend on primary histology, molecular features of the tumor, and status of systemic disease. Systemic therapy may be considered when there is an asymptomatic lesion detected on screening and if targetable mutations are present, such as BRAF in melanoma, EGFR/ALK in lung cancer, and HER2 in breast cancer. Retrospective data show that chemotherapy improves progression-free survival but not overall survival [55]. Corticosteroids are used to treat symptomatic edema, and anticonvulsants are warranted only if there is a history of seizures.

Areas of Uncertainty

Data on treatment of dural metastases are sparse, and even retrospective studies often exclude patients with dural metastases who do not have concurrent intraparenchymal metastases. Alternatively, they are grouped with intra-axial and leptomeningeal metastases, and application of study results to isolated dural-based metastases is problematic. In the era of effective targeted therapies and immunotherapy, additional studies are needed to determine the efficacy of these treatments in comparison to surgery and radiation, particularly for small, asymptomatic lesions.

Conclusions and Recommendations

Dural-based metastases are rare and may occur with intraparenchymal or calvarial metastases. They confer poor prognosis and can lead to significant morbidity. If small and asymptomatic, they may be closely monitored in a patient receiving active systemic therapy. Radiation therapy, either fractionated, hypofractionated, or radiosurgery, is the standard of care for dural-based metastases with symptoms limited to pain and not requiring urgent decompression. Large lesions causing symptoms related to mass effect or edema may be surgically resected and then treated with postoperative fractionated radiation therapy.

Leptomeningeal Disease

Case Vignette

Case 5

A 79-year-old woman presents with several months of progressive gait unsteadiness and falls. MRI brain shows extensive basilar-predominant leptomeningeal enhancement as well as hydrocephalus. She undergoes lumbar puncture, which shows normal opening pressure, elevated total protein, eight nucleated cells, normal glucose, and negative cytology. Systemic imaging shows bilateral FDG-avid pulmonary nodules. She undergoes a biopsy of a pulmonary nodule, which shows well-differentiated neuroendocrine tumor. A ventriculoperitoneal shunt is placed with improvement of gait unsteadiness.

Introduction

Leptomeningeal disease (LMD), also known as carcinomatous meningitis or leptomeningeal carcinomatosis, occurs when tumor cells seed the cerebral spinal fluid (CSF), often via hematogenous spread. It occurs in approximately 5–8% of patients with solid tumors and 5–15% of patients with hematologic malignancies [59]. The most common solid tumors to metastasize to the leptomeninges are lung, breast, and melanoma. Prognosis is poor with an average survival <2–4 months, although response to treatment varies across histologies.

Evidence Base

Diagnosis

Clinical presentation of LMD may be nonspecific but generally depends on the location of involvement. Common findings include seizure, cranial nerve dysfunction (particularly diplopia, facial droop, changes in hearing), and spinal nerve dysfunction (including radicular pain, bowel/bladder dysfunction, limb weakness). CSF resorption may be impaired, leading to increased intracranial pressure causing headache and pulsatile tinnitus. Given the frequently nonspecific presentation, index of suspicion must be high. Diagnostic evaluation should consist of gadolinium-enhanced magnetic resonance imaging (MRI) of the brain and total spine as well as lumbar puncture with cytology. MRI often shows irregular and nodular leptomeningeal enhancement (Fig. 14.7). If clinical suspicion is high, an abnormal MRI is sufficient to make the diagnosis. A lumbar puncture may reveal CSF pleocytosis, elevated protein, and hypoglycorrhachia. Flow cytometry increases the sensitivity of CSF evaluation in the setting of hematologic malignancies [60]. Care should be taken to exclude infectious meningitis or encephalitis in immunocompromised cancer patients.

Management

Optimum therapy for LMD is poorly defined, given lack of prospective, randomized trials. A palliative ventriculoperitoneal shunt should be considered in the setting of elevated opening pressure on lumbar puncture or signs and symptoms of increased ICP. Data supporting the use of intrathecal and systemic chemotherapy primarily

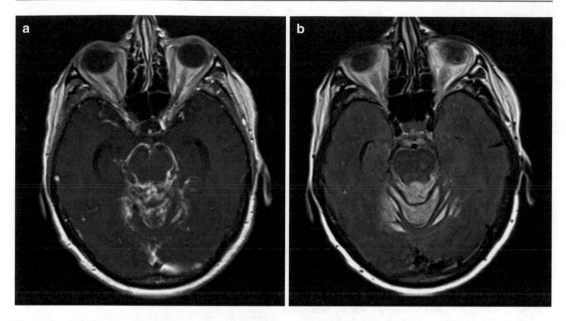

Fig. 14.7 Gadolinium-enhanced brain MRI shows enhancement along the cerebellar folia and ambient cisterns (**a**). There is also associated sulcal FLAIR hyperintensity (**b**)

come from retrospective trials. Six randomized clinical trials conducted in LMD all focus on intrathecal (IT) therapy with agents including methotrexate, cytarabine, liposomal cytarabine, and thiotepa [61–66]. Only one study compared IT chemotherapy to standard therapy without IT treatment and found no difference in survival or neurologic response in breast cancer patients treated with IT methotrexate [65]. IT chemotherapy is generally associated with increased treatment-related neurotoxicity, particularly aseptic meningitis. Importantly, series often excluded patients with poor performance status or deemed too sick for treatment, which may constitute a significant proportion of patients at presentation. While the ability to cross the blood–brain barrier (BBB) is a concern for systemic therapy, there may be a breakdown of the BBB in the setting of LMD, and a number of chemotherapies have been shown to achieve therapeutic levels in the CSF. Unlike IT administration, systemic therapy does not depend on CSF flow and is able to penetrate bulky, nodular disease. The agent used should be guided by primary histology, and chemotherapies that have been reported to have efficacy include high-dose methotrexate, high-dose cytarabine, capecitabine, thiotepa, high-

dose etoposide, and temozolomide [59]. Overall, the role of systemic versus intrathecal chemotherapy may depend on primary histology, with little added value of intrathecal therapy in studies conducted primarily in patients with lymphoma and breast cancer.

The role of whole-brain radiation therapy (WBRT) is primarily palliative. Retrospective studies in breast and lung cancer patients show no improvement in survival, although radiation may lead to rapid symptom improvement [67, 68]. While the entire craniospinal axis might be considered the target volume, irradiation of the entire neuraxis is typically not recommended due to significant myelo and neurologic toxicity but may be considered in patients with highly radiosensitive tumors, such as seminoma, leukemia, or lymphoma. Involved-field radiation may be used to treat sites of bulky, symptomatic disease in the brain or spine. Whole-brain radiotherapy (WBRT) with a total dose of 30 Gy in 3-Gy fractions is commonly used [69]. A hypofractionated course of 20 Gy in 4-Gy fractions may be considered in patients with poor prognosis or less likely to tolerate treatment. The meningeal space should be included in planning. One retrospective series found that in non-small-cell lung cancer patients, favorable performance status, longer time to LMD, and absence of concurrent intraparenchymal metastases were found to be predictors of a favorable response to WBRT [70]. Notably, there is an increased risk of leukoencephalopathy when radiation is combined with certain chemotherapeutic agents, particularly methotrexate. A recent retrospective series of 16 patients who underwent SRS for focal LMD demonstrated a median actuarial overall survival of 10 months from date of SRS [71]. Seven patients developed distant LMD at a median time of 7 months.

Future Directions

Significant advances have been made in using targeted therapies to treat many malignancies, including BRAF/MEK inhibition for melanoma, tyrosine kinase inhibitors for EGFR/ALK-mutant lung cancer, and HER2-directed therapy for HER2-positive breast cancer. Many newer targeted agents cross the blood–brain barrier (BBB) and have been shown to have some response in LMD, most notably osimertinib for EGFR-mutant lung adenocarcinoma [72]. Multiple studies are also underway to evaluate the efficacy of immunotherapy (pembrolizumab, ipilimumab + nivolumab) for LMD with promising preliminary results [73].

Conclusions and Recommendations

LMD is a devastating complication of cancer with few effective therapies. Cranial and spinal nerve dysfunction and headache are common presenting symptoms, and gadolinium-enhanced MRI and CSF evaluation are useful in making the diagnosis. Treatment is focused on palliation, and data supporting the use of intrathecal and systemic chemotherapy are mixed and dependent on primary histology. There are emerging data for the use of targeted agents and immunotherapy with promising results. WBRT and involved field radiation have not been shown to improve survival but may lead to rapid symptom improvement.

Key Points

- Leptomeningeal metastasis carries a poor prognosis, and index of suspicion should be high in cancer patients as the clinical presentation is often nonspecific.
- Treatment has traditionally been directed toward symptom palliation, including whole-brain radiotherapy or involved field radiation targeting bulky, symptomatic sites of disease.
- Small, isolated foci of leptomeningeal carcinoma may be reasonably palliated with stereotactic radiosurgery to avoid the sequelae of WBRT.

References

1. Laigle-Donadey F, Taillibert S, Martin-Duverneuil N, Hildebrand J, Delattre JY. Skull-base metastases. J Neurooncol. 2005;75(1):63–9.
2. Gupta SR, Zdonczyk DE, Rubino FA. Cranial neuropathy in systemic malignancy in a VA population. Neurology. 1990;40(6):997–9.
3. Mitsuya K, Nakasu Y, Horiguchi S, Harada H, Nishimura T, Yuen S, et al. Metastatic skull tumors: MRI features and a new conventional classification. J Neurooncol. 2011;104(1):239–45.
4. Harrison RA, Nam JY, Weathers SP, DeMonte F. Intracranial dural, calvarial, and skull base metastases. Handb Clin Neurol. 2018;149:205–25.
5. Maroldi R, Farina D, Battaglia G, Maculotti P, Nicolai P, Chiesa A. MR of malignant nasosinusal neoplasms. Frequently asked questions. Eur J Radiol. 1997;24(3):181–90.
6. McAvoy CE, Kamalarajab S, Best R, Rankin S, Bryars J, Nelson K. Bilateral third and unilateral sixth nerve palsies as early presenting signs of metastatic prostatic carcinoma. Eye (Lond). 2002;16(6):749–53.
7. Moris G, Roig C, Misiego M, Alvarez A, Berciano J, Pascual J. The distinctive headache of the occipital condyle syndrome: a report of four cases. Headache. 1998;38(4):308–11.
8. Svare A, Fossa SD, Heier MS. Cranial nerve dysfunction in metastatic cancer of the prostate. Br J Urol. 1988;61(5):441–4.
9. Greenberg HS, Deck MD, Vikram B, Chu FC, Posner JB. Metastasis to the base of the skull: clinical findings in 43 patients. Neurology. 1981;31(5):530–7.
10. McDermott RS, Anderson PR, Greenberg RE, Milestone BN, Hudes GR. Cranial nerve deficits in patients with metastatic prostate carcinoma:

clinical features and treatment outcomes. Cancer. 2004;101(7):1639–43.

11. Vikram B, Chu FC. Radiation therapy for metastases to the base of the skull. Radiology. 1979;130(2):465–8.

12. Fossati P, Vavassori A, Deantonio L, Ferrara E, Krengli M, Orecchia R. Review of photon and proton radiotherapy for skull base tumours. Rep Pract Oncol Radiother. 2016;21(4):336–55.

13. Iwai Y, Yamanaka K. Gamma Knife radiosurgery for skull base metastasis and invasion. Stereotact Funct Neurosurg. 1999;72(Suppl 1):81–7.

14. Miller RC, Foote RL, Coffey RJ, Gorman DA, Earle JD, Schomberg PJ, et al. The role of stereotactic radiosurgery in the treatment of malignant skull base tumors. Int J Radiat Oncol Biol Phys. 1997;39(5):977–81.

15. Xu KM, Quan K, Clump DA, Ferris RL, Heron DE. Stereotactic ablative radiosurgery for locally advanced or recurrent skull base malignancies with prior external beam radiation therapy. Front Oncol. 2015;5:65.

16. Phan J, Pollard C, Brown PD, Guha Thakurta N, Garden AS, Rosenthal DI, et al. Stereotactic radiosurgery for trigeminal pain secondary to recurrent malignant skull base tumors. J Neurosurg. 2018;130(3):812–21.

17. Chow E, Harris K, Fan G, Tsao M, Sze WM. Palliative radiotherapy trials for bone metastases: a systematic review. J Clin Oncol. 2007;25(11):1423–36.

18. Steenland E, Leer JW, van Houwelingen H, Post WJ, van den Hout WB, Kievit J, et al. The effect of a single fraction compared to multiple fractions on painful bone metastases: a global analysis of the Dutch Bone Metastasis Study. Radiother Oncol. 1999;52(2):101–9.

19. Posner JB. Cancer involving cranial and peripheral nerves. In: Davis F, editor. Neurologic complications of cancer. Philadelphia: F.A. Davis Co.; 1995. p. 172–84.

20. Ransom DT, Dinapoli RP, Richardson RL. Cranial nerve lesions due to base of the skull metastases in prostate carcinoma. Cancer. 1990;65(3):586–9.

21. Konstantinidis L, Rospond-Kubiak I, Zeolite I, Heimann H, Groenewald C, Coupland SE, et al. Management of patients with uveal metastases at the Liverpool Ocular Oncology Centre. Br J Ophthalmol. 2014;98(1):92–8.

22. Shields CL, Shields JA, Gross NE, Schwartz GP, Lally SE. Survey of 520 eyes with uveal metastases. Ophthalmology. 1997;104(8):1265–76.

23. Demirci H, Shields CL, Chao AN, Shields JA. Uveal metastasis from breast cancer in 264 patients. Am J Ophthalmol. 2003;136(2):264–71.

24. Mathis T, Jardel P, Loria O, Delaunay B, Nguyen AM, Lanza F, et al. New concepts in the diagnosis and management of choroidal metastases. Prog Retin Eye Res. 2019;68:144–76.

25. Jardel P, Sauerwein W, Olivier T, Bensoussan E, Maschi C, Lanza F, et al. Management of choroidal metastases. Cancer Treat Rev. 2014;40(10):1119–28.

26. Amer R, Pe'er J, Chowers I, Anteby I. Treatment options in the management of choroidal metastases. Ophthalmologica. 2004;218(6):372–7.

27. Kreusel KM, Bechrakis NE, Wiegel T, Krause L, Foerster MH. Incidence and clinical characteristics of symptomatic choroidal metastasis from lung cancer. Acta Ophthalmol. 2008;86(5):515–9.

28. Caujolle JP, Mammar H, Chamorey E, Pinon F, Herault J, Gastaud P. Proton beam radiotherapy for uveal melanomas at nice teaching hospital: 16 years' experience. Int J Radiat Oncol Biol Phys. 2010;78(1):98–103.

29. Bellmann C, Fuss M, Holz FG, Debus J, Rohrschneider K, Volcker HE, et al. Stereotactic radiation therapy for malignant choroidal tumors: preliminary, short-term results. Ophthalmology. 2000;107(2):358–65.

30. Cho KR, Lee KM, Han G, Kang SW, Lee JI. Gamma knife radiosurgery for cancer metastasized to the ocular choroid. J Korean Neurosurg Soc. 2018;61(1):60–5.

31. Kamran SC, Collier JM, Lane AM, Kim I, Niemierko A, Chen YL, et al. Outcomes of proton therapy for the treatment of uveal metastases. Int J Radiat Oncol Biol Phys. 2014;90(5):1044–50.

32. Shields CL, Shields JA, De Potter P, Quaranta M, Freire J, Brady LW, et al. Plaque radiotherapy for the management of uveal metastasis. Arch Ophthalmol. 1997;115(2):203–9.

33. Rudoler SB, Shields CL, Corn BW, De Potter P, Hyslop T, Curran WJ Jr, et al. Functional vision is improved in the majority of patients treated with external-beam radiotherapy for choroid metastases: a multivariate analysis of 188 patients. J Clin Oncol. 1997;15(3):1244–51.

34. Kocher M, Soffietti R, Abacioglu U, Villa S, Fauchon F, Baumert BG, et al. Adjuvant whole-brain radiotherapy versus observation after radiosurgery or surgical resection of one to three cerebral metastases: results of the EORTC 22952-26001 study. J Clin Oncol. 2011;29(2):134–41.

35. O'Neill BP, Iturria NJ, Link MJ, Pollock BE, Ballman KV, O'Fallon JR. A comparison of surgical resection and stereotactic radiosurgery in the treatment of solitary brain metastases. Int J Radiat Oncol Biol Phys. 2003;55(5):1169–76.

36. Shaw E, Scott C, Souhami L, Dinapoli R, Kline R, Loeffler J, et al. Single dose radiosurgical treatment of recurrent previously irradiated primary brain tumors and brain metastases: final report of RTOG protocol 90-05. Int J Radiat Oncol Biol Phys. 2000;47(2):291–8.

37. Hatiboglu MA, Chang EL, Suki D, Sawaya R, Wildrick DM, Weinberg JS. Outcomes and prognostic factors for patients with brainstem metastases undergoing stereotactic radiosurgery. Neurosurgery. 2011;69(4):796–806; discussion.

38. Hussain A, Brown PD, Stafford SL, Pollock BE. Stereotactic radiosurgery for brainstem metastases: survival, tumor control, and patient outcomes. Int J Radiat Oncol Biol Phys. 2007;67(2):521–4.

39. Kased N, Huang K, Nakamura JL, Sahgal A, Larson DA, McDermott MW, et al. Gamma knife radiosurgery for brainstem metastases: the UCSF experience. J Neurooncol. 2008;86(2):195–205.

40. Kawabe T, Yamamoto M, Sato Y, Barfod BE, Urakawa Y, Kasuya H, et al. Gamma Knife surgery for patients with brainstem metastases. J Neurosurg. 2012;117(Suppl):23–30.

41. Kilburn JM, Ellis TL, Lovato JF, Urbanic JJ, Bourland JD, Munley MT, et al. Local control and toxicity outcomes in brainstem metastases treated with single fraction radiosurgery: is there a volume threshold for toxicity? J Neurooncol. 2014;117(1):167–74.

42. Koyfman SA, Tendulkar RD, Chao ST, Vogelbaum MA, Barnett GH, Angelov L, et al. Stereotactic radiosurgery for single brainstem metastases: the cleveland clinic experience. Int J Radiat Oncol Biol Phys. 2010;78(2):409–14.

43. Lin CS, Selch MT, Lee SP, Wu JK, Xiao F, Hong DS, et al. Accelerator-based stereotactic radiosurgery for brainstem metastases. Neurosurgery. 2012;70(4):953–8; discussion 8.

44. Lorenzoni JG, Devriendt D, Massager N, Desmedt F, Simon S, Van Houtte P, et al. Brain stem metastases treated with radiosurgery: prognostic factors of survival and life expectancy estimation. Surg Neurol. 2009;71(2):188–95; discussion 95, 95–6.

45. Peterson HE, Larson EW, Fairbanks RK, MacKay AR, Lamoreaux WT, Call JA, et al. Gamma knife treatment of brainstem metastases. Int J Mol Sci. 2014;15(6):9748–61.

46. Sengoz M, Kabalay IA, Tezcanli E, Peker S, Pamir N. Treatment of brainstem metastases with gamma-knife radiosurgery. J Neurooncol. 2013;113(1):33–8.

47. Shuto T, Fujino H, Asada H, Inomori S, Nagano H. Gamma knife radiosurgery for metastatic tumours in the brain stem. Acta Neurochir. 2003;145(9):755–60.

48. Trifiletti DM, Lee CC, Kano H, Cohen J, Janopaul-Naylor J, Alonso-Basanta M, et al. Stereotactic radiosurgery for brainstem metastases: an international cooperative study to define response and toxicity. Int J Radiat Oncol Biol Phys. 2016;96(2):280–8.

49. Mayo C, Yorke E, Merchant TE. Radiation associated brainstem injury. Int J Radiat Oncol Biol Phys. 2010;76(3 Suppl):S36–41.

50. Foote KD, Friedman WA, Buatti JM, Meeks SL, Bova FJ, Kubilis PS. Analysis of risk factors associated with radiosurgery for vestibular schwannoma. J Neurosurg. 2001;95(3):440–9.

51. Clark BG, Souhami L, Pla C, Al-Amro AS, Bahary JP, Villemure JG, et al. The integral biologically effective dose to predict brain stem toxicity of hypofractionated stereotactic radiotherapy. Int J Radiat Oncol Biol Phys. 1998;40(3):667–75.

52. Kluger HM, Chiang V, Mahajan A, Zito CR, Sznol M, Tran T, et al. Long-term survival of patients with melanoma with active brain metastases treated with pembrolizumab on a phase II trial. J Clin Oncol. 2019;37(1):52–60.

53. Long GV, Atkinson V, Lo S, Sandhu S, Guminski AD, Brown MP, et al. Combination nivolumab and ipilim-

54. Margolin K, Ernstoff MS, Hamid O, Lawrence D, McDermott D, Puzanov I, et al. Ipilimumab in patients with melanoma and brain metastases: an open-label, phase 2 trial. Lancet Oncol. 2012;13(5):459–65.

55. Nayak L, Abrey LE, Iwamoto FM. Intracranial dural metastases. Cancer. 2009;115(9):1947–53.

56. Laigle-Donadey F, Taillibert S, Mokhtari K, Hildebrand J, Delattre JY. Dural metastases. J Neurooncol. 2005;75(1):57–61.

57. Newton HB. Skull and dural metastases. In: Schiff D, Kesari S, Wen PY, editors. Cancer neurology in clinical practice. Totowa: Humana Press; 2008. p. 145–61.

58. Flannery T, Kano H, Niranjan A, Monaco EA, Flickinger JC, Lunsford LD, et al. Stereotactic radiosurgery as a therapeutic strategy for intracranial metastatic prostate carcinoma. J Neurooncol. 2010;96(3):369–74.

59. Wang N, Bertalan MS, Brastianos PK. Leptomeningeal metastasis from systemic cancer: review and update on management. Cancer. 2018;124(1):21–35.

60. Bromberg JE, Breems DA, Kraan J, Bikker G, van der Holt B, Smitt PS, et al. CSF flow cytometry greatly improves diagnostic accuracy in CNS hematologic malignancies. Neurology. 2007;68(20):1674–9.

61. Hitchins RN, Bell DR, Woods RL, Levi JA. A prospective randomized trial of single-agent versus combination chemotherapy in meningeal carcinomatosis. J Clin Oncol. 1987;5(10):1655–62.

62. Grossman SA, Finkelstein DM, Ruckdeschel JC, Trump DL, Moynihan T, Ettinger DS. Randomized prospective comparison of intraventricular methotrexate and thiotepa in patients with previously untreated neoplastic meningitis. Eastern Cooperative Oncology Group. J Clin Oncol. 1993;11(3):561–9.

63. Glantz MJ, Jaeckle KA, Chamberlain MC, Phuphanich S, Recht L, Swinnen LJ, et al. A randomized controlled trial comparing intrathecal sustained-release cytarabine (DepoCyt) to intrathecal methotrexate in patients with neoplastic meningitis from solid tumors. Clin Cancer Res. 1999;5(11):3394–402.

64. Glantz MJ, LaFollette S, Jaeckle KA, Shapiro W, Swinnen L, Rozental JR, et al. Randomized trial of a slow-release versus a standard formulation of cytarabine for the intrathecal treatment of lymphomatous meningitis. J Clin Oncol. 1999;17(10):3110–6.

65. Boogerd W, van den Bent MJ, Koehler PJ, Heimans JJ, van der Sande JJ, Aaronson NK, et al. The relevance of intraventricular chemotherapy for leptomeningeal metastasis in breast cancer: a randomised study. Eur J Cancer. 2004;40(18):2726–33.

66. Shapiro WR, Schmid M, Glantz M, Miller JJ. A randomized phase III/IV study to determine benefit and safety of cytarabine liposome injection for treatment of neoplastic meningitis. J Clin Oncol. 2006;24(18_suppl):1528.

67. Morris PG, Reiner AS, Szenberg OR, Clarke JL, Panageas KS, Perez HR, et al. Leptomeningeal metastasis from non-small cell lung cancer: survival and the

impact of whole brain radiotherapy. J Thorac Oncol. 2012;7(2):382–5.

68. Gani C, Müller AC, Eckert F, Schroeder C, Bender B, Pantazis G, et al. Outcome after whole brain radiotherapy alone in intracranial leptomeningeal carcinomatosis from solid tumors. Strahlenther Onkol. 2012;188(2):148–53.

69. Souchon R, Feyer P, Thomssen C, Fehm T, Diel I, Nitz U, et al. Clinical recommendations of DEGRO and AGO on preferred standard palliative radiotherapy of bone and cerebral metastases, metastatic spinal cord compression, and leptomeningeal carcinomatosis in breast cancer. Breast Care (Basel). 2010;5(6):401–7.

70. Ozdemir Y, Yildirim BA, Topkan E. Whole brain radiotherapy in management of non-small-cell lung carcinoma associated leptomeningeal carcinomato-

sis: evaluation of prognostic factors. J Neurooncol. 2016;129(2):329–35.

71. Wolf A, Donahue B, Silverman JS, Chachoua A, Lee JK, Kondziolka D. Stereotactic radiosurgery for focal leptomeningeal disease in patients with brain metastases. J Neurooncol. 2017;134(1):139–43.

72. Yang JC-H, Cho BC, Kim D-W, Kim S-W, Lee J-S, Su W-C, et al. Osimertinib for patients (pts) with leptomeningeal metastases (LM) from EGFR-mutant non-small cell lung cancer (NSCLC): updated results from the BLOOM study. J Clin Oncol. 2017;35(15_suppl):2020.

73. Brastianos PK, Prakadan S, Alvarez-Breckenridge C, Lee EQ, Tolaney SM, Nayak L, et al. Phase II study of pembrolizumab in leptomeningeal carcinomatosis. J Clin Oncol. 2018;36(15_suppl):2007.

Salvage/Reirradiation/ Retreatment

David Roberge

Case Vignettes

Case 1

A 67-year-old presents with a new diagnosis of lung adenocarcinoma (without EGFR or ALK mutations). The final staging is T2N2M1 (AJCC 8th edition) with a single focus of extra-thoracic disease in the form of a small left parietal brain metastasis. His GPA score was 3.0 with an expected median overall survival (OS) of 26.5 months [1].

In July 2014 (Fig. 15.1a), the patient is treated with radiosurgery—21 Gy in a single fraction. Later in 2014, the patient receives concurrent chemoradiation for his intrathoracic disease.

In May 2015 (Fig. 15.1c, d), the patient is treated with radiosurgery for a new metastasis (previously noted as a millimetric anomaly on the FLAIR sequence of the previous MRI (Fig. 15.1b)). Two additional metastases are treated—one in December 2015 (Fig. 15.1e) and July 2016.

After initially responding, the left occipital lesion progresses in volume and is removed during a November 2016 craniotomy (Fig. 15.1f–h). The surgical specimen is compatible with viable

D. Roberge (✉)
Département de Radiologie, Radio-Oncologie et Médecine Nucléaire, Université de Montréal, Montreal, QC, Canada
e-mail: david.roberge.chum@ssss.gouv.qc.ca

adenocarcinoma and the patient is treated with adjuvant radiosurgery to the tumor bed (Fig. 15.1h).

The patient has a pachymeningeal recurrence which is not controlled by subsequent radiosurgery and WBRT (Fig. 15.1i–k). The patient died in 2018, 44 months after his initial diagnosis, of uncontrolled intracranial metastases.

Case 2

A 54-year-old Asian man presents with in early 2018 with diffusely metastatic lung adenocarcinoma. His extracranial disease includes malignant pleural effusions and bone metastases. Despite only having a mild headache and no focal neurological symptoms, the patient had extensive intracranial metastases. More than ten metastases were seen, including three metastases of more than 20 mm and a brainstem lesion (Fig. 15.2a). A fluorescence in situ hybridization test using an ALK gene testing kit revealed a 2p23 ALK translocation. The patient had a performance status of 90% and a GPA of 3.0 with an expected median OS of 26.5 months.

The patient started alectinib. Both the intracranial and extracranial disease responded dramatically (Fig. 15.2b). After 8 months of treatment, a single right parietal metastasis grew rapidly from 6 to 16 mm (Fig. 15.2c). This single metastasis was treated with radiosurgery (single fraction

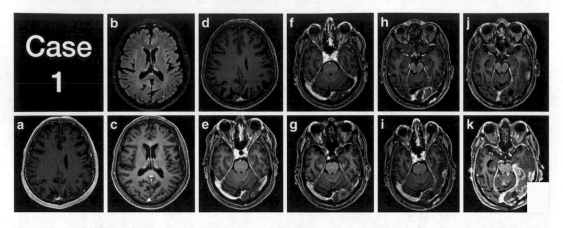

Fig. 15.1 Axial MRI images for Case 1. Initial metastasis (**a**) and subsequent metastases (**b–e**). Response (**f**), local (**g**) recurrence and surgical resection (**h**) of an occipital lesion. Subsequent pachymeningeal recurrence (**j, k**)

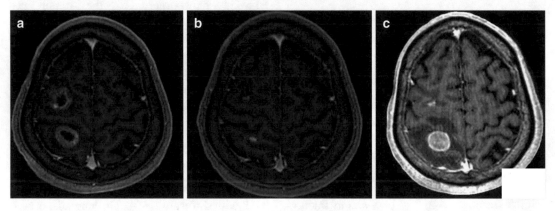

Fig. 15.2 (**a–c**) Axial MRI images for Case 2. Response to initial targeted therapy (**b**) and subsequent oligoprogression (**c**)

20 Gy) and the tyrosine kinase therapy was maintained. The patient remains alive and neurologically intact 9 months from his original diagnosis.

Case 3

A 68-year-old presents in the summer of 2016 with impaired gait. Imaging reveals a 31 mm left frontal metastasis with important vasogenic edema and a slight midline shift (Fig. 15.3a). Staging total body FDG PET scan identifies a metabolically active lesion in the left lung with associated FDG avid mediastinal lymph nodes. His GPA score is calculated to be 2.0 with an expected median OS of 13.7 months.

The patient has a performance status of no more than 70% and elects not to undergo craniotomy. He is treated with single fraction radiosurgery at a reduced dose of 15 Gy.

It was decided to address his extra-cranial disease with cytotoxic chemotherapy. The brain metastasis dramatically responded but after 1 year had nodular regrowth (Fig. 15.3b). In addition to regrowth of the original metastasis, there was the appearance of a new right parietal lesion (Fig. 15.3c). The previously treated lesion had a T2/T1 ratio greater than 0.6. One year after the initial radiosurgery, the patient was treated with repeat single fraction radiosurgery to the initial lesion (15 Gy) and radiosurgery to the new metastasis (21 Gy).

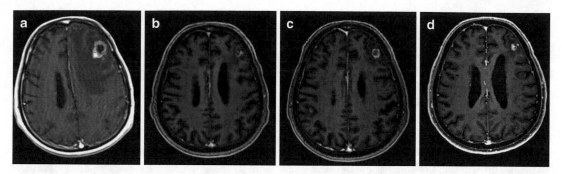

Fig. 15.3 (**a–d**) Axial MRI images for Case 3. Response to initial (**b**) and repeat (**d**) radiosurgery

The patient has since switched from chemotherapy to a single agent checkpoint inhibitor and remains well with controlled intra and extracranial disease 29 months since his initial diagnosis (Fig. 15.3d).

Introduction

The treatment of recurrent brain metastases is more prevalent and more complex than ever. Contributing to this trend are the improving survival of patients with brain metastases, the decreasing use of WBRT, and the discovery of new targets for systemic therapy.

The most common primary cancer associated with brain metastases remains non-small-cell lung (NSCLC). Non-small-cell lung cancer exemplifies the increase in survival from the diagnosis of metastatic brain disease—overall survival having improved from a median of 7 months to a median of 12 months over the past two decades [1]. This patient population also illustrates the decreasing use of WBRT—from approximately 40% to approximately 20% over the same period [2]. Both factors combined explain the substantial increase in episodes of care related to brain metastases.

Not only are more treatments being delivered for brain metastases, but the clinical scenarios are changing. For example, the use of radiosurgery as an adjuvant to surgical resection has resulted in an apparent increase in pachymeningeal recurrences [3]. The molecular landscape is also becoming more complex—just as physicians familiarize themselves with the favorable prognosis and unique therapeutic options for ALK or EGFR-mutated NSCLC cancers, findings of ROS1 and BRAF mutations are defining new subgroups of patients amenable to targeted therapies.

There is little high-level evidence to guide treatment in these various presentations of recurrent disease—many of the treatment decisions are informed by data from the up-front setting. Within such a heterogenous and changing patient population, widely applicable randomized trials are not forthcoming.

Evidence Base

Diagnosis of Recurrence

Recurrent brain metastases will occur in the form of new parenchymal metastases, pachymeningeal disease, growth/recurrence of a treated lesion or leptomeningeal seeding. The recurrences will often be asymptomatic lesions discovered on imaging. Symptoms of recurrence will be more likely for meningeal failures and progression of larger previously treated metastases.

Recurrent brain metastases are a common occurrence. In a patient previously treated with radiosurgery, the rate of distant brain failure will be approximately 50% at 1 year [4]. Of patients with larger metastases treated with a single radiosurgery dose of 15 Gy, approximately half will fail locally [5]. The local failure rate will be similar following resection and tumor bed radiosurgery [6]. In many patients, these risks will combine to further reduce the initial intracranial control rate.

The speed at which metastases grow is variable but may be correlated with histology. The average growth velocity is typically higher in melanoma. For the most common diagnosis, NSCLC, the median doubling time is approximately 2 months [7].

One can consider the risk of failure and the expected growth rate in choosing the frequency of MRI imaging but in practice most patients will initially be followed with a standard imaging schedule—a contrast MRI every 2–3 months. The frequency of the follow-up will then typically decrease as the progression-free interval increases.

The imaging diagnosis of a new metastasis will most often be straightforward and not require a confirmatory test beyond a contrast-enhanced MRI. The diagnosis of progression of a metastasis previously treated with radiosurgery will be more complex. In this case, the differential diagnosis will often include radiation necrosis. Beyond resection of the imaging abnormality, there is no perfect test to differentiate necrosis from progression. Individual institutions have developed expertise in various advanced diagnostic modalities, whether SPECT, PET, MR spectroscopy, MR perfusion imaging or delayed contrast extravasation imaging (TRAM) [8–10]. In those centers without a specific expertise, the simple ratio of the T2 nodule to the T1 contrast area is often a helpful addition to qualitative appreciation of the images and clinical acumen. A low ratio (<0.3) will be suggestive of radiation necrosis [11]. In general practice, a minority of patients will undergo craniotomy and most patients will be managed with a combination of patience and clinical judgment with therapy oriented to the most probable diagnosis.

Beyond cranial imaging and an occasional CSF sampling or spinal MRI for suspected leptomeningeal disease, it will be important to update the extracranial staging of the patient and clarify if the cancer presents any actionable mutations. In many cases, a mutational work-up may not have been performed at the time of primary diagnosis or the mutational landscape may have since changed. In some cases, the initial diagnostic

specimen may be insufficient for further genetic testing or the patient may have had therapy known to select for new mutations. A brain biopsy will almost never be indicated for the sole purpose of profiling the tumor but a new biopsy or serum analysis may be indicated. This was seen with regard to the T790M EGFR mutation which could be detected in the serum with high specificity—a test of decreasing utility as osimertinib is now commonly prescribed to patients without this specific exon 20 mutation [12].

Treatment of New Metastases

The second-line treatment of brain metastases has not been the specific subject of randomized trials. Small numbers of cases with brain recurrences were included in selected drug trials and trials looking to reduce the toxicity of WBRT [13, 14]. These trials offer no specific guidance as to the best treatment modality or sequence of treatment in patients with recurrence.

For those patients not having been treated with up-front WBRT, the treatment paradigm is informed by the results of trials in the up-front setting. Patients with a small number of small metastases are treated with radiosurgery and those patients with more extensive disease are more likely to receive salvage whole-brain radiotherapy. This approach is supported by retrospective series and the patient outcomes are in keeping with those seen after initial treatment of brain metastases. Beyond the simple number of brain metastases, other patient and disease factors enter into the decision to choose radiosurgery or WBRT. Total tumor volume or the velocity at which new metastases are appearing may be more informative than a simple count of the number of new lesions [15, 16].

In those patients having previously been treated with WBRT, there will be a tolerance to treating a larger number of metastases with salvage radiosurgery. It is interesting to note that the initial safety data for single fraction radiosurgery of metastases and the RTOG dosing guidelines (15 Gy for lesions 31–40 mm, 18 Gy for lesions 21–30 mm and 24 Gy for lesions 1–20 mm) are derived from a phase I trial in which all patients had received prior radiation (either WBRT or conformal radiotherapy) [17]. Thus, although the rate of toxicity will be slightly higher in patients with prior WBRT, there is no need to reduce the dose of salvage radiosurgery. When a radiosurgical treatment is felt to be unreasonable, repeated WBRT has been shown to be safe in retrospective series. A repeat course of WBRT has generally been prescribed to a lower total dose and with a lower dose per fraction—20 Gy in ten fractions would be typical [18]. Although hippocampal-sparing and memantine use have not been studied in patients treated with two courses of WBRT, it will be reasonable to employ these strategies when possible. Modern volumetric intensity modulated radiotherapy also makes it possible to differentially increase the dose to macroscopic tumor—a reasonable strategy when a low total dose of 20 Gy in ten fractions is used [19].

As with parenchymal brain metastases, the treatment of leptomeningeal recurrences will be similar in the recurrent setting as it is in the upfront setting. In this situation, the available evidence base is even weaker than for parenchymal brain metastases. On a case-by-case basis, varied treatment options will be considered as monotherapy or in combination:

- Radiosurgery
- Local radiotherapy to symptomatic sites
- Whole-brain radiotherapy
- Intrathecal or intraventricular therapy
- Systemic therapy
- Supportive care

The treatment of tumor bed recurrences is challenging. Early retrospective data is emerging to support consideration of focal treatment to pachymeningeal recurrences as an alternative to WBRT [3]. This remains an area where even retrospective data is scant.

Diagnosis and Management

A reasonable treatment algorithm is presented in Fig. 15.4. The algorithm presented reflects the complexity of the varied scenarios of recurrent disease. Because of this complexity and the

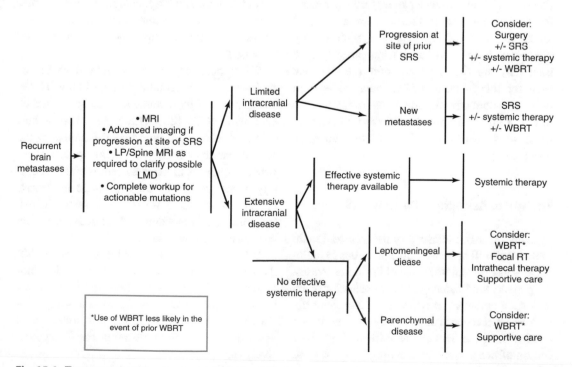

Fig. 15.4 Treatment algorithm for recurrent brain metastases

lack of high-level data, the recommendations contain much leeway for clinical judgment. In summary, limited new metastases (whether in number, velocity or total volume) should typically be addressed with SRS and more extensive disease addressed with systemic therapy when an effective agent is available and WBRT (or supportive care) when such an agent is not available.

The other available treatment modalities will find niche indications. A craniotomy may be indicated for a symptomatic progressive tumor in a patient with otherwise controlled disease. Intrathecal trastuzumab (Herceptin) may be reasonable in a patient with HER-2 positive leptomeningeal disease [20]. Focal palliative radiation may be used to alleviate a cranial nerve palsy and a patient with extensive posterior fossa disease despite prior WBRT may be well served by partial brain reirradiation [21].

The proposed algorithm, as well as current guidelines addressed in the "Guidelines" section of this chapter, do not address the situations of oligo-persistence or oligo-recurrence of intracranial disease. What should one do in a case such as that of our Case 2 when a patient initially treated for diffuse metastatic disease with a tyrosine kinase inhibitor subsequently progresses at only one site of disease? Although it appears logical to treat only the site of progression, the evidence base for this is lacking. The situation is even more uncertain when a patient has complete resolution of all but a limited number of metastases. In those situations, may it be more prudent to observe?

Technical Aspects of Repeat SRS

In many regards, radiosurgery for recurrent brain metastases will be technically analogous to radiosurgery as up-front treatment of brain metastases. As patients are treated over many years for many lesions, an element of risk will be unnecessarily re-treating a metastasis or leaving a new lesion untreated. These risks can be mitigated by registration of every previous planning image set and

transferring the previous target volumes to the current image set. Every visible metastasis should thus be segmented either as a current GTV or a prior target volume.

When applying radiosurgery to a lesion for a second time, there are no standard dosing guidelines. Depending on many factors, including the time since the original treatment and the use of prior WBRT, doses may be similar or slightly lower than those used for unirradiated tumors. At retreatment, single fraction radiosurgery is a reasonable choice for most small lesions. Although it remains to be demonstrated whether fractionation improves the therapeutic ratio, it will frequently be used for the larger target volumes [22].

Technical Aspects of Salvage WBRT

Whether or not a patient has received prior WBRT, hippocampal avoidance should be considered when using salvage WBRT. Little is known of the benefits or partial hippocampal avoidance, but it is probable that unilateral sparing of the dominant hippocampus is useful. Other normal structures segmented include: eyes, lenses, optic chiasm, optic nerves, and middle/inner ears.

When possible, the maximum dose to the avoidance volume should be kept below 16 Gy and as much of the volume as possible should be kept below 9 Gy [23]. These plans will be best delivered with volumetric IMRT. Contouring the optic apparatus will help avoid hot spots in these structures. Doses to the eyes, lenses and the auditory apparatus will be minimized. In healthcare systems where most WBRT is delivered in five fractions, the hippocampal dose constraints can be scaled down by a third.

When delivering a second course of WBRT, the total dose will typically be reduced—commonly to 20 Gy in ten fractions. In these cases, a boost volume to the visible metastases plus a margin can be created (30 Gy is a conservative boost dose) and the hippocampi can be aggressively spared.

Areas of Uncertainty

Many areas of uncertainty remain in the management of brain metastases. A dilemma which is common to many primary tumor histologies is the appropriate indication for WBRT (vs. repeated SRS). Should WBRT use be based on the number of new metastases, the velocity at which they appear, the total volume of the lesions, the performance status of the patient? These decisions are made more complex as the cognitive toxicity of WBRT is reduced through hippocampal avoidance and the use of prophylactic memantine [13, 24]. Although prospective evidence is lacking, WBRT is more commonly considered when new metastases appear at a rate of greater than one per month.

In cancer types for which new systemic agents are showing greater activity against brain metastasis, an evolving dilemma is the relative roles of repeated radiation treatments vs. a trial of systemic therapy (Table 15.1). The cancers in which this is the most topical are: HER-2 positive breast cancer, ALK/EGFR/ROS1 mutated NSCLC, melanoma amenable to immunotherapy and the growing range of BRAF mutated cancers. A widely referenced retrospective series has suggested that better outcomes are achieved when systemic agents are added to radiation rather than used in lieu of radiation [25]. In addition to being subject to the usual biases of retrospective series, this finding does not address issues of timing,

quality of life or the relevance to newer, more active, agents.

Future Directions

The volume of patients requiring salvage treatment for brain metastases is increasing with the improving prognosis of patients with advanced cancer. The relative role of radiosurgery and WBRT is being defined in most clinical scenarios of up-front brain metastases—whether in patients with more than five metastases or having undergone surgical resection [6, 24]. As fewer patients receive WBRT at diagnosis, it will become feasible to conduct trials of WBRT in the recurrent setting.

As previously noted, for many patients with either targetable mutations or diseases amenable to immune checkpoint inhibitors, there is an increasing role for systemic therapy of brain metastases. A necessary area of investigation is in demonstrating an incremental benefit to adding upfront radiation to an active systemic regimen and optimizing the combination. In those patients treated with immune checkpoint inhibitors, the sequencing of the treatments may matter. The oft described, infrequently observed abscopal effect may be more often observed when radiation is fractionated and inserted within a course of immunotherapy. Although current evidence suggests that most systemic therapies appear safe

Table 15.1 Examples of potential systemic treatments for recurrent brain metastases

Cancer	Agents	Radiological response rate	Response duration (months)
HER-2 positive breast cancer	Neratinib + Capecitabine	49% [31]	5.5
ALK-mutated NSCLC	Crizotinib, Ceritinib, Alectinib, Brigatinib	44% (95% CI 33–55%) [32]	14.6 (range 8–22)
EGFR-mutated NSCLC	Osimertinib	91% [14]	Not reached (12.4 months median f/u)
Melanoma	Nivolumab + Ipilimumab	55% [33]	Not reached (14 months median f/u)
BRAF-mutated melanoma	Dabrafenib + trametinib	43% [34]	5.8
BRAF-mutated NSCLC	Dabrafenib	33% [35]	5.5

when delivered with SRS, the potential added toxicity of varied combinations of systemic agents and radiosurgery will need to be addressed continuously as more patients are treated with newer agents [26].

Up until now treatment of brain metastases has focused on surgery, radiation and, increasingly, systemic agents. New physical treatment modalities—notably in the form of alternating electric field (so-called tumor treating fields) may disrupt these paradigms. Tumor treating fields (TTF) as an antimitotic therapy have demonstrated clinical activity in primary CNS cancer. A Phase 3 trial of adjuvant TTF is currently accruing for non-small-cell lung cancer with newly diagnosed brain metastases amenable to radiosurgery. Should this trial be positive, it is likely that the adoption of this treatment will be limited in the upfront setting and TTF may thus find a place in the management of recurrent brain metastases from lung cancer.

Guidelines

As previously emphasized, patients with brain metastases represent a heterogeneous patient population. This makes it difficult to describe the nuances of clinical decision making within guidelines. The problem is compounded when prior treatment is introduced as a variable. Whereas some guidelines avoid addressing recurrent disease altogether, the following are summaries of guidelines where recurrent intracranial metastases are addressed.

NCCN (National Comprehensive Cancer Network)

The 2019 NCCN guidelines (https://www.nccn. org/professionals/physician_gls/pdf/cns.pdf) provide general guidance for recurrences after treatment of limited or extensive brain metastases.

For those patients with local recurrence at the site of a treated brain metastases, local treatment can once again be considered (surgery, single fraction or fractionated radiosurgery). For more voluminous recurrences, WBRT can be considered if not previously used.

For distant brain recurrences, WBRT (if not previously administered), surgery and focal radiation can be considered based on the number and size of the brain metastases.

For patients initially treated for more extensive brain metastases, the options are similar with supportive care preferred in those patients with progressive extracranial disease for which no systemic treatment is available.

In each case, systemic therapy can be considered. The list of potential agents is more extensive in the recurrent setting and focuses mainly on lung cancer, breast cancer, and melanoma. Although some more traditional cytotoxic agents can be considered (such as topotecan for small-cell cancer), most options are targeted agents or immunotherapy. Newer drugs offer improvements in CNS response, whether it be capecitabine/neratinib or osimertinib.

AANS (American Association of Neurological Surgeons) [27]

The AANS guidelines were published in 2009 and reflect a lack of high-quality evidence, which persists 10 years later: "Since there is insufficient evidence to make definitive treatment recommendations in patients with recurrent/ progressive brain metastases, treatment should be individualized based on a patient's functional status, extent of disease, volume/number of metastases, recurrence or progression at original versus nonoriginal site, previous treatment and type of primary cancer, and enrollment in clinical trials is encouraged. In this context, the following can be recommended depending on a patient's specific condition: no further treatment (supportive care), reirradiation (either WBRT and/or SRS), surgical excision or, to a lesser extent, chemotherapy."

ASCO (American Society of Clinical Oncology) [28]

In 2018, the ASCO updated guidelines for the management of patients with HER-2 positive breast cancer and brain metastases. The recommendations for patients with progressive intracranial disease despite initial radiation therapy are general and include consideration of SRS, surgery, WBRT or systemic therapy. For patients who have diffuse recurrence, best supportive care is also listed as an option.

EANO (European Association of Neuro-Oncology)

The 2017 EANO guidelines include specific recommendations for the management of recurrent brain metastasis and the use of systemic therapy [29]. Recognized is the role surgery can perform in differentiating between radiation necrosis and tumor progression as well as its potential role in the salvage of limited disease in selected patients (younger age, high performance status, controlled systemic disease) with tumors in accessible locations. The potential for SRS after prior SRS or WBRT is mentioned.

With regard to medical therapy, the following recommendations are included:

- Conventional chemotherapy may be the initial treatment for patients with brain metastases from chemosensitive tumors, like SCLC or breast cancer, especially when small and/or asymptomatic.
- No targeted agents are currently registered for the treatment of brain metastases from any solid tumors.
- Patients with brain metastases from NSCLC harboring activating EGFR mutations or ALK rearrangements can derive benefit from the use of specific TKIs.
- Continuous HER2 blockade should be offered to patients with CNS metastases of HER2 positive breast cancer.
- Patients with brain metastases from HER2 positive breast cancer can derive benefit from the use of lapatinib, alone or associated with capecitabine.

- Patients with melanoma and brain metastases can derive benefit from targeted agents either ipilimumab or BRAF inhibitors.
- Patients with renal cell carcinoma and brain metastases can derive benefit from multitarget TKIs, in particular sunitinib.
- Pausing of treatment with novel systemic agents during radiotherapy to the brain should be considered to minimize the risk of unexpected toxicities.

As an editorial point, the reported objective response rate of intracranial metastases from primary renal cell carcinoma was 0% (out of 16 evaluable patients) in the only prospective trial of sunitinib in this patient population [30].

Conclusions and Recommendations

In conclusion, the treatment or recurrent brain metastases is complex. There is often more than one reasonable treatment option.

The most important overall recommendations are to recognize that many patients will have extended survival, to involve patients in treatment decisions and to stay up to date with advances in systemic therapy as well as available clinical trials. If the critical mass of physicians is available, a multidisciplinary brain metastasis tumor board will be an ideal forum to discuss and debate management issues.

References

1. Sperduto PW, Yang TJ, Beal K, Pan H, Brown PD, Bangdiwala A, et al. Estimating survival in patients with lung cancer and brain metastases: an update of the graded prognostic assessment for lung cancer using molecular markers (Lung-molGPA). JAMA Oncol. 2017;3(6):827–31.
2. Sperduto PW, Yang TJ, Beal K, Pan H, Brown PD, Bangdiwala A, et al. The effect of gene alterations and tyrosine kinase inhibition on survival and cause of death in patients with adenocarcinoma of the lung and brain metastases. Int J Radiat Oncol Biol Phys. 2016;96(2):406–13.
3. Prabhu RS, Soltys SG, Turner BE, Marcrom S, Fiveash JB, Foreman PM, et al. Timing, presentation, and patterns of failure of leptomeningeal disease

after surgical resection and radiosurgery for brain metastases: a multi-institutional analysis. J Clin Oncol. 2018;36(15_suppl):2070.

4. Prabhu RS, Press RH, Boselli DM, Miller KR, Lankford SP, McCammon RJ, et al. External validity of two nomograms for predicting distant brain failure after radiosurgery for brain metastases in a bi-institutional independent patient cohort. J Neurooncol. 2018;137(1):147–54.

5. de Azevedo Santos TR, Tundisi CF, Ramos H, Maia MA, Pellizzon AC, Silva ML, et al. Local control after radiosurgery for brain metastases: predictive factors and implications for clinical decision. Radiat Oncol. 2015;10:63.

6. Roberge D, Brown P. SRS versus WBRT for resected brain metastases – Authors' reply. Lancet Oncol. 2017;18(10):e560.

7. Yoo H, Nam BH, Yang HS, Shin SH, Lee JS, Lee SH. Growth rates of metastatic brain tumors in nonsmall cell lung cancer. Cancer. 2008;113(5):1043–7.

8. Lohmann P, Kocher M, Ceccon G, Bauer EK, Stoffels G, Viswanathan S, et al. Combined FET PET/MRI radiomics differentiates radiation injury from recurrent brain metastasis. Neuroimage Clin. 2018;20:537–42.

9. Zach L, Guez D, Last D, Daniels D, Grober Y, Nissim O, et al. Delayed contrast extravasation MRI: a new paradigm in neuro-oncology. Neuro Oncol. 2015;17(3):457–65.

10. Chuang MT, Liu YS, Tsai YS, Chen YC, Wang CK. Differentiating radiation-induced necrosis from recurrent brain tumor using MR perfusion and spectroscopy: a meta-analysis. PLoS One. 2016;11(1):e0141438.

11. Dequesada IM, Quisling RG, Yachnis A, Friedman WA. Can standard magnetic resonance imaging reliably distinguish recurrent tumor from radiation necrosis after radiosurgery for brain metastases? A radiographic-pathological study. Neurosurgery. 2008;63(5):898–903; discussion 4.

12. Sim WC, Loh CH, Toh GL, Lim CW, Chopra A, Chang AYC, et al. Non-invasive detection of actionable mutations in advanced non-small-cell lung cancer using targeted sequencing of circulating tumor DNA. Lung Cancer. 2018;124:154–9.

13. Brown PD, Pugh S, Laack NN, Wefel JS, Khuntia D, Meyers C, et al. Memantine for the prevention of cognitive dysfunction in patients receiving whole-brain radiotherapy: a randomized, double-blind, placebo-controlled trial. Neuro Oncol. 2013;15(10):1429–37.

14. Reungwetwattana T, Nakagawa K, Cho BC, Cobo M, Cho EK, Bertolini A, et al. CNS response to osimertinib versus standard epidermal growth factor receptor tyrosine kinase inhibitors in patients with untreated EGFR-mutated advanced non-small-cell lung cancer. J Clin Oncol. 2018:JCO2018783118. https://doi.org/10.1200/JCO.2018.78.3118.

15. Farris M, McTyre ER, Cramer CK, Hughes R, Randolph DM 2nd, Ayala-Peacock DN, et al. Brain metastasis velocity: a novel prognostic metric predictive of overall survival and freedom from whole-brain radiation therapy after distant brain failure following upfront radiosurgery alone. Int J Radiat Oncol Biol Phys. 2017;98(1):131–41.

16. Hirshman BR, Wilson B, Ali MA, Proudfoot JA, Koiso T, Nagano O, et al. Superior prognostic value of cumulative intracranial tumor volume relative to largest intracranial tumor volume for stereotactic radiosurgery-treated brain metastasis patients. Neurosurgery. 2018;82(4):473–80.

17. Shaw E, Scott C, Souhami L, Dinapoli R, Bahary JP, Kline R, et al. Radiosurgery for the treatment of previously irradiated recurrent primary brain tumors and brain metastases: initial report of radiation therapy oncology group protocol (90-05). Int J Radiat Oncol Biol Phys. 1996;34(3):647–54.

18. Guo S, Balagamwala EH, Reddy C, Elson P, Suh JH, Chao ST. Clinical and radiographic outcomes from repeat whole-brain radiation therapy for brain metastases in the age of stereotactic radiosurgery. Am J Clin Oncol. 2016;39(3):288–93.

19. Hsu F, Carolan H, Nichol A, Cao F, Nuraney N, Lee R, et al. Whole brain radiotherapy with hippocampal avoidance and simultaneous integrated boost for 1–3 brain metastases: a feasibility study using volumetric modulated arc therapy. Int J Radiat Oncol Biol Phys. 2010;76(5):1480–5.

20. Ferrario C, Davidson A, Bouganim N, Aloyz R, Panasci LC. Intrathecal trastuzumab and thiotepa for leptomeningeal spread of breast cancer. Ann Oncol. 2009;20(4):792–5.

21. Choi JH. Outcomes following re-irradiation for symptomatic brain metastasis. J Cancer Sci Ther. 2015;7(10):308–11.

22. Rana N, Pendyala P, Cleary RK, Luo G, Zhao Z, Chambless LB, et al. Long-term outcomes after salvage stereotactic radiosurgery (SRS) following in-field failure of initial SRS for brain metastases. Front Oncol. 2017;7:279.

23. Gondi V, Pugh SL, Tome WA, Caine C, Corn B, Kanner A, et al. Preservation of memory with conformal avoidance of the hippocampal neural stem-cell compartment during whole-brain radiotherapy for brain metastases (RTOG 0933): a phase II multi-institutional trial. J Clin Oncol. 2014;32(34):3810–6.

24. Roberge D, Brown PD, Whitton A, O'Callaghan C, Leis A, Greenspoon J, et al. The future is now-prospective study of radiosurgery for more than 4 brain metastases to start in 2018! Front Oncol. 2018;8:380.

25. Magnuson WJ, Lester-Coll NH, Wu AJ, Yang TJ, Lockney NA, Gerber NK, et al. Management of brain metastases in tyrosine kinase inhibitor-naive epidermal growth factor receptor-mutant non-small-cell lung cancer: a retrospective multi-institutional analysis. J Clin Oncol. 2017;35(10):1070–7.

26. Kim JM, Miller JA, Kotecha R, Xiao R, Juloori A, Ward MC, et al. The risk of radiation necrosis following stereotactic radiosurgery with concurrent systemic therapies. J Neurooncol. 2017;133(2):357–68.

27. Robinson PD, Kalkanis SN, Linskey ME, Santaguida PL. Methodology used to develop the AANS/CNS management of brain metastases evidence-based clinical practice parameter guidelines. J Neurooncol. 2010;96(1):11–6.

28. Ramakrishna N, Temin S, Chandarlapaty S, Crews JR, Davidson NE, Esteva FJ, et al. Recommendations on disease management for patients with advanced human epidermal growth factor receptor 2-positive breast cancer and brain metastases: ASCO clinical practice guideline update. J Clin Oncol. 2018;36(27):2804–7.

29. Soffietti R, Abacioglu U, Baumert B, Combs SE, Kinhult S, Kros JM, et al. Diagnosis and treatment of brain metastases from solid tumors: guidelines from the European Association of Neuro-Oncology (EANO). Neuro Oncol. 2017;19(2):162–74.

30. Chevreau C, Ravaud A, Escudier B, Amela E, Delva R, Rolland F, et al. A phase II trial of sunitinib in patients with renal cell cancer and untreated brain metastases. Clin Genitourin Cancer. 2014;12(1):50–4.

31. Freedman RA, Gelman RS, Melisko ME, Anders CK, Moy B, Blackwell KL, et al. TBCRC 022: phase II trial of neratinib + capecitabine for patients (Pts) with human epidermal growth factor receptor 2 (HER2+) breast cancer brain metastases (BCBM). J Clin Oncol. 2017;35(15_suppl):1005.

32. Petrelli F, Lazzari C, Ardito R, Borgonovo K, Bulotta A, Conti B, et al. Efficacy of ALK inhibitors on NSCLC brain metastases: a systematic review and pooled analysis of 21 studies. PLoS One. 2018;13(7):e0201425.

33. Tawbi HA, Forsyth PA, Algazi A, Hamid O, Hodi FS, Moschos SJ, et al. Combined nivolumab and ipilimumab in melanoma metastatic to the brain. N Engl J Med. 2018;379(8):722–30.

34. Geukes Foppen MH, Boogerd W, Blank CU, van Thienen JV, Haanen JB, Brandsma D. Clinical and radiological response of BRAF inhibition and MEK inhibition in patients with brain metastases from BRAF-mutated melanoma. Melanoma Res. 2018;28(2):126–33.

35. Planchard D, Kim TM, Mazieres J, Quoix E, Riely G, Barlesi F, et al. Dabrafenib in patients with BRAF(V600E)-positive advanced non-small-cell lung cancer: a single-arm, multicentre, open-label, phase 2 trial. Lancet Oncol. 2016;17(5):642–50.

Part II

Technical: Treatment Planning and Delivery

General Techniques for Radiosurgery

Mark Ruschin, Arjun Sahgal, Lijun Ma, Lei Wang, Ermias Gete, and Alan Nichol

Case Vignette

A lung cancer patient with no prior brain radiation and good performance status presents with 17 brain metastases ranging in diameter from 3 mm up to 1.8 cm (Fig. 16.1). The decision is made to treat the patient using stereotactic radiosurgery (SRS). Is there an optimal technology for SRS to use for treating the patient?

When deciding what technology to use for multiple brain metastases SRS, the factors to consider range from technical/dosimetric issues to administrative/financial ones. From a dosimetric perspective, the ability to tightly conform the dose to the target and minimize the dose to normal tissue is of high concern. The dosimetric

interplay between targets for a given technology and planning system dictates how tightly the dose is contained around each target. However, in addition to plan quality, the dosimetric and mechanical accuracy of the treatment delivery is paramount to its success. Knowledge of the quality assurance (QA) recommendations and guidelines and how they apply to multiple metastases is essential.

This chapter summarizes the major types of SRS technology, including a technical description of each, a review of current evidence as to

M. Ruschin (✉) · A. Sahgal
Department of Radiation Oncology, Sunnybrook Health Sciences Centre, Odette Cancer Centre, University of Toronto, Toronto, ON, Canada
e-mail: Mark.Ruschin@sunnybrook.ca

L. Ma
Department of Radiation Oncology, University of California San Francisco, San Francisco, CA, USA

L. Wang
Department of Radiation Oncology, Stanford University, Palo Alto, CA, USA

E. Gete
Medical Physics, BC Cancer, Vancouver Centre, Vancouver, BC, Canada

A. Nichol
Department of Radiation Oncology, BC Cancer, Vancouver, BC, Canada

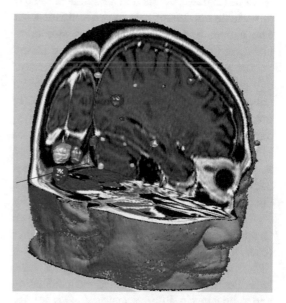

Fig. 16.1 3D rendering of a patient with 17 brain metastases

© Springer Nature Switzerland AG 2020
Y. Yamada et al. (eds.), *Radiotherapy in Managing Brain Metastases*,
https://doi.org/10.1007/978-3-030-43740-4_16

the dosimetric advantages and disadvantages of each for treating multiple metastases, and an overview of the guidelines and recommendations for best practices and QA.

Technical Overview of Major Technologies

The three major categories of state-of-the-art SRS treatment apparatus consist of (i) Gamma Knife (GK, Elekta AB, Stockholm, Sweden); (ii) robotic multi-leaf collimator (MLC)-based X-band CyberKnife (CK, Accuray, Sunnyvale, US) system, and (iii) high-definition (HD) MLC-based S-band linear accelerator (linac) systems.

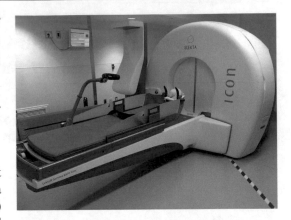

Fig. 16.2 Gamma Knife Icon system at the Sunnybrook Odette Cancer Center. The unit is equipped with a retractable 90 kV CBCT unit mapped in submillimeter stereotactic coordinates for treatment setups. Shown is the retracted position of the CBCT arm

The Gamma Knife (GK) SRS System

In 2006, GK underwent a major redesign resulting in the GK Perfexion (PFX), which consisted of a larger treatable field-of-view, a stationary collimator cap, and robotically driven sources that align to the desired collimator setting [1]. Furthermore, the sources were divided into eight sections (called "sectors") that facilitated the use of variable collimator size for a given isocenter. The patient positioning system was also completely redesigned and became robotically driven.

The most recent development in GK technology occurred in 2015 with the integration of an onboard stereotactic cone-beam CT (CBCT) image-guidance system, resulting in a new system named the GK Icon (GKI), as shown in Fig. 16.2. This development has been realized primarily for delivering image-guided frameless SRS and hypofractionated (2–5 treatments with a dose per fraction of ≥5 Gy) GK treatments [2, 3].

Because Co-60 beamlets possess well-known energy spectra with two distinctive gamma rays (energies 1.17 MeV and 1.33 MeV), the output factors and beamlet profiles of GK SRS have been determined with Monte Carlo calculation and validated via different measurements [4]. By simply adjusting the prescription isodose level, small lesions of 1 mm in size have been routinely and precisely targeted via frame-based GK SRS,

including focal areas within the brain tissue for functional disorders such as trigeminal neuralgia and refractory tremor.

One of the workflow changes in the current system is the ability to preplan based on the diagnostic MRI. Once the patient is simulated in the frame, then the preplanning image is co-registered to the stereotactic planning CT or MRI and the treatment plan superimposed based on the stereotactic reference coordinates. The shots can then be adjusted to account for the actual patient position within the frame system, which may be rotated with respect to the pre-planning image set. The key to the success of such an approach, given that the couch can only translate but cannot rotate in 6 degrees of freedom (6 DOF) to compensate for rotations, is that the dose distribution of an individual shot is invariant to small translation offset or rotational errors due to the simultaneous exposure of 192 beams around the head focused at the isocenter. Thus, translational or rotational errors can accurately be corrected for via a simple mathematical transformation of shot locations. For the GKI, online adaptive patient-positioning detection and immediate 3D dose review are based on the GKI CBCT imaging studies with again real-time interactive replanning before a treatment delivery. GKI clinical data are forthcoming to define the accuracy of the stereotactic CBCT functionality in targeting small lesions and hypo-fractionation for larger lesions.

CyberKnife (CK)

CyberKnife (CK) is an X-band compact 6 MV linear accelerator mounted on a robotic arm [5–7]. The robotic arm is capable of moving with 6DOF following a predefined path that allows for both isocentric and non-isocentric treatments. At each position or node of the beam irradiation, the robotic arm can also tilt the linear accelerator to direct multiple beams toward a target. As a result, nodal-centric rather than isocentric beams are predominantly employed for CK treatments. This is helpful for treating multiple brain metastases where any lesion may be targeted from a given node on a path of robotic motion. Another distinct feature of robotic CK delivery is that any translation less than 1 cm, and/or rotations of 1–2 degrees, in the target positioning can be rapidly compensated by manipulating the robotic arm instead of realigning and repeating setting up of the patient [7, 8].

In terms of beam collimation, the original CK system was equipped with detachable physical cones ranging from 0.5 cm to 6 cm in diameter. In order to facilitate rapid collimator switching, an Iris collimator system was introduced where the diameter of the cone may be adjusted automatically during the treatment delivery [9]. The Iris collimator possesses two banks of 12 tungsten–copper alloy segments to form a projected field of 12-sided polygon to mimic a circular cone. The polygon varies from 0.5 cm and 6 cm in maximum dimensions similar to the physical cones. To minimize uncertainties in the output factor determinations, the size of an Iris-collimator-defined field is generally limited to 7 mm or larger. By default, one robotic path is programmed for the Iris collimator due to its capability of varying beam apertures.

For the latest CK M6 model, an interchangeable multi-leaf collimator (MLC) system has become available. The MLC system consists of 26 MLC leaf pairs, and each leaf width is 3.85 mm specified at a source-to-axis distance of 80 cm, resulting in a maximum rectangle field size of 10 cm × 11.5 cm at a source-to-axis distance of 80 cm. The smallest MLC field is restricted to approximately 0.8 cm × 0.8 cm for the reason of maintaining dosimetric reliability similar to the Iris collimator. The intra-leaf MLC transmission is on the order of 0.5%, and each leaf is made from tungsten 9.0 cm thick. Most MLC-based CK treatments were designed for larger lesions with the goal of improving treatment delivery efficiency. The MLC system also enables conventionally fractionated CK treatments. Depending on the disease site and the treatment fractionation scheme (conventional, single- or hypofractionated treatments), current users have the flexibility of selecting physical cones, Iris collimator or MLC for a treatment. A robotic collimator changer has also been developed to minimize the downtime of collimator switching for a treatment (Fig. 16.3). In terms of online target localization, CK primarily relies on a pair of stereoscopic X-ray imaging to detect the target and align the radiation unit.

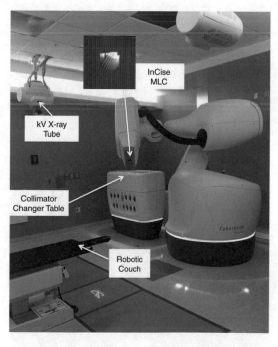

Fig. 16.3 The CyberKnife M6 model with the MLC attached to the gantry. The collimator changer table is shown next to the main unit. Two stereoscopic X-ray sources mounted on the ceiling are also shown

Linac

Linear accelerator radiosurgery started with treatment of a single metastasis per isocenter using cones and head frames. Initially, it was suitable only for oligometastatic disease, because the treatment times were intolerably long for many patients with more than three metastases. The technique became more efficient with the introduction of high-definition MLCs. Frameless SRS became feasible with improvements in imaging methods for setup verification and the introduction of couches capable of 6DOF setup correction. New linear accelerators with higher dose rates and flattening-filter free (FFF) modes have shortened the overall treatment times, making the treatment of more metastases feasible in a single visit for many patients. SRS delivered to a single metastasis per isocenter offers high accuracy and can be delivered with narrow margins because the isocenter is in the center of each metastasis and rotational setup variation has minimal effect on accurate dose delivery. The drawback of this approach of treating at one isocenter per metastasis is that the treatment duration scales with the number of metastases treated.

A new generation of digitally controlled linacs coupled with on-board image guidance, 6-DOF robotic couch, beam modulation with fast leaf-motion, FFF X-ray beams (Fig. 16.4), and advanced software for treatment planning allowing for volumetric modulated arc therapy (VMAT) has enabled rapid treatment of multiple

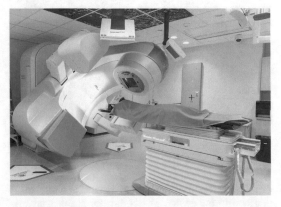

Fig. 16.4 Truebeam STX linear accelerator with ExacTRAC setup verification equipment

intracranial lesions simultaneously with a single isocenter.

The treatment duration increases as the amount of modulation and the number of monitor units increase for plans with numerous metastases, but the additional time required for patients with 15, as opposed to 3 metastases, is not substantially greater. Patient comfort and higher throughput are advantages of this short beam on time. An important issue for this planning technique is the high demand for setup accuracy. Even small rotational uncertainties are magnified as the distance between the isocenter and the metastasis increases. A rotational uncertainty of one degree can cause a translational uncertainty of 2 mm for brain metastases that are near the skull and distant from the isocenter [10]. When metastases are clustered, the isocenter can be placed within the cluster to minimize this effect. However, when metastases are widely distributed in the brain, and multiple couch positions are used to deliver the treatment, this issue must be managed with planning target volume (PTV) margins. The staff at each center must establish the optimal margins for their own process. One strategy to minimize the risk of radionecrosis is to use variable margins that increase in magnitude with increase in target distance from the isocenter [11].

In linac-based SRS, the high degree of dose conformality is typically achieved with non-coplanar arcs that employ either the dynamic conformal arc (DCA) or the volumetric-modulated arc therapy (VMAT) technique [12, 13]. The non-coplanar arcs delivered with VMAT and DCA use multiple couch positions and dynamic delivery in which the linac gantry and multileaf collimators (MLCs) move during treatment. In order to achieve the required dosimetric and spatial accuracy at all time during treatment, it is important that the linac's mechanical and dosimetric accuracy is maintained during dynamic deliveries and for all couch angle positions [14].

The introduction of Varian's TrueBeam (2010) along with the PerfectPitch (2013) has dramatically shifted the SRS paradigm, especially when it comes to the SRS treatment of multiple brain metastases [15]. TrueBeam is a new generation of linear accelerators whose advanced control system enables it to move all of its degrees of freedom of motion with high degree of accuracy while the beam is on [16]. When operated in FFF mode, TrueBeam can produce beams with dose rate of up to 24 Gy/min at the linac isocenter, reducing treatment time, while its high-definition multileaf collimator (HDMLC) can produce highly conformal dose distributions [17]. The linac's on-board imaging system and the PerfectPtich 6 DOF couch are fully integrated with the overall operation of the linac, allowing for a reliable and accurate patient positioning prior to treatment [18]. Elekta markets a similar design of linear accelerator called Versa HD for stereotactic applications [19].

Evidence Base

SRS treatment planning studies have shown that, despite substantial differences in delivery methods and planning strategies, PFX, linac, and CK have similar dose fall-off characteristics in single-target SRS. In terms of physical characteristics, PFX has a reported steep dose fall-off (penumbra) in the cranial-caudal direction: 1.6 mm (80–20%) for a 4 mm "shot." In other directions, modern modalities have reported similar penumbrae: 2.2 mm for CK for a 5-mm diameter field; 2.8 mm for PFX (axially); and 2.5–3 mm for narrow 6MV-linac MLC-defined fields. Translating these penumbrae into a composite plan is a complex issue involving overlapping shots (PFX) or beamlets (VMAT), in particular for multiple targets, as discussed below. In general, the literature supports all modalities as having somewhat equivalent dose fall-off for a single beam. Multiple studies have compared treatments of multiple brain metastases across modalities [20–26]. CK has been noted to compare favorably against conventional linac-based treatments. However, studies have noted that the peripheral normal brain dose was somewhat higher for the CK versus GK treatments [20, 22, 24, 27]. How such a difference would translate into potential discrepancy in the clinical outcome remains unclear. In practice, a user needs to examine peripheral dose surrounding individual lesions, as well as the dose to the whole brain, to ensure safe treatment.

In the absence of a definitive conclusion as to which system confers a dosimetric or clinical advantage, the focus should be on ensuring robust and accurate delivery, as treating multiple targets is a complex technique. Three relevant issues for SRS are (1) planning considerations, (2) small field dosimetry, and (3) targeting accuracy.

Treatment Planning Considerations

GammaKnife

Planning GKRS remains primarily a manual process, with the user placing isocenters (or "shots") in each individual target and selecting the appropriate collimator settings, weights, and prescription isodose level to obtain a conformal dose distribution. Larger targets often require multiple isocenters, but there is little time penalty involved in adding additional low-weight isocenters as the couch is accurately robotically driven to each isocenter. For multiple targets that are well spread out, there is almost no contribution of dose from one target to the next. For closer-spaced targets, the dose spread must be taken into account, which becomes challenging the closer the targets are to each other. In general, the dose distributions around each target are well separated due to rapid dose fall off with GK. Figure 16.5 shows the case from Fig. 16.1 with isodose lines shown on several slices.

As each target is treated sequentially, the total treatment time for multiple metastases can be long. One approach to reduce the time burden to the patient is to group metastases into smaller clusters and spread out how many days the treatment lasts. This is possible now with the Icon system and mask-based immobilization. For the case presented above, the treatment was divided into four days: Day1 (77 min) + Day2 (86 min) + Day3 (44 min) + Day4 (37 min) = 4 hours of treatment time over 4 days. A radiobiological advantage of this approach is that the normal tissue dose effectively receives a

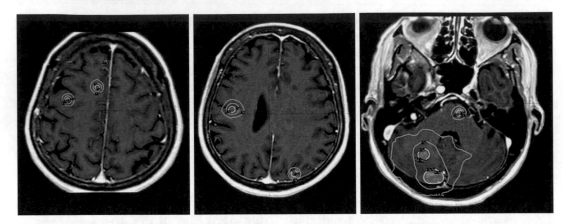

Fig. 16.5 Sample axial slices of the Gamma Knife treatment plan for case shown in Fig. 16.1. The yellow isodose line is the prescription dose (18 Gy in these cases except one lesion in the brainstem getting 15 Gy). The outer green isodose lines show 9 Gy and 4.5 Gy (i.e., 50% and 25%). As can be seen for the small (3–4 mm) targets, there is negligible dosimetric interplay between them. For adjacent larger targets (>2 cm) as on the far right, the 50% and 25% isodose lines can encompass both while sparing the smaller targets a few centimeters away

fractionated treatment while each target still receives the full SRS prescription. Another advantage of this approach is that combined hypofractionated and single-fraction targets can be accommodated [28]. It should be noted that this 17-target was particularly challenging involving both large and small targets in close proximity to each other, with varying prescription levels.

CyberKnife

Specific to the treatment of multiple brain metastases, lesion size generally dictates which type of collimator to use. If the size of the target is small (<1 cm), then the physical cones are typically used to sharpen the peripheral dose distributions. A recent study has shown that MLC-based treatments typically produce less conformal treatment plans versus fixed-cone-based treatments for small-sized lesions [29]. For lesions > = 1 cm in diameter, the Iris collimator or the MLC system is preferred for the sake of improving treatment delivery efficiency. If there is a mixture of small and large brain lesions, then fixed cones with up to 3 sizes are typically used instead to prevent swapping the collimator during treatment. A mixture of brain metastases of variable sizes also poses treatment planning challenges. If some of these targets are prescribed to the same dose, then they may be grouped together and planned as a composite target, adopting the same approach as a single-target treatment planning. However, if the targets are different in size, then the prescription dose levels may vary significantly across different targets. Inter-target dose interplay effect may also vary significantly as the number and sizes of these targets increase [8, 9].

Careful setting of dose-volume constraints is needed during treatment plan optimization. Normal tissue tuning structures such as concentric shell structures surrounding individual targets are often applied to improve dose conformity, as well as dose gradient surrounding the target. In addition, lowering the maximum contributing MU per node prevents excess dose being delivered along a limited number of directions, which results in more beams over a greater angular span.

When planning a high number of brain lesions (n > 5), a two-step approach has been reported to minimize the dose interplay effects among the targets [30]. In the first step, a user may group targets of similar size together and plan accordingly. In the second step, relative weightings between different groups of targets are iteratively optimized to produce a composite treatment plan.

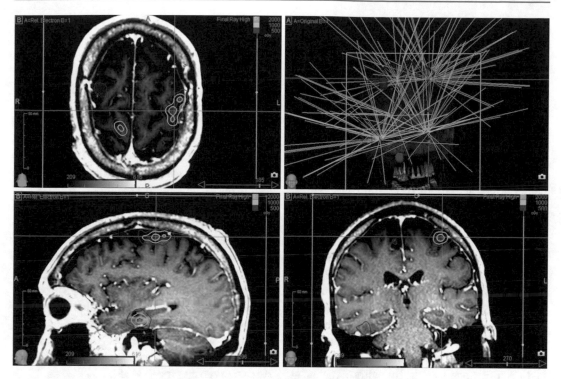

Fig. 16.6 Example of CK treatment of four metastatic brain lesions. For the case, 20 Gy was prescribed to 70% of the maximum dose for all the lesions. In addition, 10 Gy and 5 Gy isodose lines are also shown. Note the merging of low-level isodose lines when the targets are close with each other. A total of 178 beams with 7.5 mm cone were employed. The estimated treatment time for these four lesions was 59 min

It has been shown that the two-step approach enhances peripheral dose fall-off and improves normal brain sparing of the treatment [30]. The latest CK planning system Precision 1.1 has implemented the functionality of grouping and optimizing multiple brain metastases over several treatment sessions. An example case is shown in (Fig. 16.6), where four brain metastases of less than 1.0 cm are planned for treatment. The total treatment planning process for the case took approximately 1 hour, and total treatment time for the treatment was estimated to be 59 minutes.

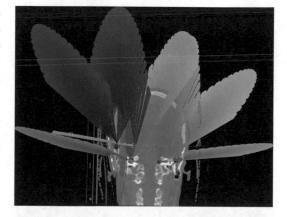

Fig. 16.7 Multi-isocenter, dynamic conformal arc plan for three brain metastases

Linac

There are two broad categories of planning and delivery SRS approaches using linacs: multiple isocenter versus single isocenter. Traditionally, multiple isocenters were used, with each target being positioned at the isocenter and treated sequentially much like in GK. For each isocenter/target, a series of 3–6 non-coplanar arcs were typically used to attain a conformal plan with a steep dose gradient (see Fig. 16.7).

Historically, stereotactic cones were used, with the diameter of cone selected to match the target. With the introduction of MLCs, centers began first investigating conformal arc techniques and then dynamic conformal arc techniques where the MLC aperture varies as a function of gantry angle to match the projected shape of the target.

More recently, however, there has been a substantial interest and uptake of a single isocenter approach to treating multiple targets, which is possible due to the MLCs. Initially, dynamic conformal off-axis apertures were investigated in which the shape of the MLC-defined field changes to match the shape of the target at all gantry angles. More recently, centers are using VMAT approaches in which the planning systems' inverse optimizer generates plans that involve modulated fields to attain conformal dose to the tumor and control normal tissue dose between tumors. The isocenter is thus positioned centrally within the head, and using a limited number of (often noncoplanar) arcs, a modulated VMAT plan can be optimized to treat all of the targets in as little a treatment time as possible, shown graphically in Fig. 16.8.

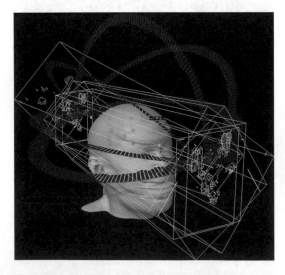

Fig. 16.8 Single-isocenter, volumetric-modulated arc therapy plan for nine brain metastases

Small Field Dosimetry

The dosimetry of small photon fields is challenging due to several factors including occlusion of the radiation source, lateral electronic disequilibrium, and perturbation of the photon field by the detector [31]. Doblado et al. showed in 2007 the importance of the choice of the detector in small field dosimetry [32]. They observed response differences for the various detectors for field sizes less than 3.0 cm, with deviations in excess of 50% for very small fields less than 10 mm when inappropriate detectors such as large volume ionization chambers are used. Consequently, accurate measurement of the standard dosimetric quantities required for the commissioning of an SRS treatment planning systems (TPS) requires extra attention to details and should only be performed by specialized physicists. In the past decade, a steady progress has been made in the development of detectors that are suitable for small field dosimetry [33–35].

Currently, AAPM Task Group 51 protocol [36] and its update [37], as well as the IAEA TRS-398 [38], form the basic formalism for clinical reference dosimetry. These protocols require reference conditions (10 cm × 10 cm field size, 100 cm source to axis or source to surface distance, etc.) and do not encompass such delivery units as CyberKnife, which cannot produce these. In such cases, the proposed remedy is to use a so-called machine-specific reference field (MSR field), which is an intermediate stationary field deliverable by the specific unit that most closely resembles the reference conditions [39]. The larger the differences between the MSR field and the reference field and reference conditions (i.e., calibration conditions of the detector), the larger the potential differences in the beam quality and variations in detector response. It is the qualified medical physicist's responsibility first to ensure use of appropriate reference-caliber detectors for the given MSR field and second to make sure to apply appropriate beam quality correction factors to account for differences between the MSR and the reference field/conditions.

The introduction of a comprehensive protocol [39, 40] for reference dosimetry of small fields has now made it possible to apply the necessary correction factors that account for factors such as detector's size and lack of charged particle equilibrium in a consistent manner. When the procedures outlined in the small field dosimetry protocol are followed, and with a careful choice of detectors, it is presently possible to measure basic dosimetric parameters of small fields with an accuracy of on the order of <2% for fields as small as 1 cm [39].

GammaKnife

GammaKnife perhaps poses the largest challenge for reference dosimetry. Since the calibration of each individual source is impractical and of limited use, an appropriate MSR field would be the largest diameter collimator helmet (e.g., 16 mm for GK Icon) with all sources in the beam-on position. Detector selection should be carefully considered balancing the need for a small-volume detector with sensitivity and accuracy.

CyberKnife

Besides machine-specific quality assurance (QA) tests such as the automatic quality assurance test to ensure submillimeter targeting accuracy, patient-specific QA tests involving multiple metastases treatments may be performed in a solid water phantom with embedded fiducials or in a head phantom. Point dose verification and two-dimensional isodose film measurements may be taken to match the dose distributions with those predicted in the treatment planning system. Independent treatment plan monitor unit (MU) calculation checks are recommended and can be performed via commercially available software (e.g., MUcheck, Oncology Data System, OK, USA) to verify the beam path and associated MU settings prior to the treatment delivery. For CyberKnife, the 60-mm diameter fixed collimator (80 cm from the source) provides a relatively flat and uniform field that normally is recommended as the MSR field.

Linac

The VMAT-based single isocenter technique for the treatment of multiple metastases presents its own unique challenges. In addition to the basic dosimetric quantities that are essential for the commissioning of a TPS, empirical parameters are required to model the dynamic radiation fields that are used in VMAT deliveries. For example, Varian's Eclipse AAA algorithm requires a quantity called the dosimetric leaf gap (DLG) that is used in the modeling of the rounded shape of the MLC tip. These parameters are fine-tuned by comparing measurement with calculations from the TPS in an iterative fashion during beam commissioning.

Dosimetric verification measurements for single-isocenter VMAT plans are made complicated by the fact that the measurements are performed at off-axis locations, and the effective field sizes of the radiation field are small. Detector arrays that are routinely used for dose verification of conventional VMAT plans are not suitable for SRS dose measurements because of inadequate sampling, yielding 1 or 2 point measurements where the tumors are located. Typically, point dose measurements are performed with compact solid-state detectors, requiring multiple positioning of the phantom for each target-dose measurement. While absolute dose measurements with films are prone to systematic errors, their high spatial resolution makes them invaluable in ascertaining the spatial accuracy of the dose delivery of SRS treatments (Fig. 16.9). Once the TPS is commissioned, dose verification for patient-specific QA can be performed with less cumbersome methods such as fluence-based measurements using the Linac's electronic portal imaging system or independent dose calculation with Monte Carlo.

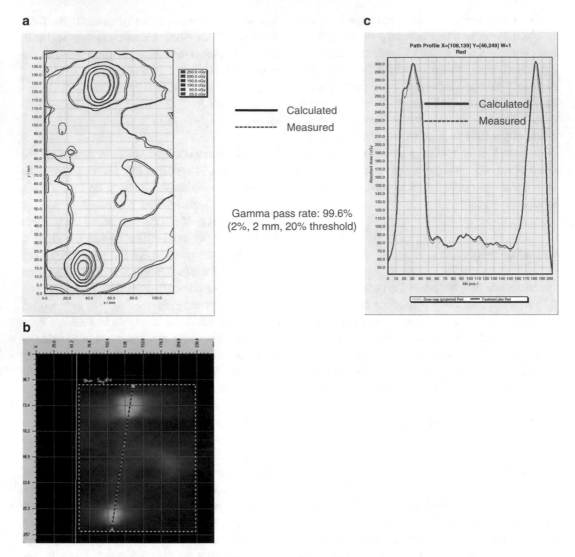

Fig. 16.9 (**a**) Comparison of calculated isodose distributions with film measurement of a single-isocenter noncoplanar VMAT plan used in the treatment of multiple brain metastases. (**b**) Film measurement (**c**) Dose profile comparison between measurement and calculation across the line shown in (**b**) [unpublished]

Unlike the dose calculation algorithms employed by commercial treatment planning systems, the Monte Carlo method calculates dose from first principles and is considered the gold standard in dosimetry, especially for dose calculation involving complex deliveries [39]. At the BC Cancer – Vancouver, an in-house Monte Carlo dose verification system, which is based on the EGSnrc code [41], is used for independent dose calculation of complex VMAT deliveries. Figure 16.10 shows an example of a dose distribution comparison between Eclipse AAA and Monte Carlo calculations for a multiple-met SRS VMAT plan containing five non-coplanar arcs.

Targeting Accuracy

GammaKnife

The hallmark of GK-SRS has traditionally been the Leksell stereotactic frame, which is surgically

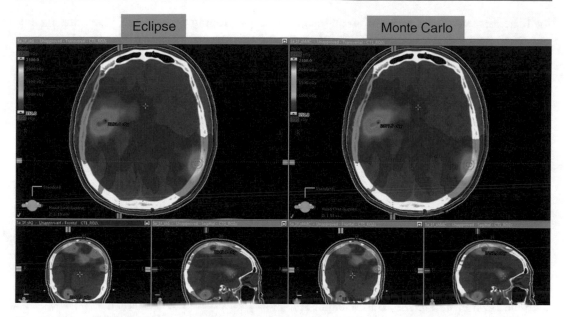

Fig. 16.10 Dose distribution comparison between Eclipse AAA and Monte Carlo calculations for a multiple-met SRS VMAT plan containing five non-coplanar arcs [unpublished]

mounted to the patient head and provides both the localization coordinate system, as well as rigid immobilization. More recently, frameless SRS on GK has been made possible with the integration of a CBCT image-guided unit on the GK Icon system. However, regardless of whether frame or mask, the main advantage of the GK is the mechanical precision with which it can target a fixed point. In the most recent GK Icon model, the collimator cap is a stationary object, and all 192 beams simultaneously converge at the focal spot. Furthermore, the patient positioning system has been reported to have a precision of <0.3 mm across the treatable field of view [42].

CyberKnife

To visualize small brain metastases, high-definition 2D digitally reconstructed radiographs (DRRs) are first created from thin-cut planning CT scans to serve as the reference images for the alignment. The slice thickness of the planning CT is typically acquired at 1.0 mm to achieve adequate DRR resolution and minimize the systematic uncertainties for target localizations. Submillimeter accuracy in tracking any lesion

located inside the skull has been demonstrated [7, 43]. Since the patient is immobilized with a mask, frequent imaging during the treatment delivery on the order of every 30–45 seconds is recommended in order to timely track and validate the locations of individual lesions. Frequent imaging is especially important for small brain metastases as misalignment of 1–2 mm may cause the beam to completely miss the target. End-to-end testing using radiochromic film in a head phantom typically yields a maximum targeting error of <1 mm.

Linac

The mechanical accuracy of a linac is affected by the weight of the gantry head (that causes sag) and the couch runout, as well as the MLC leaf position calibration. TG-142 requires that the isocenter accuracy for SRS units to be <1 mm [14].

The Winston Lutz (WL) test [44] is a standard method for measuring the combined effect of the gantry, collimator, MLC, and couch on the isocenter accuracy. The test is done with a metal ball bearing (BB) that is mounted on the treatment couch. The BB is precisely aligned with the linac isocenter, and a series of portal images of a small field defined by the MLC are taken at various gantry, couch, and collimator positions to measure the alignment of the BB with respect to the treatment field. In addition to the standard WL test, the rotational accuracy of the couch (floor rotation, pitch, and roll) needs to be quantified for the entire range of couch rotation, as these affect the targeting accuracy for off-axis targets. Studies have shown that the angular accuracy of the TrueBeam couch is within 0.1 degrees [45].

Besides the isocenter accuracy test, all the links in the process chain for patient positioning (OBI, 6DOF couch, and patient immobilization) need to be verified and periodically monitored with the Hidden Target Test using an anthropomorphic Head Phantom. The Hidden Target Test mimics the image-guided radiotherapy (IGRT) workflow from CT simulation through treatment delivery and is used to quantify the systematic uncertainty of target positioning. Traditionally, this test is done for isocentric targets.

With the introduction of the single isocenter SRS technique for the treatment of multiple metastases, it has become necessary to measure the positioning accuracy of plans that include off-axis targets. At the BC Cancer – Vancouver, targeting accuracy for single-isocenter multiple target plans is tested using an anthropomorphic Head Phantom. In this test, six radio-opaque markers are inserted at different locations within the phantom, and the test is performed using treatment fields with multiple ports exposing each target. Figure 16.11 shows a comparison of the DRR of a lateral treatment field that exposes the six targets with the corresponding portal image. By comparing the DRR with respect to the portal image, it is possible to quantify the accuracy of the patient positioning system at different locations from the isocenter.

Areas of Uncertainty and Future Directions

There is yet to be any conclusive evidence to support one technology over another in terms of clinical outcomes. Some of the directions being investigated to improve efficiency or efficacy include the following:

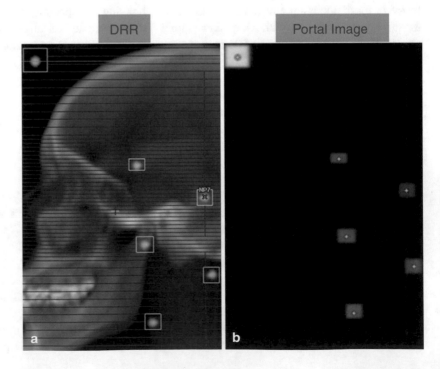

Fig. 16.11 Images of a lateral field (**a**) DRR and (**b**) portal image from hidden target test on an anthropomorphic head phantom: This is a single-isocenter, multi-metastases plan with the isocenter placed at the center of Target #3. The blue stars on the portal image show the center of the BBs. [unpublished]

GammaKnife

GammaKnife treatments tend to be long for multiple metastases. However, with the flexibility now afforded by the Icon system, the treatment can be divided into multiple sessions. This has been hypothesized to incur a radiobiological advantage in that the normal tissue throughout the brain can receive a fractionated schedule while each tumor receives the full radiosurgical dose in a single fraction [28]. Together with advanced automated planning techniques, including a continuous treatment-couch path optimization, more rapid and highly tailored plans for patients with multiple metastases are continuously being developed on the GammaKnife platform [46–48].

CyberKnife

CK treatments of multiple brain metastases primarily use non-coplanar non-isocentric beams with patient immobilized in a thermoplastic mask. The latest CK M6 system has significantly expanded its accessible beam angles, especially from the posterior directions compared to the previous CK models. The introduction of InCise MLC system has improved the treatment delivery efficiency of large lesions (e.g., >1 cm). Since brain metastases of a treatment session can range from a few millimeters to a few centimeters in size, as illustrated in the Case Vignette, further improvements in the high-definition MLC system such as the leaf width and leaf positioning accuracy would expand its applications in the treatments of small lesions. Another area of development is versatile quality assurance tools and process that can accommodate all three collimation systems of the current CK system for treating multiple brain metastases.

Linac

One of the advantages of treating multiple metastases from a single isocenter position is the rapid treatment delivery. However, to generate high-quality SRS plans for cases with numerous (5+) brain metastases using conventional VMAT treatment, planning algorithms, shell structures, considerable planning skills, computational resources, sometimes avoidance structures and lengthy planning time may be required. Convenience for the patient is counterbalanced by challenges for the radiation oncologists and dosimetrists. However, improved methods of planning these cases are commercially available and are entering routine use.

Elements™

BrainLAB is an important supplier of hardware and software for SRS. It makes an orthogonal X-ray imaging system for setup verification at any couch angle and a six degree-of-freedom couch for correcting translational and rotational positional offsets (ExacTRAC™). For many years, they have provided dedicated software for traditional linear accelerator SRS, where the isocenter is placed in the center of each metastasis. This new software, Elements Cranial SRS™, uses lightly modulated dynamic conformal arcs to deliver treatment to multiple metastases from a single isocenter position. Some of the planning innovations include optimizing fixed collimator angles for each arc, treating a subset of the metastases at different couch angles, and limiting the width of leaf openings so that only one metastasis is between open leaves. A planning comparison for 10 cases with multiple brain metastases for VMAT SRS, multi-isocenter dynamic arcs, and single-isocenter dynamic arcs, planned with Elements, showed that the gradient index and V12 were improved with Elements planning and that the conformity indices were similar with the three techniques [49].

HyperArc™

Varian Medical Systems has developed a dedicated VMAT algorithm optimized for single-isocenter multiple-metastasis SRS, called HyperArc, which uses collimator angle optimization to improve the quality of plans. A planning study comparing 15 cases planned with VMAT SRS, CyberKnife, and HyperArc SRS demonstrated faster treatment times with VMAT and HyperArc, but no significant differences in Paddick conformity or gradient indices [50]. Two planning studies with 20 or more single-isocenter, multiple-metastasis cases showed that HyperArc SRS achieved a statistically significant improvement of conformity index and gradient index over conventional VMAT SRS [51, 52].

New Concepts

Dynamic modification of the MLC collimator angle during treatment delivery is an area of active research. By adding this additional degree of freedom to single-isocenter, multiple-metastasis planning using dynamic conformal arcs, the monitor units required to deliver a plan can be reduced by 50% without any sacrifice of plan quality [53].

MLCs

Current Varian stereotactic MLCs were optimized for single-target stereotactic treatments and concentric-target conventional radiation treatment. They are designed with 2.5 mm leaves spanning the central 8 cm of the fields. However, for single-isocenter, multiple-metastases treatments, the quality of the dose distributions diminish for the targets located in the periphery of the brain because more of the dose to these lesions is delivered by 5 mm MLC leaves. One solution is to choose a few isocenters carefully, so the multiple metastases are never outside the high-definition leaves [54]. However, this increases both planning time and treatment delivery time. A hardware solution is to increase the number, speed, and accuracy of the central narrow leaves in multileaf collimators, which would improve dose delivery for single-isocenter, multiple-metastasis

SRS. Elekta Versa HD has 160 pairs of MLC leaves, and each has a leaf width of 5 mm [19].

Guidelines

Regardless of technology, the success of an SRS program hinges on a thorough and ongoing quality assurance (QA) program to ensure that the treatment unit is in compliance with the recommendations of the treatment unit manufacturer and within specified clinical tolerances based on international and national guidelines and recommendations [14, 55–58].

Quality assurance (QA) tasks for the CK M6 system follow TG135 guidelines including the minimum equipment tolerance levels as specified in the AAPM-RSS medical physics practice guideline [59], which cover mechanical checks, radiation characteristics checks, imaging/tracking system checks, as well as collimator checks [60].

The accuracy and precision for which the narrow beams of radiation in SRS target the lesion should be well characterized and routinely tested for sub-millimeter targeting accuracy. For MLC-based delivery of multiple metastases treating off-axis, specialized QA devices may be needed to verify the accuracy of radiation field placement throughout the angular range of gantry, collimator, and couch angles [61, 62]. A positional end-to-end test for delivery accuracy is recommended that encompasses as much as the workflow as possible, from MRI, through to target delineation and treatment delivery.

For reference, dosimetry recent recommendations as per TRS-483 using machine-specific reference (MSR) fields apply [39]. The differential detector response at small fields relative to the MSR field must be taken into account using Monte Carlo calculated corrections. Additionally, proper alignment and orientation of the detector with respect to the field are also important to consider in relative small field dosimetry.

Key Points

- The SRS technologies for treating brain metastases are continuously evolving.
- All of the existing technologies have advantages and disadvantages that must be considered when a clinical team is evaluating which to use for their patients.
- As the number of patients with brain metastases is likely to increase, as well as the patients' longevity, efficiency of technology may become a high priority.
- On the other hand, one cannot understate how complex the technologies are, despite the ability of the vendors to automate and streamline processes.
- A fundamental understanding of the physical basis of the technology, including how accurate small radiation fields are at delivering dose, is becoming increasingly important as the technologies become more conformal and more precise over time.

References

1. Lindquist C, Paddick I. The Leksell Gamma Knife Perfexion and comparisons with its predecessors. Neurosurgery. 2007;61(3 Suppl):130–40; discussion 40-1.
2. Zeverino M, Jaccard M, Patin D, Ryckx N, Marguet M, Tuleasca C, et al. Commissioning of the Leksell Gamma Knife® Icon™. Med Phys. 2017;44(2):355–63.
3. Sarfehnia A, Ruschin M, Chugh B, Yeboah C, Becker N, Cho YB, et al. Performance characterization of an integrated cone-beam CT system for dedicated gamma radiosurgery. Med Phys. 2018;45(9):4179–90.
4. Pappas EP, Moutsatsos A, Pantelis E, Zoros E, Georgiou E, Torrens M, et al. On the development of a comprehensive MC simulation model for the Gamma Knife Perfexion radiosurgery unit. Phys Med Biol. 2016;61(3):1182–203.
5. Adler JR Jr, Murphy MJ, Chang SD, Hancock SL. Image-guided robotic radiosurgery. Neurosurgery. 1999;44(6):1299–306; discussion 306-7.
6. Andrews DW, Bednarz G, Evans JJ, Downes B. A review of 3 current radiosurgery systems. Surg Neurol. 2006;66(6):559–64.

7. Chang SD, Main W, Martin DP, Gibbs IC, Heilbrun MP. An analysis of the accuracy of the CyberKnife: a robotic frameless stereotactic radiosurgical system. Neurosurgery. 2003;52(1):140–6; discussion 6-7.
8. Yu C, Main W, Taylor D, Kuduvalli G, Apuzzo ML, Adler JR Jr. An anthropomorphic phantom study of the accuracy of Cyberknife spinal radiosurgery. Neurosurgery. 2004;55(5):1138–49.
9. van de Water S, Hoogeman MS, Breedveld S, Nuyttens JJ, Schaart DR, Heijmen BJ. Variable circular collimator in robotic radiosurgery: a time-efficient alternative to a mini-multileaf collimator? Int J Radiat Oncol Biol Phys. 2011;81(3):863–70.
10. Winey B, Bussiere M. Geometric and dosimetric uncertainties in intracranial stereotactic treatments for multiple nonisocentric lesions. J Appl Clin Med Phys. 2014;15(3):122–32.
11. Chang J. Incorporating the rotational setup uncertainty into the planning target volume margin expansion for the single isocenter for multiple targets technique. Pract Radiat Oncol. 2018;8(6):475–83.
12. Otto K. Volumetric modulated arc therapy: IMRT in a single gantry arc. Med Phys. 2008;35(1):310–7.
13. Solberg TD, Boedeker KL, Fogg R, Selch MT, DeSalles AA. Dynamic arc radiosurgery field shaping: a comparison with static field conformal and noncoplanar circular arcs. Int J Radiat Oncol Biol Phys. 2001;49(5):1481–91.
14. Klein EE, Hanley J, Bayouth J, Yin FF, Simon W, Dresser S, et al. Task Group 142 report: quality assurance of medical accelerators. Med Phys. 2009;36(9):4197–212.
15. Schmidhalter D, Fix MK, Wyss M, Schaer N, Munro P, Scheib S, et al. Evaluation of a new six degrees of freedom couch for radiation therapy. Med Phys. 2013;40(11):111710.
16. Scorsetti M, Alongi F, Castiglioni S, Clivio A, Fogliata A, Lobefalo F, et al. Feasibility and early clinical assessment of flattening filter free (FFF) based stereotactic body radiotherapy (SBRT) treatments. Radiat Oncol. 2011;6:113.
17. Dhabaan A, Elder E, Schreibmann E, Crocker I, Curran WJ, Oyesiku NM, et al. Dosimetric performance of the new high-definition multileaf collimator for intracranial stereotactic radiosurgery. J Appl Clin Med Phys. 2010;11(3):3040.
18. Zhang Q, Driewer J, Wang S, Li S, Zhu X, Zheng D, et al. Accuracy evaluation of a six-degree-of-freedom couch using cone beam CT and IsoCal phantom with an in-house algorithm. Med Phys. 2017;44(8):3888–98.
19. Thompson CM, Weston SJ, Cosgrove VC, Thwaites DI. A dosimetric characterization of a novel linear accelerator collimator. Med Phys. 2014;41(3):031713.
20. Ma L, Nichol A, Hossain S, Wang B, Petti P, Vellani R, et al. Variable dose interplay effects across radiosurgical apparatus in treating multiple brain metastases. Int J Comput Assist Radiol Surg. 2014;9(6):1079–86.
21. Slosarek K, Bekman B, Wendykier J, Grzadziel A, Fogliata A, Cozzi L. In silico assessment of the dosi-

metric quality of a novel, automated radiation treatment planning strategy for linac-based radiosurgery of multiple brain metastases and a comparison with robotic methods. Radiat Oncol. 2018;13(1):41.

22. Zhang I, Antone J, Li J, Saha S, Riegel AC, Vijeh L, et al. Hippocampal-sparing and target volume coverage in treating 3 to 10 brain metastases: a comparison of Gamma Knife, single-isocenter VMAT, CyberKnife, and TomoTherapy stereotactic radiosurgery. Pract Radiat Oncol. 2017;7(3):183–9.

23. Ma L, Petti P, Wang B, Descovich M, Chuang C, Barani IJ, et al. Apparatus dependence of normal brain tissue dose in stereotactic radiosurgery for multiple brain metastases. J Neurosurg. 2011;114(6):1580–4.

24. Sio TT, Jang S, Lee SW, Curran B, Pyakuryal AP, Sternick ES. Comparing gamma knife and cyberknife in patients with brain metastases. J Appl Clin Med Phys. 2014;15(1):4095.

25. Thomas EM, Popple RA, Wu X, Clark GM, Markert JM, Guthrie BL, et al. Comparison of plan quality and delivery time between volumetric arc therapy (RapidArc) and Gamma Knife radiosurgery for multiple cranial metastases. Neurosurgery. 2014;75(4):409–17; discussion 17-8.

26. Potrebko PS, Keller A, All S, Sejpal S, Pepe J, Saigal K, et al. GammaKnife versus VMAT radiosurgery plan quality for many brain metastases. J Appl Clin Med Phys. 2018;19(6):159–65.

27. Eaton DJ, Lee J, Paddick I. Stereotactic radiosurgery for multiple brain metastases: results of multicenter benchmark planning studies. Pract Radiat Oncol. 2018;8(4):e212–e20.

28. Kelly DA. Treatment of multiple brain metastases with a divide-and-conquer spatial fractionation radiosurgery approach. Med Hypotheses. 2014;83(4):425–8.

29. Jang SY, Lalonde R, Ozhasoglu C, Burton S, Heron D, Huq MS. Dosimetric comparison between cone/Iris-based and InCise MLC-based CyberKnife plans for single and multiple brain metastases. J Appl Clin Med Phys. 2016;17(5):184–99.

30. Ma L, Sahgal A, Hwang A, Hu W, Descovich M, Chuang C, et al. A two-step optimization method for improving multiple brain lesion treatments with robotic radiosurgery. Technol Cancer Res Treat. 2011;10(4):331–8.

31. Das IJ, Ding GX, Ahnesjö A. Small fields: non-equilibrium radiation dosimetry. Med Phys. 2008;35(1):206–15.

32. Sánchez-Doblado F, Hartmann GH, Pena J, Roselló JV, Russiello G, Gonzalez-Castaño DM. A new method for output factor determination in MLC shaped narrow beams. Phys Med. 2007;23(2):58–66.

33. Lárraga-Gutiérrez JM, Ballesteros-Zebadúa P, Rodríguez-Ponce M, García-Garduño OA, de la Cruz OO. Properties of a commercial PTW-60019 synthetic diamond detector for the dosimetry of small radiotherapy beams. Phys Med Biol. 2015;60(2):905–24.

34. De Coste V, Francescon P, Marinelli M, Masi L, Paganini L, Pimpinella M, et al. Is the PTW 60019 microDiamond a suitable candidate for small field reference dosimetry? Phys Med Biol. 2017;62(17):7036–55.

35. Carrasco P, Jornet N, Jordi O, Lizondo M, Latorre-Musoll A, Eudaldo T, et al. Characterization of the Exradin W1 scintillator for use in radiotherapy. Med Phys. 2015;42(1):297–304.

36. Almond PR, Biggs PJ, Coursey BM, Hanson WF, Huq MS, Nath R, et al. AAPM's TG-51 protocol for clinical reference dosimetry of high-energy photon and electron beams. Med Phys. 1999;26(9):1847–70.

37. McEwen M, DeWerd L, Ibbott G, Followill D, Rogers DW, Seltzer S, et al. Addendum to the AAPM's TG-51 protocol for clinical reference dosimetry of high-energy photon beams. Med Phys. 2014;41(4):041501.

38. Andreo P, Huq MS, Westermark M, Song H, Tilikidis A, DeWerd L, et al. Protocols for the dosimetry of high-energy photon and electron beams: a comparison of the IAEA TRS-398 and previous international codes of practice. International Atomic Energy Agency. Phys Med Biol. 2002;47(17):3033–53.

39. Vatnisky S, Meghzifene A, Christaki K, Palmans H, Andrew P, Saiful Huq M, et al. IAEA TRS-483. Dosimetry of small fields used in external beam radiotherapy: an international code of practice for reference and relative dose determination. International Atomic Energy Agency. 2017.

40. Alfonso R, Andreo P, Capote R, Huq MS, Kilby W, Kjäll P, et al. A new formalism for reference dosimetry of small and nonstandard fields. Med Phys. 2008;35(11):5179–86.

41. Rogers DWO, Kawrakow I, Seuntjens JP, Walters BRB, Mainegra-Hing E. NRC user codes for EGSnrc. National Research Council Canada. Institute for National Measurement Standards.

42. Ma L, Chiu J, Hoye J, McGuiness C, Perez-Andujar A. Quality assurance of stereotactic alignment and patient positioning mechanical accuracy for robotized Gamma Knife radiosurgery. Phys Med Biol. 2014;59(23):N221–6.

43. Okamoto H, Hamada M, Sakamoto E, Wakita A, Nakamura S, Kato T, et al. Log-file analysis of accuracy of beam localization for brain tumor treatment by CyberKnife. Pract Radiat Oncol. 2016;6(6):e361–e7.

44. Lutz W, Winston KR, Maleki N. A system for stereotactic radiosurgery with a linear accelerator. Int J Radiat Oncol Biol Phys. 1988;14(2):373–81.

45. Wilson B, Gete E. Machine-specific quality assurance procedure for stereotactic treatments with dynamic couch rotations. Med Phys. 2017;44(12):6529–37.

46. Cevik M, Shirvani Ghomi P, Aleman D, Lee Y, Berdyshev A, Nordstrom H, et al. Modeling and comparison of alternative approaches for sector duration optimization in a dedicated radiosurgery system. Phys Med Biol. 2018;63(15):155009.

47. Ghobadi K, Ghaffari HR, Aleman DM, Jaffray DA, Ruschin M. Automated treatment planning for a dedicated multi-source intracranial radiosurgery treatment unit using projected gradient and grassfire algorithms. Med Phys. 2012;39(6):3134–41.

48. Vandewouw MM, Aleman DM, Jaffray DA. Robotic path finding in inverse treatment planning for stereotactic radiosurgery with continuous dose delivery. Med Phys. 2016;43(8):4545.

49. Gevaert T, Steenbeke F, Pellegri L, Engels B, Christian N, Hoornaert MT, et al. Evaluation of a dedicated brain metastases treatment planning optimization for radiosurgery: a new treatment paradigm? Radiat Oncol. 2016;11:13.

50. Slosarek K, Bekman B, Wendykier J, Grządziel A, Fogliata A, Cozzi L. In silico assessment of the dosimetric quality of a novel, automated radiation treatment planning strategy for linac-based radiosurgery of multiple brain metastases and a comparison with robotic methods. Radiat Oncol. 2018;13(1):41.

51. Ruggieri R, Naccarato S, Mazzola R, Ricchetti F, Corradini S, Fiorentino A, et al. Linac-based VMAT radiosurgery for multiple brain lesions: comparison between a conventional multi-isocenter approach and a new dedicated mono-isocenter technique. Radiat Oncol. 2018;13(1):38.

52. Ohira S, Ueda Y, Akino Y, Hashimoto M, Masaoka A, Hirata T, et al. HyperArc VMAT planning for single and multiple brain metastases stereotactic radiosurgery: a new treatment planning approach. Radiat Oncol. 2018;13(1):13.

53. MacDonald RL, Thomas CG, Syme A. Dynamic collimator trajectory algorithm for multiple metastases dynamic conformal arc treatment planning. Med Phys. 2018;45(1):5–17.

54. Ballangrud Å, Kuo LC, Happersett L, Lim SB, Beal K, Yamada Y, et al. Institutional experience with SRS VMAT planning for multiple cranial metastases. J Appl Clin Med Phys. 2018;19(2):176–83.

55. Benedict SH, Yenice KM, Followill D, Galvin JM, Hinson W, Kavanagh B, et al. Stereotactic body radiation therapy: the report of AAPM Task Group 101. Med Phys. 2010;37(8):4078–101.

56. Kirkby C, Ghasroddashti E, Angers CP, Zeng G, Barnett E. COMP report: CPQR technical quality control guideline for medical linear accelerators and multileaf collimators. J Appl Clin Med Phys. 2018;19(2):22–8.

57. Vandervoort E, Patrocinio H, Chow T, Soisson E, Nadeau DB. COMP report: CPQR technical quality control guidelines for CyberKnife ((R)) technology. J Appl Clin Med Phys. 2018;19(2):29–34.

58. Berndt A, van Prooijen M, Guillot M. COMP report: CPQR technical quality control guidelines for Gamma Knife radiosurgery. J Appl Clin Med Phys. 2018;19:365.

59. Halvorsen PH, Cirino E, Das IJ, Garrett JA, Yang J, Yin F, Fairobent LA. AAPM-RSS medical physics practice guideline 9.a. for SRS-SBRT. J Appl Clin Med Phys. 2017;18:10–21.

60. Dieterich S, Cavedon C, Chuang CF, Cohen AB, Garrett JA, Lee CL, et al. Report of AAPM TG 135: quality assurance for robotic radiosurgery. Med Phys. 2011;38(6):2914–36.

61. Gao J, Liu X. Off-Isocenter Winston-Lutz tEST for stereotactic radiosurgery/stereotactic body radiotherapy. Int J Med Phys. 2016;5:154–61.

62. Du W, Gao S, Wang X, Kudchadker RJ. Quantifying the gantry sag on linear accelerators and introducing an MLC-based compensation strategy. Med Phys. 2012;39(4):2156–62.

Single-Isocenter, Multiple Metastasis Treatment Planning

17

Evan M. Thomas, Richard A. Popple,
Elizabeth Covington, and John B. Fiveash

Background and History of Multiple Metastasis Treatment

Historically, metastatic cancer conferred a very limited prognosis upon a patient, particularly if their cancer had metastasized to the brain. Metastases to the brain are among the most clinically significant, where even a very small tumor can be associated with substantial disability. In recent years however, advances in systemic therapies, particularly immunotherapy and targeted molecular therapies, have markedly improved the prognosis and durable survival in patients with advanced malignancy. In fact, the three types of primary malignancy responsible for most brain metastases (lung cancer, breast cancer, and melanoma) have arguably seen the greatest advances in systemic therapy. Though a few of the latest-generation agents have demonstrated activity in the brain, the response they confer extracranially often far exceeds that observed intracranially. As these patients live longer on systemic agents with greater extracranial than intracranial activity, they exhibit an increased likelihood of experiencing brain metastases.

In patients with multiple metastases, stereotactic radiosurgery (SRS) has become an increasingly utilized mainstay of therapy. This is due in large part to multiple randomized trials demonstrating the superiority of SRS over whole-brain radiation therapy (WBRT) in preserving cognition but also due to increasing availability of technology capable of delivering SRS. Modh et al. [1] reviewed the proportional utilization of SRS in comparison with WBRT for patients with intracranial metastases between 2004 and 2014 and demonstrated that the fraction of patients receiving SRS grew from 7% in 2004 to 37% in 2014. In 2017, the NCCN guidelines for brain metastases only recommended SRS for patients with one to three metastases. As of the 2019 edition [2], the guidelines still categorize patients into those with limited versus extensive brain metastasis but include SRS as an option for either group of patients and as the preferred option for those with limited brain metastasis.

All these factors have led to peaking interest from neuro-oncologists, neurosurgeons, and radiation oncologists in the ability to treat increasing numbers of brain metastases in a single session. In this chapter, we will review the history and evolution of the treatment of multiple brain metastases and then discuss and demonstrate the most modern techniques for the most efficient form of treatment, single-isocenter treatment.

E. M. Thomas (✉) · R. A. Popple · E. Covington
J. B. Fiveash
Department of Radiation Oncology, University of Alabama at Birmingham, Birmingham, AL, USA
e-mail: ethomas@uab.edu

© Springer Nature Switzerland AG 2020
Y. Yamada et al. (eds.), *Radiotherapy in Managing Brain Metastases*,
https://doi.org/10.1007/978-3-030-43740-4_17

Single-Isocenter Treatment of Multiple Metastases

Origins

Very soon after the development of the multi-leaf collimator (MLC) and the advent of intensity-modulated radiation therapy (IMRT), radiation oncologists realized the potential of treating multiple targets simultaneously with a single isocenter. The potential benefits of not needing to employ a separate isocenter and set of beams for each target were immediately obvious. The earliest published efforts to design a plan to treat multiple targets in the brain with a single isocenter was in 1996 with the Peacock planning system [3], but this technique would not be widely utilized for some time. Although a rotational IMRT algorithm had been developed by Cedric Yu at the University of Maryland at about the same time [4], both computing power and software platforms were not sufficiently advanced enough for the technology to be widely integrated. In 2008, Karl Otto published an improved algorithm to solve the problem of determining the optimal fluence map for a dynamic multi-leaf collimation in concert with gantry rotation. The technique was dubbed volumetric modulated arc therapy (VMAT) [5]. By this time, the exponential increase in available CPU speed predicted by Moore's law had rendered widely available the computing power needed for VMAT optimization and dose calculation on a clinically viable timescale. VMAT was quickly adopted for single-target radiosurgery plans. The potential increase in efficiency for treating multiple targets with a single isocenter even more efficiently rapidly attracted efforts to employ single-isocenter VMAT to multiple targets [6, 7]. In 2009, Mayo et al. described their initial experiences using RapidArc™ VMAT for intracranial radiosurgery, including treatment of a patient with two metastases, and a sagacious prediction that "the ability to treat multiple lesions simultaneously will have a significant impact on care patterns for patients with metastatic lesions."

In 2010, Clark et al. [8] of the University of Alabama at Birmingham (UAB) published the first full paper demonstrating dosimetric and delivery feasibility of VMAT for single-isocenter multiple metastasis radiosurgery. In 2012, Clark et al. published a recipe or class solution for the technique that has since been requested and circulated in its original and updated form to hundreds of institutions across the world, many of whom still currently employ the methodology. The technique was initially developed for the Eclipse™ (Varian Medical Systems, Palo Alto, CA) treatment planning software platform but has been adapted with varying degrees of success for other platforms as well, including Pinnacle™ (Phillips, Amsterdam, Netherlands) [9] and Raystation (RaySearch Laboratories, Stockholm, Sweden) [10].

Adoption of single-isocenter, multiple metastasis treatment with VMAT grew rapidly thereafter, particularly in centers without access to a dedicated radiosurgery platform. Until 2014, however, for multiple metastasis treatments, most neurosurgeons and radiation oncologists still regarded multi-isocenter planning with Gamma Knife-based treatment to be superior to Linac SRS treatments, including those performed with single-isocenter VMAT. Small-case number dosimetry comparisons published by Ma et al. [11, 12] had shown Gamma Knife treatments to be markedly superior to single-isocenter VMAT on the Novalis Tx™ (Varian Medical Systems, Palo Alto, USA) platform with respect to gradient and low-isodose spill. In 2014, however, Thomas et al. published a larger, more robust comparison of Gamma Knife and single-isocenter VMAT with the UAB technique. This work showed that across 28 cases with up to 9 metastases, well-planned single-isocenter VMAT plans were of equivalent quality to their GK counterparts across all metrics, including moderate and low-isodose spill as shown in Fig. 17.1. These disparate results highlight the importance of meticulous attention to technical detail in planning VMAT to achieve optimal plans.

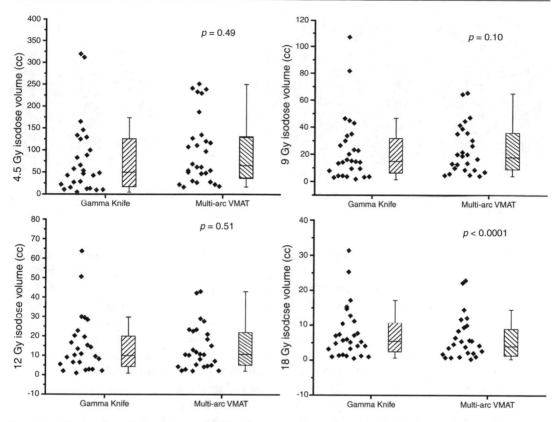

Fig. 17.1 Distributions of V4.5, V9, V12, and V18Gy levels for Gamma Knife and single-isocenter VMAT SRS plans of multiple metastasis cases. (From Thomas et al. [13] Reprinted with permission from Oxford University Press)

Advantages of Single-Isocenter Treatment Planning

The principal advantage of single-isocenter treatment is efficiency of delivery [13]. It had long been known that coplanar beam arrangements produced unsatisfactory dose spill in the axial plane, even for a single target. For Gamma Knife treatments, which inherently leverage beam angles from nearly the entirety of the upper half of the 4pi space, this was not a problem. However, for each additional target, at least one new isocenter and at least one additional shot were required. For larger or complex shaped targets, often several shots were necessary. Treatment of more than a few lesions could take several hours. For single-isocenter VMAT, treatment time is generally independent on the number of lesions unless additional arcs are added.

For multiple-isocenter radiosurgery plans on a gantry-based Linac, either with cones or with dynamic conformal treatment, a dosimetrically favorable plan requires beams from at least one noncoplanar angle in addition to those from the axial plane. Thus, for each target, at least one table shift and one table rotation would be required.

For CyberKnife™ (Accuray Inc., Sunnyvale, USA) SRS plans utilizing cones, dosimetrically favorable plans require at least several nodes but usually many more nodes per target. Multiple metastasis radiosurgery plans with >200 nodes are not uncommonly encountered [14]. Some more modern CyberKnife configurations utilize a small MLC [Incise™ (Accuray Inc)] rather than cones. This could in theory eliminate some required beam angles for multiple metastasis radiosurgery plans, but currently, only dosimetric

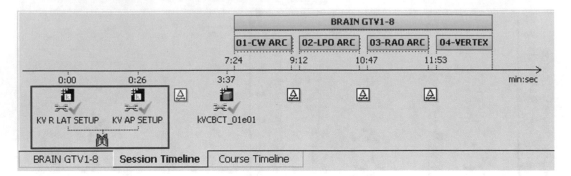

Fig. 17.2 Plan delivery synopsis for patient with eight metastases treated with single-isocenter SRS on a Varian Edge in 10MV flattening-filter free mode

feasibility [15] and no clinical studies have been published.

Single-isocenter VMAT plans require only the initial table shift for exact alignment of the patient, and then one to three table rotations to access each non-axial arc angle – regardless of the number of targets being treated. When coupled with flattening filter-free (FFF) high-dose rate delivery, treatments become extremely efficient. On Varian linear accelerators, native FFF delivery is available on the Edge™ and TrueBeam STx™ platforms, with dose rates of up to 1400 MU/min and 2400MU/min for 6MV and 10MV beams, respectively. The Versa HD™ is currently the only Elekta linear accelerator with FFF delivery and has identical dose rate delivery capability.

The degree of field modulation (number of MLC patterns and monitor units for a given field) determines the final MU count for each field and ultimately the plan. But in general, most 360° fields delivered in FFF mode require 1–2 minutes to complete and most 180° fields require 30 to 60 seconds. The amount of time required in between each field depends on the number of fields in a given plan, and whether or not a room entry is required for each couch adjustment, and, if so, how quickly the process of table rotation can be executed.

At our institution (UAB), all intracranial SRS plans are delivered in single-isocenter with 10MV beam in FFF mode at 2400 MU/min. Total beam-on time is 1–4 minutes, and the total treatment time for most plans is 10–20 minutes depending mainly on the number of fields used

(2–4) but also patient setup compliance and any patient motion detected by optical surface monitoring. Any detected motion prompts the therapist to halt the treatment, bring the couch back to 0°, and repeat cone beam CT (CBCT) alignment. Figure 17.2 demonstrates the treatment delivery for a patient with eight metastases. Total treatment time from initiation of first kV image was about 13 minutes.

Minimizing delivery time reduces patient treatment anxiety, increases patient comfort and satisfaction with treatment, minimizes likelihood of intra-treatment interruption due to patient motion [16, 17], and reduces likelihood of patient noncompliance with sequential treatments in fractionated SRS plans.

Potential Pitfalls of Single-Isocenter Planning

The potential efficiency advantages of single- over multi-isocenter planning and delivery are obvious for any center that offers intracranial radiosurgery. There are, however, pitfalls of which the radiosurgery team needs to be aware; and precautions and workflow need to be in place to mitigate the risk thereof.

The principal hazard is a geometric risk because of patient misalignment, whether translational or rotational, that will result in under-treatment of one or more targets and potentially deliver excessive dose to a critical structure. For a target near a critical organ at risk, misalignment could also result in exposure of that organ to high-isodose volume than was unintended, engendering an increased risk of injury. Multiple works have examined in particular the risk, occurrence frequency, and dosimetric consequence of rotational misalignment in single-isocenter multiple target radiosurgery plans. Roper et al. [18] undertook what is probably the most thorough dosimetric analysis. Their study evaluated the implications of simulated rotational errors of 0.5°, 1.0°, and 2.0° about all axes (pitch, roll, and yaw) on the D95% (dose received by 95% of PTV) of two targets within each of 50 SRS plans. They found that target D95% decreased proportionally with both the degree of misalignment and the distance from the isocenter. Figure 17.3a shows a plot of the D95% versus target center distance to isocenter by degree of misalignment. Figure 17.3b shows an illustrative case with dose cloud and DVH of the loss in coverage associated with 2.0° rotational error.

Multiple techniques exist to manage and prevent positional error and/or uncertainty. They can roughly be divided into accurate positional setup, motion prevention, motion monitoring, and motion mitigation. Although these are discussed in further detail elsewhere in this text, an overview is provided here due to the high impact of uncertainty on single-isocenter treatments. The most important and mandatory step is of course

maximal elimination of all positional error (translational and rotation) via proper imaging and table adjustment during initial setup. Fortunately for the intracranial radiosurgeon, very little anatomic variation is typically observed in the time scales normally found between simulation and treatment; additionally, CBCT on the modern radiosurgery platform usually provides excellent depiction of bony anatomy landmarks for automatic and manual registration between CBCT and simulation CT. The planning and treating physician should of course be mindful of the clinical scenarios when anatomic variation can arise. A few of the principals to keep in mind are cyst cavities, rapidly growing tumors (e.g., metastases from, e.g., an aggressive squamous cell carcinoma of the lung), and evolving edema (either worsening or improving). For these scenarios, a margin (which in this case would be appropriately designated a CTV) can be added.

Once positional uncertainty has been eliminated in the initial setup, prevention of motion during treatment with robust immobilization is the next step. The gold standard for many years had been the stereotactic frame, secured with pins screwed into the skull, but advances in polymers have facilitated the development of a number of moldable, noninvasive immobilization apparatuses. Babic et al. [19] performed a cone beam CT-based analysis of the intrafraction

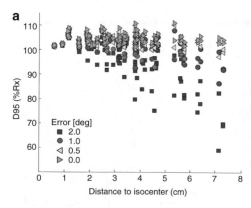
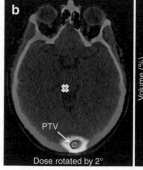
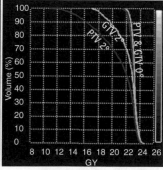

Fig. 17.3 Loss of target coverage secondary to rotational misalignment. (**a**) D95 plotted as a function of PTV distance to isocenter and stratified by rotational error. Ideal values for D95 and V95 are 100% and 100%, respectively. (**b**) Substantial loss in target coverage for a 0.78-cc planning target volume (PTV) at 7.3 cm from isocenter when

rotated by 2.0°. The other PTV, not shown, is in a different plane. A cross denotes the transaxial position of the isocenter. Dose-volume histogram data are reported for the gross target volume (GTV) and PTV at 0.0 and 2.0. (From Roper et al. [18] Reprinted with permission from Elsevier) motion of SRS and fSRT patients immobilized with either a frame-based or frameless solution. Their SRS patients were immobilized with either a Cosman-Roberts-Wells (CRW) frame (Integra-Radionics, Burlington, MA, USA) or a noninvasive PinPoint system (Aktina Medical, Congers, NY, USA); the fSRT patients were immobilized with one of either a noninvasive Gill-Thomas-Cosman (GTC) relocatable frame (Integra-Radionics, Burlington, MA, USA) or a noninvasive PinPoint system, Uniframe mask (WFR/Aquaplast Corp., Avondale, PA, USA), or an Orfit mask (Orfit Industries, Wijnegem, Belgium). For SRS patients, mean 3D intrafraction motion (defined as difference between pre- and posttreatment cone beam CT) was 0.45 ± 0.33 mm for noninvasive PinPoint system and 0.30 ± 0.21 mm for CRW invasive frame. The intrafraction motion for all immobilization strategies tested is shown in Fig. 17.4.

Detection of intrafraction motion is the next step in managing the effects of positional error. There are multiple intrafraction motion monitoring strategies that have been deployed with platforms on which single-isocenter SRS is utilized. The simplest is continuous visual inspection of the patient by the treating therapist and physician via a video monitor. While large magnitude motions may be seen, visual inspection via video monitor is unlikely to reliably discern motions

that are clinically meaningful during a radiosurgery treatment. The authors do not recommend such an approach in the absence of a validated immobilization solution with submillimeter robustness. The foremost technologies for intrafraction motion monitoring during treatment are serial intrafraction kV imaging and surface imaging. The former, utilized by the ExacTrac™ (BrainLab, Munich, Germany) and CyberKnife systems, employs registration of kV images acquired from multiple angles during treatment with congruent DRRs from the treatment planning CT to detect misalignment. Surface imaging technologies such as those used in the AlignRT™ (VisionRT, London, England) or IDENTIFY (humediQ/Varian Medial Systems, Palo Alto, CA) systems use multiple cameras to generate a real-time 3D mesh grid of a reference surface and then monitor for change in the surface map. Another surface imaging technology that BrainLab has recently incorporated uses a thermal camera to generate a three-dimensional surface heat contour profile, which is monitored for changes. With a short treatment time, approximately 5% or fewer patients will require repositioning with repeat CBCT due to motion during treatment. At UAB the median intrafraction motion from the beginning to end of treatment is approximately 0.3 mm (real-time delta as measured by surface imaging) [20].

Fig. 17.4 Magnitude of intrafraction motion 3D error as calculated from the vector difference between pre- and the posttreatment CBCTs for several invasive and non-immobilization options. (From Babic S, et al. [19]. Reprinted with permission under terms of Creative Commons Attribution License)

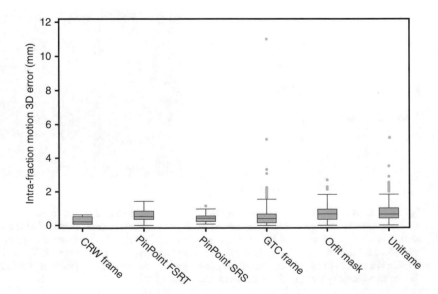

Mitigation with margin is the final strategy for positional uncertainty. Addition of a PTV margin can be employed when a sufficiently robust immobilization and monitoring solution is not available. The addition of a margin is not without cost to plan quality, which is further discussed later in the chapter.

Island Blocking

In most VMAT optimization algorithms, the medial aspect of each collimator leaf pair is set to align itself with the lateral edge of a target. In this manner, leaf positions tracking a lesion along each of its projections throughout an arc are easily obtained. The "island-blocking" phenomenon occurs when a pair of targets is aligned collinearly with the orientation of the collimator leaves and a given leaf pair is open for two targets instead of just one. This results in the normal tissue in between the two targets receiving undesired and unnecessary exposure to the uncollimated beam. Figure 17.5 depicts an example of the occurrence in a patient with eight metastases.

As treatment planning software designers became aware of the phenomenon, updates to the optimization algorithm deployment largely allevi-

ated this phenomenon. Planners without access to the most up-to-date software may have to rely on alternative techniques when this situation is encountered. The phenomenon and mitigation tactics are discussed in great detail in Yuan et al. [21].

Strategies to employ are listed below and are individually discussed in greater detail later:

- Additional noncoplanar arcs
- Collimator angle adjustment/optimization
- Increased penalization of healthy brain tissue in cost function
- Addition of dose-limiting tuning structure "walls" in between targets in close proximity

Techniques in Single-Isocenter Multiple Metastasis Planning

Currently, all single-isocenter multiple metastasis techniques can only be employed on a gantry based-linear accelerator outfitted with a multi-leaf collimator. Furthermore, these techniques should only be used on a platform that allows delivery of noncoplanar fields. Single-isocenter treatments

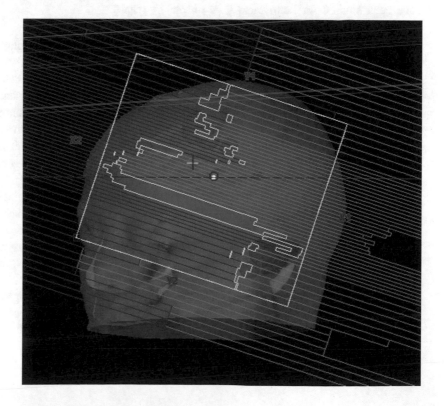

Fig. 17.5 Depiction of "island-blocking" phenomenon characterized by a leaf-pair or leaf-pair block open between two targets, unnecessarily exposing the healthy tissue in between the targets. The example shown here in a treatment for a patient with eight metastases was mitigated by the use of additional noncoplanar beams and dose-limiting tuning "wall" structures in between the closest targets

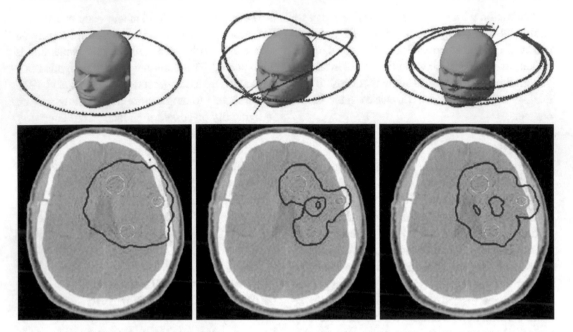

Fig. 17.6 Coplanar versus noncoplanar plan delivery quality. Arc geometry and isodose lines of three treatment planning scenarios with three tumors in same axial plane 3 cm apart [are shown]. (Left) Single-arc/single-isocenter, (Middle) triple-arc/single-isocenter, and (Right) triple-arc/triple-isocenter. White indicates target volume; green, 100% isodose lines; and red, 50% isodose lines. (From Clark et al. [8] Reprinted with permission from Elsevier)

have been studied for brain metastasis on platforms without the capability of noncoplanar delivery such as the TomoTherapy (Accuray) system and the newer MR-Linacs [MRIdian (Viewray Technologies, Oakwood Village, United States) and Unity (Elekta)], but (as noted in Fig. 17.6 from Clark et al.'s single-isocenter feasibility treatise) the quality of plans (VMAT or IMRT) with fields confined to the axial plane is demonstrably inferior to their noncoplanar counterparts [22].

We consider the following prerequisites obligatory for the generation of a high-quality single-isocenter multiple metastasis radiosurgery plan:

- Modern gantry-based linear accelerator capable of at least 6MV beam energy with reliable output factor
- Multi-leaf collimator with central leave shadow thickness no greater than 5 mm
- Capability to deliver noncoplanar beams via couch rotation of up to 90°

IMRS

Intensity-modulated radiosurgery (IMRS) refers to the use of an array of static but intensity-modulated fields for intracranial radiosurgery. The development and rapid deployment in the 1990s of the multi-leaf collimator allowed the generation of significantly more conformal treatment plans. There was prompt interest in its application for intracranial targets. The technique was extensively utilized for fractionated treatment of larger, solitary intracranial targets, but the larger central leaf widths of early MLCs prevented the techniques' widespread adoption for multiple metastasis plans with targets smaller than about 1 centimeter. Nevertheless, some centers did utilize a single-isocenter technique to treat multiple metastases, but this approach has largely been abandoned in favor of noncoplanar VMAT because of its favorable dosimetry and high efficiency.

VMAT

As referred to previously, Clark et al. [22] elucidated a robust technique for treatment of multiple intracranial targets that has been used to treat up to 27 metastases in a single session at our institution [23].

The planning methodology is outlined here but provided in detail in its most updated format for the readers in Appendix 17.1. Plans consist of two to four VMAT arcs, one 360-degree axial arc, and up to three 180° noncoplanar half arcs at couch angles of 45, 90, and 315° (IEC convention). The collimator angle is rotated out of the angle of rotation of the gantry. Further adjustment of the collimator angle for each arc is often advantageous in eliminating or reducing the effect of the island-blocking phenomenon on normal tissue spill. Multiple investigators have independently developed scripted techniques to optimize the jaw and collimator settings for multiple metastases for this purpose. Yuan et al. showed across ten multiple metastasis plans of variable target distribution and geometry that the use of jaw tracking (when primary and secondary jaws of a Linac aperture collimate to the outer MLC boundaries), optimization of the collimator angle, and employment of a highly weighted low-dose constraint consistently result in meaningful reduction in normal tissue low-dose spill as shown in Fig. 17.7 [24–26].

Most treatment planning software inverse-optimization implementations are outfitted with a normal tissue objective (NTO), designed to penalize the spill of dose into tissue not designated as a target by the user in the form of a GTV, CTV, or PTV. There is often an "automatic" NTO that has a default priority by which nontarget

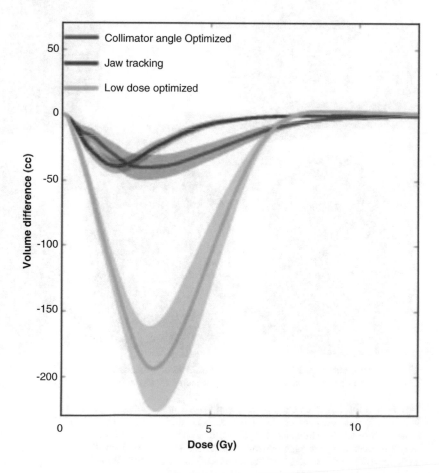

Fig. 17.7 Mean difference between dose volume histograms for normal brain for each parameter. Negative numbers indicate that collimator angle optimization, jaw tracking, or a low-dose objective reduces the volume of normal brain at the given dose. The bands indicate the 95% confidence intervals

tissue is penalized within the optimizer and a "manual" or "custom" NTO. Largely, the classic NTO functionality works well for a target or contiguous targets encompassed by normal tissue, but these NTOs were not designed for the multiple targets found in multiple metastasis SRS plans requiring a sharp gradient in between each, sometimes situated less than a centimeter from each other. A viable solution for the inadequacy of the NTO was to use tuning structures to assist the planner in communicating to the optimizer the goal of rapid dose falloff around each radio-

surgery target. Clark et al. exploited a nested array of concentric shells around each of the targets constructed via the treatment planning software's Boolean operator contouring functionality. Each successive shell structure around the targets penalizes a sequentially reduced dose level to enforce the planner's desire for isotropic rapid falloff around each target (unless another nearby target or organ at risk is present); this concept is demonstrated in Fig. 17.8.

For a constraint-based inverse-optimized plan, the dose falloff will only be penalized unto the

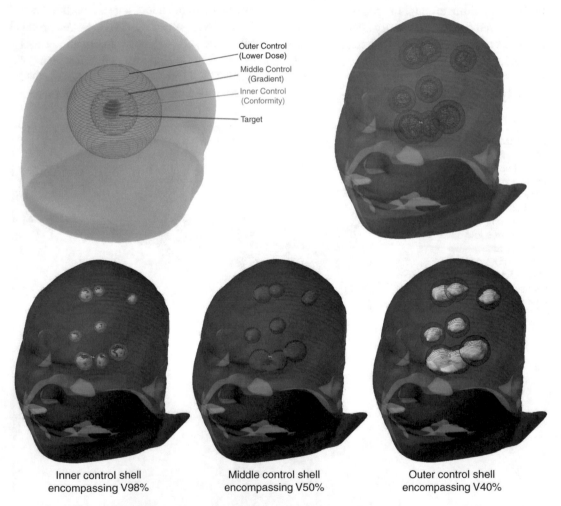

Outer Control
(Lower Dose)

Middle Control
(Gradient)

Inner Control
(Conformity)

Target

Inner control shell
encompassing V98%

Middle control shell
encompassing V50%

Outer control shell
encompassing V40%

Fig. 17.8 (Top left) Depiction of concentric shells utilized to progressively penalize dose falloff at sequentially reduced dose levels. The inner shell emphasizes conformity by containing the high-isodose spill. The middle shell constrains the gradient/moderate-isodose spill. The outer shell constrains the lower-isodose level spill.

Additional shells could of course be added for further or more refined falloff constraint. (Top right) Example of concentric cells applied to a case with eight metastases. (Bottom) Illustration of each shell and the isodose level it constrained in this single-isocenter plan lowest isodose level accorded the largest shell structure unless an additional constraint is added to penalize the very low-isodose spill. At some dose level depending on the number and size of targets, the isodose curves will no longer be discretely quantized around the targets and will become contiguous with each other. If the planner considers the dose spill at lower levels than they are penalizing in the shell structures clinically relevant, he or she must include additional shells at lower levels or include an additional constraint. The planner may constrain a dose-volume threshold or a quantity such as the mean dose to the healthy brain tissue. Either method can perform effectively. The most effective means of constraining low-dose spill has not been established and likely depends on specific optimization algorithm and target number, volume, and distribution. Figure 17.9 shows an example case wherein five metastases were treated with single-isocenter VMAT, with the use of different low-dose constraint criteria compared.

The final consideration of the treatment planning step in development of a single-isocenter multiple metastasis case is the normalization. In multiple-isocenter plans (Gamma Knife (GK) or Linac cone-based), a separate normalization can be undertaken to each isocenter, for each separate target. For multi-isocenter plans, specifically for Gamma Knife plans, each target was typically normalized to a given prescription isodose line. Because there is negligible variation between the fluence of an unplugged shot with a given collimator size, the isodose line associated with optimum gradient is well known, and simplest targeting would be normalized accordingly (e.g., ~50% isodose line for a 4 mm GK shot). In single-isocenter VMAT plans, however, only one normalization can be performed, globally. Therefore, the planner must consider how the normalized fluence will affect the coverage of each of the targets in the plan. Prior to normalization, if one target is overcovered with respect to the rest of the tar-

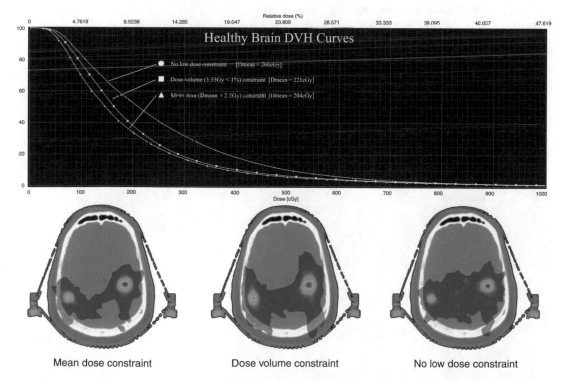

Fig. 17.9 Comparison of the 3.33Gy dose spill for a five metastasis single-isocenter VMAT case between a plan using (left) a mean dose constraint, (middle) a dose-volume constraint to the healthy brain tissue, and (right) no low-dose constraint

gets, that target will remain overcovered after normalization. This at the very least will result in increased low- and moderate-isodose spill around that target, and any nearby organs at risk may receive higher than intended exposure.

The plan will exhibit an optimum balance of coverage with healthy tissue exposure when the entire volume of each target receives exactly or near exactly its prescription dose, as shown in Fig. 17.10.

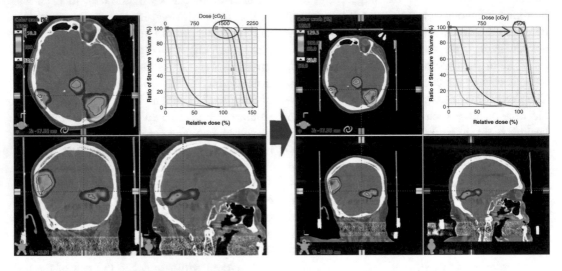

Plan quality for 3 target multi met case

Without & with uniform DVH coverage

Rx =15Gy		
	Non-uniform DVH coverage	Uniform DVH coverage
RTOG CI (L Occip)	1.37	1.04
RTOG CI (Midbrain)	1.18	1.09
RTOG CI (R Occip)	1.64	1.10
Overall plan RTOG CI	1.43	1.06
Healthy brain V12Gy	36.3cc	22.1cc
Healthy brain mean dose	188cGy	164cGy
Healthy brain V25%	358cc	277cc

Fig. 17.10 Comparison of plans for a three target multiple metastasis case (left) without and (right) with uniform DVH coverage. (Bottom) Table shows plan quality improvements associated with ensuring uniform DVH coverage

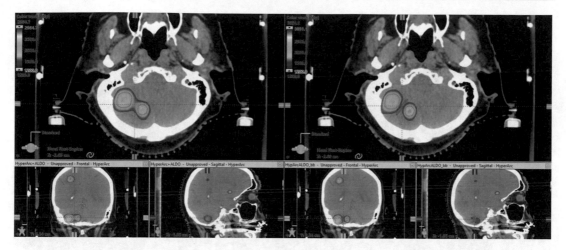

Fig. 17.11 Demonstration of use of a bridge-breaker structure to reduce V12Gy bridging between adjacent structures

Other VMAT Planning Considerations

Bridging

If a plan exhibits "bridging" at an isodose level that the planner considers to be clinically relevant (e.g., the 12Gy isodose line), the planner may wish to reoptimize the plan utilizing a strategy to disrupt the bridging at that level, which can significantly reduce the volume of tissue receiving that dose. Reviewing the beam's-eye view through each arc can help establish whether there is "island blocking" occurring between two targets. If this is the case, then adjustment of the collimator angle may resolve the bridging. If not, the planner can consider the use of a "bridge breaker" tuning structure (shown in Fig. 17.11). This structure is typically a discoid- or wall-shaped structure that is drawn between two targets when undesired bridging is occurring. The structure is then penalized heavily at a dose level below which the bridging was observed. This forces the optimizer to identify alternative fluence patterns to meet the given optimization criteria.

Limiting of Hotspots/Heterogeneity

A surprisingly still controversial topic within single-isocenter VMAT radiosurgery is the question of whether the dose heterogeneity (hotspot) within a target should be constrained. Neurosurgeons and radiation oncologists who trained with a Gamma Knife almost never limit the hotspot beyond selection of the prescription isodose line that produces optimum falloff at the desired level of coverage. This routinely results in hotspots of approximately 200% of the prescription dose at the center of the target. Inversely optimized plans in modern radiosurgery planning platforms rarely exceed Dmax >170% left to their own devices. Some radiation oncologists, however, only feel comfortable with radiosurgery plans whose hotspots are constrained in a similar fashion to conventionally fractionated treatments (Dmax <110%). We strongly caution against this practice, because limiting the hotspot within a target pushes dose outside of the target and worsens the moderate- and low-isodose spillage in a radiosurgery plan. This phenomenon is demonstrated in Fig. 17.12.

While this practice may be sensible when treating large volumes with healthy tissue distributed throughout a PTV, one is hard-pressed to identify a cogent rationale for doing so in a radiosurgery plan for brain metastases, particularly in a metastasis where the hotspot will be located in malignant and possibly hypoxic tissue.

No homogeneity constraint   Homogeneity constraint (*D*max <120%)

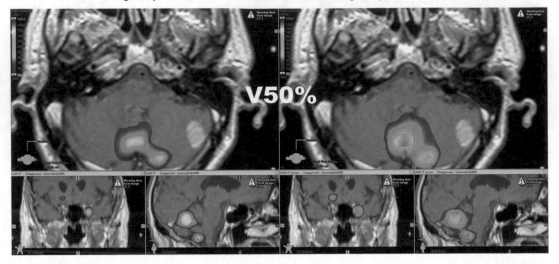

Fig. 17.12 Penalizing the hotspot worsens plan quality. Shown is dose color wash for 50% isodose line for an eight metastasis SRS plan, without a constraint on the hotspot (left) and with a constraint on the hotspot (right). For this case, constraining the hotspot increased the PIV50% by 87% and increased the mean dose to healthy brain tissue by 27%

Single-Isocenter Dynamic Conformal Arc

Another recently developed technique for treating multiple metastases with a single isocenter is single-isocenter dynamic conformal arc (SIDCA). The SIDCA technique was described in 2014 by Huang et al. [27] of Henry Ford Hospital. In a single-isocenter DCA plan, each individual target is treated by a group of conformal arcs. The MLCs are shaped to conform to the projection of target structure, with only one MLC pair being allowed to treat a given lesion at a time. If a given couch and collimator angle result in two targets sharing a leaf pair, the leaf pair will only conform to one, and additional arcs are included to treat the untargeted metastasis. In this manner, SIDCA obligately avoids plans exhibiting the island-blocking phenomenon. Although a single isocenter is used, each lesion can still be normalized separately since a discrete set of fields are treating it independently of other arcs and other lesions. Figure 17.13 illustrates the arc geometry and collimator configuration that would be associated with a SIDCA plan for an eight-metastasis case.

Dynamic conformal arc plans are for the most part forward-optimized and therefore considerably less computationally intensive and quicker to calculate than their VMAT counterparts. There is much less inter-planner variability, as the only meaningful variables that can be adjusted are the collimator angle, arc angles, and prescription normalization values for each target. An optimal solution for these is trivial.

Automated Multiple Metastasis Treatment Planning Solutions

Multiple Metastasis Elements (MME)™

Multiple Metastasis Elements™ is a treatment planning software module by BrainLab within the iPlan™ RT platform specifically designed for single-isocenter conformal arc treatment of multiple metastases. Figure 17.13 demonstrates a typical schema for a MME plan. The software is designed to assess the arrangement of a group of contoured metastases and automatically generate a forward-optimized array of noncoplanar arcs and collimator and collimator angles for a

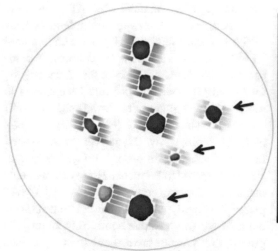

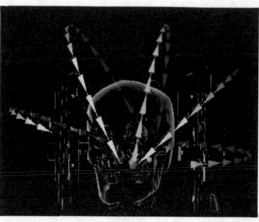

Fig. 17.13 Single-isocenter dynamic conformal arc (SIDCA). In this case, all eight tumors are covered with a field of multi-leaf collimator (left). Three tumors (arrows) are irradiated by "return" arc in this case. All tumors are irradiated by one multi-arc group. Each tumor is targeted by some of the ten arcs, five arcs by "go" and "return," in this case (right). (Figure from Mori et al. [28] and reused without modification under terms of Creative Commons Open Access License)

single-isocenter dynamic conformal arc plan. As illustrated in the diagram, during an arc sweep, all metastases are treated unless one or more metastases are collinear with the collimator angle, in which case only target is treated by that leaf block and the arc is swept in the reverse direction to treat the other collinear target. This technique seeks to solve the island-blocking problem at some expense to efficiency.

HyperArc

HyperArc™ (Varian) is a treatment planning software module within the Eclipse platform designed to streamline and automate single-isocenter VMAT treatment of multiple metastases. Akin to Elements, once targets are designated, the HyperArc module will place an isocenter at the centroid of the targets and offer the planner a selection of two to five (Fig. 17.14) noncoplanar partial arcs that facilitate high-quality treatment but also allow automated movement of the table and delivery of the arcs. To ensure collision-free delivery, Hyper Arc requires the use of the Encompass™ (Qfix, Avondale, PA)

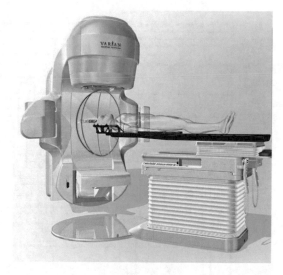

Fig. 17.14 Depiction of the possible arc angles utilized in a HyperArc VMAT SRS treatment

immobilization system. As VMAT is a rotational intensity-modulated treatment, the optimization process is inverse and a full-dose grid calculation follows the optimization. Optimization and calculation require between 5 and 30 minutes depending on the resolution of the dose grid selected and the hardware capabilities of the workstation on which the optimization is being carried out. An example of a HyperArc plan is shown in greater detail in the case example section.

Comparison of Single-Isocenter Treatment Planning Solutions

Both the BrainLab Elements and Varian HyperArc software are examples of automated VMAT single-isocenter planning and consistently generate high-quality radiosurgery plans for multiple brain metastasis cases. Much of the inter-planner variability is removed by such automated VMAT strategies. Two interinstitutional case series comparisons have been performed assessing their relative performances for multiple metastasis cases. A multi-institutional case series [29] between Rutgers, Thomas Jefferson University, and University of Pennsylvania compared

Gamma Knife, manual VMAT planning, HyperArc, and Elements for multiple metastasis SRS cases and found that HyperArc and manual VMAT planning yield superior conformity compared to Gamma Knife (except for <1 cm targets, for which GK was similar) and Elements. The relationships among the lower-isodose spill regions are shown below (Fig. 17.15) in a box plot. In their study, HyperArc demonstrated favorable mean brain dose, V12Gy, V6Gy, and V3Gy compared to Elements. However, Elements plans were superior to manually planned VMAT plans. This study did compare gradient indices, but as there was variable conformity among the groups, those results are difficult to interpret (see Chap. 19).

Another multi-institution study between Thomas Jefferson University and the University of Alabama at Birmingham compared Elements (v1.5) directly with manual VMAT in Eclipse by an expert planner. This study found that manual

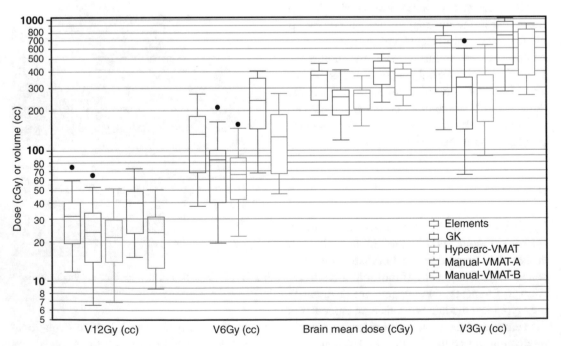

Fig. 17.15 Comparison of moderate- and low-isodose spill volumes between Gamma Knife, BrainLab Elements, Varian HyperArc, and manual VMAT plan for multiple

metastasis SRS cases. (From Vergalasova I, et al. [29]. Reproduced with permission under terms of Creative Commons Attribution License)

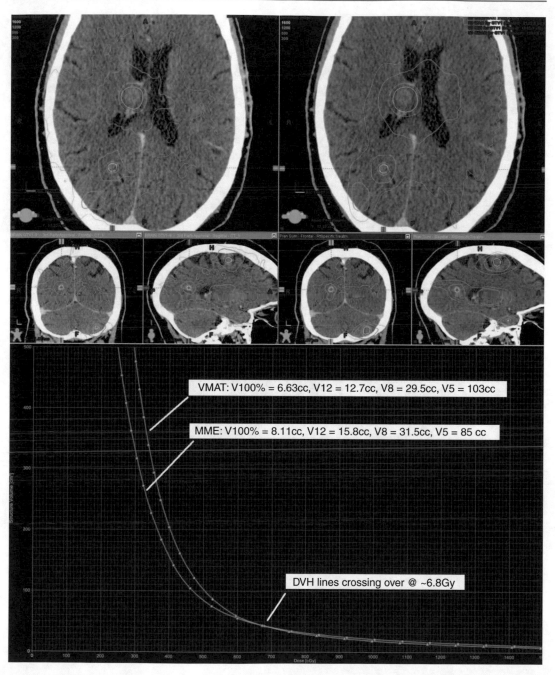

Fig. 17.16 Side-by-side comparison (top left, VMAT; top right, Elements) of dose distributions on axial, sagittal, and coronal CT slice for each target of a representative case having five brain metastases with a total PTV volume of 6.24 cc prescribed 16 Gy. (Bottom) DVH of normal brain tissue for each plan in this case. The DVH lines crossed over at 6.8 Gy

VMAT plans exhibited superior conformity and moderate isodose spill (V12Gy), but Elements plans exhibited better isodose spill in the low-dose regions. Isodose curves and DVH are shown in Fig. 17.16. In both studies, the computer-optimized techniques (manual VMAT, HyperArc) produce more conformal plans than the 3D arc technique (Elements).

Case Vignette

A patient presents with eight intracranial metastases for which radiosurgery in a single fraction is planned. You plan to give 21 Gy to each lesion. You have a TrueBeam STx, with 10MV FFF capability, which is equipped with a HD-MLC with central leaf functional width of 2.5 mm. You have the capability to deliver the SRS treatment with either VMAT or SIDCA. What would a plan look like for each case? What would the plan quality be? What would be the beam-on time?

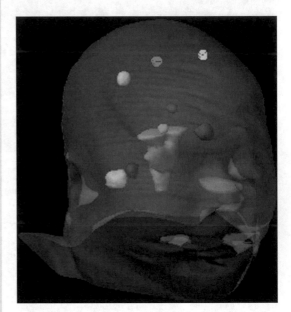

VMAT (RapidArc)

1. Use the Boolean function to create a composite structure of all targets. (Ensure all targets are designated as high-resolution targets.)

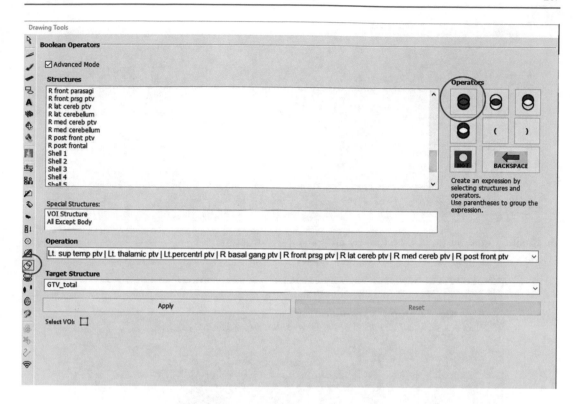

2. Create at least three tuning shell structures around the composite GTV (as described in Appendix 17.1, Section 1.5) by creating a margin around the composite GTV. Starting from the outer expansion, remove each volume from the larger one around it (including the GTV from the inner shell), using the Crop or Boolean function.

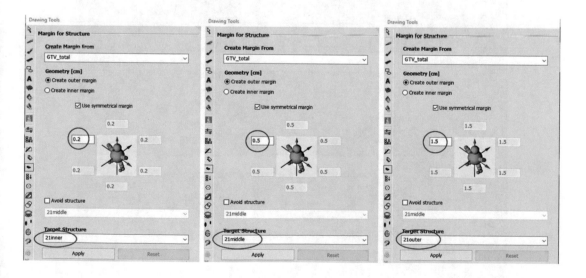

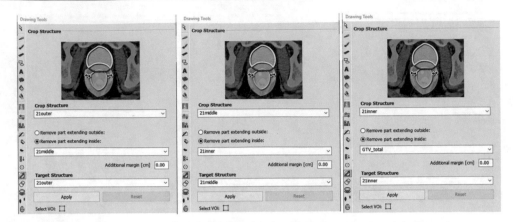

3. Create a healthy brain structure by cropping the "composite GTV" out of the brain structure.

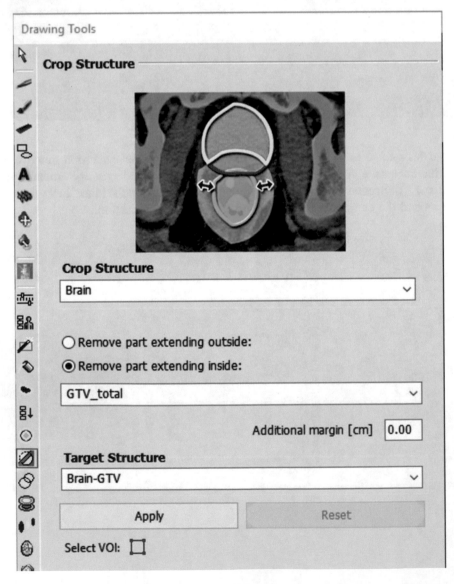

4. Set up your field geometry by utilizing two or more arcs according to Appendix 17.1, Section 2.1. For this case with eight metastases, four arcs were selected. (Note that in his figure, length of the red bar at each control indicates the amount of fluence at that point.)

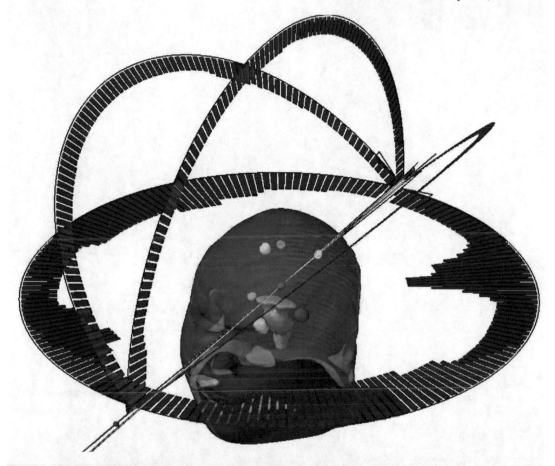

Group	Field ID	Technique	Machine/Energy	MLC	Field Weight	Scale	Gantry Rtn [deg]	Coll Rtn [deg]	Couch Rtn [deg]
I	Field 1	SRS ARC-I	Edge_2613 - 10X-FFF	VMAT	2.105	IEC61217	181.0 CW 179.0	45.0	0.0
I	Field 2	SRS ARC-I	Edge_2613 - 10X-FFF	VMAT	0.688	IEC61217	179.0 CCW 0.0	45.0	315.0
I	Field 3	SRS ARC-I	Edge_2613 - 10X-FFF	VMAT	0.707	IEC61217	0.0 CCW 181.0	45.0	45.0
I	Field 4	SRS ARC-I	Edge_2613 - 10X-FFF	VMAT	0.724	IEC61217	181.0 CW 0.0	45.0	90.0

5. Ensure calculation grid is set to high resolution (0.1–0.125 cm). Designate a floor constraint for each target, a ceiling constraint for each tuning shell, and either a ceiling or mean dose constraint to the healthy brain tissue.

👁	ID/Type	cm³	Vol [%]	Dose[cGy]	Actual Dose [cGy]	Priority	gEUD a	
	Lower	0.2	100.0	2100		50		x
☑	R basal gang ptv	0.3						
	Lower	0.3	100.0	2100		50		x
☑	R front prsg ptv	0.2						
	Lower	0.2	100.0	2100		50		x
☑	R lat cereb ptv	2.5						
	Lower	2.5	100.0	2100		50		x
☑	R med cereb ptv	0.8						
	Lower	0.8	100.0	2100		50		x
☑	R post front ptv	0.7						
	Lower	0.7	100.0	2100		50		x
▣	21inner	9.1						
	Upper	0.0	0.0	2058		50		x
▣	21middle	24.8						
	Upper	0.0	0.0	1050		50		x
▣	21outer	84.9						
	Upper	0.0	0.0	840		50		x
▣	Brain	1170.1						
	Upper	12.9	1.1	350		125		x

6. During optimization, adjust the priorities of the target constraints such that target coverage is homogenous among all the targets (Appendix 17.1, Section 3.6.2.1).

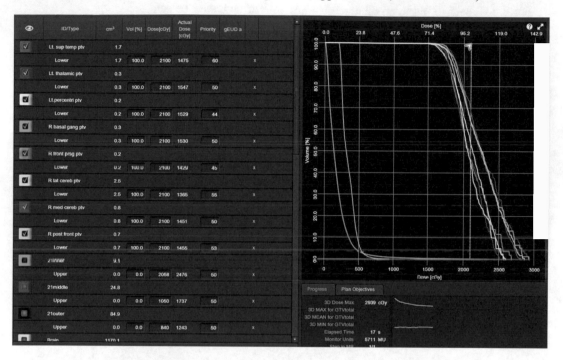

7. Normalize to desired level of coverage. We prefer to normalize such that 100% of prescription dose covers 99% of target volume.

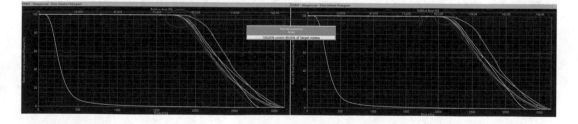

8. Evaluate plan by desired metrics.

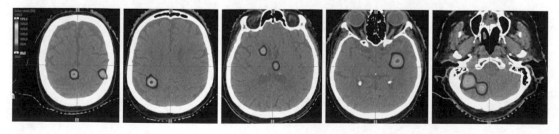

VMAT (HyperArc)

1. For the HyperArc plans, no tuning structures are required. Once targets are contoured, a HyperArc plan is added and the target prescriptions are designated and the desired field arrangement selected.

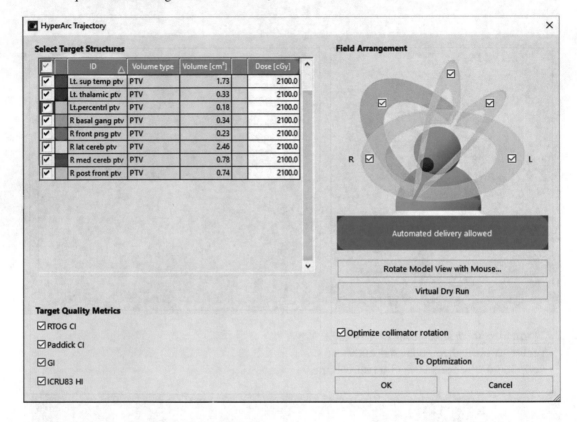

2. SRS NTO (normal tissue objective) replaces the functionality of the tuning structures, and ALDO (automatic low-dose objective) automatically homogenizes the target coverage among multiple structures.

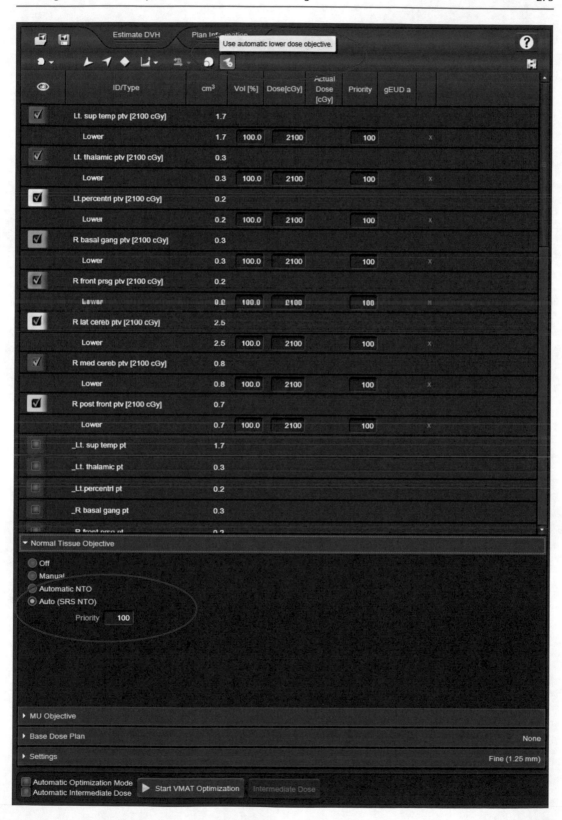

3. After dose calculation, minimal normalization is normally necessary but is sometimes nontrivial if heavily weighted OARs are included in the cost function. Our practice is typically to normalize such that 100% of target dose is delivered to 99% of composite target volume, but if one target is undercovered with respect to the rest and the planner does not desire to replan for uniform coverage, the least covered target can be selected as the normalization target, which will ensure every target is covered.

	Primary Reference Point			Plan Normalization Mode	Plan Normalization Value [%]
ID	Planned Dose per Fraction [cGy]		Planned Total Dose [cGy]		
GTV_total	2100.0		2100.0	100.00% covers 99.00% of Target Volume	92.6

4. After normalization, the final step is plan review and calculation of any quality metrics the planner deems of interest. In addition to target coverage, we typically evaluate the conformity, the R50 (V50%/V100%), a surrogate for radione-crosis risk (largest contiguous V12 region in a single-fraction plan), and any high- to moderate-isodose bridging between nearby targets. HyperArc will display the RTOG CI, Paddick CI, Paddick GI, and ICRU heterogeneity index.

| Fields | Dose | Field Alignments | Plan Objectives | Optimization Objectives | Dose Statistics | Reference Points | Calculation Models | Plan Sum | | | | | | | |

Show DVH	Structure	Approval ...	Plan	Course	Volume [c...	Dose Cove...	Sampling ...	Min Dose ...	Max Dose ...	Mean Dos...	Dose Level...	RTOG CI	Paddick CI	GI	ICRU83 HI
☑	Lt. sup temp ...	Unapproved	PS6	HyperArc	1.7	100.0	100.1	88.7	136.6	112.8	2100.0	0.98	0.79	4.18	0.31
☑	Lt. thalamic p...	Unapproved	PS6	HyperArc	0.3	100.0	100.7	88.0	130.2	112.7	2100.0	1.25	0.63	5.31	0.22
☑	R basal gang ...	Unapproved	PS6	HyperArc	0.3	100.0	99.2	87.0	128.0	109.7	2100.0	1.11	0.58	5.65	0.23
☑	R lat cereb ptv	Unapproved	PS6	HyperArc	2.5	100.0	100.5	83.5	124.5	109.5	2100.0	0.98	0.77	4.44	0.26
☑	R front prsg p...	Unapproved	PS6	HyperArc	0.2	100.0	99.8	92.2	129.4	110.3	2100.0	1.26	0.62	5.72	0.22
☑	R med cereb ...	Unapproved	PS6	HyperArc	0.8	100.0	100.6	83.2	132.6	111.4	2100.0	1.07	0.74	5.42	0.37
☑	R post front p...	Unapproved	PS6	HyperArc	0.7	100.0	100.0	89.9	127.7	110.2	2100.0	1.02	0.71	5.56	0.25
☑	Lt.percentrl ptv	Unapproved	PS6	HyperArc	0.2	100.0	99.9	91.1	133.8	112.6	2100.0	1.23	0.60	6.71	0.24

Appendix 17.1

Updated Institutional Systematic Treatment Planning Technique for Single-Isocenter VMAT Radiosurgery at the University of Alabama at Birmingham
(v. 2019)

1. *Contouring*
    1.1. Contour all normal structures, including the brain, optic nerves, and brainstem.
    1.2. Contour each GTV and label as GTV1, GTV2, GTV3, etc.
    1.3. Using Boolean operations, create a GTV_total; for example, for three targets "GTV_total" = "GTV1" OR ("GTV2" OR "GTV3").
        1.3.1. *Note: previous versions of this guide erroneously used the Boolean operator AND instead of OR.
    1.4. Using Boolean operations, create a structure for healthy brain tissue, i.e., "BRAIN" SUBTRACT "GTV_TOTAL."
    1.5. Create control structures as volumetric shells surrounding the target. In a stepwise fashion, create structures, and use the "margin for structure" function as follows:
        1.5.1.1. "inner control" = GTV_total + 0.2 cm.
        1.5.1.2. "middle control" = GTV_total + 0.5 cm.
        1.5.1.3. "outer control" = GTV_total + 1.5 cm.
        1.5.1.4. Shell sizes in original Technique are listed below, but we have found the smaller shells in general superior for all plans.
            1.5.1.4.1. "inner control" = GTV_total + 0.5 cm.
            1.5.1.4.2. "middle control" = GTV_total + 1.0 cm.
            1.5.1.4.3. "outer control" = GTV_total + 3.0 cm.
        1.5.2. Boolean operation: "outer control" = "outer control" SUB "middle control."

1.5.3. Boolean operation: "middle control" = "middle control" SUB "inner control."

1.5.4. Boolean operation: "inner control" = "inner control" SUB "GTV_total."

1.5.5. Crop any control structures outside the body using Boolean operations.

1.6. *If a plan contains multiple prescriptions, for optimal recipe performance, there should be a separate GTV_total and set of shell structures for each prescription level* (e.g., *GTV_total_18, Outer18, Middle18, Inner18,* etc.).

1.7. If plan contains targets in close proximity, dose "bridging" may occur. This is when the dose cloud at a given isodose level connects two targets. This is only problematic at moderate- to high-isodose levels (e.g., >9 Gy in an 18Gy single-fraction plan).

1.7.1. To mitigate this, create an arbitrary structure in between the two "bridged" targets, and add an optimization criterion that does not permit any of the structure to receive > the dose level of concern less 1 Gy (e.g., if 9Gy level is of concern: upper constraint, 0% of structure receiving 8Gy). If this does not alleviate bridging, increase priority of this structure or lower control dose in constraint.

1.8. For DVH calculation of conformity indices, create evaluation structures using the "margin for structure" function as before:

$$"GTV1\_eval" = GTV1 + 1.0\,cm, "GTV2\_eval" = GTV2 + 1.0\,cm, etc.$$

1.8.1. For a single target, this is not necessary; the prescription isodose volume of the BODY structure may be used for conformity calculation, or Eclipse will calculate the RTOG CI automatically in the dose statistics tab.

1.9. For maximum accuracy (and possibly for increased plan quality for plans with very small targets), right click on each target structure and select "high-resolution segment."

1.9.1. In the External Beam Planning window, select Calculation Models, click Edit next to the appropriate Volume Dose Algorithm, and change the dose grid resolution to 0.1 cm from 0.25 cm. (Note that this will significantly increase the time required for calculation – using Acuros algorithm will mitigate time increase.)

2. *Isocenter and Field Geometry*

2.1. Consider arc geometries as follows (Fig. 17.17) (they are ordered for optimal delivery):

Arc number	Field	Arc length (°)	Table rotation (°)	Collimator angle (°)	Arc direction	Gantry angle (°)	Stop angle (°)
1	1	360	0	45	CW	181	179
2	1	360	0	45	CW	181	179
	2	180	315/45/90[a]	45	CCW	180	0
3	1	360	0	45	CW	181	179
	2	180	315	45	CCW	180	0
	3	180	45	315	CCW	0	180
4	1	360	0	45	CW	181	179
	2	180	315	45	CCW	179	0
	3	180	45	315	CCW	0	181
	4	180	90	45	CW	181	0

[a]Choosing a 315° or 45° instead of a 90° couch kick for this arc forces some of the exit dose to spill out the sides of the head instead of into the body. Please note some Linacs may be configured with default table rotation to be 180° instead of 0°

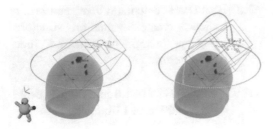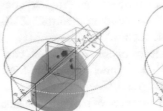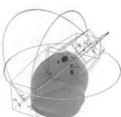

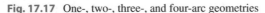

Fig. 17.17 One-, two-, three-, and four-arc geometries

2.2. Place isocenter at the geometric center of GTV_total by right-clicking a field and selecting "Align grouped fields to structure [GTV_total]."

   2.2.1. If this places the isocenter too close to a large target such that a small target is not within space covered by leaves, the isocenter can be manually adjusted so that all targets are within the field.

3. *Plan Optimization and Normalization*

   3.1. If available, enable jaw tracking.

   3.2. Each individual GTV (not the composite) receives the lower objective: 100% of the target to receive 100% of the prescription dose; default priority = 50 (this can be adjusted to 100 according to planner preference, but if done, adjust other priorities in similar proportion).

   3.3. What you prioritize most in the plan should get the highest optimization priority; normalization will scale the dose so that adequate target coverage occurs.

   3.4. For a plan with no critical OARs and in which low-dose spill to healthy tissue is to be minimized, each control structure receives the following upper objective:

   3.4.1. Inner control: 0% of the structure to receive 98% of the prescription dose; priority = 50.

   3.4.2. Middle control: 0% of the structure to receive 50% of the prescription dose; priority = 50.

   3.4.3. Outer control: 0% of the structure to receive 40% of the prescription dose; priority = 50.

   3.4.4. Healthy brain: 1% of the structure to receive one-sixth of the prescription dose; priority = 125 (in our experience, this is typically about the point where the healthy tissue DVH curve's inflection point should be, which corresponds to the modal dose on the healthy brain's DDH curve).

   3.4.4.1. Note that weighting this priority to such a high value will lead to a lower plan normalization value (and thus a higher degree of normalization). If the value becomes such that you are uncomfortable with the level of post-calculation MU scaling, then reduce the priority of this criterion.

   3.4.4.2. Further note that these priority values are surrogates for weighting coefficients in the mathematical expression being optimized. They are proportional.

3.5. Additional dose constraint objectives may be needed if sensitive adjacent normal structures are within the region of the control structures (e.g., brainstem, optic nerves, chiasm, etc.). If not nearby, control structures will adequately serve as constraints on limiting dose to these organs.

   3.5.1. For example, if the brainstem overlaps the inner control shell, consider the following additional constraint – brainstem: 0% of the structure to receive 800 cGy; priority = 75. Priority must be ≥ priority of control structure with which organ at risk overlaps or optimization algorithm will not take objective into consideration as desired.

3.6. For multiple target plans with identical prescriptions, low-isodose spill is minimized when prescription isodose coverage is homogeneous across all targets. This is because normalization occurs for the entire plan and not for each target independently, as in a Gamma Knife plan.

   3.6.1. On the DVH, homogenous target coverage will appear as all target DVH lines superimposing one another at the prescription isodose point (Fig. 17.18).

      3.6.1.1. Note: homogenous target coverage is not to be confused with plan homogeneity (minimizing hot spots within tumor volume).

   3.6.2. We have found that plan quality can be increased by freezing the optimization on the first step of the first level and waiting for the optimization to stabilize (indicated by a leveling out of the line for each structure in the optimization line graph). Increase or decrease the priority of each structure's cost function as needed to achieve homogeneous target coverage. Once reached, unfreeze the optimization from the first level.

      3.6.2.1. If the plan finishes and DVH shows heterogeneous coverage, one can reinitiate optimization and "Continue the previous optimization." The optimization will start frozen in the final level. Cost function priorities can also be adjusted here

to achieve the desired homogeneity of coverage.

3.7. Normalize plan for desired coverage. We utilize a normalization that delivers 100% of the prescription to 99–100% of the GTV_total, and ensure that each target has received appropriate coverage.

3.8. For plans with targets of differing prescriptions, ensuring each target receives sufficient coverage but not excessive coverage can sometimes require additional effort.

   3.8.1. During the initial optimization, freeze the optimization at the first or second level of the multilevel resolution optimization and pick one target as an anchor.

   3.8.2. For each other target, adjust the priority of its optimization constraint such that its DVH curve is covering a dose the same percentage difference from the anchor curve as the percentage difference between the two targets' respective prescription doses.

      3.8.2.1. For example, prescription dose for target A is 18 Gy and is 24 Gy for target B ($\Delta = 6$ Gy or 25%). Target A is designated as the anchor target. If, during the initial phase of the optimization, target A's DVH curve indicates 100% coverage at 12 Gy, then adjust target B's optimization constraint priority such that its curve indicates 100% coverage at 12 + 25% or 15Gy. Thus, when the post-optimization plan-wide normalization is performed, each target should have roughly 100% coverage at its respective prescription dose.

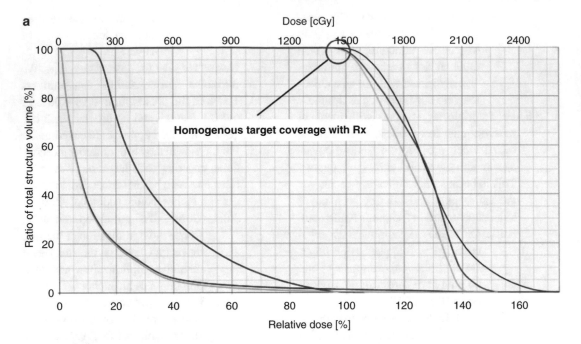

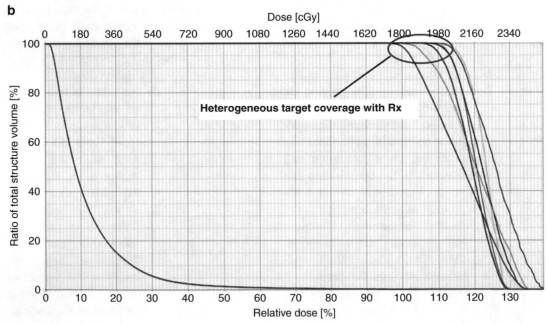

Fig. 17.18 Homogeneous (**a**) and heterogeneous (**b**) target coverage with 100% prescription dose

4. *Plan Evaluation*
  4.1. Calculate the conformity index (CI) of each target by using the evaluation structures.
    4.1.1. Ensure that 100% isodose line is not extending outside of evaluation structures (if it does, you do

not have a very good plan) or overlapping with another target's 100% isodose line.
    4.1.2. RTOG CI = 100% isodose line of eval structure divided by the target volume; for example: CI for GTV1 = 100% isodose line for

"GTV1_eval" divided by the volume of GTV1.

4.1.2.1. CI can also be calculated by the Eclipse treatment planning software, but the current software version will not accurately compute the CI if the plan contains more than one target; in such cases, the individual target 100% isodose volume can be obtained by extracting the prescription volume from each evaluation structure.

4.2. Evaluate the high- to moderate-dose falloff.

4.2.1. Paddick gradient index (GI) or the R50% of the plan

4.2.1.1. GI = volume of 50% isodose line ($V_{50\%}$) divided by the volume of the 100% prescription isodose line (PIV).

4.2.1.2. R50% = volume of 50% isodose line ($V_{50\%}$) divided by the total target volume (GTV_total).

4.2.1.3. Note that Eclipse will calculate a gradient measure which is a different definition than the above calculated GI.

4.2.1.4. Also note that the Paddick GI cannot be used to accurately compare the dose falloff between plans with different conformity indices. This is because different conformity indices indicate different 100% prescription isodose volumes.

4.2.2. For comparing the high- to moderate-isodose falloff between two radiosurgery plans of differing conformities, we recommend comparing either:

4.2.2.1. AUC-DVH – the area under the DVH curve in the region of interest (e.g., 9 to 18Gy)

4.2.2.1.1. This can be done easily in by exporting the DVH at a sufficiently fine-dose resolution (e.g., 1cGy) to excel and utilizing the trapezoidal rule for numerical integration.

4.2.2.2. R50% – volume of 50% isodose line ($V_{50\%}$) divided by the total target volume (GTV_total)

References

1. Modh A, Burmeister C, Elshaikh M, Siddiqui F, Siddiqui S, Shah M. Radiation utilization trends in the treatment of brain metastases from non-small cell lung cancer. Int J Radiat Oncol Biol Phys. 2017;99(2):E94.
2. Network NCC. Central Nervous System Cancers (Version 1.2019) [03/15/2019]. Available from: https://www.nccn.org/professionals/physician_gls/pdf/cns.pdf.
3. Woo SY, Grant WH III, Bellezza D, Grossman R, Gildenberg P, Carpenter LS, et al. A comparison of intensity modulated conformal therapy with a conventional external beam stereotactic radiosurgery system for the treatment of single and multiple intracranial lesions. Int J Radiat Oncol Biol Phys. 1996;35(3):593–7.
4. Yu CX. Intensity-modulated arc therapy with dynamic multileaf collimation: an alternative to tomotherapy. Phys Med Biol. 1995;40(9):1435–49.
5. Otto K. Volumetric modulated arc therapy: IMRT in a single gantry arc. Med Phys. 2008;35(1):310–7.
6. Lagerwaard F, Verbakel W, van der Hoorn E, Slotman B, Senan S. Volumetric modulated arc therapy (RapidArc) for rapid, non-invasive stereotactic radiosurgery of multiple brain metastases. Int J Radiat Oncol Biol Phys. 2008;72(1):S530.

7. Kang J, Ford EC, Smith K, Wong J, McNutt TR. A method for optimizing LINAC treatment geometry for volumetric modulated arc therapy of multiple brain metastases. Med Phys. 2010;37(8):4146–54.

8. Clark GM, Popple RA, Young PE, Fiveash JB. Feasibility of single-isocenter volumetric modulated arc radiosurgery for treatment of multiple brain metastases. Int J Radiat Oncol Biol Phys. 2010;76(1):296–302.

9. McDonald D, Schuler J, Takacs I, Peng J, Jenrette J, Vanek K. Comparison of radiation dose spillage from the Gamma Knife Perfexion with that from volumetric modulated arc radiosurgery during treatment of multiple brain metastases in a single fraction. J Neurosurg. 2014;121(Suppl 2):51–9.

10. Han EY, Kim G-Y, Rebueno N, Yeboa DN, Briere TM. End-to-end testing of automatic plan optimization using RayStation scripting for hypofractionated multimetastatic brain stereotactic radiosurgery. Med Dosim. 2019;44(4):e44–50.

11. Ma L, Nichol A, Hossain S, Wang B, Petti P, Vellani R, et al. Variable dose interplay effects across radiosurgical apparatus in treating multiple brain metastases. Int J Comput Assist Radiol Surg. 2014;9(6):1079–86.

12. Ma L, Petti P, Wang B, Descovich M, Chuang C, Barani IJ, et al. Apparatus dependence of normal brain tissue dose in stereotactic radiosurgery for multiple brain metastases. J Neurosurg. 2011;114(6):1580–4.

13. Thomas EM, Popple RA, Wu X, Clark GM, Markert JM, Guthrie BL, et al. Comparison of plan quality and delivery time between volumetric arc therapy (RapidArc) and Gamma Knife radiosurgery for multiple cranial metastases. Neurosurgery. 2014;75(4):409–18.

14. Jang SY, Lalonde R, Ozhasoglu C, Burton S, Heron D, Huq MS. Dosimetric comparison between cone/Iris-based and InCise MLC-based CyberKnife plans for single and multiple brain metastases. J Appl Clin Med Phys. 2016;17(5):184–99.

15. Ermiş E, Blatti-Moreno M, Leiser D, Cihoric N, Schmidhalter D, Henzen D, et al. Dose analysis of InCise 2 multi leaf collimator and IRIS-based stereotactic radiotherapy plans for brain and liver tumors. Biomed Phys Eng Express. 2019;5(3):035007.

16. Hoogeman MS, Nuyttens JJ, Levendag PC, Heijmen BJ. Time dependence of intrafraction patient motion assessed by repeat stereoscopic imaging. Int J Radiat Oncol Biol Phys. 2008;70(2):609–18.

17. Kim J, Hsia A, Xu Z, Ryu S. Motion likelihood over spine radiosurgery treatments—an intrafraction motion analysis. Int J Radiat Oncol Biol Phys. 2017;99(2):E678.

18. Roper J, Chanyavanich V, Betzel G, Switchenko J, Dhabaan A. Single-isocenter multiple-target stereotactic radiosurgery: risk of compromised coverage. Int J Radiat Oncol Biol Phys. 2015;93(3):540–6.

19. Babic S, Lee Y, Ruschin M, Lochray F, Lightstone A, Atenafu E, et al. To frame or not to frame? Cone-beam CT-based analysis of head immobilization devices specific to linac-based stereotactic radiosurgery and radiotherapy. J Appl Clin Med Phys. 2018;19(2):111–20.

20. Covington EL, Fiveash JB, Wu X, Brezovich I, Willey CD, Riley K, et al. Optical surface guidance for sub-millimeter monitoring of patient position during frameless stereotactic radiotherapy. J Appl Clin Med Phys. 2019;20(6):91–8.

21. Yuan Y, Thomas EM, Clark GM, Fiveash JB, Popple RA, editors. Factors influencing normal brain dose for single-isocenter multi-target radiosurgery. AAPM 55th annual meeting & exhibition; 2013 Aug 4–8; Indianapolis, IN.

22. Clark GM, Popple RA, Prendergast BM, Spencer SA, Thomas EM, Stewart JG, et al. Plan quality and treatment planning technique for single isocenter cranial radiosurgery with volumetric modulated arc therapy. Pract Radiat Oncol. 2012;2(4):306–13.

23. Thomas EM FC-G, Dempsey K, Riley K, Fiveash JB, Popple RA, Bredel M. Treatment of 27 brain metastases with single-isocenter VMAT radiosurgery: a case report. 13th international stereotactic radiosurgery society congress; Montreaux, Switzerland, 2017.

24. Yuan Y, Thomas EM, Clark GA, Markert JM, Fiveash JB, Popple RA. Evaluation of multiple factors affecting normal brain dose in single-isocenter multiple target radiosurgery. J Radiosurg SBRT. 2018;5(2):131–44.

25. Wu Q, Snyder KC, Liu C, Huang Y, Zhao B, Chetty IJ, et al. Optimization of treatment geometry to reduce normal brain dose in radiosurgery of multiple brain metastases with single–Isocenter volumetric modulated arc therapy. Sci Rep. 2016;6:34511.

26. Huang Y, Yue H, Wang M, Li S, Zhang J, Liu Z, et al. Fully automated searching for the optimal VMAT jaw settings based on Eclipse Scripting Application Programming Interface (ESAPI) and RapidPlan knowledge-based planning. J Appl Clin Med Phys. 2018;19(3):177–82.

27. Huang Y, Chin K, Robbins JR, Kim J, Li H, Amro H, et al. Radiosurgery of multiple brain metastases with single-isocenter dynamic conformal arcs (SIDCA). Radiother Oncol. 2014;112(1):128–32.

28. Mori Y, Kaneda N, Hagiwara M, Ishiguchi T. Dosimetric study of automatic brain metastases planning in comparison with conventional multi-isocenter dynamic conformal arc therapy and gamma knife radiosurgery for multiple brain metastases. Cureus. 2016;8(11):e882.

29. Vergalasova I, Liu H, Alonso-Basanta M, Dong L, Li J, Nie K, et al. Multi-institutional dosimetric evaluation of modern day stereotactic radiosurgery (SRS) treatment options for multiple brain metastases. Front Oncol. 2019;9:483.

Dose Tolerances in Brain Metastasis Management

Giuseppe Minniti, Claudia Scaringi, and Barbara Tolu

Introduction

The clinical management of patients with brain metastases has changed substantially in the last years, with a shift away from whole-brain radiation therapy (WBRT) to stereotactic radiosurgery (SRS). Currently, SRS alone is the recommended treatment for patients with a limited number (up to five) of brain metastases. Its efficacy has been demonstrated in randomized trials that report a local control of approximately 75% or more at 1 year and survival benefit similar to that observed with the use of SRS plus WBRT but lower risk of long-term neurotoxicity [1–4].

According to Radiation Therapy Oncology Group (RTOG) 90-05 guidelines [5], small lesions ≤20 mm can be treated with up to 24 Gy to the margin of the lesion, those between 21 and 30 mm with 18 Gy, and those between 31 and 40 mm with 15 Gy. As shown in the study, single-fraction SRS was effective at both controlling tumor growth and sparing normal tissue, although the ability to deliver an effective and safe dose was limited for tumors larger than 2–3 cm

In the last years, multi-fraction SRS (nominally 2–5 fractions), also called hypofractionated SRS, fractionated SRS, multidose SRS, multi-session SRS, or hypofractionated stereotactic radiotherapy, has been employed as an alternative to single-fraction SRS with the aim to provide an improved balance of tumor control and normal brain toxicity, particularly for larger lesions and for those located in proximity or within critical brain areas, since high single doses are perceived to carry higher risks of neurological complications. Using doses of 24–35 Gy given in 3–5 fractions, several retrospective studies have reported a local control from 70% to 90% at 1 year, with a relatively low risk of brain tissue damage in the range of 2–10% [6–12].

The linear-quadratic (LQ) model is generally used to compare the biologically effective dose (BED) of different fractionation schedules given a specific α/β ratio, total dose (D), and dose/fractionation (d) according to the formula $BED = D[1 + d/(\alpha/\beta)]$ [13]; however, its application for doses above 8–10 Gy, as used for multi-fraction SRS, remains controversial [14]; thus, different models have been created. Joiner et al. [15] have proposed the linear-quadratic-cubic model, in which BEDs are calculated by adding an additional term proportional to the cube of dose to the formula of the linear-quadratic

G. Minniti (✉)
Department of Medicine, Surgery and Neuroscience, University of Siena, Siena, Italy

Radiation Oncology Unit, UPMC Hillman Cancer Center, San Pietro Hospital, Rome, Italy
e-mail: minnitig@upmc.edu

C. Scaringi · B. Tolu
Radiation Oncology Unit, UPMC Hillman Cancer Center, San Pietro Hospital, Rome, Italy

© Springer Nature Switzerland AG 2020
Y. Yamada et al. (eds.), *Radiotherapy in Managing Brain Metastases*,
https://doi.org/10.1007/978-3-030-43740-4_18

model; according to this model, three fractions of 8.5–9 Gy for larger lesions, which correspond to 20–22 Gy given in a single fraction, are potentially associated with higher efficacy and lower risk of radiation necrosis than single-fraction doses of 15–18 Gy used for equivalent volumes.

In clinical practice, minimizing radiation-induced normal tissue damage in the normal brain is a key objective of SRS; for both single-fraction and multi-fraction SRS, brain tissue dose constraints include several structures, e.g., the brainstem, cranial nerves, cochlea, and motor and sensory cortex. In this chapter, we have summarized current clinical evidences of radiation tolerance to cranial SRS of the brain. The impact of dose, volume, fractionation, and other relevant clinic-pathologic variables is discussed.

Evidence Base

SRS plays a fundamental role in the treatment of brain metastases, but it is associated with the risk of inducing harmful effects on the healthy tissues surrounding the lesion. It is therefore important to quantify this risk so as to be able to reduce treatment-related toxicity. In the clinical case illustrated below (Case Vignette 1), a patient

with breast cancer received SRS for intracranial progression of her disease. Four lesions <2 cm in size received single-fraction SRS, and one lesion >3 cm in size was treated with multi-fraction SRS. According to the above considerations, the choice of dose and fractionation was largely based on minimizing the risk of neurological toxicity.

Clinical recommendations for the dose tolerance limits of normal tissues for patients receiving SRS treatments to the brain come from the "Quantitative Analysis of Normal Tissue Effects in the Clinic" or QUANTEC papers [16–19] published in 2010 by a joint American Association of Physics in Medicine (AAPM) and American Society of Therapeutic Radiology and Oncology (ASTRO) committee. The QUANTEC papers essentially present a critical review of the existing literature on radiation dose/volume/outcome for normal tissue, providing recommendations on dose-volume limits of normal tissue toxicity for 16 anatomic sites and type of irradiation, including the use of SRS in the brain. However, data of tolerance doses to multi-fraction SRS are quite limited, and dose constraints remain not validated. A summary on normal tissue constraints for single-dose SRS and multi-fraction SRS is shown in Tables 18.1 and 18.2.

Table 18.1 Summary of normal tissue constrains following single-fraction radiosurgery (SRS)

Organ	Type of radiation	Dose toxicity	Dose volume parameters	Toxicity	References
Brain	Single-fraction SRS	V12 <5–10 cc (<20)	Rapid rise when V12 >10 cc	Symptomatic necrosis	QUANTEC [16, 17, 21, 22, 33]
Brainstem	Single-fraction SRS	Dmax <12.5 (<5)	Risk for dose to one-third of brainstem 12.5 Gy (1%), 14.2 Gy (13%), 16 Gy (61%), and 17.5 (94%)	Permanent neurological deficit or necrosis	QUANTEC [36]
Optic nerve/ chiasm	Single-fraction SRS	Dmax <8 Gy (<3), Dmax 8–12 Gy (<10), Dmax >12 Gy (>10),	Low risk for dose <12 Gy to 2–4 mm3	Optic neuropathy	QUANTEC [18, 43, 44]
Spinal cord	Single-fraction SRS	Dmax <13 Gy (<1)		Myelopathy	QUANTEC [19]
Cavernous sinus cranial nerves	Single-fraction SRS	Dmax 16–18 Gy (<4)		Permanent cranial nerve deficit	[40, 41]

Table 18.2 Unvalidated normal tissue dose constraints for multi-fraction radiosurgery (SRS)

Organ	Type of radiation	Dose (toxicity rate %)	Dose volume parameters	Toxicity (Grade 3)	References
Brain	3-fraction SRS	27 Gy in 3 fractions (5–10)	5% for $V_{18} \leq 30.2$ ml 14% for $V_{18} > 30.2$ ml	Symptomatic necrosis	[6, 7]
Brainstem	3-fraction SRS, 5-fraction SRS	18 Gy (6 Gy/fx) to <1 ml (<3%) 26 (5.2 Gy/fx) to <1 ml (<3%)	Dmax 23 Gy (7.67 Gy/fx) Dmax 31 Gy (6.2 Gy/fx)	Permanent cranial deficit or necrosis	[39]
Optic nerve/ chiasm	3-fraction SRS, 5-fraction SRS	15 (5 Gy/fx) to 0.2 ml (<3%) 20 (4.0 Gy/fx) to 0.2 ml (<3%)	Dmax 19.5 Gy (6.5 Gy/fx) Dmax 25 Gy (5 Gy/fx)	Optic neuropathy	[39, 50]
Cochlea	3-fraction SRS, 5-fraction SRS		Dmax 20 Gy (6.67 Gy/fx) Dmax 25 Gy (5 Gy/fx)	Hearing loss	[39]
Spinal cord	3-fraction SRS, 5-fraction SRS	18 (6 Gy/fx) to 0.25 ml (<1%) 22.5 (4.5 Gy/fx) to 0.25 ml (<1%)	Dmax 22.5 Gy (6.67 Gy/fx) Dmax 30 Gy (6 Gy/fx)	Myelopathy	[19, 39]

Normal Tissue Dose Constraints of the Central Nervous System

Normal Brain Parenchyma

In SRS of brain lesions, normal tissue toxicity appears to be a function of dose, volume, and proximity to eloquent sensitive brain structures. The end point for assessing radiation-induced complications in the brain is typically the development of brain radiation necrosis which is associated with the presence of different degrees of neurological deficits in up to one-third of patients [16–23]. Other measures have included steroid usage, preservation of performance status, and neurocognitive function [2, 4]. Factors correlated with the development of radiation-induced brain necrosis are the radiation dose, the target volume, and the volume of the normal brain irradiated to various doses.

The diagnosis of radiation necrosis is challenging [24]. Surgical exploration including biopsy is the gold standard for the histological confirmation of radiation necrosis or tumor progression. Using conventional magnetic resonance imaging (MRI), the areas of radiation necrosis appear in T2-weighted sequences as hyperintensity of the white matter and in T1-weighted sequences as increases in tumor contrast enhancement or as space-occupying enhancing lesions with a central necrotic area, although the predictive of these features is low [25]. Integration of "conventional"

with advanced MRI techniques, such as diffusion-weighted imaging, MR spectroscopy, and MR perfusion, may be helpful to differentiate tumor progression from radiation necrosis [26, 27]. In addition to advanced MRI techniques, positron-emission tomography (PET), especially using amino acid analogues, such as ^{11}C methionine (MET), ^{18}F fluoroethyl-tyrosine (FET), and, more recently, ^{18}F fluoro-dihydroxy-phenylalanine (F-DOPA), has emerged as a promising technique with high sensitivity and specificity in the differential diagnosis of radiation necrosis and recurrence after SRS [28–31]. Thus, the variable rate of brain necrosis following radiation in the brain reported in different published studies may, at least in part, reflect the different diagnostic accuracy of various assessment techniques.

In the RTOG 90-05 dose-escalation study of SRS to recurrent brain metastases and primary tumors in patients who previously received whole- or partial-brain irradiation, the rates of late toxicities resulting in irreversible severe neurological symptoms were 10% for lesions <2 cm receiving 24 Gy, 14% for those 2.1–3 cm receiving 18 Gy, and 20% for those 3.1–4 cm receiving 15 Gy [5]. In another RTOG trial (RTOG 95-08) including 333 patients with brain metastases who were randomized to receive SRS plus WBRT or WBRT alone, grade 3 and 4 acute and late toxicities were observed in 3% and 6% of patients who received SRS using the dose constraints developed in RTOG 90-05 [32].

In several published studies, a common powerful independent predictive factor for the development of radiation necrosis is the volume of normal brain receiving 10 Gy (V_{10}) or 12 Gy (V_{12}) [17, 21, 22, 33]. Based on the review of these results, QUANTEC recommendations indicate a risk of symptomatic radionecrosis up to 20% for V_{12} of 5–10 cm^3. In a series of 63 patients with a total of 173 brain metastases treated with single-fraction SRS, Blonigen et al. [21] have reported a significant risk of radiation necrosis up to 68.8% for V_{10} Gy >14.5 cm^3 and V_{12} Gy >10.8 cm^3, respectively. In contrast, no cases of radiation necrosis were observed for V_{10} Gy <0.68 cm^3 and V_{12} Gy <0.5 cm^3. In another series of 206 patients with 310 metastases who underwent single-fraction SRS at the University of Rome Sapienza Sant'Andrea Hospital between September 2006 and January 2010 for one to four brain metastases, the 1-year rates of radiation necrosis were 0% for V_{12} <3.3 cm^3, 16% for V_{12} of 3.3–5.9 cm^3, 24% for V_{12} of 6.0–10.9 cm^3, and 51% for V_{12} >10.9 cm^3 [22].

These findings have important clinical implication in daily practice. When RTOG-recommended radiosurgery doses are applied to spherical lesions of 2, 3, and 4 cm in diameter, corresponding to volumes of 4.3, 14.1, and 33.4 cm^3, the calculated V_{12} are about 21, 57, and 101 cm^3, respectively, resulting in a significant risk of radiation necrosis. In addition, the rapid increase of neurological complications as the V_{12} increases beyond 5–10 cm^3 suggests that margins of 1–2 mm applied to the gross tumor volume (GTV) to generate a planning target volume (PTV) may result in an unacceptable risk of radiation necrosis even when treating small lesions; in general, the target volume will double when adding 1 mm GTV-to-PTV margin to a lesion of 8 mm or 2 mm margin to a lesion of 15 mm in size. This means that GTV-to-PTV expansions of 0, 1, and 2 mm to a lesion of 1.5 cm^3 receiving a single dose of 24 Gy result in PTVs of 1.5, 2.1, and 2.8 cm^3 and V_{12} of 3.8, 7.7, and 11.4 cm^3, respectively, potentially causing a significant increase in the risk of radiation necrosis.

Multi-fraction SRS is usually utilized in the treatment of large brain metastases when high-dose single-fraction SRS would result in unacceptable risks of severe neurological toxicity. Using radiation

doses of 24–35 Gy given in 3–5 fractions, several studies report a relatively low risk of symptomatic radiation necrosis in the range of 2–10% [6–12]; however, there is little systematic reporting on normal tissue dose constraints for hypofractionated regimens using fraction sizes in the 6–9 Gy range. Minniti et al. [6] have reported the clinical outcomes of 289 patients with brain metastases >2.0 cm in size who received single-fraction SRS (16–18 Gy) or multi-fraction SRS (3 × 9 Gy given in 3 consecutive days) at the University of Rome Sapienza between 2008 and 2014. Cumulative local control rates were 90% after multi-fraction SRS and 77% after single-fraction SRS at 12 months ($p = 0.01$), with a 12-month risk of developing radiation brain necrosis of 18% and 9% ($p = 0.01$), respectively. For patients receiving multi-fraction SRS, the volume of normal brain receiving doses of 18 Gy (V_{18}) was the most significant predictor of brain necrosis; the incidence was 5% for V_{18} ≤30 cm^3 and 14% for V_{18} >30 cm^3 ($p = 0.04$). According to quartiles distribution, the 12-month risk of developing brain necrosis was 0%, 6%, 13%, and 24% for volumes <22.8 cm^3, 22.8–30.2 cm^3, 30.3–41.2 cm^3, and >41.2 cm^3, respectively.

Brainstem

The brainstem is comprised of the midbrain, pons, and medulla. For single-fraction SRS, maximum brainstem doses of 12–14 Gy are associated with a rate of neurological complications <5%, although this risk significantly increases for doses >15 Gy given in single fraction [34–38]. In QUANTEC review of radiation-associated brainstem toxicity, Mayo et al. [36] calculated a risk of normal tissue complication probability of 1%, 13%, 61%, and 94% for partial volume irradiation of one-third of the brainstem to doses of 12.5, 14.2, 16, and 17.5 Gy, respectively, although lower risks of complications may be predicted when the same doses are delivered to a small partial volume (<1%). In a large retrospective study of 547 patients with 596 brainstem metastases treated receiving SRS with a median marginal dose of 16 Gy, local control was 81.8% at 1 year [38]. Forty-four patients (7.4%) developed grades 3–4 toxicity as a result of treatment at any time point in follow-up. Increasing tumor volume, increasing margin dose, and prior WBRT were associated with increased odds of severe toxicity after SRS ($p < 0.001$, $p = 0.049$, and $p = 0.002$, respectively). Currently, no definitive conclusions can be drawn regarding dose-volume effects on brainstem dose tolerance after single-fraction SRS; although single radiation doses to small brainstem volumes up to 20 Gy have been used to treat brainstem metastases with a low reported rate of complication, caution should be used in routine clinical practice when delivering doses to the brainstem >16 Gy.

There is little normal tissue dose constraints data for the multi-fraction SRS of the brainstem. In general, a risk of permanent neurological deficits <3% is predicted when lesions treated with 3-fraction or 5-fraction SRS receive a maximum point dose of 23 Gy and 31 Gy and maximum doses of 18 and 26 Gy to a brainstem volume <1 cm^3 [36, 40] (Table 18.2). Since most data are extrapolated from iso-effect curves for brainstem toxicity using various radiobiologic models, dose-volume metrics to predict toxicity of multi-fraction SRS to the brainstem should be used with caution.

Optic Pathway and Other Skull Base Structures

The optic nerves and chiasm may receive a substantial dose of radiation during SRS of brain metastases, especially for those located at the base of the skull; for cases at the anterior skull base, the optic apparatus is frequently the dose-limiting structure. The optic nerves and chiasm are thin (<5 mm diameter), and visualization is best performed using thin-cut (≤2 mm) T1- or T2-weighted magnetic resonance imaging. The primary end point for radiation-induced optic neuropathy (RION) is visual impairment, defined by visual acuity and the size/extent of visual fields.

The tolerance of the optic nerves and chiasm to single-fraction SRS is still unclear. In a few studies, a risk of RION up to 2% and >10% has been reported for patients receiving a maximum dose of 8–10 Gy and 12–15 Gy to the anterior optic pathway [40–44]; however, this risk appears to remain low when doses of 10–12 Gy are delivered to small portions (2–4 mm^3) of the optic apparatus [43].

There is little known about the tolerance of the cranial nerves of the cavernous sinus. Several series of SRS for primary skull base tumors after SRS report an incidence of 1–6% of cranial nerve deficits for doses in the range of 13–18 Gy [40, 41]. Although a precise tolerance dose of cranial nerves in the cavernous sinus after single-fraction SRS cannot be defined, data from several studies support the concept that doses to the cavernous sinus of up to 16–18 Gy are associated with low toxicity.

There is limited evidence relating the tolerance of the optic pathway to multi-fraction SRS [39, 45]. Retrospective series of skull base tumors [45–50] or brain metastases in close proximity to optic pathway receiving 21 Gy in 3 fractions or 25 Gy in 5 fractions report severe visual disorder in less than 1% of patients; however, in most studies no dosimetric details were provided. In a study of 34 patients who underwent multi-fraction SRS (5 × 5 Gy) at the University of Rome Sapienza, Sant'Andrea Hospital for a skull base metastasis compressing or in close proximity to optic nerves and chiasm, no optic neuropathy was observed for doses >25 Gy to <33% of the optic chiasm and 27.5–28.5 Gy to a small volume (0.01–0.06 cm^3) at a median follow-up of 13 months [50]. Although studies indicate that 5 × 5 Gy or 3 × 7 Gy schedules are associated to a low risk of RION and other cranial nerve deficits, further studies need to better evaluate the dose-volume constraints of optic chiasm and nerves for multi-fraction SRS.

For brain metastases located in the temporal lobe, the hippocampi should be contoured in an effort to reduce the potential negative neurocognitive effect of high dose of radiation to the hippocampal region; the principle of this approach is acknowledged, but there is currently insufficient evidence to support recommendations on hippocampal sparing in general during single-fraction or fractionated SRS.

Combined Systemic Therapies and Brain Irradiation

Limited data are available on the safety profile of combining chemotherapy or systemic agents with WBRT. Tsao et al. [51] conducted a Cochrane systematic review on the efficacy and toxicity of WBRT for the treatment of newly diagnosed multiple brain metastases. Data from nine fully published phase III trials examining the use of WBRT alone versus WBRT and chemotherapy reported an increase in toxicity with no survival benefit with the addition of a variety of chemotherapy agents, including cisplatin, vinorelbine, carboplatin, gemcitabine, topotecan, and temozolomide [51–59]. A few phase II/III trials have evaluated the use of concurrent targeted agents or immunotherapy and WBRT in patients with brain metastases [59–64]. A few trials assessing the combination of epidermal growth factor receptor (EGFR) tyrosine kinase inhibitors (TKIs) erlotinib or gefitinib with WBRT have shown that combined treatments are well tolerated, but they did not result in significant survival benefit [59–62]; however, participants were not tested for EGFR mutation, and any possible beneficial effect of EGFR TKIs in these populations remains undefined. Similarly, WBRT and concurrent targeted therapies BRAF and MEK inhibitors or immunotherapy with CTLA-4 checkpoint inhibitors [63, 64] are not apparently associated with increased toxicity, although robust evidences based on large clinical trials are not available.

As up-front SRS has been increasingly used for patients with brain metastases, several retrospective series have evaluated the efficacy and toxicity of combined SRS and systemic therapies [65–79]. For patients with human epidermal growth factor receptor 2-positive (HER2+) breast cancer and those with EGFR-mutant non-small cell lung cancer (NSCLC), the use of concomitant SRS and TKI therapy has been associated with survival benefits and a low risk of radiation necrosis [65–68]; however, no correlation between dose-volume parameters and the development of brain necrosis was reported. In patients with BRAF-mutated melanoma, a few retrospective studies have shown that BRAF/MEK inhibitors and concurrent SRS are associated with improved local control with acceptable safety profile [69–72], although an increased development of intratumoral hemorrhages has been reported [69–72]. SRS and checkpoint inhibitors given concurrently, typically within 4 weeks of SRS, are associated with improved intracranial control and similar neurological toxicity compared

to those reported after nonconcurrent therapy following either single-fraction or multi-fraction SRS [73–79]. Of note, patients treated with SRS and immunotherapy, in the first 12 weeks after treatment, may present on conventional imaging a transient enlargement of the treated lesions in up to 50% of cases which resolves in a few weeks; these alterations are indicated by the term pseudoprogression [74–79] (Fig. 18.1). The Immunotherapy Response Assessment in Neuro-oncology (iRANO) criteria have been recently proposed for neuro-oncology patients receiving immunotherapy, as the correct interpretation of imaging following administration of immunotherapy plays an essential role in patients' follow-up [80]. The iRANO working committee recommends that if follow-up images do not confirm progression, compared to the scan first revealing progressive changes, but instead show stable or reduced tumor burden, in the absence of increased corticosteroid dosing, treatment should be continued. Overall, combined SRS with target agents or immunotherapy is associated with improved control without a significant increase of neurological toxicity; however, in absence of large prospective studies, no definitive conclusions can be drawn about the safety of combined treatments.

Reirradiation

SRS is frequently employed in patients with progressive brain disease after prior irradiation. A few studies report the risk of neurological toxicity after reirradiation [5, 81–85]. As shown in the RTOG 90-05 study [5], the risk of irreversible severe neurological toxicity following single-fraction SRS after prior partial-brain irradiation or WBRT increases with the volume of irradiated lesions (see above). A rate of symptomatic radiation necrosis leading to grade 3 or 4 toxicity has been reported in 13–24% of patients receiving either single-fraction SRS (15–20 Gy) or multi-fraction SRS (3 × 7–8 Gy) [81–85]. Although retrospective studies support the efficacy of a second course of SRS with acceptable neurological toxicity, the risk of radiation necrosis after repeat SRS remains largely undetermined, and currently there is no satisfactory model to predict

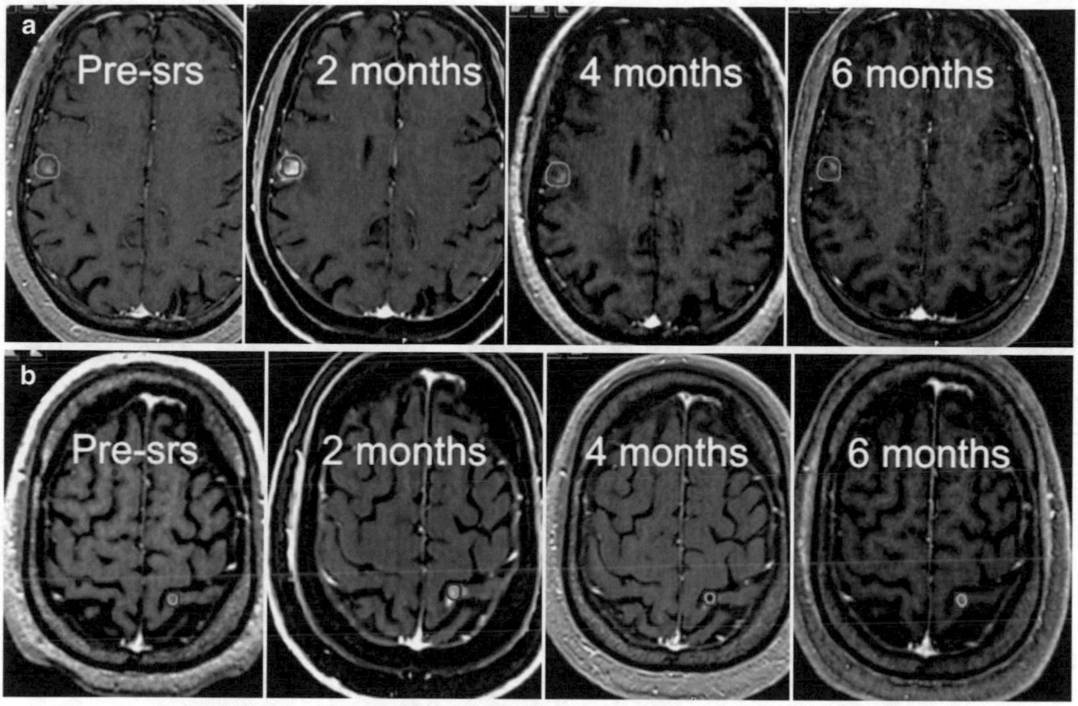

Fig. 18.1 Representative axial postcontrast T1-weighted magnetic resonance images in two patients with brain metastases from melanoma (**a**) and NSCLC (**b**) treated with frameless linear accelerator (Linac)-based single-fraction stereotactic radiosurgery (SRS, dose, 22 Gy; GTV-to-PTV expansion 1 mm) combined with nivolumab. A transient enlargement of lesions at T1 postcontrast (gadolinium) sequences occurring 2 months after SRS that resolved within 6 months was interpreted as pseudoprogression

the risk of radiation-induced toxicity. Although multi-fraction SRS is frequently used for larger recurrent brain metastases over single-fraction SRS, no clinical recommendation for the dose tolerance limits for repeat SRS can be drawn.

Areas of Uncertainty

Several issues regarding the dose tolerance of the normal brain to the radiation treatment of brain metastases remain undetermined. Currently, models predicting the risk for radiation-induced complications following either single-fraction or multi-fraction SRS are limited and should be improved, for example, by incorporation of both patient- and treatment-specific factors. In addition, the applicability of the LQ to calculate the BED of different SRS schedules has been questioned because the LQ model is considered to overestimate the effect of high single doses.

Based on clinical trials showing no difference in survival and better cognitive and quality of life (QOL) outcomes for patients receiving SRS alone over SRS plus WBRT, SRS alone has become the preferred strategy for the treatment of patients with limited brain metastases. With the widespread adoption of radiosurgery techniques, there has been an increasing use of SRS alone for patients with more than five brain metastases. The patient described in Case Vignette 2 received up-front SRS for ten brain metastases from a NSCLC; subsequently, he received WBRT as salvage treatment for progressive intracranial disease. A few studies have shown similar survival rates in patients receiving SRS for more than five metastases versus one to four metastases with a similar safety profile [86–89]; however, the risk of neurocognitive decline for such patients has not been evaluated in prospective studies. Models predicting the risk of long-term neurological toxicity, including the location, the number, and total volume of metastases, are needed.

As reported in the phase III RTOG 0614 and phase II RTOG 0933, the use of memantine and intensity-modulated radiation therapy (IMRT) planning for hippocampus sparing has demonstrated cognitive benefits in patients receiving WBRT [90–93]. The NRG Oncology phase III trial CC001 of WBRT plus memantine with or without hippocampal avoidance has enrolled 518 patients who were randomized to receive WBRT plus memantine versus hippocampal-avoidant WBRT plus memantine (30 Gy in 10 fractions) [93]. The primary end point was the time to neurocognitive decline. At a median follow-up of 7.9 months for alive patients, risk of cognitive failure was significantly lower after hippocampal-avoidant WBRT plus memantine versus WBRT plus memantine (adjusted hazard ratio, 0.74; 95% CI, 0.58 to 0.95; P = .02). This difference was attributable to less deterioration in executive function at 4 months and learning and memory at 6 months, respectively). The present results raise the question of the optimal approach for patients with more than five to ten metastases. Additional data on the impact of SRS alone or WBRT with hippocampal sparing are needed according to the location, size, number, and total volume of brain metastases. In this regard, there are ongoing trials (ClinicalTrials. gov: NCT01592968 and NCT02353000) enrolling patients with 4–10 or 15 brain metastases to WBRT or SRS with primary end points of local tumor control, cognitive function, or quality of life (QOL).

As noted in the QUANTEC papers, data on neurological toxicity following multi-fraction SRS using 5–9 Gy per fraction is scarce. In clinical practice, hypofractionated regimens are often used for larger brain metastases as an alternative to single-fraction SRS with the aim to maintain high local control and avoid radiation-induced toxicity; however, no prospective studies have compared these different approaches. Using common dose-volume parameters, e.g., V12 for single-fraction SRS and V18 for 3-fraction SRS, it would be helpful to have validate models predicting dose tolerance limits for normal brain tissue/structure toxicity following biologically equivalent radiosurgical treatments.

Additional data on the impact of combining radiation with systemic treatments, either target agents or immunotherapy, on the dose-volume outcome are needed. Specifically, future randomized trials are needed to assess the superiority of fractionated versus single-fraction SRS in combination with systemic agents in terms of radiation-induced toxicity, local control, and quality of life in patients affected by brain metastases.

Finally, studies of SRS for brain metastases should systematically report SRS techniques, prescription doses, treated volumes, location of lesions, dosimetric parameters, the use of concomitant systemic agents, and clinical outcomes, either local control or neurological toxicity, with the aim of developing appropriate models for predicting radiation-induced toxicity and converting hypofractionated doses in single doses.

Conclusions and Recommendations

Single-fraction SRS and multi-fraction SRS represent an effective treatment for brain metastases associated with a relatively low risk of long-term neurological toxicity. Currently, SRS alone is the recommended treatment for patients with up to five brain metastases, yielding an equivalent survival but a lower risk of long-term neurotoxicity compared with SRS plus WBRT. For both single-fraction and multi-fraction SRS, dose and fractionation are chosen with the aim to effectively control tumor growth and minimize the risk of radiation-induced brain necrosis. As for RTOG guidelines, recommended single SRS doses are 24 Gy, 18 Gy, and 15 Gy for lesions ≤20, 21–30 mm, and 31–40 mm, respectively; however, as the tumor size becomes larger, the ability to safely deliver an adequate dose to larger lesions is limited; specifically, QUANTEC data on dose-volume toxicity in the brain indicates that the rate of neurological toxicity increases rapidly for V12 exceeding 5–10 cm^3. In practice, every lesion >2.5–3 cm in size treated with single-fraction SRS would exceed this dose tolerance limits of normal brain tissue when RTOG-recommended doses are applied. For such cases, multi-fraction SRS, typically 3 or 5 fractions, is frequently employed with the aim of reducing the risk of radiation-induced toxicity. With the same rationale, multi-fraction SRS is frequently employed for large postoperative resection cavity, previously irradiated lesions, or those in close proximity to critical structures, such as optic apparatus or brainstem SRS. However, a clear dose-volume toxicity following multi-fraction SRS has not been established, and its superiority over single-fraction SRS for large lesions remains to be demonstrated in large prospective studies.

SRS alone is frequently employed in patients with up to ten metastases with no reported significant increase of toxicity compared with those receiving SRS for two to four brain metastases; however, in the absence of randomized studies, there are no robust data to recommend its use over WDRT. When WBRT is utilized, the use of IMRT planning for hippocampal sparing and concomitant and sequential memantine should be considered.

> **Key Points**
> - Use SRS for patients with up to five brain metastases.
> - Consider multi-fraction SRS as an alternative to single-fraction SRS for large brain metastases (more than 2–3 cm in maximum size) or those in close proximity to critical structures, such as optic apparatus or brainstem SRS.
> - Consider SRS alone in selected patients with up to ten brain metastases.
> - WBRT remains an effective strategy for patients with more than five to ten metastases. The use of memantine and IMRT planning for hippocampus sparing limits the neurocognitive decline in patients receiving WBRT.
> - V12 is a strong factor for predicting the risk of radiation necrosis after single-fraction SRS.
> - A close MRI follow-up is mandatory in patients receiving SRS alone because of the high risk of distant brain progression.
> - For patients receiving SRS and immunotherapy, a transient enlargement of

> irradiated lesions may occur within 12 weeks from the treatment, the so-called pseudoprogression. Early imaging findings of confirmation of radiographic progression should be sought no sooner than 3 months after initial radiographic suspect of progression.

Case Vignettes

Case 1

A 72-year-old patient with a history of breast cancer, for which she had undergone surgery and chemotherapy, 2 years after diagnosis presented with left-sided deficits suggesting the presence of brain metastases. The contrast-enhanced MRI showed five brain lesions: four lesions were less than 2 cm in size, and one was more than 3.0 cm. SRS was suggested and a simulation computed tomography (CT) scan with a thermoplastic mask at 1.25 mm slice-thickness was performed. After fusion of CT and MR scans, GTVs were outlined together with organs at risk (OARs). No GTV-to-PTV margin expansion was given for all lesions. SRS doses were delivered with volumetric modulated arc therapy (VMAT) on the Varian TrueBeam STx. The largest lesion received multi-fraction SRS, 3×9 Gy, over 3 consecutive days; the other four lesions received single-fraction SRS at a dose of 22 Gy (Fig. 18.2a). Dexamethasone at doses of 4 mg per day was continued during the treatment and then gradually stopped in a few days. No acute or long-term toxicity SRS-related side effects were observed. On subsequent follow-up, MRI showed a complete or partial response of all the treated lesions (Fig. 18.2).

Case 2

A 56-year-old patient presented to our attention with a history of an advanced NSCLC metastatic to liver and adrenal gland. He was firstly treated

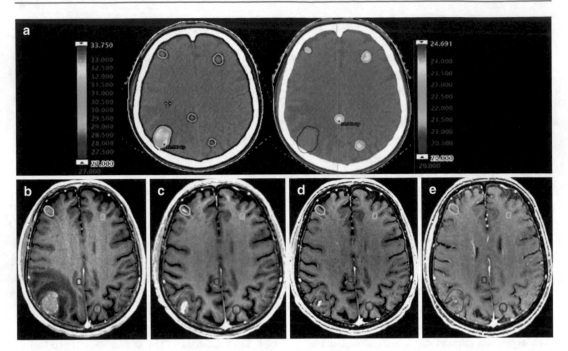

Fig. 18.2 Linac-based stereotactic radiosurgery (SRS) volumetric modulated arc technique (VMAT) treatment plan for a patient presenting with five brain metastases. Four lesions received single-fraction SRS (22 Gy) and one lesion (blue contour) with multi-fraction SRS (27 Gy in three fractions over 3 consecutive days). Dose distribution to target volumes for either multi-fraction (left) or single-fraction SRS (right) is displayed in panel (**a**). Pretreatment (**b**) and posttreatment (**c–e**) MRI, T1 gadolinium-enhanced axial images, at 2 months (**c**), 6 months (**d**), and 12 months (**e**) show a complete radiologic response

with platinum-based chemotherapy (6 cycles). After an initial partial response, a CT detected progressive disease (small multiple lung nodules in both sides of the lung). Chemotherapy was suspended and immunotherapy (nivolumab) was initiated. At 6 months following initiation of immunotherapy, further investigation with CT and MRI showed the presence of eleven brain lesions 5–20 mm in size. All lesions received frameless SRS to a dose of 22 Gy in a single fraction using a single-isocenter dynamic conformal arc (DCA) technique for multiple targets (Fig. 18.3).

Because extracranial disease remained stable, immunotherapy was continued. An MRI was performed at 2 months showing an important dimensional shrinking of most of the lesions, with some of them disappearing completely (Fig. 18.4). Further MRI scans performed at 4 and 6 months showed stable intracranial disease. At 9 months, a CT scan showed extracranial and cranial disease progression, with the appearance of multiple and widespread brain lesions distant from the initial SRS sites. The patient died of progressive intracranial disease 4 months after receiving WBRT.

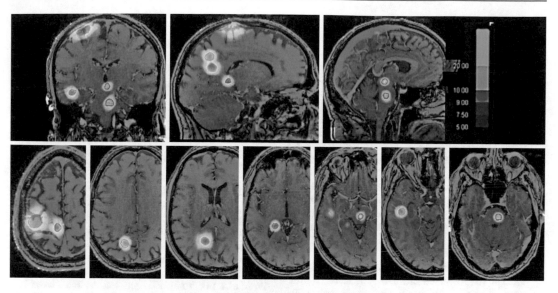

Fig. 18.3 Linac-based stereotactic radiosurgery (SRS) treatment plan for eleven brain metastases from NSCLC. All lesions were treated at a dose of 22 Gy in a single ses- sion using a single-isocenter dynamic conformal arc tech- nique for multiple targets. The total treated tumor volume was 4.7 cm^3

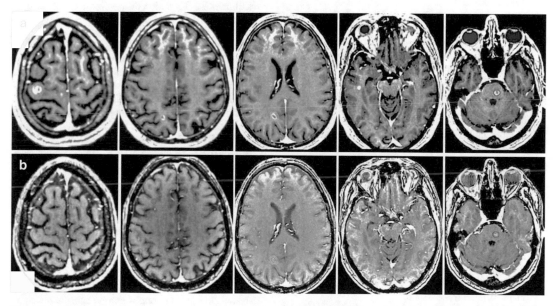

Fig. 18.4 NSCLC brain metastases response to stereo- tactic radiosurgery (SRS): (**a**) before SRS, (**b**) after SRS. All lesions received single-fraction SRS at a dose of 22 Gy (see Fig. 18.3 for details). Representative axial postcontrast T1-weighted magnetic resonance images obtained 2 months following SRS show a complete or a partial response of all treated lesions

References

1. Aoyama H, Shirato H, Tago M, Nakagawa K, Toyoda T, Hatano K, et al. Stereotactic radiosurgery plus whole-brain radiation therapy vs stereotactic radiosurgery alone for treatment of brain metastases: a randomized controlled trial. JAMA. 2006;295(21):2483–91.
2. Chang EL, Wefel JS, Hess KR, Allen PK, Lang FF, Kornguth DG, et al. Neurocognition in patients with brain metastases treated with radiosurgery or radiosurgery plus whole-brain irradiation: a randomised controlled trial. Lancet Oncol. 2009;10(11):1037–44.
3. Kocher M, Soffietti R, Abacioglu U, Villà S, Fauchon F, Baumert BG, et al. Adjuvant whole-brain radiotherapy versus observation after radiosurgery or surgical resection of one to three cerebral metastases: results of the EORTC 22952-26001 study. J Clin Oncol. 2011;29(2):134–41.
4. Brown PD, Jaeckle K, Ballman KV, Farace E, Cerhan JH, Anderson SK, et al. Effect of radiosurgery alone vs radiosurgery with whole brain radiation therapy on cognitive function in patients with 1–3 brain metastases: a randomized clinical trial. JAMA. 2016;316(4):401–9. Erratum in: JAMA. 2018;320(5):510.
5. Shaw E, Scott C, Souhami L, Dinapoli R, Kline R, Loeffler J, et al. Single dose radiosurgical treatment of recurrent previously irradiated primary brain tumors and brain metastases: final report of RTOG protocol 90-05. Int J Radiat Oncol Biol Phys. 2000;47(2):291–8.
6. Minniti G, Scaringi C, Paolini S, Lanzetta G, Romano A, Cicone F, et al. Single-fraction versus multifraction (3 × 9 Gy) stereotactic radiosurgery for large (>2 cm) brain metastases: a comparative analysis of local control and risk of radiation-induced brain necrosis. Int J Radiat Oncol Biol Phys. 2016;95:1142–8.
7. Minniti G, D'Angelillo RM, Scaringi C, Trodella LE, Clarke E, Matteucci P, et al. Fractionated stereotactic radiosurgery for patients with brain metastases. J Neuro-Oncol. 2014;117:295–301.
8. Aoyama H, Shirato H, Onimaru R, Kagei K, Ikeda J, Ishii N, et al. Hypofractionated stereotactic radiotherapy alone without whole brain irradiation for patients with solitary and oligo brain metastasis using noninvasive fixation of the skull. Int J Radiat Oncol Biol Phys. 2003;56(3):793–800.
9. Ernst-Stecken A, Ganslandt O, Lambrecht U, Sauer R, Grabenbauer G. Phase II trial of hypofractionated stereotactic radiotherapy for brain metastases: results and toxicity. Radiother Oncol. 2006;81(1):18–24.
10. Murai T, Ogino H, Manabe Y, Iwabuchi M, Okumura T, Matsushita Y, et al. Fractionated stereotactic radiotherapy using CyberKnife for the treatment of large brain metastases: a dose escalation study. Clin Oncol (R Coll Radiol). 2014;26(3):151–8.
11. Kim JW, Park HR, Lee JM, Kim JW, Chung HT, Kim DG, et al. Fractionated stereotactic gamma knife radiosurgery for large brain metastases: a retrospective, single center study. PLoS One. 2016;11:e0163304.
12. Lehrer EJ, Peterson JL, Zaorsky NG, Brown PD, Sahgal A, Chiang VL, et al. Single versus multifraction stereotactic radiosurgery for large brain metastases: an international meta-analysis of 24 trials. Int J Radiat Oncol Biol Phys. 2019;103(3):618–30.
13. Fowler JF. 21 years of biologically effective dose. Br J Radiol. 2010;83(991):554–68.
14. Kirkpatrick JP, Meyer JJ, Marks LB. The linear-quadratic model is inappropriate to model high dose per fraction effects in radiosurgery. Semin Radiat Oncol. 2008;18(4):240–3.
15. Joiner M. Quantifying cell kill and survival. In: Joiner M, Van der Kogel A, editors. Basic clinical radiobiology. 4th ed. London: Hodder Arnold; 2009. p. 102–19.
16. Lawrence YR, Li XA, el Naqa I, Hahn CA, Marks LB, Merchant TE, et al. Radiation dose-volume effects in the brain. Int J Radiat Oncol Biol Phys. 2010;76(3 Suppl):S20–7.
17. Marks LB, Yorke ED, Jackson A, Ten Haken RK, Constine LS, Eisbruch A, et al. Use of normal tissue complication probability models in the clinic. Int J Radiat Oncol Biol Phys. 2010;76(3 Suppl):S10–9.
18. Mayo C, Martel MK, Marks LB, Flickinger J, Nam J, Kirkpatrick J. Radiation dose-volume effects of optic nerves and chiasm. Int J Radiat Oncol Biol Phys. 2010;76(3 Suppl):S28–35.
19. Kirkpatrick JP, van der Kogel AJ, Schultheiss TE. Radiation dose-volume effects in the spinal cord. Int J Radiat Oncol Biol Phys. 2010;76(3 Suppl):S42–9.
20. Kirkpatrick JP, Marks LB, Mayo CS, Lawrence YR, Bhandare N, Ryu S. Estimating normal tissue toxicity in radiosurgery of the CNS: application and limitations of QUANTEC. J Radiosurg SBRT. 2011;1:95–107.
21. Blonigen BJ, Steinmetz RD, Levin L, Lamba MA, Warnick RE, Breneman JC. Irradiated volume as a predictor of brain radionecrosis after linear accelerator stereotactic radiosurgery. Int J Radiat Oncol Biol Phys. 2010;77(4):996–1001.
22. Minniti G, Clarke E, Lanzetta G, Osti MF, Trasimeni G, Bozzao A, et al. Stereotactic radiosurgery for brain metastases: analysis of outcome and risk of brain radionecrosis. Radiat Oncol. 2011;6:48.
23. Williams BJ, Suki D, Fox BD, Pelloski CE, Maldaun MV, Sawaya RE, et al. Stereotactic radiosurgery for metastatic brain tumors: a comprehensive review of complications. J Neurosurg. 2009;111(3):439–48.
24. Chao ST, Ahluwalia MS, Barnett GH, Stevens GH, Murphy ES, Stockham AL, et al. Challenges with the diagnosis and treatment of cerebral radiation necrosis. Int J Radiat Oncol Biol Phys. 2013;87(3):449–57.
25. Dequesada IM, Quisling RG, Yachnis A, Friedman WA. Can standard magnetic resonance imaging reliably distinguish recurrent tumor from radiation necrosis after radiosurgery for brain metastases? A radiographic-pathological study. Neurosurgery. 2008;63:898–904.

26. Vellayappan B, Tan CL, Yong C, Khor LK, Koh WY, Yeo TT, et al. Diagnosis and management of radiation necrosis in patients with brain metastases. Front Oncol. 2018;8:395.

27. Verma N, Cowperthwaite MC, Burnett MG, Markey MK. Differentiating tumor recurrence from treatment necrosis: a review of neuro-oncologic imaging strategies. Neuro-Oncology. 2013;15(5):515–34.

28. Galldiks N, Stoffels G, Filss CP, Piroth MD, Sabel M, Ruge MI, et al. Role of O-(2-(18)F-fluoroethyl)-L-tyrosine PET for differentiation of local recurrent brain metastasis from radiation necrosis. J Nucl Med. 2012;53(9):1367–74.

29. Terakawa Y, Tsuyuguchi N, Iwai Y, Yamanaka K, Higashiyama S, Takami T, et al. Diagnostic accuracy of 11C methionine PET for differentiation of recurrent brain tumors from radiation necrosis after radiotherapy. J Nucl Med. 2008;49(5):694–9.

30. Cicone F, Minniti G, Romano A, Papa A, Scaringi C, Tavanti F, et al. Accuracy of F-DOPA PET and perfusion-MRI for differentiating radionecrotic from progressive brain metastases after radiosurgery. Eur J Nucl Med Mol Imaging. 2015;42(1):103–11.

31. Langen KJ, Galldiks N. Update on amino acid PET of brain tumours. Curr Opin Neurol. 2018;31(4):354–61.

32. Andrews DW, Scott CB, Sperduto PW, Flanders AE, Gaspar LE, Schell MC, et al. Whole brain radiation therapy with or without stereotactic radiosurgery boost for patients with one to three brain metastases: phase III results of the RTOG 9508 randomised trial. Lancet. 2004;363(9422):1665–72.

33. Korytko T, Radivoyevitch T, Colussi V, Wessels BW, Pillai K, Maciunas RJ, et al. 12 Gy gamma knife radiosurgical volume is a predictor for radiation necrosis in non-AVM intracranial tumors. Int J Radiat Oncol Biol Phys. 2006;64(2):419–24.

34. Meeks SL, Buatti JM, Foote KD, Friedman WA, Bova FJ. Calculation of cranial nerve complication probability for acoustic neuroma radiosurgery. Int J Radiat Oncol Biol Phys. 2000;47(3):597–602.

35. Foote KD, Friedman WA, Buatti JM, Meeks SL, Bova FJ, Kubilis PS. Analysis of risk factors associated with radiosurgery for vestibular schwannoma. J Neurosurg. 2001;95(3):440–9.

36. Mayo C, Yorke E, Merchant TE. Radiation associated brainstem injury. Int J Radiat Oncol Biol Phys. 2010;76(3 Suppl):S36–41.

37. Lin CS, Selch MT, Lee SP, Wu JK, Xiao F, Hong DS, et al. Accelerator-based stereotactic radiosurgery for brainstem metastases. Neurosurgery. 2012;70(4):953–8.

38. Trifiletti DM, Lee CC, Kano H, Cohen J, Janopaul-Naylor J, Alonso-Basanta M, et al. Stereotactic radiosurgery for brainstem metastases: an international cooperative study to define response and toxicity. Int J Radiat Oncol Biol Phys. 2016;96(2):280–8.

39. Timmerman RD. An overview of hypofractionation and introduction to this issue of seminars in radiation oncology. Semin Radiat Oncol. 2008;18(4):215–22.

40. Tishler RB, Loeffler JS, Lunsford LD, Duma C, Alexander E 3rd, Kooy HM, et al. Tolerance of cranial nerves of the cavernous sinus to radiosurgery. Int J Radiat Oncol Biol Phys. 1993;27(2):215–21.

41. Leber KA, Berglöff J, Pendl G. Dose-response tolerance of the visual pathways and cranial nerves of the cavernous sinus to stereotactic radiosurgery. J Neurosurg. 1998;88(1):43–50.

42. Stafford SL, Pollock BE, Leavitt JA, Foote RL, Brown PD, Link MJ, et al. A study on the radiation tolerance of the optic nerves and chiasm after stereotactic radiosurgery. Int J Radiat Oncol Biol Phys. 2003;55(5):1177–81.

43. Leavitt JA, Stafford SL, Link MJ, Pollock BE. Long-term evaluation of radiation-induced optic neuropathy after single-fraction stereotactic radiosurgery. Int J Radiat Oncol Biol Phys. 2013;87(3):524–7.

44. Pollock BE, Link MJ, Leavitt JA, Stafford SL. Dose-volume analysis of radiation-induced optic neuropathy after single-fraction stereotactic radiosurgery. Neurosurgery. 2014;75(4):456–60.

45. Hiniker SM, Modlin LA, Choi CY, Atalar B, Seiger K, Binkley MS, et al. Dose-response modeling of the visual pathway tolerance to single-fraction and hypofractionated stereotactic radiosurgery. Semin Radiat Oncol. 2016;26(2):97–104.

46. Adler JR Jr, Gibbs IC, Puataweepong P, Chang SD. Visual field preservation after multisession cyberknife radiosurgery for perioptic lesions. Neurosurgery. 2006;59(2):244–54.

47. Killory BD, Kresl JJ, Wait SD, Ponce FA, Porter R, White WL. Hypofractionated CyberKnife radiosurgery for perichiasmatic pituitary adenomas: early results. Neurosurgery. 2009;64(2 Suppl): A19–25.

48. Iwata H, Sato K, Tatewaki K, Yokota N, Inoue M, Baba Y, et al. Hypofractionated stereotactic radiotherapy with CyberKnife for nonfunctioning pituitary adenoma: high local control with low toxicity. Neuro-Oncology. 2011;13(8):916–22.

49. Liao HI, Wang CC, Wei KC, Chang CN, Hsu YH, Lee ST, et al. Fractionated stereotactic radiosurgery using the Novalis system for the management of pituitary adenomas close to the optic apparatus. J Clin Neurosci. 2014;21(1):111–5.

50. Minniti G, Esposito V, Clarke E, Scaringi C, Bozzao A, Falco T, et al. Fractionated stereotactic radiosurgery for patients with skull base metastases from systemic cancer involving the anterior visual pathway. Radiat Oncol. 2014;9:110.

51. Tsao MN, Xu W, Wong RK, Lloyd N, Laperriere N, Sahgal A, et al. Whole brain radiotherapy for the treatment of newly diagnosed multiple brain metastases. Cochrane Database Syst Rev. 2018;1:CD003869.

52. Guerrieri M, Wong K, Ryan G, Millward M, Quong G, Ball DL. A randomised phase III study of palliative radiation with concomitant carboplatin for brain metastases from non-small cell carcinoma of lung. Lung Cancer. 2004;46(1):107–11.

53. Knisely J, Berkey B, Chakravarti A, Yung AWK, Curran WJ, Robins HI, et al. A phase III study of conventional radiation therapy plus thalidomide versus conventional radiation therapy for multiple brain metastases (RTOG 0118). Int J Radiat Oncol Biol Phys. 2008;71(1):79–86.

54. Lee DH, Han J-Y, Kim HT, Yoon SJ, Pyo HR, Cho KH, et al. Primary chemotherapy for newly diagnosed nonsmall cell lung cancer patients with synchronous brain metastases compared with whole-brain radiotherapy administered first. Results of a randomized pilot study. Cancer. 2008;113(1):143–9.

55. Mornex F, Thomas L, Mohr P, Hauschild A, Delaunay MM, Lesimple T, et al. A prospective randomized multicentre phase III trial of fotemustine plus whole brain irradiation versus fotemustine alone in cerebral metastases of malignant melanoma. Melanoma Res. 2003;13(1):97–103.

56. Neuhaus T, Ko Y, Muller RP, Grabenbauer GG, Hedde JP, Schueller H, et al. A phase III trial of topotecan and whole brain radiation therapy for patients with CNS-metastases due to lung cancer. Br J Cancer. 2009;100(2):291–7.

57. Postmus PE, Haaxma-Reiche H, Smit EF, Groen HJ, Karnicka H, Lewinski T, et al. Treatment of brain metastases of small-cell lung cancer: comparing teniposide and teniposide with whole-brain radiotherapy–a phase III study of the European Organization for the Research and Treatment of Cancer Lung Cancer Cooperative Group. J Clin Oncol. 2000;18(19):3400–8.

58. Robinet G, Thomas P, Breton JL, Léna H, Gouva S, Dabouis G, et al. Results of a phase III study of early versus delayed whole brain radiotherapy with concurrent cisplatin and vinorelbine combination in inoperable brain metastasis of non-small-cell lung cancer: Groupe Français de Pneumo-Cancérologie (GFPC) Protocol 95-1. Ann Oncol. 2001;12(1):59–67.

59. Sperduto PW, Wang M, Robins HI, Schell MC, Werner-Wasik M, Komaki R, et al. A phase 3 trial of whole brain radiation therapy and stereotactic radiosurgery alone versus WBRT and SRS with temozolomide or erlotinib for non-small cell lung cancer and 1–3 brain metastases: radiation Therapy Oncology Group 0320. Int J Radiat Oncol Biol Phys. 2013;85(5):1312–8.

60. Ushio Y, Arita N, Hayakawa T, Mogami H, Hasegawa H, Bitoh S, et al. Chemotherapy of brain metastases from lung carcinoma: a controlled randomized study. Neurosurgery. 1991;28(2):201–5.

61. Pesce GA, Klingbiel D, Ribi K, Zouhair A, von Moos R, Schlaeppi M, et al. Outcome, quality of life and cognitive function of patients with brain metastases from non-small cell lung cancer treated with whole brain radiotherapy combined with gefitinib or temozolomide. A randomised phase II trial of the Swiss Group for Clinical Cancer Research (SAKK 70/03). Eur J Cancer. 2012;48(3):377–84.

62. Welsh JW, Komaki R, Amini A, Munsell MF, Unger W, Allen PK, et al. Phase II trial of erlotinib plus concurrent whole-brain radiation therapy for patients with brain metastases from non-small-cell lung cancer. J Clin Oncol. 2013;31(7):895–902.

63. Jiang T, Su C, Li X, Zhao C, Zhou F, Ren S, et al. EGFR TKIs plus WBRT demonstrated no survival benefit other than that of TKIs alone in patients with NSCLC and EGFR mutation and brain metastases. J Thorac Oncol. 2016;11(10):1718–28.

64. Anker CJ, Grossmann KF, Atkins MB, Suneja G, Tarhini AA, Kirkwood JM. Avoiding severe toxicity from combined BRAF inhibitor and radiation treatment: consensus guidelines from the Eastern Cooperative Oncology Group (ECOG). Int J Radiat Oncol Biol Phys. 2016;95(2):632–46.

65. Williams NL, Wuthrick EJ, Kim H, Palmer JD, Garg S, Eldredge-Hindy H, et al. Phase 1 study of ipilimumab combined with whole brain radiation therapy or radiosurgery for melanoma patients with brain metastases. Int J Radiat Oncol Biol Phys. 2017;99(1):22–30.

66. Yang WC, Xiao F, Shih JY, Ho CC, Chen YF, Tseng HM, et al. Epidermal growth factor receptor mutation predicts favorable outcomes in non-small cell lung cancer patients with brain metastases treated with stereotactic radiosurgery. Radiother Oncol. 2018;126(2):368–74.

67. Robin TP, Camidge DR, Stuhr K, Nath SK, Breeze RE, Pacheco JM, et al. Excellent outcomes with radiosurgery for multiple brain metastases in ALK and EGFR driven non-small cell lung cancer. J Thorac Oncol. 2018;13(5):715–20.

68. Yomo S, Oda K. Impacts of EGFR-mutation status and EGFR-TKI on the efficacy of stereotactic radiosurgery for brain metastases from non-small cell lung adenocarcinoma: a retrospective analysis of 133 consecutive patients. Lung Cancer. 2018;119:120–6.

69. Parsai S, Miller JA, Juloori A, Chao ST, Kotecha R, Mohammadi AM, et al. Stereotactic radiosurgery with concurrent lapatinib is associated with improved local control for HER2-positive breast cancer brain metastases. J Neurosurg. 2019;8:1–9.

70. Ly D, Bagshaw HP, Anker CJ, Tward JD, Grossmann KF, Jensen RL, et al. Local control after stereotactic radiosurgery for brain metastases in patients with melanoma with and without BRAF mutation and treatment. J Neurosurg. 2015;123(2):395–401.

71. Gallaher IS, Watanabe Y, DeFor TE, Dusenbery KE, Lee CK, Hunt MA, et al. BRAF mutation is associated with improved local control of melanoma brain metastases treated with gamma knife radiosurgery. Front Oncol. 2016;6:107.

72. Xu Z, Lee CC, Ramesh A, Mueller AC, Schlesinger D, Cohen-Inbar O, et al. BRAF V600E mutation and BRAF kinase inhibitors in conjunction with stereotactic radiosurgery for intracranial melanoma metastases. J Neurosurg. 2017;126(3):726–34.

73. Mastorakos P, Xu Z, Yu J, Hess J, Qian J, Chatrath A, et al. BRAF V600 mutation and BRAF kinase inhibitors in conjunction with stereotactic radiosurgery for intracranial melanoma metastases: a multicenter retrospective study. Neurosurgery. 2019;84(4):868–80.

74. Mathew M, Tam M, Ott PA, Pavlick AC, Rush SC, Donahue BR, et al. Ipilimumab in melanoma with limited brain metastases treated with stereotactic radiosurgery. Melanoma Res. 2013;23(3):191–5.

75. Kiess AP, Wolchok JD, Barker CA, Postow MA, Tabar V, Huse JT, et al. Stereotactic radiosurgery for melanoma brain metastases in patients receiving ipilimumab: safety profile and efficacy of combined treatment. Int J Radiat Oncol Biol Phys. 2015;92(2):368–75.

76. Ahmed KA, Abuodeh YA, Echevarria MI, Arrington JA, Stallworth DG, Hogue C, et al. Clinical outcomes of melanoma brain metastases treated with stereotactic radiosurgery and anti-PD-1 therapy, anti-CTLA-4 therapy, BRAF/MEK inhibitors, BRAF inhibitor, or conventional chemotherapy. Ann Oncol. 2016;27(12):2288–94.

77. Qian JM, Yu JB, Kluger HM, Chiang VL. Timing and type of immune checkpoint therapy affect the early radiographic response of melanoma brain metastases to stereotactic radiosurgery. Cancer. 2016;122(19):3051–8.

78. Patel KR, Chowdhary M, Switchenko JM, Kudchadkar R, Lawson DH, Cassidy RJ, et al. BRAF inhibitor and stereotactic radiosurgery is associated with an increased risk of radiation necrosis. Melanoma Res. 2016;26(4):387–94.

79. Chen L, Douglass J, Kleinberg L, Ye X, Marciscano AE, Forde PM, et al. Concurrent immune checkpoint inhibitors and stereotactic radiosurgery for brain metastases in non-small cell lung cancer, melanoma, and renal cell carcinoma. Int J Radiat Oncol Biol Phys. 2018;100(4):916–25.

80. Minniti G, Anzellini D, Reverberi C, Cappellini GCA, Marchetti L, Bianciardi F, et al. Stereotactic radiosurgery combined with nivolumab or ipilimumab for patients with melanoma brain metastases: evaluation of brain control and toxicity. J Immunother Cancer. 2019;7(1):102.

81. Okada H, Weller M, Huang R, Finocchiaro G, Gilbert MR, Wick W, et al. Immunotherapy response assessment in neuro-oncology: a report of the RANO working group. Lancet Oncol. 2015;16(15):e534–42.

82. Minniti G, Scaringi C, Paolini S, Clarke E, Cicone F, Esposito V, et al. Repeated stereotactic radiosurgery for patients with progressive brain metastases. J Neuro-Oncol. 2016;126(1):91–7.

83. McKay WH, McTyre ER, Okoukoni C, Alphonse-Sullivan NK, Ruiz J, Munley MT, et al. Repeat stereotactic radiosurgery as salvage therapy for locally recurrent brain metastases previously treated with radiosurgery. J Neurosurg. 2017;127(1):148–56.

84. Koffer P, Chan J, Rava P, Gorovets D, Ebner D, Savir G, et al. Repeat stereotactic radiosurgery for locally recurrent brain metastases. World Neurosurg. 2017;104:589–93.

85. Rana N, Pendyala P, Cleary RK, Luo G, Zhao Z, Chambless LB, et al. Long-term outcomes after salvage stereotactic radiosurgery (SRS) following in-field failure of initial SRS for brain metastases. Front Oncol. 2017;7:279.

86. Balermpas P, Stera S, Müller von der Grün J, Loutfi-Krauss B, Forster MT, Wagner M, et al. Repeated in-field radiosurgery for locally recurrent brain metastases: feasibility, results and survival in a heavily treated patient cohort. PLoS One. 2018;13(6):e0198692.

87. Yamamoto M, Serizawa T, Shuto T, Akabane A, Higuchi Y, Kawagishi J, et al. Stereotactic radiosurgery for patients with multiple brain metastases (JLGK0901): a multi-institutional prospective observational study. Lancet Oncol. 2014;15(4):387–95.

88. Greto D, Scoccianti S, Compagnucci A, Arilli C, Casati M, Francolini G, et al. Gamma knife radiosurgery in the management of single and multiple brain metastases. Clin Neurol Neurosurg. 2016;141:43–7.

89. Yamamoto M, Serizawa T, Higuchi Y, Sato Y, Kawagishi J, Yamanaka K, et al. A multi-institutional prospective observational study of stereotactic radiosurgery for patients with multiple brain metastases (JLGK0901 study update): irradiation-related complications and long-term maintenance of mini-mental state examination scores. Int J Radiat Oncol Biol Phys. 2017;99(1):31–40.

90. Knoll MA, Oermann EK, Yang AI, Paydar I, Steinberger J, Collins B, et al. Survival of patients with multiple intracranial metastases treated with stereotactic radiosurgery: does the number of tumors matter? Am J Clin Oncol. 2018;41(5):425–31.

91. Brown PD, Pugh S, Laack NN, Wefel JS, Khuntia D, Meyers C, et al. Memantine for the prevention of cognitive dysfunction in patients receiving whole-brain radiotherapy: a randomized, double-blind, placebo-controlled trial. Neuro-Oncology. 2013;15(10):1429–37.

92. Gondi V, Pugh SL, Tome WA, Caine C, Corn B, Kanner A, et al. Preservation of memory with conformal avoidance of the hippocampal neural stem-cell compartment during whole-brain radiotherapy for brain metastases (RTOG 0933): a phase II multi-institutional trial. J Clin Oncol. 2014;32(34):3810–6.

93. Brown PD, Gondi V, Pugh S, Tome WA, Wefel JS, Armstrong TS, et al. For NRG Oncology. Hippocampal avoidance during whole-brain radiotherapy plus memantine for patients with brain metastases: Phase III trial NRG Oncology CC001. J Clin Oncol. 2020;38:1019–29.

Evaluation of the Quality of a Radiosurgery Plan

19

Evan M. Thomas, Richard A. Popple, and John B. Fiveash

Background

Radiosurgery has long established itself as a safe, viable, and cost-effective alternative to invasive resection or ablation of tissue within the central nervous system. The applications and roles of radiosurgery continue to grow at an extraordinarily rapid pace. The current generation of radiation oncologists and neurosurgeons are now completing training in an era where familiarity with the principles and practice of radiosurgery is a requisite and expected component of their vocational skills.

The evaluation of the quality of a radiosurgery plan is the most expedient way to consider not only the clinical efficacy of the treatment but its likelihood of associated toxicity as well. A consistent evaluation of one's own radiosurgery plans and comparison to others is the most useful heuristic for treatment quality improvement.

Evaluation of radiosurgery plan quality with numerical indices is an attempt to quantify a plan's ability to maximize its likelihood of achieving its intent and minimizing unintended effects. Different clinical scenarios may entail different clinical objectives. A very large number of indices have been developed; each has advantages and disadvantages compared to others in certain scenarios. It is up to the planner to understand the clinician's objectives in a given plan and select a metric that most appropriately surrogates that objective.

Dose-Volume Metrics

Numerical indices used for evaluation of a radiosurgery plan are derived from dose-volume metrics. The metrics that are used in the indices to be considered here are defined in Table 19.1.

Conformity Indices

A conformity (or conformality) index is designed to be surrogate for how closely the prescription dose aligns with the target. In an absolutely ideal plan, the prescription dose would exactly encompass the target volume, and for most conformity indices as they are designed, the ideal value would be one. However, there are a number other aspects of prescription dose coverage the planner may want to capture in a metric, such as the maximum or minimum dose within a target, the geometric alignment with the prescription isodose cloud with the target, and the degree of protection of nearby critical organs. The Shaw or RTOG

E. M. Thomas (✉) · R. A. Popple · J. B. Fiveash
Department of Radiation Oncology, University of Alabama at Birmingham, Birmingham, AL, USA
e-mail: ethomas@uab.edu

© Springer Nature Switzerland AG 2020
Y. Yamada et al. (eds.), *Radiotherapy in Managing Brain Metastases*,
https://doi.org/10.1007/978-3-030-43740-4_19

Table 19.1 List of various plan quality descriptors used in metrics and indices in this chapter

Metric	Description
TV	Target volume – volume of actual target coverage is designated for, whether gross tumor volume (GTV) or planning target volume (PTV)
$TV_{<PI}$	Volume of target receiving less than the prescription dose
PIV	Prescription isodose volume – volume receiving at least the prescription dose
TV_{PIV}	Amount of the target volume receiving the prescription dose
HTV_{PI}	Volume of healthy (nontarget) tissue receiving at least the prescription dose
$PIV_{50\%}$	Volume receiving at least half of the prescription dose
V12Gy[cc]	Volume receiving at least 12 Gy in cm^3
D_{Rx}	Prescribed dose
D_{max}	Maximum dose with a given volume
D_{min}	Minimum dose with a given volume
D_{mean}	Mean dose of a given volume
ID	Integral dose (product of the mean dose to a structure and its volume)

conformity index is the simplest and is defined as the ratio of the volume of tissue receiving the prescription dose divided by the target volume. Figure 19.1 illustrates three scenarios in which the ideal value for the RTOG conformity index fails to capture various aspects in which a plan would be not conformal. Because of this, a large number of alternative compound conformity indices have been developed which ascribe to capture other metrics of plan quality.

Shaw/RTOG

$$RTOG\,CI = \frac{PIV}{TV}$$

From the 1993 original RTOG radiosurgery guidelines [2], this is the simplest and most commonly utilized conformity index. Simply, it is the prescribed treated volume divided by the target volume. As noted in Fig. 19.1, it can erroneously suggest good conformity in several scenarios, but

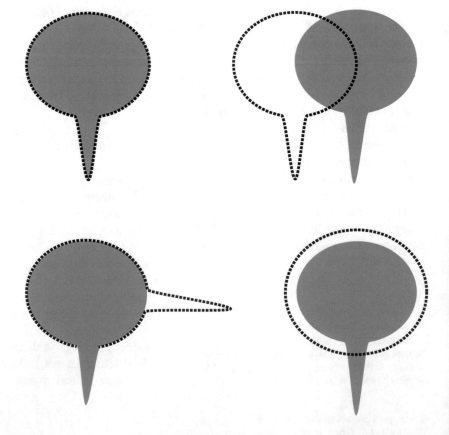

Fig. 19.1 Four possibilities for which the PV/TV ratio is equal to 1. (From Feuvret et al. [1] Reprinted with permission from Elsevier)

most modern treatment planning systems are robust to these errors. Some of these erroneous scenarios led proposals for alternative definitions to account for situations where the target was not covered. The larger a target is, the more easily a planner should be able to achieve a conformity index approaching unity. This value is <1 for undercovered plans and >1 for overcovered plans.

ICRU

$$ICRU\,CI = \frac{TV}{PIV} = RTOG\,CI^{-1}$$

The inverse of the Shaw/RTOG conformity index was originally proposed by Dr. Dave Larson. It can be used as a matter of preference but has no discrete advantage. This value is >1 for undercovered plans and <1 for overcovered plans.

Radiation Conformity Index or Undertreatment Ratio

$$RCI = \frac{TV_{PIV}}{TV} \quad OR \quad RCI = \frac{TV}{TV_{PIV}}$$

This metric was first reported by Knöös et al. [3] for use in conventional radiotherapy but appropriated by Paddick [4] for inclusion in the Paddick CI as a radiosurgical metric. It is the first use of the quantity representing the portion of the target volume receiving the prescription isodose line. It was initially described by the authors in conference proceedings [5] as TV_{PIV}/TV but in publication later reported as TV/TV_{PIV} to suit the author preference of having the metric decrease toward unity as the plan became more conformal. It is later referred to as the "undertreatment ratio" by Paddick [4] and simply "conformity index" by Lomax [6].

Overtreatment Ratio or Selectivity Index or Healthy Tissues Conformity Index

Healthy tissues conformity index

$$\left(selectivity\,index\right) = \frac{TV_{PIV}}{PIV}$$

This measure was first described by Paddick [4] as the "overtreatment ratio" and is a component of the Paddick CI. It was later used and

described by Regis et al. [7] as the "selectivity index." Finally, it was renamed and employed by Lomax et al. [6] as "healthy tissues conformity index" to quantify irradiation of healthy tissue by taking the proportion of the target volume receiving both the prescription isodose volume and the prescription isodose volume. As the target volume receiving prescription isodose is only an indirect measure of healthy tissue irradiation, this measure is not particularly efficient at representing its surrogate.

Paddick CI/Conformation Number

$$Paddick\,CI = \frac{TV_{PIV}^2}{TV \times PIV}$$

Ian Paddick proposed this metric in 2000 [4], after noting aforementioned shortcomings in the RTOG conformity index. It is in fact a composite product of his previously described quantities, the overtreatment ratio and the undertreatment ratio. Its ideal value is 1 but is always <1 and approaches unity in increasing plan quality from below. It simultaneously surrogates target overcoverage, undercoverage, and/or misalignment of prescription dose with the target as shown in Fig. 19.2. One downside is that by incorporating all three, one is unable to immediately attribute the source of a plan's imperfections from this value alone. Although not readily output by most treatment planning systems by default, the index is easy to calculate or script and highly useful. Additionally, the index can be thought of as a quality score from 0 to 100, e.g., a plan with PCI = 0.95 can be thought of as 95% conformal plan, which can facilitate more rapid intuiting to a new planner.

New Conformity Index (NCI)/ Nakamura's CI

$$NCI = \frac{TV \times PIV}{TV_{PIV}^2} = Paddick\,CI^{-1}$$

This index is the inverse of the Paddick CI [8]. It has no practical benefit over the Paddick CI except that some planners may prefer their indices approach unity from >1 rather than <1.

Treatment plan	Parameters	RTOG PIV/TV	RCI TV_{PIV}/TV	HTCI/SI TV_{PIV}/PIV	Paddick CI $\dfrac{TV_{PIV} \times TV_{PIV}}{TV \times V_{RI}}$
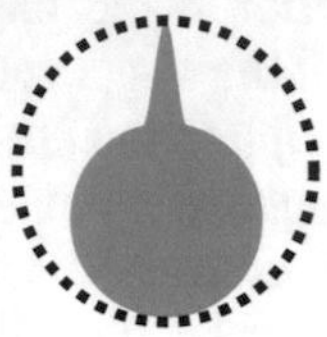	Tv = 5 cm³ PIV = 10 cm³ TV_{PIV} = 5 cm³	2	1	0.50	0.50
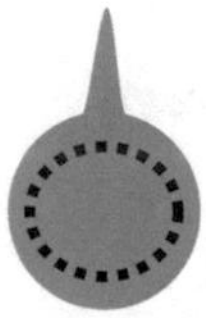	Tv = 5 cm³ PIV = 3 cm³ TV_{PIV} = 3 cm³	0.60	0.60	1	0.60
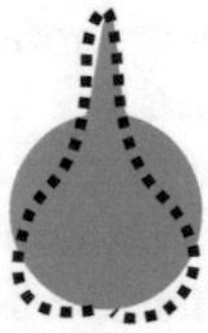	Tv = 5 cm³ PIV = 5 cm³ TV_{PIV} = 4 cm³	1	0.80	0.80	0.64
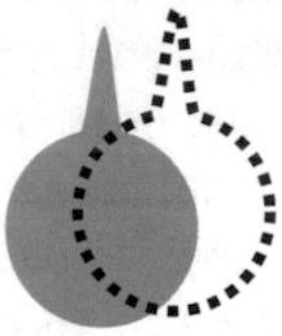	Tv = 5 cm³ PIV = 5 cm³ TV_{PIV} = 2.5 cm³	1	0.50	0.50	0.25
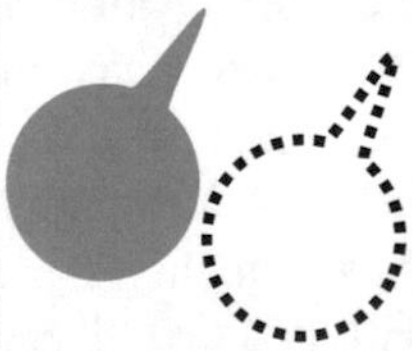	Tv = 5 cm³ PIV = 5 cm³ TV_{PIV} = 0 cm³	1	0	0	0
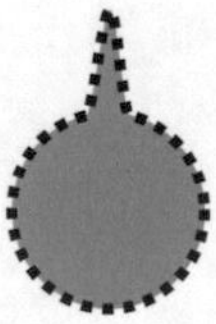	Tv = 5 cm³ PIV = 5 cm³ TV_{PIV} = 5 cm³	1	1	1	1

Fig. 19.2 Comparison of previous conformity indices with the 2000 Paddick Conformity Index. (From Feuvret et al. [1] Reprinted with permission from Elsevier)

Geometric Conformity Index

$$g = LUF + OHTF$$

$$LUF = \frac{TV_{<PI}}{TV}$$

$$HTOF = \frac{HTV_{PI}}{TV}$$

where LUF denotes the lesion underdose volume (or volume of target not receiving the prescription dose) and HTOF represents the healthy tissue overdose volume factor (volume of nontarget tissue receiving the prescription dose).

The geometric conformity index was designed by the Saint-Anne, Lariboisiere, Tenon (SALT) [9] group in their effort to quantify global treatment quality, particularly their cohort of arteriovenous malformations (AVM) treated with radiosurgery. For this index, geometric conformity is optimal at minimum values as it is the

sum of two indices that each captures an aspect of plan deficiency.

COnformal INdex (COIN)

$$COIN = CN \times \prod_{i=1}^{N_{CO}} \left[1 - \frac{V_{COref,i}}{V_{COi}} \right]$$

N_{CO} : Number of critical organs (CO)
V_{COref} : CO volume receiving reference dose
V_{COi} : Critical organ volume (Fig. 19.3)

Baltas et al. [10] integrated the conformation number with an additional index to assess not only the conformity of the prescription dose but with a penalty factor for adjacent organs at risk receiving a reference dose. It was originally suited for brachytherapy but is equally applicable to EBRT or SRS. The reference dose for the critical organs may not need to be identical to the pre-

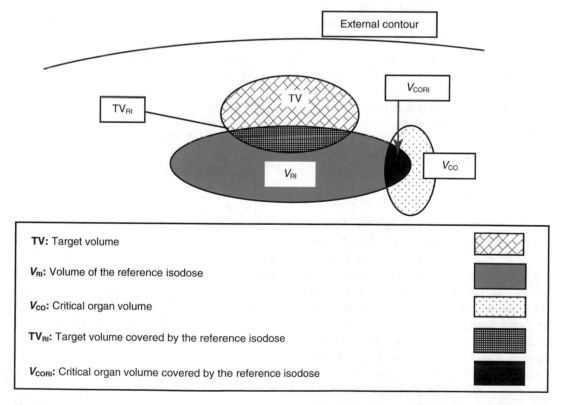

Fig. 19.3 Illustration of the volumes used in the COIN index. (From Feuvret et al. [1] Reprinted with permission from Elsevier)

scription dose. For instance, a radiosurgery plan to an optic chiasm meningioma could use a prescription dose of 14 Gy in the conformation number side of the calculation and a reference dose of 8 Gy in the critical organ indexed product.

Gradient Indices

Gradient indices generally measure some aspect of dose falloff around the target especially the steepness between the prescription isodose and one-half the prescription isodose. More simply a gradient index is a measure of the compactness of the moderate isodose volume.

UF Gradient Index

$$CGIg = 100 - [100 \times \left(R_{Eff,50\%Rx} - R_{Eff,Rx} \right) - 0.3cm]$$

where REff, 50%Rx and REff,Rx are the radii of spheres having volumes PIV50% and PIV, respectively. The UF gradient index was the first gradient index proposed to evaluate the steepness of the falloff between the prescription isodose line and half prescription isodose line. Its principal disadvantages are the difficulty in calculation of effective isodose curve radii in certain treatment planning systems and its assumption of isotropic falloff in all directions.

Paddick/Dose Gradient Index

$$Paddick\,GI = \frac{PIV_{50\%}}{PIV}$$

The Paddick GI is perhaps the most commonly utilized of the gradient indices. It was proposed by Paddick in 2006 [11] as a means of simplifying the computation of a metric of dose falloff. He found the requirement to compute effective radii of isodose volumes too cumbersome for routine use. The Paddick GI is easy to compute but is not so useful in interplan comparison. If two plans have an identical $PIV_{50\%}$, because the PIV is the denominator, a plan with worse conformity will spuriously appear to have better gradient. Conversely, improving a plan's conformity will falsely suggest a worse gradient

index even though $PIV_{50\%}$ is the same. This effect is illustrated in Fig. 19.4. Plans differing in conformity should not be compared using this common gradient index.

R50% or Falloff Index (FI)

$$FI = \frac{PIV_{50\%}}{TV}$$

The R50% was first widely used as metric of plan quality in the RTOG 0915 study comparing SBRT schedules for medically inoperable non-small cell lung cancer patients. It has the advantage over the Paddick gradient index of not being dependent on the quality of conformity in a given plan.

Coverage

Minimum Coverage

$$Coverage = \frac{D_{min}}{D_{Rx}}$$

Coverage is another metric from the original RTOG radiosurgery guidelines. Obviously, the minimum dose in the target should be as close to the prescription as possible.

Homogeneity

Homogeneity (RTOG)

$$Homogeneity = \frac{D_{max}}{D_{Rx}}$$

The homogeneity index as defined by RTOG is the ratio of dmax to the prescription dose. By convention it was considered a minor protocol violation if it was >2 and a major violation if it was >5. Some centers penalize this metric in an attempt keep the target dmax with 120% of the prescription dose. This can be done but comes at the expense of the plan's gradient or falloff. For metastases, there is simply no reason to do it.

Energy Index (Yomo)

$$EI = \frac{ID}{TV \times D_{Rx}}$$

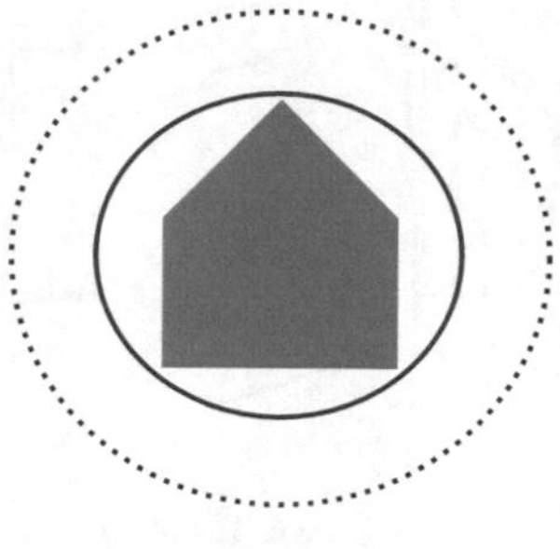

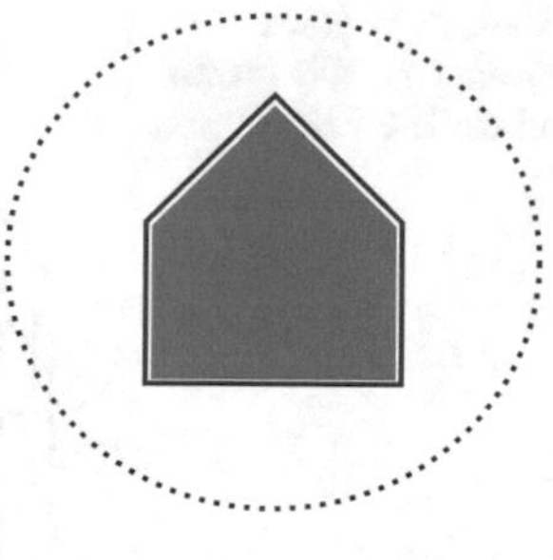

Parameters	TV = 1.5	TV = 1.5
	PIV= 2.25	PIV = 1.55
	PIV 50% = 0.0	PIV 50% = 9.0
RTOG CI	1.5	1.03
Paddick CI	0.67	0.97
Paddick GI	4	5.81
R50%	6	6

Fig. 19.4 Gradient index for dose distributions having the same PIV50% but different conformity indices. Solid red line represents the prescription dose and the dashed blue line half of the prescription dose. Notice that though the plan on the right is a more conformal plan, with the same PIV50%, it has a worse Paddick GI

The energy index [12] is another metric to assess the degree of heterogeneity within the target. This metric incorporates the integral dose of the target and is very sensitive to under- or over-dosing of the target.

Other Useful Indices

AUC-DVH

$$\mathrm{AUC}_{100\%-50\%} = \int_{\mathrm{Rx}_{50\%}}^{\mathrm{Rx}_{100\%}} V_{\mathrm{structure}} \delta \mathrm{dose}$$

The AUC-DVH is metric used to quantify not just the ratio of a dose-volume in a specific point to the prescription isodose volume but all the dose volumes in between. It is useful for further characterizing the dose falloff performance of a given radiosurgery plan. In this example, it uses the 50% isodose volume and the prescription isodose volume [13] and is a more robust falloff metric than the R50% or gradient index for assessing the totality of clinically consequential dose when comparing plans, but it can also be used for any two points along the DVH (Fig. 19.5).

Fig. 19.5 Illustration depicting the area under the DVH curve for two radiosurgery plans between the 9Gy (50%) and the 18Gy (Rx) levels

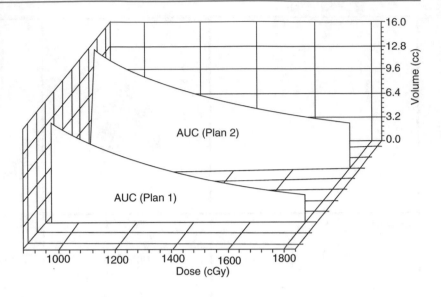

Efficiency Index

$$\eta_{50\%} = \frac{\text{Useful Energy}}{\text{Total Energy}} = \frac{\text{Integral Dose}_{TV}}{\text{Integral Dose}_{50\%PIV}} = \frac{\int_{D_{min}}^{D_{max}} TV \delta \text{dose}}{\int_{PIV_{50\%}}^{D_{max}} V \delta \text{dose}}$$

$$G\eta_{12Gy} = \frac{\text{Integral Dose}_{TV1} + \text{Integral Dose}_{TV2}}{\text{Global Integral Dose}_{12Gy}}$$

$$OAR\eta_{50\%} = \frac{\text{Integral Dose}_{OAR}}{\text{Integral Dose}_{50\%PIV}}$$

The efficiency index is a recently proposed metric which has not been widely employed yet but is unique in that it attempts to capture and quantify the proportion of all dose "doing good" versus the dose "doing harm." It amalgamates conformity, gradient, and mean dose into a single metric [14]. One can see the theoretical utility of a metric which encompasses three of the most arguably meaningful aspects of plan quality; however work remains necessary to validate the index against previously established plan quality and efficacy/toxicity outcome relationships.

Twelve Gray Isodose Volume (V12Gy)

The volume of tissue receiving 12 Gy has been the most commonly proposed predictor of radio-necrosis in the brain. Initially studied in Gamma

Knife radiosurgery for arteriovenous malformations [15], the V12Gy has also been found to correlate with radionecrosis in treatments to both benign and malignant tumors [16] and LINAC SRS as well [17]. When this volume exceeds 10–15 cc in a given location, a higher likelihood of toxicity exists. Some investigators have attempted to exclude the target from this calculation. The principle problem with this metric is that it is closely associated with the target volume, a known predictor of radiation toxicity. Figure 19.6 shows V12Gy vs. target volume demonstrating a direct linear relationship for 18 Gy prescription on both LINAC and Gamma Knife platforms when treating multiple metastases. It is clinically easier to make prescription decisions based upon target volume or target diameter before the treatment plan is available.

A second issue with the use of V12 is the (mis) application in multiple metastases plans. The most common V12-based models of toxicity treated a single target (e.g., AVM). The radiation necrosis estimates from V12 for an entire plan of multiple

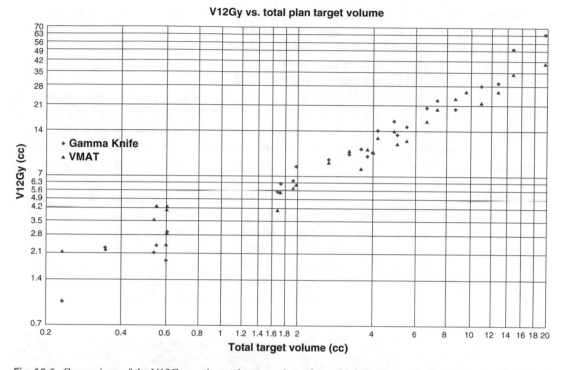

Fig. 19.6 Comparison of the V12Gy vs. the total target volume for multiple metastases in Gamma Knife and LINAC SRS plans

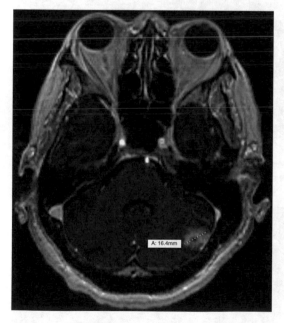

Fig. 19.7 Axial MRI slice of patient with ten metastases, the largest measuring 16.4 mm in the left cerebellum. Ten total metastases are present (others not shown) resulting in a high V12Gy on the radiosurgery plan, but all tumors are less than 2 cm. Caution is urged in extrapolating single target V12 models of toxicity to multiple target plans. This case should be safe for single fraction radiosurgery despite a high total V12

tumors should not be simply extrapolated from single target models. Consider the case in Fig. 19.7 with ten metastases. The largest metastasis is in the left cerebellum and measures ~16 mm in greatest diameter with a volume of 2.6 cc. The total target volume for all tumors is 5.3 cc, but the single fraction radiosurgery plan has a total V12 of 16 cc. This patient has a lower risk of radiation injury compared to a patient with the same total target volume from a single tumor. This patient has a high V12 but does not require does reduction or hypofractionation.

Case Vignettes

Organ Avoidance Is a Treatment Planning Goal

Case 1
Radiation treatment plans can generally be categorized as having a primary goal of either three-dimensional conformity or organ avoidance. The treatment of brain metastases generally has a primary goal of conformity where all the tissue sur-

rounding the tumor is equally at risk. If a tumor is very close to a sensitive structure, conformity in all directions is less important than the high dose to the nearby critical structure. In brain radiosurgery, this might be the optic structures or brainstem in selected cases. If organ avoidance is the primary determinant of plan quality, the prior metrics focused on conformity and gradient indices may be compromised. An example case is shown in Fig. 19.8 of a renal cell metastasis in the fourth ventricle (target in magenta). This patient had prior whole-brain RT and was prescribed 30 Gy in five fractions (yellow isodose line) to the growing fourth ventricular mass. Although the RTOG conformity index was still good at 1.3, the gradient index was poor at 8.3. Forcing organ avoidance is generally detrimental to the gradient index. In this case the dose level of the gradient (3 Gy × 5 fractions, 15 Gy shown in green isodose line) may be less clinically relevant than the small volume receiving 25–30 Gy.

Case 2

In this next case, a 68-year-old female presents with intermittent spells of patchy hypoesthesia on the right side of her face. MR reveals a 1.8 cm ring-enhancing lesion just above the pontine-medullary junction. CT chest showed an intact lump in the left breast as well as a left axillary lymph node. The lymph node was excisionally biopsied and positive for metastatic breast cancer. The patient's receptor status is still pending. She was placed on dexamethasone 4 mg PO TID by the referring physician with some resolution of her symptoms. Her performance status is excellent and she has no other major medical comorbidities (Fig. 19.9).

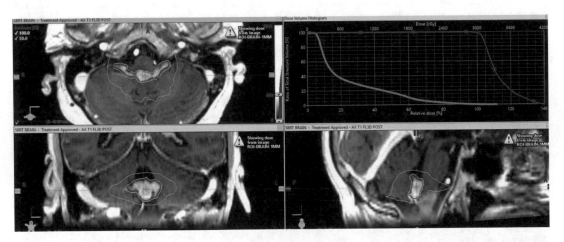

Fig. 19.8 An organ avoidance treatment plan for fourth ventricular metastasis to deliver 30 Gy in five fractions. This plan prioritizes sparing the brainstem at high isodose levels over conformity and gradient

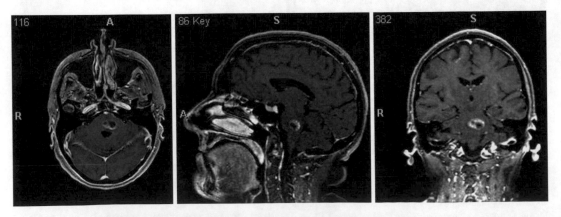

Fig. 19.9 Brainstem metastasis with different treatment planning goals compared to Case 1 in Fig. 19.8

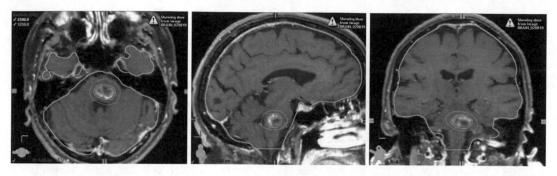

Fig. 19.10 Radiosurgery plan with conformity as the primary goal since the target is nearly equally surrounded by sensitive tissue. The prescription isodose is shown in yellow. The green line represents 50% of the prescription dose

Questions:

1. How should this case be managed?
2. What are reasonable dose fractionation schemes for this lesion?
3. Is this a conformity or organ avoidance plan?
4. What are the relevant plan quality indices to evaluate for this case?

The lesion is obviously non-operable and potentially life-limiting in short order with expectant management. Given its size, the lesion is candidate for either single fraction or fractionated radiosurgery. For this patient, the decision was made to more conservatively proceed with fractionated radiosurgery to the lesion. A dose scheme of 25 Gy/5fx was selected and was prescribed such that 100% of the prescription dose was delivered to 99% of the target volume. Other reasonable dose schemes include 15–18 Gy/1fx, 24–27 Gy/3fx, and 25–30 Gy/5fx. A multi-noncoplanar arc plan for a gantry-based linear accelerator was developed. As the lesion is encompassed by a critical organ at risk (brainstem), tissue is equally important in all directions; therefore the goal is minimize dose falloff from the prescription in all directions, making this a conformity plan. Contrast the goals of this case to the one shown in Fig. 19.8 even though both of these plans are dose-limited by the brainstem. Relevant plan quality indices for this patient would include one or more conformity indices, a measure of the gradient, and a surrogate for radionecrosis risk, as well. The isodose curves of the plan are shown below. V12Gy is the most common surrogate for radionecrosis for single fraction treatments; we review V18Gy for five-fraction plans (Fig. 19.10).

$$TV = 2.53\,cc$$

$$PIV = 2.67\,cc$$

$$PIV_{50\%} = 8.71$$

$$TV_{100\%} = 2.51$$

$$D_{max} = 34.4\,Gy$$

$$D_{min} = 23.5\,Gy$$

$$\text{Brainstem } D_{0.1cc} = 25.5\,Gy$$

$$\text{Brainstem } V18_{Gy} = 2.6\,cc$$

$$\text{RTOG CI} = \frac{PIV}{TV} = 1.06$$

$$\text{Paddick CI} = \frac{TV_{PIV}^2}{TV \times PIV} = 0.93$$

$$\text{Paddick GI} = \frac{PIV_{50\%}}{PIV} = 3.26$$

$$FI = \frac{PIV_{50\%}}{TV} = 3.44$$

$$\text{Coverage} = \frac{D_{min}}{D_{Rx}} = 94\%$$

$$\text{Homogeneity} = \frac{D_{max}}{D_{Rx}} = 1.37$$

$$EI = \frac{ID}{TV \times D_{Rx}} = 1.14$$

$$OAR\,\eta_{50\%} = \frac{\text{Integral Dose}_{OAR}}{\text{Integral Dose}_{50\%PIV}} = \frac{\text{Integral Dose}_{Brainstem}}{\text{Integral Dose}_{50\%PIV}} = 1.55$$

Authors' Recommendations

Despite a great deal of literature on the various metrics of radiosurgery plan quality, there remains a paucity of data correlating any clinical outcome to any metric of plan quality. As shown in Fig. 19.11, the achievable conformity varies by target volume such that the conformity index for small tumors will be higher than for larger tumors. This is observed in both LINAC and Gamma Knife platforms. A plan with a large tumor with an excellent conformity index may have a high V12Gy volume and exhibit elevated risk of radiation injury. Conversely, very small tumors with a RTOG conformity index >2 are typically very safe to treat.

The authors recommend that upon evaluating a radiosurgery plan, the clinician first visually assesses the plan's isodose curves through the sequence of relevant axial slices, then the concordance between the prescription dose and the target, the rapidity of the dose falloff from the prescription dose to either the half prescription dose or whatever clinically significant OAR dose may be relevant for a nearby critical structure, and finally the low-dose spill.

In our clinical practice, upon reviewing a radiosurgery plan, we display the 100% (prescription) and 50% prescription dose isocurves over the relevant imaging. We do not specify a predefined isodose line for the prescription but rather prescribe to the line that best covers the target. Portions of the target typically receive 130–160% of the peripheral prescription for single isocenter multiple target plans treated with VMAT. This normalization scheme differs from the common Gamma Knife practice of preselecting the 50% isodose volume to receive the prescription. The following metrics are then evaluated:

- RTOG conformity.
- R50% (<4 for TV >2 cm, <5–6 for 0.5 < TV <2.0 cc, <7–10 for TV < 0.5 cc).

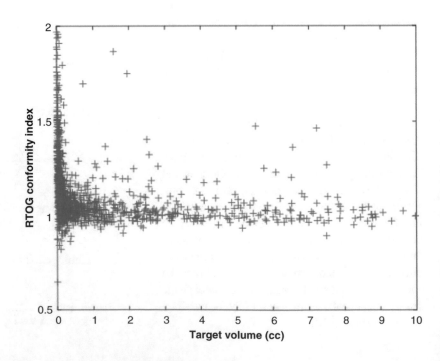

Fig. 19.11 Comparison of the RTOG conformity index with the tumor volume of targets treated in multiple metastases LINAC SRS plans. The achievable conformity for very small tumors will be higher than larger tumors. Note should be made that outliers over 1 cc on this graph generally represent cases where tumors were geometrically close together and there was unavoidable dose spill. (Data from R. Popple)

- V12Gy [(for single fx, V66% for fSRS plans) if V12 > 10 cc contiguous volume, consider an fSRS treatment].
- Mean dose to healthy brain (ALARA, but consider replan if not <3 Gy for single fraction).
- Homogeneity of the plan is generally not considered beneficial in the treatment of intact metastases and may be detrimental to other metrics.

Key Points

- Well-executed radiosurgery is an important and effective component of oncologic and benign condition care for patients with CNS disease.
- A number of plan quality metrics are available to assess how well a radiosurgery plan is designed.
- Knowledge of plan quality metrics is critical to the design and implementation of high-quality radiosurgery.

References

1. Feuvret L, Noël G, Mazeron J-J, Bey P. Conformity index: a review. Int J Radiat Oncol Biol Phys. 2006;64(2):333–42.
2. Shaw E, Kline R, Gillin M, Souhami L, Hirschfeld A, Dinapoli R, et al. Radiation Therapy Oncology Group: radiosurgery quality assurance guidelines. Int J Radiat Oncol Biol Phys. 1993;27(5):1231–9.
3. Knöös T, Kristensen I, Nilsson P. Volumetric and dosimetric evaluation of radiation treatment plans: radiation conformity index. Int J Radiat Oncol Biol Phys. 1998;42(5):1169–76.
4. Paddick I. A simple scoring ratio to index the conformity of radiosurgical treatment plans. J Neurosurg. 2000;93(Suppl 3):219–22.
5. Knoos T, Kristensen I, Nilsson P, editors. Results from clinical practice of 3D conformal radiotherapy at Lund University Hospital. Proceedings of the twelfth international conference on the use of computers in radiation therapy. Madison: Medical Physics Publishing; 1997.
6. Lomax NJ, Scheib SG. Quantifying the degree of conformity in radiosurgery treatment planning. Int J Radiat Oncol Biol Phys. 2003;55(5):1409–19.
7. Régis J, Hayashi M, Porcheron D, Delsanti C, Muracciole X, Peragut JC. Impact of the model C and automatic positioning system on gamma knife radiosurgery: an evaluation in vestibular schwannomas. J Neurosurg. 2002;97(Supplement 5):588–91.
8. Nakamura JL, Verhey LJ, Smith V, Petti PL, Lamborn KR, Larson DA, et al. Dose conformity of gamma knife radiosurgery and risk factors for complications. Int J Radiat Oncol Biol Phys. 2001;51(5):1313–9.
9. Lefkopoulos D, Dejean C, El-Balaa H, Platoni K, Grandjean P, Foulquier J-N, et al. Determination of dose-volumes parameters to characterise the conformity of stereotactic treatment plans. In: The use of computers in radiation therapy. Heidelburg, Germany: Springer; 2000. p. 356–8.
10. Baltas D, Kolotas C, Geramani K, Mould RF, Ioannidis G, Kekchidi M, et al. A conformal index (COIN) to evaluate implant quality and dose specification in brachytherapy. Int J Radiat Oncol Biol Phys. 1998;40(2):515–24.
11. Paddick I, Lippitz B. A simple dose gradient measurement tool to complement the conformity index. J Neurosurg. 2006;105(Supplement):194–201.
12. Yomo S, Tamura M, Carron R, Porcheron D, Régis J. A quantitative comparison of radiosurgical treatment parameters in vestibular schwannomas: the Leksell Gamma Knife Perfexion versus Model 4C. Acta Neurochir. 2010;152(1):47–55.
13. Thomas EM, Popple RA, Wu X, Clark GM, Markert JM, Guthrie BL, et al. Comparison of plan quality and delivery time between volumetric arc therapy (RapidArc) and Gamma Knife radiosurgery for multiple cranial metastases. Neurosurgery. 2014;75(4):409–18.
14. Dimitriadis A, Paddick I. A novel index for assessing treatment plan quality in stereotactic radiosurgery. J Neurosurg. 2018;129(Suppl1):118–24.
15. Flickinger JC, Lunsford LD, Kondziolka D, Maitz AH, Epstein AH, Simons SR, et al. Radiosurgery and brain tolerance: an analysis of neurodiagnostic imaging changes after gamma knife radiosurgery for arteriovenous malformations. Int J Radiat Oncol Biol Phys. 1992;23(1):19–26.
16. Korytko T, Radivoyevitch T, Colussi V, Wessels BW, Pillai K, Maciunas RJ, et al. 12 Gy gamma knife radiosurgical volume is a predictor for radiation necrosis in non-AVM intracranial tumors. Int J Radiat Oncol Biol Phys. 2006;64(2):419–24.
17. Blonigen BJ, Steinmetz RD, Levin L, Lamba MA, Warnick RE, Breneman JC. Irradiated volume as a predictor of brain radionecrosis after linear accelerator stereotactic radiosurgery. Int J Radiat Oncol Biol Phys. 2010;77(4):996–1001.

Image Guidance for Frameless Radiosurgery Including Surface Mapping

Guang Li, Yoshiya Yamada, and Åse Ballangrud

With the recent advent of image-guided radio-therapy (IGRT) and surface-guided radiotherapy (SGRT), treatment accuracy has been substantially improved [1–3]. Such improvements are critical to deliver cranial radiosurgery treatment plans that require high precision due to high dose-per-fraction to the planning tumor volume (PTV) and a sharp dose falloff gradient outside the PTV. By following careful calibration and well-developed procedures, IGRT provides sub-millimeter accuracy for interfractional patient setup and SGRT delivers real-time intra-fractional patient motion monitoring during treatment.

Although the invasive frame-based stereotactic radiosurgery (SRS) technique provides high-precision treatments for patients with brain metastasis, it has some limitations in clinical implementation and workflow. For instance, the use of an invasive frame demands that the entire treatment from simulation and planning to delivery be completed within 1 day. The time constraint becomes a limiting factor on how many lesions can be treated in one setting. In addition, the invasive frame-based technique cannot be applied to treat a patient with hypofractionated radiotherapy (SRT). In the following, we discuss the limitations of the frame-based technique and advantages of frameless SRS and SRT techniques through a clinical case; describe detailed IGRT/SGRT techniques that were developed for frameless SRS/SRT treatment, including system requirements, calibration and treatment procedures, and the uncertainties involved; and then provide recommendations and future perspectives.

Case Vignette

Case 1: A Patient Needs Both Single-Fraction and Hypofractionated Radiotherapy

A 66-year-old female presents with eight cranial metastases from a primary large cell neuroendocrine lung cancer. Pretreatment magnetic resonance images (MRI) are shown in Fig. 20.1. Physical examination was non-focal and the patient was neurologically intact. The patient was concerned about the potential effects of whole-brain radiation on neurocognitive function and opted for stereotactic radiosurgery. Although the patient had other sites of extracranial metastases, the brain was the only site of active disease. Prescription dose and fractionation for each lesion were determined based on lesion volume, location, and proximity to other lesions that

G. Li (✉) · Å. Ballangrud
Department of Medical Physics, Memorial Sloan Kettering Cancer Center, New York, NY, USA
e-mail: LiG2@mskcc.org

Y. Yamada
Department of Radiation Oncology, Memorial Sloan Kettering Cancer Center, New York, NY, USA

© Springer Nature Switzerland AG 2020
Y. Yamada et al. (eds.), *Radiotherapy in Managing Brain Metastases*,
https://doi.org/10.1007/978-3-030-43740-4_20

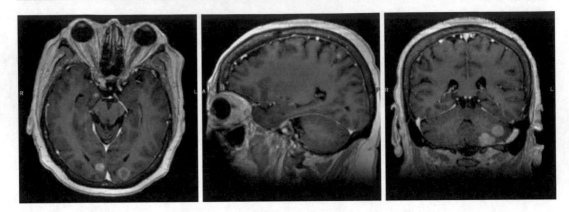

Fig. 20.1 Pretreatment MR images showing six out of the eight metastatic lesions

would be targeted for treatment. The treating radiation oncologist prescribed 1800 cGy × 1 to two lesions, 2100 cGy × 1 to four lesions, and 900 cGy × 3 to two lesions. One single-fraction SRS plan was generated to treat six lesions and a separate SRT plan to treat two lesions in 3 fractions. Frameless immobilization combined with image guidance for patient positioning and optical surface monitoring during treatment was used to facilitate treatment. The single-fraction plan was delivered in the same treatment session as the first fraction of the hypofractionated plan. The remaining fractions were delivered daily, completing treatment in 3 days. At last follow-up, 26 months after treatment, the brain remains locally controlled, and the patient has no discernable radiation-related toxicity.

The frameless immobilization and image-guided setup provide a flexible solution for patients that need different fractionation to some lesions to safely deliver the cranial radiation. However, if a patient were treated using the invasive frame for the SRS plan, the patient would be simulated, planned, and treated in two separate processes: one simulation with the invasive frame and one in a noninvasive head mask. Furthermore, the two treatments would be treated sequentially, increasing the overall treatment visits. In contrast, the frameless immobilization provides not only patient comfort and convenience but also additional clinical treatment options, possibly with fewer treatment visits.

Recent developments in more effective systemic therapies have become important for patients with multiple cranial metastases. For example, checkpoint inhibitors show promising intracranial efficacy in patients with brain metastasis from melanoma and non-small lung cancer [4, 5]. The management of brain metastasis has become increasingly individualized pending the patient's performance status, primary cancer types, and genotypes. The results of several studies have shown that instead of delivering whole-brain radiation, focal radiation of the metastatic lesions provides improved cognition for these patients [6–8]. Whole-brain radiation is no longer the standard of care for all patients with multiple brain metastasis. New treatment planning and delivery techniques are needed to meet these new clinical needs. The use of a noninvasive immobilization system along with image-guided setup and motion monitoring provides the flexibility needed to customize SRS and SRT treatments to meet the new clinical standards.

Background and Motivation

Conventional invasive frame-based SRS has been the standard of care for brain metastatic lesions treated on a linear accelerator (LINAC), providing high geometric accuracy (≤1.0 mm) [9–11]. The stereotactic technique involves a complex clinical procedure where a head frame is fixated with four surgical screws into a patient's skull by a neurosurgeon prior to computed tomography (CT) simulation. The head frame serves as head fixation as well as an external fiducial reference system for stereotactic patient positioning at treatment. Following CT simulation, the patient will wait in the radiation oncology clinic until a patient-specific treatment plan is generated, reviewed and approved by the treating radiation oncologist, and passed through physics second check. The stereotactic technique requires quality assurance (QA) of the invasive frame and reference frames used during simulation and treatment as well as the LINAC prior to treatment. The wall lasers are used for positioning of the patient for stereotactic setup, and prior to treatment, the coincidence of the laser isocenter to the LINAC megavoltage radiation isocenter must be verified using the Winston-Lutz test [12, 13]. The time from simulation to treatment is often 4–6 h making it a long day for the patient. The treatment planning time, the time it takes to perform the QA, and the treatment delivery time increase by each additional lesion that is targeted when using traditional planning techniques with one isocenter for each lesion. The combined plan preparation and treatment time increase by approximately 1–1.5 h for each additional lesion. Therefore, the clinical staff is under stress with a stringent time constraint to create, approve, verify, and deliver the radiation in a timely manner.

There is also a lack of flexibility in the invasive frame stereotactic system. For patients who have undergone surgical resection of the metastases prior to radiation treatment, mounting the invasive frame can be challenging. Occasionally the combination of the patient's anatomy and the location of the lesion to be treated make it difficult to place the invasive frame in a position that finally will allow for stereotactic setup. Because many cancer patients live longer owing to improved systemic therapies, a flexible system is needed to provide repeated cranial radiosurgery, often to multiple cranial metastases. Noninvasive immobilization devices have been used in the past [14–19], but without the use of a robotic couch, image-guided setup, and motion monitoring, providing insufficient accuracy for radiosur-

gery. Early efforts in the frameless approach have been reported [20, 21] aiming to provide fractionated treatment with improved accuracy.

With cranial radiosurgery becoming the standard of care for patients with multiple brain metastases, there is a need for a frameless immobilization and positioning system providing the same high geometric accuracy as the invasive frame systems. A frameless immobilization system will open for high-precision fractionated treatments. Because a frameless immobilization system may not provide the same level of immobilization during treatment as the frame-based head fixation, patient motion monitoring during treatment is crucial for frameless cranial radiosurgery. A radiosurgery plan on a LINAC will include multiple couch and gantry angles, complicating the option for motion monitoring. At many couch angles, the on-board imaging (OBI) system installed on the LINAC gantry will not clear from a collision with the couch and the patient. Therefore, an independent floor-mounted noncoplanar X-ray-based imaging system is frequently used for cranial radiosurgery [22]. Such X-ray systems provide bony match verification with submillimeter accuracy at manually determined time points but not continuous monitoring. Alternatively, a video-based optical surface imaging (OSI) system can provide real-time (3–4 Hz frame rate) imaging. These systems use three ceiling-mounted camera pods, and, at any given moment, at least two pods will avoid blocking by the gantry and will map the patient's facial surface area. The OSI monitoring systems use an uncovered, open area of the patient's face as a surrogate to infer the tumor position, taking advantage of the rigid anatomy of the head that provides a fixed relationship between the surface and the radiation target. The OSI systems cannot be used if closed face masks are used for immobilization as the skin surrogate is not available. Motion monitoring is performed by matching the real-time OSI images to a reference surface either obtained from the planning CT external contour or acquired after the patient is positioned for treatment using cone-beam computed tomography (CBCT). A LINAC equipped with image-guided technologies is shown in Fig. 20.2.

Fig. 20.2 A linear accelerator (LINAC) with image-guided technologies, including (**a**–**c**) a ceiling-mounted camera system for optical surface imaging (OSI), (**d**, **e**) a kilovoltage (kV) imaging system for cone-beam computed tomography (CBCT), (**f**) a megavoltage (MV) electronic portal imaging detector (EPID), and (**g**) a couch extension on (**h**) a robotic couch for six-dimensional (6D) patient positioning adjustments

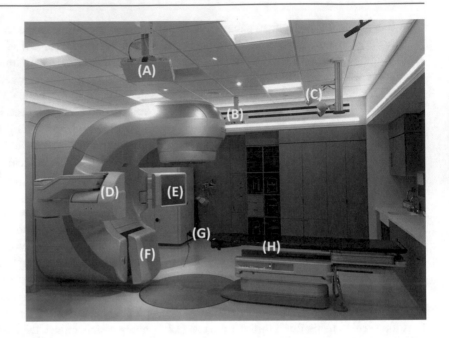

Image-Guided Frameless Radiosurgery

Selecting Immobilization and Monitoring System

Because the invasive frame stereotactic system must provide both accurate patient positioning and fixation, patient motion is very limited during treatment. It is important to consider the following factors together: (1) availability of a 6D robotic couch for accurate positioning with CBCT setup, (2) availability of motion monitoring systems (continuous motion monitoring during treatment for beam gating or periodic verifications), and (3) selecting a patient immobilization system that provides sufficient motion restriction and works with the motion monitoring system.

Certain immobilization systems reproduce the simulated position by utilizing a mouth guard, whereas other systems provide couch extension that is used for pitch/roll adjustments [18, 23]. It is highly recommended to use a 6D robotic couch to facilitate patient setup with improved accuracy and shortened setup time. Alternatively, a rotationally adjustable couch extension may be used to manually minimize the rotational error with

real-time OSI guidance. If only the 3D translational shifts determined by a CBCT-to-CT registration are applied, any remaining rotational errors may affect the motion monitoring accuracy. When the residual rotational errors are significant, the translational and rotational motions may become tangled making it difficult to interpret the errors. Therefore, the conventional 3D patient setup does not provide sufficient accuracy for SRS treatment.

It is important to set appropriate clinical tolerance level for setup accuracy, both on translational and rotational residual shifts. For instance, if a plan is for one lesion with the isocenter placed inside the lesion, residual rotational errors may have a small effect on the accuracy of the delivered dose. However, if one isocenter is used with a volumetric-modulated arc therapy (VMAT) plan to treat multiple lesions distributed within the brain, a small residual rotational error may cause a substantial setup error for a lesion farther away from the isocenter. This will be discussed in more detail in the section for uncertainties and future directions.

An OSI system with three camera pods is ideal for frameless SRS motion monitoring during treatment (Fig. 20.2). The OSI system requires mapping of the patient's face, and therefore an immobilization system with an open face should be utilized [24], as shown in Fig. 20.3. If a robotic 6D couch, or rotationally adjustable couch extension, is unavailable, it is important to select an immobilization system that can precisely reproduce the simulated head position at time of treatment. Without a 6D couch, the patient treatment setup may take significant time to achieve the desired accuracy.

Some cranial immobilization systems use a couch extension for manual correction of rotations [23, 24]. These systems utilize an open-face mask and a custom head support, which forms a clamshell to hold the patient's head in position and has an extension board that provides manual pitch and roll adjustment. When used together with the OSI system, it will significantly shorten the setup time by registering the outer structure from planning CT to the OSI surface and by correcting the head rotation first (<0.5°), followed by couch translational shifts (<0.5 mm) [18, 23]. This will bring the patient position within the range that can be corrected by a robotic couch. When CBCT is acquired, all rotational and translational shifts based on CBCT match to CT are applied by using a 6D robotic couch, a new OSI system reference image is acquired in this final treatment position for motion monitoring during treatment.

Description of a Frameless Image-Guided Radiosurgery Procedure

At CT simulation, a custom immobilization system is made by the simulation therapists. In the example shown in Fig. 20.3, a head mold covers the posterior skull all the way to the vertex of the

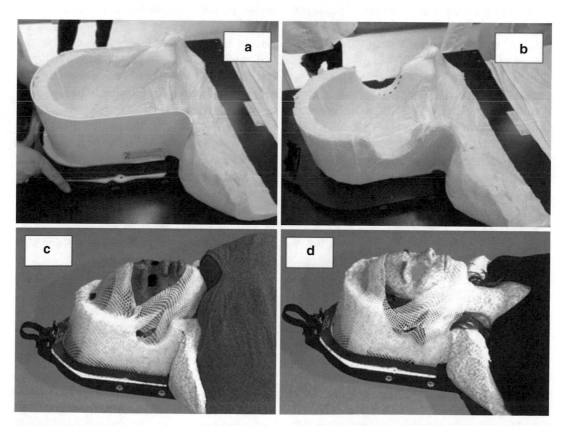

Fig. 20.3 A frameless stereotactic radiosurgery (SRS) immobilization system with a customized head mold and open-face mask allowing optical surface imaging (OSI) to view the face for real-time motion monitoring. The chin and forehead are leveled. (Courtesy of Dr. Li, published in J App Clin Med Phys [23])

head and up to the ears laterally. After the mold is hardened, a thermal plastic open-face mask is applied to the patient anteriorly and locked to the couch extension board, completing the clamshell assembly. A neutral head position (the forehead and chin are roughly aligned horizontally) provides a larger visible skin surface, improving the signal-to-noise ratio for OSI monitoring.

The OSI setup is prepared using the external contour from simulation CT and the plan isocenter as the references, where a region of interest (ROI) is defined that typically covers the open-face area, excluding the lips/mouth.

The sim-to-treatment schedule for frameless radiosurgery can follow the same process as other image-guided treatment plans due to the elimination of the invasive head frame. The planning techniques can be VMAT, dynamic conformal arc (DCA), or multiple static beams [25].

The LINAC QA required for image-guided radiosurgery includes the isocenter congruence test between the CBCT imaging system and megavoltage (MV) treatment beam and daily calibration of the OSI system to verify the isocenter. The two-level calibration process is used to achieve higher accuracy than one-level calibration, together with the OSI-MV beam isocenter congruence check as the monthly calibration [26]. A daily QA is performed in the morning by the radiation therapists and reviewed by a physicist.

At time of treatment, the patient is immobilized in the head mold with the open-face mask on the couch extension, attached to a robotic 6D couch. The OSI system is used as a guide when adjusting the pitch and roll on the couch extensions. This ensures that the patient is positioned within the range that can be corrected with the robotic couch. The entire process takes less than 1 min inside the treatment room. The OSI is continuously monitoring while a CBCT is acquired, followed by a bony match registration by a therapist, verification by a physicist, and approval by an attending physician. The difference between the initial OSI-guided setup and the final CBCT registration is usually less than 2 mm. Once the CBCT shifts are applied, a new reference OSI image is acquired to establish the treatment position with the ROI automatically mapped to the

new reference image. This new ROI is used for position verification at different couch angles by capturing a static image and for motion monitoring using the real-time delta (RTD) during the treatment. The static image has larger field of view (FOV) than the RTD image, which only reconstructs the ROI image, leading to a higher frame rate for continuous motion monitoring. Through a motion management interface (MMI) with a LINAC, radiation beam will be held if the patient motion exceeds the set clinical tolerance until the motion falls back within the tolerance.

Should the static OSI verification at a treatment couch angle produce a deviation from the initial post-CBCT reference greater than 1.0 mm, a simple method to distinguish patient motion from couch-angle dependency error is to move back the couch to zero and recapture a static OSI verification image. If the static OSI verification image is in agreement with the pretreatment image, then the patient has not moved and the deviation is caused by technical factors of the camera system. Any discrepancy between the OSI verification images at couch zero indicates that the patient has moved and a new CBCT is acquired to reposition the patient. The frequency of false indication of patient motion has been significantly reduced with the use of a 6D couch which minimizes any initial head rotation at the setup and with the use of the two-level (3D) calibration instead of the one-level (2D) plate calibration. The experience from our clinic with the above-described immobilization, setup, and monitoring technique is that less than 2% of the patients will move 1.0 mm or more during treatment.

In summary, the OSI system allows for (1) quick in-room patient setup with initial surface alignment, (2) establishing a new OSI reference image for motion monitoring after the CBCT setup, (3) verification of the patient position at each planned couch angle, and (4) real-time OSI motion monitoring at 3–4 Hz frame rate during treatment. The combination of the flexible open-face immobilization system [24], a 6D robotic couch to correct the CBCT 6D shifts, and an OSI system for motion monitoring provides the geometric accuracy needed for cranial radiosurgery [23], including multiple-lesion treatments with a single isocenter [25]. Although the new frameless immobilization systems provide good patient fixation, patient compliance is needed to avoid a prolonged treatment [24]. Real-time motion monitoring is necessary to catch the outliers that do move during treatment [25].

Geometric Uncertainties in Image-Guided Radiosurgery

Possible geometric uncertainties in a frameless SRS delivery includes (1) imaging system uncertainties, (2) motion monitoring uncertainty, and (3) operator variations. The procedures for commissioning and calibration of the imaging systems are discussed below, whereas training and credentialing of the clinical staff is discussed at the end of this section.

OSI System Commissioning, Calibration, and QA

The OSI system was initially developed for breast cancer treatment where the skin is a good surrogate for the target [27–29]. The systems have since been adapted to provide sufficient spatial and temporal accuracy for frameless radiosurgery, and the QA procedures have been developed to ensure adequacy [18]. The OSI system commissioning, monthly calibration, and routine daily QA are of paramount importance to ensure the system meets the requirement for frameless SRS. The recent development and clinical application of the two-level plate calibration method, the advance camera optimization (ACO) technique, and the OSI-MV isocenter congruence check have greatly reduced the number of false positive in patient motion, facilitating smooth frameless SRS treatment [26, 30, 31].

System Characterization and Commissioning

The special accuracy and frame rate of the OSI system must be determined before a clinical application. The spatial accuracy is best determined using a head phantom mounted on a high-precision platform to control the phantom motion, as shown in Fig. 20.4a. Because this platform allows 0.1 mm motion increment in one horizontal direction, the experiment was performed with the couch at 0° and 90°, to cover the two dimensions, while the third vertical dimension can be controlled by the couch. The accuracy of this platform has been reported [27]. Motion detection was tested by running the RTD, comparing with a reference image captured at the initial setting. The results are shown in Fig. 20.4b, c.

Typically, a radiosurgery radiation plan contains noncoplanar beams, and it is therefore important to evaluate couch-angle dependency of the OSI system. In the OSI commissioning process, it is highly recommended to include the couch-angle dependency test, ensuring that the system provides a similar accuracy of motion detection at all couch angles. After a system calibration, a head phantom experiment is conducted to check the phantom image alignment at a couch angle in reference to the image captured at couch zero, with couch rotation from 0° to ±90° at the interval of 10°. By changing from the one- to two-level plate calibration (discussed next), the error as function of couch angle is reduced to approximately 0.5–1.0 mm.

Testing of a possible OSI baseline drift in the RTD should be included in the commissioning to demonstrate the stability of the real-time imaging system. For the new high-definition (HD) camera system using low heat-emitting LED as the light source for sparkle pattern projection, the baseline drift is reduced to an amplitude of −0.3 mm in the vertical direction in the first 5–10 min. In summary, the above two commissioning tests provide the baseline error of a new OSI system, serving as the guideline for clinical error assessment for frameless SRS treatments.

OSI Calibration Procedures

There are three methods available to calibrate the OSI system, depending on the accuracy requirement for the intended clinical use. The first two methods use a calibration plate, which is a 1×1 m^2 white board with an array of circular block dots and a crosshair, indicating the center

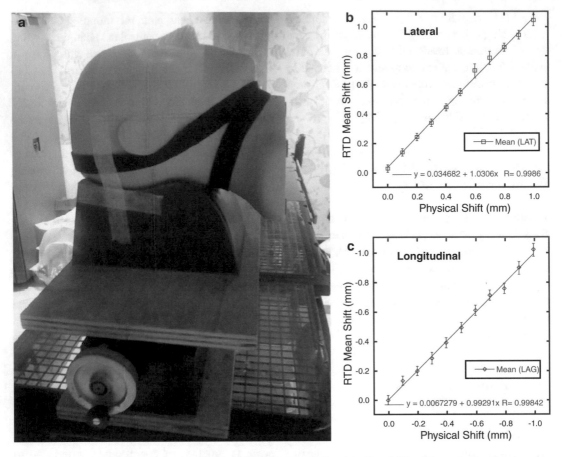

Fig. 20.4 Setup of a head phantom experiment to determine the motion detection ability of the optical surface imaging (OSI) system using its real-time delta (RTD) detection mode. (Courtesy of Dr. Li; published in Med Phys [18])

of the plate. The plate is precisely placed at the LINAC isocenter by aligning the light-projected crosshair from the gantry to the plate crosshair so that the OSI isocenter can be determined. The dot array will provide necessary data for 3D surface image reconstruction based on the law of sine within the triangle between the two cameras in a pod and one point on the surface such as the center of a black dot. The difference between the two methods is one level vs. two level of plate positions. Unlike the one-level calibration, the two-level one is a true 3D calibration, providing a calibration condition close to the actual clinical imaging condition, where the patient's skin surface is above the isocenter in a deep-seated tumor. Therefore, applying the two-level calibration procedure is recommended.

A third calibration method is to fine-tune the OSL isocenter position by using a large cube

phantom ($15 \times 15 \times 15$ cm^3) that provides a large surface and contains five internal radiopaque markers. By minimizing the deviation of the OSI isocenter with the megavoltage (MV) radiation isocenter, the uncertainty of the OSI system becomes less dependent of couch angle because the OSI rotational transformation has a more accurate rotation center. If the calibration is not performed, the deviation of the OSI isocenter will be amplified at a couch rotation, the so-called couch angle dependency, in addition to the couch walk and OSI partial-view uncertainties.

System QA and Annual Preventive Maintenance (PM)

Routine QA includes daily consistency check and monthly calibration. The daily QA is performed by therapists and verified by physicists. If the daily QA is consistently meeting the requirement, the calibration period can be extended to quarterly or semiannually. According to the service contract, an annual PM service should be performed by an engineer from the vendor. After the service, or a system upgrade, the system should be recalibrated. An ad hoc calibration is needed when a daily QA fails, likely due to the corruption of the calibration file or a physical shift of the ceiling-mounted OSI camera pods.

X-Ray Imaging QA

The congruence of the imaging isocenter and radiation isocenter must be checked and within a tight tolerance for image-guided patient positioning for radiosurgery. CBCT is the clinical standard for patient setup for radiosurgery patients, using the skull bone to register the CBCT to the planning CT image. The CBCT is acquired in the treatment room using an on-board imager (OBI) with a kilovoltage (kV) beam perpendicular to the treatment megavoltage (MV) beam. The alignment of the kV and MV isocenters is crucial to produce accurate IGRT treatment because this uncertainty is transparent to clinical users. The verification and/or adjustment of the kV CBCT and MV treatment isocenters must be performed by a physicist in the LINAC QA process under the guideline from AAPM (American Associate of Physicists in Medicine) task groups 104 [32] and 142 [33]. A daily QA to check the isocenter consistency is performed by a therapist in the morning and reviewed by a physicist before treatment starts.

Once the immobilization system and setup procedure are established, an end-to-end test must be performed to demonstrate the treatment accuracy, following the exact clinical procedure from simulation to treatment. An anthropomorphic head phantom with radiochromic films inserted in the center can be used to determine geometric and dosimetry accuracy. The phantom is scanned in CT by the therapist, target structures contoured, planned and checked by the physicist, and positioned and treated by the therapist, mimicking a real clinical treatment. The film is analyzed by the physicist. Geometric accuracy

must be within 1 mm. The end-to-end test is completed for all LINACs used for the frameless cranial radiosurgery.

Uncertainties in OSI Real-Time Motion Monitoring

Outer Structure from Planning CT

Prior studies have investigated if the optical surface can be used to tack motion relevant for lesion inside the brain [34]. Questions have been raised whether a minor change on a patient face within the ROI would matter. For instance, what if a patient blinks or makes a face? Eye blinking effect can be ignored, because (1) eyelid thickness is thin and areas are small compared with the ROI and (2) opened eyes often produce holes in the image that do not contribute to the alignment. The tightness of the mask, due to the hardening of the mask (shrinks ~1 mm after 24 h), makes it difficult for a patient to move the facial skin without extra effort.

In some cases, the outer structure from the planning CT does not serve as a good surrogate for the isocenter position. Some patients experience facial swelling in the period from simulation to treatment, making OSI pre-alignment unreliable. This can be visually identified and avoided by drawing a temporary ROI on the mask for the pre-CBCT alignment. After the patient is positioned using CBCT with bony alignment, a new OSI reference image is captured and used for motion monitoring.

OSI Resolution and Frame Rate for Motion Monitoring

It is important to have continuous monitoring to capture a possible patient motion during treatment, as the patient motion is rather random. For the OSI system, the frame rates are affected by image capture speed and image reconstruction speed. The former is within 50 ms, including data saving, whereas the latter is much longer depending on the size of the ROI and OSI spatial resolution. For the clinical SRS procedure, the highest resolution should be used to provide the best spatial accuracy for SRS treatment, and the

ROI size should be as large as possible within the open-face area. Under these conditions, the frame rate is about 3–4 frames per second (fps), with an imaging-related latency of 250 ms. Ideally, an automatic beam hold should be applied, but manual beam hold may be sufficient and used, given the high restriction of the head immobilization.

The OSI systems communicate with the LINAC via the motion management interface (MMI), and automatic beam hold can be triggered once the RTD exceeds the set tolerance. When MMI is enabled for OSI beam gating, the OSI workstation will be "booked" for the entire treatment day regardless of whether the OSI will be used for SGRT, preventing preparation of new starts on that OSI workstation.

Staff Training and Credentialing

The high accuracy required for image-guided frameless SRS prompts training programs for all staff involved, including physicians, physicists, therapists, and nurses. Although the image-guided process is similar to non-SRS treatments, it is important that everyone understands the extra accuracy needed. Because most of the changes from frame-based to frameless SRS are related to utilizing IGRT and SGRT techniques, training is mostly focused on the technical changes and updates for physicians, physicists, and therapists. For physicists, the emphasis is on the IGRT patient setup and SGRT motion monitoring, together with their tolerances, including required SRS daily QA, surface ROI preparation, DICOM and on-site references, as well as handling of OSI false positive and patient motion. An SRS physicist acts as the supervisor for the SRS treatment.

To implement the staff training and credentialing, a credential committee comprised of experienced physicians, physicists, therapists, and nurses may be established. Training programs with initial and periodic training should be developed for all staff to follow, so that the quality of frameless radiosurgery can be maintained in the clinic.

Recommendations and Future Directions

In summary, development of a frameless SRS procedure using IGRT and SGRT requires careful selection of an immobilization system; detailed workflow for simulation, planning, and treatment; daily QA for the imaging systems to ensure required SRS precision; and training of all personnel involved.

A detailed clinical workflow is necessary for a successful implementation of a frameless SRS/SRT program. A complete dry run with end-to-end testing must be completed with all involved staff to iron out possible issues that may come up along the process from the beginning to the end. For example, when the head immobilization is made prior to CT simulation, it is important that the patient's face and forehand are horizontally leveled to ensure optimal motion monitoring with the OSI system because the three ceiling-mounted cameras are inferior-anterior to the patient. To expedite the patient setup, the treatment couch position should be acquired based on the marking on the immobilization device, as indicated as isocenter shifts in the setup instruction before the patient enters the treatment room. After the patient is positioned in the head mold, the couch can be moved to the treatment position directly. The rotational shifts should be first minimized with OSI guidance and then the translational shifts. During CBCT acquisition, RTD motion monitoring should be kept on, so that the patient can be monitored during CBCT acquisition and registration. Simultaneously, the camera system can be warmed up and stabilized (the baseline drift reaches the plateau), ready for treatment. At the end of treatment, a final check of head position at couch zero with OSI is recommended. These are key example steps in the workflow that can be optimized to ensure a smooth SRS treatment. Hypofractionated treatment may be preferable for some patients, due to either the location and size of the lesion, prior brain radiation courses, or concurrent systemic treatment, using the exact same workflow, immobilization, plan type, and setup and motion monitoring for treatment. By doing so, the PTV margin can be reduced from 3 to

2 mm. The IGRT/SGRT offers a flexible solution, and a workflow for same-day frameless SRS/SRT can also be worked out if there is a need for fast turnover.

Image-guided setups using CBCT and surface-guided real-time motion monitoring using OSI provide adequate geometric accuracy for frameless radiosurgery. This opens the possibility to deliver a single-fraction treatment to some lesions and hypofractionated treatment to other lesions in the same treatment course. With increased flexibility, treatment can be customized depending on the number of brain lesions, the volume of the lesions, and the location of all lesions relative to each other and to organs at risk. The treatment planning time is currently the limiting factor for fast aim to treatment for multiple-lesion VMAT SRS on a LINAC. Better dose calculation algorithms may simplify the planning process [25], better optimizers may shorten the planning time and generate better plans, and better tools for tracking new and treated lesions on consecutive magnetic resonance images (MRIs) for retreatments could still significantly improve the SRS planning using LINACs.

Key Points

- Development of a frameless SRS procedure using IGRT and SGRT requires careful selection of an immobilization system; detailed workflow for simulation, planning, and treatment; daily QA for the imaging systems to ensure required SRS precision; and training of all personnel involved.
- A complete dry run with end-to-end testing must be completed with all involved staff to iron out possible issues that may come up along the process from the beginning to the end.
- Image-guided setups using CBCT and surface-guided real-time motion monitoring using OSI provide adequate geometric accuracy for frameless

radiosurgery and reduce uncertainties associated with frameless radiosurgery.
- Careful commissioning and ongoing quality assurance are crucial for the proper use of OSI systems.
- Staff training and credentialing is highly recommended for use with OSI systems.

References

1. Chen GT, Sharp GC, Mori S. A review of image-guided radiotherapy [published online ahead of print 2009/01/01]. Radiol Phys Technol. 2009;2(1):1–12.
2. Jaffray DA. Image-guided radiotherapy: from current concept to future perspectives. Nat Rev Clin Oncol. 2012;9(12):688–99.
3. Li G, Mageras G, Dong L, Mohan R. Image-guided radiation therapy. In: Khan FM, Gerbi BJ, editors. Treatment planning in radiation oncology. 4th ed. Philadelphia: Lippincott Williams & Wilkins; 2016. p. 229–58.
4. Murphy B, Walker J, Bassale S, et al. Concurrent radiosurgery and immune checkpoint inhibition: improving regional intracranial control for patients with metastatic melanoma [published online ahead of print 2018/12/18]. Am J Clin Oncol. 2019;42(3):253–7.
5. Kamath SD, Kumthekar PU. Immune checkpoint inhibitors for the treatment of central nervous system (CNS) metastatic disease. Front Oncol. 2018;8:414.
6. Kirkpatrick JP, Wang Z, Sampson JH, et al. Defining the optimal planning target volume in image-guided stereotactic radiosurgery of brain metastases: results of a randomized trial. Int J Radiat Oncol Biol Phys. 2015;91(1):100–8.
7. Savitz ST, Chen RC, Sher DJ. Cost-effectiveness analysis of neurocognitive-sparing treatments for brain metastases. Cancer. 2015;121(23):4231–9.
8. Brown PD, Jaeckle K, Ballman KV, et al. Effect of radiosurgery alone vs radiosurgery with whole brain radiation therapy on cognitive function in patients with 1 to 3 brain metastases: a randomized clinical trial. JAMA. 2016;316(4):401–9.
9. Palta JR, Liu C, Li JG. Current external beam radiation therapy quality assurance guidance: does it meet the challenges of emerging image-guided technologies? Int J Radiat Oncol Biol Phys. 2008;71(1 Suppl):S13–7.
10. Friedman WA. Linear accelerator radiosurgery. In: Chin LS, Regine WF, editors. Principles and practice of stereotactic radiosurgery. New York: Springer; 2008. p. 129–40.

11. Schell MC, Bova FJ, Larson DA, et al. Stereotactic radiosurgery. AAPM Report No. 54. 1995. https://www.aapm.org/pubs/reports/RPT_54.pdf.

12. Winston KR, Lutz W. Linear accelerator as a neurosurgical tool for stereotactic radiosurgery. Neurosurgery. 1988;22(3):454–64.

13. Lutz W, Winston KR, Maleki N. A system for stereotactic radiosurgery with a linear accelerator. Int J Radiat Oncol Biol Phys. 1988;14(2):373–81.

14. Bova FJ, Buatti JM, Friedman WA, Mendenhall WM, Yang CC, Liu C. The University of Florida frameless high-precision stereotactic radiotherapy system. Int J Radiat Oncol Biol Phys. 1997;38(4):875–82.

15. Ryken TC, Meeks SL, Pennington EC, et al. Initial clinical experience with frameless stereotactic radiosurgery: analysis of accuracy and feasibility. Int J Radiat Oncol Biol Phys. 2001;51(4):1152–8.

16. Kamath R, Ryken TC, Meeks SL, Pennington EC, Ritchie J, Buatti JM. Initial clinical experience with frameless radiosurgery for patients with intracranial metastases. Int J Radiat Oncol Biol Phys. 2005;61(5):1467–72.

17. Das S, Isiah R, Rajesh B, et al. Accuracy of relocation, evaluation of geometric uncertainties and clinical target volume (CTV) to planning target volume (PTV) margin in fractionated stereotactic radiotherapy for intracranial tumors using relocatable Gill-Thomas-Cosman (GTC) frame. J Appl Clin Med Phys. 2010;12(2):3260.

18. Li G, Ballangrud A, Kuo LC, et al. Motion monitoring for cranial frameless stereotactic radiosurgery using video-based three-dimensional optical surface imaging. Med Phys. 2011;38(7):3981–94.

19. Tachibana H, Uchida Y, Shiizuka H. Technical note: determination of the optimized image processing and template matching techniques for a patient intrafraction motion monitoring system. Med Phys. 2012;39(2):755–64.

20. Shirato H, Suzuki K, Nishioka T, et al. Precise positioning of intracranial small tumors to the linear accelerator's isocenter, using a stereotactic radiotherapy computed tomography system (SRT-CT). Radiother Oncol. 1994;32(2):180–3.

21. Willner J, Flentje M, Bratengeier K. CT simulation in stereotactic brain radiotherapy–analysis of isocenter reproducibility with mask fixation. Radiother Oncol. 1997;45(1):83–8.

22. Lewis BC, Snyder WJ, Kim S, Kim T. Monitoring frequency of intra-fraction patient motion using the ExacTrac system for LINAC-based SRS treatments. J Appl Clin Med Phys. 2018;19(3):58–63.

23. Li G, Ballangrud A, Chan M, et al. Clinical experience with two frameless stereotactic radiosurgery (fSRS) systems using optical surface imaging for motion monitoring. J Appl Clin Med Phys. 2015;16(4):5416.

24. Li G, Lovelock DM, Mechalakos J, et al. Migration from full-head mask to "open-face" mask for immobilization of patients with head and neck cancer. J Appl Clin Med Phys. 2013;14(5):243–54.

25. Ballangrud A, Kuo LC, Happersett L, et al. Institutional experience with SRS VMAT planning for multiple cranial metastases. J Appl Clin Med Phys. 2018;19(2):176–83.

26. Paxton AB, Manger RP, Pawlicki T, Kim GY. Evaluation of a surface imaging system's isocenter calibration methods. J Appl Clin Med Phys. 2017;18(2):85–91.

27. Bert C, Metheany KG, Doppke K, Chen GT. A phantom evaluation of a stereo-vision surface imaging system for radiotherapy patient setup. Med Phys. 2005;32(9):2753–62.

28. Djajaputra D, Li S. Real-time 3D surface-image-guided beam setup in radiotherapy of breast cancer. Med Phys. 2005;32(1):65–75.

29. Bert C, Metheany KG, Doppke KP, Taghian AG, Powell SN, Chen GT. Clinical experience with a 3D surface patient setup system for alignment of partial-breast irradiation patients. Int J Radiat Oncol Biol Phys. 2006;64(4):1265–74.

30. Hoisak JDP, Pawlicki T. The role of optical surface imaging systems in radiation therapy. Semin Radiat Oncol. 2018;28(3):185–93.

31. Covington EL, Fiveash JB, Wu X, et al. Optical surface guidance for submillimeter monitoring of patient position during frameless stereotactic radiotherapy. J Appl Clin Med Phys. 2019;20(6):91–8.

32. Yin F, Wong J, Balter J, et al. The role of in-room kV x-ray imaging for patient setup and target localization. AAPM Task Group Report No. 104. 2009. https://www.aapm.org/pubs/reports/detail.asp?docid=104.

33. Klein EE, Hanley J, Bayouth J, et al. Task Group 142 report: quality assurance of medical accelerators. Med Phys. 2009;36(9):4197–212.

34. Cervino LI, Pawlicki T, Lawson JD, Jiang SB. Frameless and mask-less cranial stereotactic radiosurgery: a feasibility study. Phys Med Biol. 2010;55(7):1863–73.

Safety Procedures and Checklists for Radiosurgery

21

Richard A. Popple

Introduction

Radiosurgery is considered a safe treatment when delivered accurately, having a low incidence of toxicity [1, 2]. However, because of the high dose per fraction, the consequences of a delivery error can be significant.

Delivery errors in SRS can be broadly classified as dosimetric errors, geometric errors, or machine errors. Dosimetric errors occur when the delivered dose differs by a clinically significant amount from the prescribed dose. The definition of "clinically significant" is not well-defined, but reported events usually exceed a regulatory threshold such as the United States Nuclear Regulatory Commission's definition of a medical event [3]. Examples of dosimetric errors include a calibration error on a radiosurgery linac in Florida [4] and an error in the measurement of output factors in Toulouse, France [5–7]. The error in Florida was caused by an error during the calibration of the machine output. The initial calibration was not independently checked, and the error was not detected until a year later during routine review by the RPC (now IROC Houston). The miscalibration resulted in a 50% overdose to 77 patients. In France, output factors of small MLC fields (<3 cm^2) required for commissioning

of the treatment planning system were measured using a detector that was not suitable for the measurement of small radiation fields. Consequently, 145 patients received an overdose. The error was detected a year after commissioning when the vendor conducted an inter-comparison of the output factors in use at a number of clinics. The vendor discovered the discrepancy and alerted the clinic. Of 32 patients in this group treated for acoustic neuroma, 31% had trigeminal neuropathy at 12 months [5]. In contrast, for a cohort of 33 patients treated for brain metastases no morbidity was observed 3 years after the accident despite mean overdose of 61.2% (mean delivered dose 31.5 Gy), and the survival rate was similar to that reported in the literature [7].

Geometric errors occur when the dose distribution is delivered to the wrong location. Procedures directed to the wrong site are a problem common to all areas of medicine [8]. Geometric errors result in both underdose to the target and overdose to healthy tissue. Target underdosage can result in suboptimal therapeutic effect; however, a healthy tissue overdose during radiosurgery can be catastrophic because an ablative dose is delivered to healthy tissue. In a review of adverse events related to Gamma Knife radiosurgery published by the United States Nuclear Regulatory Commission, two thirds (10 of 15) of reported events had coordinate errors as a primary cause [9]. For example, a treatment was administered to the right trigeminal nerve when the intended tar-

R. A. Popple (✉)
Department of Radiation Oncology, The University of Alabama at Birmingham, Birmingham, AL, USA
e-mail: rpopple@uabmc.edu

© Springer Nature Switzerland AG 2020
Y. Yamada et al. (eds.), *Radiotherapy in Managing Brain Metastases*,
https://doi.org/10.1007/978-3-030-43740-4_21

get was the left trigeminal nerve. Similarly, in a review of the Nuclear Regulatory Commission (NRC) Radiation Event Report Notification database for the period 2005–2010, more than half (7 of 13) of the radiosurgery-related events involved treatment to the wrong site [10].

Machine errors occur when the delivery unit does not function as expected. Machine errors can be the result of either a design flaw or improper configuration of the equipment. In one well-publicized example, the secondary collimator of linear accelerator fitted with a cone was set too large, resulting in full dose radiation outside of the cone. Three patients were severely injured, and at least one is in a near vegetative state [11]. A similar accident occurred in France in which the patient developed an esophago-tracheal fistula and died of a hemorrhage following surgery [6].

This chapter will review important concepts for risk mitigation: a culture of safety, human factors engineering, and failure modes and effects analysis. Then key recommendations of the professional guidance documents will be summarized.

Concepts for Risk Mitigation

Safety Culture

The cornerstone of error reduction is a culture of safety. A robust safety culture is one that promotes trust and collaboration among team members, encourages reporting of errors, and uses error reports to improve treatment processes [12]. Establishing and maintaining a safety culture requires concrete action in addition to the statement of values. Two important actions are the establishment of a quality committee and the use of an incident learning system.

A dedicated quality committee is a multi-disciplinary team comprised of physicians, physicists, dosimetrists, therapists, nurses, IT professionals, and any other disciplines involved in the radiation therapy process. The role of the committee is to develop and implement safety initiatives, to disseminate safety and quality information, and to act as a liaison with other safety committees in the hospital or health system. The committee should meet regularly to review policies and procedures and to investigate incidents

and near-misses. The committee should have procedures to investigate serious events rapidly, typically within 24 hours. The quality committee is responsible for regular reporting to the clinic leadership of errors, trends, and safety initiatives.

The establishment of an incident learning system and policies and procedures for reporting incidents is a key element of a safety culture and is necessary for the quality committee to collect, investigate, and act upon incidents as they occur. Although clinics can establish their own internal system, there are several multi-institutional systems available. Participation in an established, multi-institutional incident learning system is advantageous for two reasons. First, the database and reporting tools are already developed. Second, participation in a multi-institutional system allows individual clinics to learn from errors made elsewhere. One such system is RO-ILS: Radiation Oncology Incident Learning System® (www.astro.org/Patient-Care-and-Research/Patient-Safety/RO-ILS), developed by ASTRO and the American Association of Physicists in Medicine (AAPM). The framework for the RO-ILS database structure was based on "Consensus recommendations for incident learning database structures in radiation oncology," developed by the AAPM Work Group on Prevention of Errors in Radiation Oncology [13]. Other incident learning systems include Radiation Oncology Safety Education and Information System (ROSEIS, roseis.estro.org) [14] and the Center for the Assessment of Radiological Sciences' Radiotherapy Incident Reporting & Analysis System (www.cars-pso.org).

Human Factors Engineering

Many of the errors in radiosurgery can be attributed to human error [4, 10, 15, 16]. However, human error is often the final causal factor in a chain of events leading to an error, rather than a root cause. Adverse events are typically the result of systems and processes that create an environment in which people make mistakes or fail to prevent them [17]. To minimize the probability of errors, radiosurgery systems and processes must be designed such that mistakes are difficult to make [17]. Task Group 100 of the American Association of Physicists in Medicine (AAPM) identified lack of standardized procedures, inadequate training, inadequate communication, hardware and software failures, inadequate resources, inadequate design specifications, and inadequate commissioning as important sources of error [15]. Human factors engineering is a methodology for the design of processes and systems that are robust against human error. It has been applied in a range of industries, such as aviation, to improve safety and reliability but only recently to healthcare [18].

A fundamental tenet of human factors engineering is that processes and systems should be designed with the consideration of human performance and behavior. Therefore, human error is the result of a deficiency in the system design rather than the root cause of a failure. There is a spectrum of strategies available to mitigate user errors; however, they are not equally effective. The strategies (also referred to as interventions) and the relative effectiveness are illustrated in Fig. 21.1. The least effective

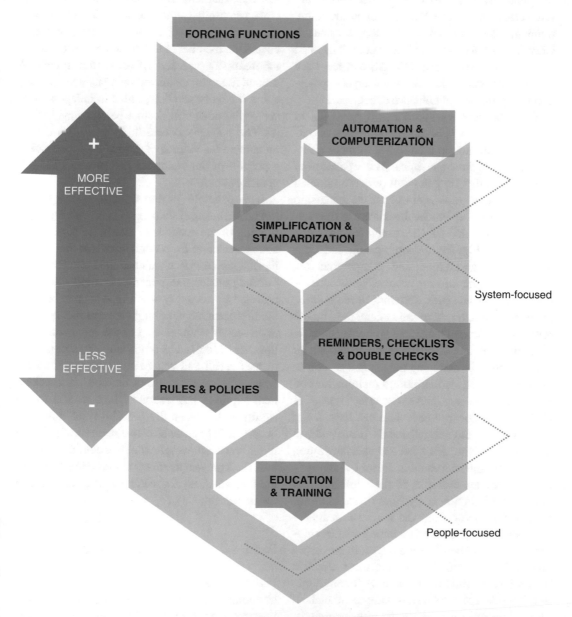

Fig. 21.1 The hierarchy of intervention effectiveness. (From Cafazzo and St-Cyr [18], with permission from Healthcare Quarterly. Copied under licence from Access Copyright). Further reproduction, distribution, or transmission is prohibited except as otherwise permitted by law

interventions are education, training, rules, and policies. These approaches require operators to be highly reliable when executing a task, that is, to recall all of the information necessary to complete the task without error. Although education, training, rules, and policies are necessary components of error-resistant processes, alone they are insufficient to address safety issues. For example, in one state database of errors, failure to follow policies and procedures was a contributing factor to 84% of events [4]. Checklists and double checks are more effective because they build upon education, training, rules, and policies by aiding user recall. Checklist use in healthcare has been demonstrated to reduce adverse events [19, 20] and has been strongly recommended for radiosurgery procedures by professional guidance documents [4].

Checklist use is an important component of risk mitigation in radiosurgery. However, checklist use should not be used in lieu of more effective risk reduction strategies. The weakness of checklists is that they are still reliant on human behavior. Organizations must have the leadership to develop and implement checklists and the vigilance to ensure that they are used. Consequently, as shown in Fig. 21.1, simplification and standardization, automation and computerization, and forcing functions are more effective at mitigating risk in complex systems. Because these strategies are inherent to the system, they do not rely on human behavior to reduce risk. Simplification and standardization accomplishes risk reduction by reducing the number of opportunities for error. Furthermore, simplification and standardization maximizes the effectiveness of checklist use because checklists can have fewer items that are better targeted to the process. More effective than simplification and standardization is software and automation. Record and verify systems are an example of the application of automation in radiotherapy. These systems eliminate human error from the entry of treatment parameters into the machine control system (provided that the parameters are correct in the record and verify system). Finally, the most effective intervention is forcing functions. A forcing function is when a process task is designed to make it impossible for a user to do the task incorrectly.

An example of a forcing function is the ubiquitous door interlock, which prevents a machine from producing radiation when the door is open.

Case Vignette – Case 1

Human Factors Engineering in the Selection of Incorrect Cone Size

A patient was prescribed 20 Gy to a single 4.7 mm diameter metastatic lesion located in close proximity to the brainstem. Treatment was planned for a linear accelerator using a 5 mm cone. One member of the treatment team misread the treatment plan and affixed a 15 mm cone. A second member, distracted by a physician asking about the daily schedule, failed to independently verify the cone size despite being trained to do so. The patient received high-dose treatment to an unintended volume of normal brain, including a portion of the brainstem that received the full prescription dose.

This example illustrates the hierarchy shown in Fig. 21.1. The system relied on the professional training of the operator to attach the correct size cone and that of the second team member to verify that the cone size matched the treatment plan. Formal policies and procedures would somewhat reduce the probability of this type of error because the first team member might have remembered to ask a second team member to check the cone size; however, policies and procedures are still subject to user recall and can be forgotten, particularly when other events cause distractions. A checklist item requiring verification of the cone size would significantly reduce the probability of this error occurring. The most effective method of preventing this error, however, would be automated interlocks that prevent treatment if the cone attached to the machine does not match the one called for in the treatment plan.

Failure Modes and Effects Analysis

Failure modes and effects analysis (FMEA) is a systematic technique for evaluating potential failures and the impact of failures on a process. The application of FMEA to radiotherapy processes was thoroughly investigated and described by the AAPM task group 100 [15]. FMEA is a multidisciplinary process that should be carried out by a team. For radiosurgery, an FMEA team should be comprised of a radiation oncologist, a medical physicist, a treatment therapist, and a simulation therapist. Other members, such as a dosimetrist, nurse, and neurosurgeon, should be included depending on the details of the planning and treatment process. Briefly, FMEA of a process comprises four steps:

1. Creation of a process map
2. Identification of failure modes
3. Assignment of occurrence, severity, and detectability to each failure mode
4. Development of preventive measures to minimize the risk.

The first steps are the development of a detailed process map followed by the assessment of possible failures in the process. The propagation of failures through the process (fault tree analysis) is evaluated to determine the effect of the failure on the outcome. Based on the fault tree analysis, the team members assign scores in three categories to each failure mode:

- Occurrence (O) – the likelihood that the failure will occur, ranging from 1 (failure unlikely, <0.01%) to 10 (more than 5% of the time)
- Severity (S) – the severity of the outcome if the failure remains undetected, ranging from 1 (minimal disturbance of clinical routine) to 10 (catastrophic)
- Detectability (D) – the likelihood that the failure will not be detected in time to prevent an event, ranging from 1 (very detectable: ≤0.01% of failures remain undetected throughout treatment) to 10 (very difficult to detect: >20% of the failures persist throughout treatment)

The product OSD is termed the risk priority number (RPN), which is a metric for the relative risk posed to the patient by each failure mode. High RPN values indicate failures that are likely to occur, are difficult to detect, and have serious consequences for the patient. The final step of the FMEA process is to rank the RPN values and design a quality management program to mitigate the failure risk. Typically, the severity of a particular failure cannot be reduced and so risk mitigation is focused on decreasing the probability of occurrence and increasing the likelihood of detection. There have been several descriptions of FMEA applied to radiosurgery described in the literature [21–24]. Along with the report of AAPM TG100, these reports are useful as guidance when doing an FMEA; however, they cannot substitute for doing an FMEA of a clinic's local process because the failure modes and corresponding risk priority numbers are strongly dependent on the details of the process under consideration.

Case Vignette – Case 2

FMEA Analysis of Radiosurgery

An FMEA applied to radiosurgery done at the University Hospital Maggiore della Carita in Novara, Italy, is summarized here [21]. The institution had several years of radiosurgery experience using a linear accelerator equipped with circular cones and a head frame immobilization. The clinic formed an FMEA working group with the aim of improving the process quality to prevent errors. The group was comprised of 8 radiation oncologists, 2 residents, 3 medical physicists, 4 radiation therapists, and a nurse.

The team identified 73 steps in the radiosurgery process and 116 possible failure modes. The mean risk priority number was 14, with a range of 1–180. The mean severity was 3.4 with a range of 1–9, indicating that some failures would be catastrophic (the team defined a severity of 9 as a near-fatal injury). The mean occurrence was 1.5 with a range of 1–4, and the mean detectability was 1.6 with a range of 1–5. This suggests that errors do not occur frequently (the team defined a detectability of 2 as 1 per 10,000 cases) and are readily detectable (the team defined a detectability of 2 as almost always detected). The team established a risk priority number of 125 as the threshold for corrective action. Two failure modes that exceeded the threshold were identified: the use of incorrect collimator size for treatment and wrong isocenter coordinates setting on the localization frame.

The effect of an incorrect collimator size can be severe, particularly if the actual collimator is too large and so the severity score assigned to this failure was 9 (near-fatal injury). Although the treatment procedures called for the collimator size to be checked by a therapist, physicist, and physician, this second check was not deemed sufficiently reliable to minimize detectability. Therefore, a bar code reader with an interface to the record and verify system was installed. This improved the detectability to the minimum score (1).

The impact of incorrect isocenter coordinates is as catastrophic as an incorrect collimator size, and so was also assigned severity score of 9. Also similar to collimator size, treatment procedures relied on a double check to verify that the coordinates were set correctly. The team implemented a second, independent check of the patient position using a surface imaging system. After the isocenter was set on the localizer frame, the surface imaging system compared an image of the patient's face with a rendering obtained from the treatment planning system. The new procedure established a 1 mm threshold for reviewing the coordinates on the localizer frame.

Several points should be taken from this case study. The first is that the institution had an ongoing quality improvement program that initiated the FMEA process. Second, the institution was committed to making changes based on the results of the FMEA analysis. The two failure modes with the highest risk priority numbers required not only process changes, but significant financial investment to mitigate the risk. Finally, note that both process changes relied on moving the process up the hierarchy of effectiveness. The collimator change moved from a policy of second checking to a forcing function: treatment cannot proceed if the bar code of the collimator does not match the treatment plan. The surface imaging system used software and automation to ensure correct isocenter placement.

Checklists and Checklist Design

A checklist is simply a list of organized items that prompt the user to consider or complete each item. Checklists are an effective risk mitigation strategy because they build on education, training, policies, and procedures by providing users an aid in recall (Fig. 21.2). One advantage of checklists, as compared to direct reference to procedures, is that instructions organized as lists are better understood than those in a paragraph format [25]. Consequently, checklist utilization is a critical element in radiosurgery and is strongly recommended by both ASTRO and AAPM [4, 26]. ASTRO recommends that the minimum elements of an SRS pretreatment checklist be comprised of

1. Verification of patient identification
2. Verification of physician and physicist review and approval of the treatment plan for the patient to be treated
3. Verification that the patient setup and target re-localization are accurate
4. Verification that the selected set of beams/arcs to be delivered are matched correctly to the patient to be treated

The development of checklist items beyond these requires an understanding of the specific treatment process. The FMEA analysis can be used to guide checklist development. The use of a checklist can be used to reduce the occurrence and increase the detectability of errors, thus reducing the risk priority number of identified failure modes. It is important to note that checklists should not be used as a substitute for process improvement. Checklists are reliant on human behavior and thus are not as effective as system-focused interventions. For example, a checklist specifying that the therapist check that the proper cone is affixed to the machine is not a substitute for a software verification that the cone attached to the delivery system matches the treatment plan.

The American Association of Physicists in Medicine has provided extensive practical guidance for checklist development in Medical

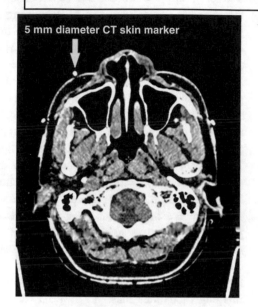

History of Present Illness
Jane Doe is an 89 year old female returning to the clinic for evaluation of right-sided facial pain. Pt developed right-sided facial pain primarily in V2 distribution 3 years ago. She ...

☑ Laterality from consult note in EHR (circle one)   ⬭Right⬯   Left

☑ Position of laterality marker (circle one)   ⬭Right⬯   Left

☑ Position of isocenter placed by physician (circle one)   ⬭Right⬯   Left

☑ Laterality according to consult note, laterality marker position, and isocenter position are consistent.

Fig. 21.2 Laterality portion of treatment planning checklist for a patient treated for right-sided trigeminal neuralgia, along with the relevant portion of neurosurgery clinic note and relevant images

Physics Practice Guideline 4.a: Development, implementation, and the use and maintenance of safety checklists [26].

Checklists are not a panacea and should be used appropriately. Checklists can be overused, resulting in users becoming overburdened completing the checklists, hindering rather than improving delivery of quality care. Furthermore, checklist overuse can result in healthcare providers becoming dependent on them, interfering with professional judgment. Therefore, checklists should have a limited number of items focused on high-risk steps for which the consequences of an error are severe. Institutions should include periodic review of checklists as part of the ongoing quality improvement process.

Case Vignette – Case 3

Use of a Checklist to Mitigate Incorrect Laterality

A patient was prescribed a treatment of 90 Gy to the right trigeminal nerve of his brain. The medical physicist imported the MR and CT images into the treatment planning system and prepared a treatment plan for the opposite (left) trigeminal nerve. The radiation oncologist reviewed and approved the treatment plan. The treatment was delivered to the incorrect trigeminal nerve with the neurosurgeon, radiation oncologist, and medical physicist present at the procedure. The error was discovered when the neurosurgeon was preparing a procedure note after treatment.

The patient had to undergo a second procedure to treat the correct side and subsequently developed left-sided facial numbness as a consequence of the treatment to the wrong side.

Incorrect laterality is one of the most common errors in the treatment of trigeminal neuralgia and the treatment process should be designed with that in mind. When imaging is done for a trigeminal procedure, the patient should be asked to point to the side of the pain and a marker placed on that side. During treatment planning, the location of the marker, the position of the isocenter designated by the radiation oncologist, and the laterality designated by the neurosurgeon should be checked for consistency. An example portion of a treatment planning checklist is shown in Fig. 21.2. At the time of treatment, the patient should be again asked to point to the side of the pain, which should be consistent with the laterality of the treatment plan and confirmed with the neurosurgeon and radiation oncologist. This step should be included in a pre-treatment time-out checklist.

Key Recommendations

The components of quality and safety in a radiosurgery program have been discussed extensively in the professional guidance literature [4, 27, 28]. These elements are summarized here, but it is strongly recommended that readers directly review the relevant literature.

Stereotactic radiosurgery requires team members with appropriate training and credentials specific to SRS. An SRS team should be comprised of, at a minimum, a radiation oncologist, medical physicist, dosimetrist, neurosurgeon, and radiation therapist. Team members must be appropriately certified or licensed and have a sufficient level of training specific to SRS, whether as part of formal training or continuing education. Team members should have well-defined roles and responsibilities.

An SRS program requires a resource commitment larger than that for conventional radiation therapy. There is limited guidance on personnel levels required for an SRS program, so it is incumbent upon clinics operating a program to evaluate staffing needs and ensure that staff are provided adequate time to carry out their tasks. Similarly, equipment needs will be dependent on the program goals. Access to MRI imaging is a prerequisite for a radiosurgery program. If treatment of arterio-venous malformations (AVMs) is a program goal, angiography will be needed. Historically, head frames have been used for patient immobilization but frameless immobilization systems are becoming more common. The treatment planning system must be able to support accurate dose calculation for small fields. This capability is typically inherent in systems dedicated to stereotactic radiosurgery but should be carefully evaluated. Particular caution is warranted when using systems designed for general purpose radiation therapy planning rather than stereotactic radiosurgery. In addition to dose calculation, the treatment planning system must have the capability to import and register the imaging modalities that will be used for target definition. In particular, not all treatment planning systems are capable of using bi-plane angiograms for planning SRS of AVMs. The delivery system should be designed with specifications and safety systems appropriate to stereotactic radiosurgery. When using image guidance for localization, the coincidence between the imaging system isocenter and the treatment delivery isocenter should meet SRS specifications (typically < 1 mm). If a frame-based system is used for both immobilization and localization, it is strongly recommended to use an image guidance system whenever possible to verify correct patient positioning. Treatment systems using cones should be equipped with the capability to verify that the correct cone has been affixed. When selecting equipment for a radiosurgery program, the corresponding quality assurance equipment should also be considered. Because of the tight mechanical tolerances and the challenges of small field dosimetry, the QA equipment used for conventional radiotherapy is insufficient to carry out a QA program for SRS. Equipment required includes phantoms for the evaluation of treatment imaging systems, tools and software for routine Winston-Lutz testing, detectors suitable for dose measurement in small fields, and, if modulated techniques are to be used, patient-specific QA equipment.

Acceptance testing and commissioning are related, but distinct, components of an SRS program. Acceptance testing is done together with the vendor to demonstrate that the equipment is operating within the stated specifications. Equipment specifications are established by the vendor and the customer during the purchasing process and should meet or exceed the recommendations of professional guidance documents for SRS systems [4, 29]. Commissioning is the process of collecting the measurements necessary to configure the system for clinical use and then testing the system to ensure that it is configured correctly. The most common measurement task is the measurement of data to characterize the radiation beam for use in commissioning the treatment planning system. Due to small field sizes, this task is particularly challenging for SRS [30] and medical physicists responsible for the collection of beam data and for the configuration of the planning system should be trained and equipped specifically for commissioning of radiosurgery systems. In addition to beam data collection and configuration of the treatment planning system, commissioning includes the integration and configuration of all systems required for the SRS treatment process. These include the localization system [31], radiation oncology information system (ROIS), image registration systems [32], CT simulation, and the image guidance systems [33, 34]. End-to-end testing is an important final step in commissioning an SRS system [28]. An independent end-to-end test is particularly valuable. The M.D. Anderson Dosimetry Laboratory (MDADL) can provide an anthropomorphic head phantom containing film and point dosimeters. The clinic using the phantom uses their standard SRS planning and delivery procedure, including localization, and then returns the phantom to the MDADL. The MDADL evaluates the measured dose distribution against the treatment planning data provided by the clinic and provides the clinic a report of the results. Excerpts of a report are shown in Fig. 21.3.

A robust quality assurance program is necessary to minimize errors in radiosurgery practice. A complete description of a QA program is beyond the scope of this chapter, so the reader is encouraged to review the literature (see, for example [4, 12, 27–29, 32, 34, 35]). However,

Description of procedure:

An anthropomorphic head phantom containing a 1.9 cm diameter spherical target was imaged and irradiated. Two TLD capsules provided dose information near the center of the target. Two orthogonal sheets of GAFChromic Dosimetry Media provided dose profiles and an evaluation of the delivered dose distribution. The results are presented in summary below and the detailed report is attached.

The typical dosimetric precision of the TLD is ±3%, and the spatial precision of the film and densitometer system is ±1 mm.

Summary of TLD and film results:

	Ratio	Criteria	Acceptable
Dose to the center of the target (TLD / Institution)	1.03	0.95 – 1.05	Yes

Film Plane	Gamma Index*	Criteria	Acceptable
Coronal	99%	≥85%	Yes
Sagittal	99%	≥85%	Yes

*Percentage of points meeting gamma-index criteria 5% and 3 mm
The phantom irradiation results listed in the table above **do meet** the criteria established by IROC Houston.

Fig. 21.3 Report excerpt summarizing the results of IROC Houston/M.D. Anderson Dosimetry Laboratory SRS head phantom irradiation. The phantom and a dose profile through the center of the target are shown in Fig. 22.2 of Chap. 22

several important items are summarized here. First, a radiosurgery program must establish and maintain a safety culture in which all team members are empowered to question and, if necessary, halt procedures when there is any question about the safety of the treatment. Such a safety culture requires trust and communication among team members. Careful attention should be paid to social hierarchies in which some team members feel they must defer to others or are concerned about retribution if they express concerns. Second, a time-out should be done before treatment is initiated. The minimum components of a time-out are verification of correct patient and correct site. A time-out can also include verification of other safety checklists. Thirdly, standard policies and procedures should be developed for all the aspects of the treatment process, including quality assurance. Policies and procedures should incorporate checklists wherever appropriate. Fourth, peer-review and independent audits should be conducted on a regular basis. Peer review includes internal and external review. Independent audits include annual evaluation of machine calibration by an external entity, such as IROC-Houston or the M.D. Anderson Accredited Dosimetry Laboratory. Finally, acceptance testing, commissioning, and quality assurance activities should be thoroughly documented.

Continuous quality improvement is essential to an SRS program and is an extension of the quality assurance program. The policies and procedures should be periodically reviewed and updated to reflect any practice changes. Tools such as statistical process control should be considered for the quantitative monitoring of QA test results [36–41].

Future Directions

As shown in Fig. 21.1, system-focused interventions are most effective at mitigating errors. Unfortunately, individual institutions have much less control over systems than they do over human behavior. Institutions can simplify and standardize their processes, but automation and forcing functions frequently require engineering

expertise and access to the software/hardware of equipment vendors. For example, automated comparison of the cone affixed to a linear accelerator to the treatment plan requires sensor hardware to detect the cone and software to check that the cone matches the plan. If a delivery system is not designed to do such a comparison, it is extremely difficult for users to build an independent automated verification system and so they must fall back on checklists. Therefore, healthcare providers must collaborate with the industry to facilitate improvements in patient safety.

Standardization and simplification across institutions will provide further error reduction. One area that is ripe for standardization is beam modeling in treatment planning systems. Incorrectly measured output factors have been implicated in a number of radiosurgery overdoses; however, the output factors do not vary significantly across treatment machines of the same model. Standardizing beam data and output factors in the treatment planning system changes the implications of a measurement error. In the current paradigm, an error in measurement during commissioning will be transferred directly to an error in patient care. For a system having standardized beam data, an error in measurement during commissioning will result in a mismatch between the planning system and the measurement, which should trigger the commissioning physicist to investigate the disagreement before proceeding. It is important to understand that standardization of this type is not a blanket solution and is subject to failure as well. Professional judgment and vigilance will still be required of physicists responsible for commissioning radiosurgery systems, because a disagreement between a measurement and the treatment planning system could be indicative of an actual problem rather than a measurement error.

Another opportunity for improvement is standardization and automation of delivery system quality assurance. There are standards for the tests and tolerances for equipment [4, 29] but the details of implementation are site-specific. There is significant potential if tests are automated because treatment delivery can be made dependent on appropriate tests being done and meeting the specification. For example, it is up to clinics to implement procedures that ensure that treatment delivery does not occur if the output of the machine is out of tolerance. There are ongoing efforts by vendors [42–45] and multi-institutional consortiums [46] to develop standardized and automated QA tools.

Key Points – Recommendations
- Develop and nurture a safety culture.
- Implement an incident learning system.
- Form a dedicated quality committee.
- Ensure that radiosurgery team members have appropriate training and credentials.
- Dedicate sufficient resources to the radiosurgery program.
- Develop procedures and checklists based on a failure modes and effects analysis (FMEA) and human factors engineering (HFE).
- Obtain independent program review on a regular basis.

References

1. Suh JH. Stereotactic radiosurgery for the management of brain metastases. N Engl J Med. 2010;362(12):1119–27.
2. Combs SE, Welzel T, Schulz-Ertner D, Huber PE, Debus J. Differences in clinical results after LINAC-based single-dose radiosurgery versus fractionated stereotactic radiotherapy for patients with vestibular schwannomas. Int J Radiat Oncol Biol Phys. 2010;76(1):193–200.
3. NRC regulations: title 10, code of federal regulations. Sect. 35.3045.
4. Solberg TD, Balter JM, Benedict SH, Fraass BA, Kavanagh B, Miyamoto C, et al. Quality and safety considerations in stereotactic radiosurgery and stereotactic body radiation therapy: executive summary. Pract Radiat Oncol. 2012;2(1):2–9.
5. Gourmelon P, Bey E, De Revel T, Lazorthes Y, Lotteries J, Lataillade JJ. The French radiation accident experience: emerging concepts in radiation burn and ARS therapies and in brain radiopathology. Radioprotection. 2008;43(5):23–6.
6. Derreumaux S, Etard C, Huet C, Trompier F, Clairand I, Bottollier-Depois JF, et al. Lessons from recent accidents in radiation therapy in France. Radiat Prot Dosim. 2008;131(1):130–5.
7. Borius PY, Debono B, Latorzeff I, Lotterie JA, Plas JY, Cassol E, et al. Dosimetric stereotactic radiosurgical accident: study of 33 patients treated for brain metastases. Neurochirurgie. 2010;56(5):368–73.
8. Stahel PF, Sabel AL, Victoroff MS, Varnell J, Lembitz A, Boyle DJ, et al. Wrong-site and wrong-patient procedures in the universal protocol era: analysis of a prospective database of physician self-reported occurrences. Arch Surg. 2010;145(10):978–84.
9. Information notice 2000–22: medical misadministrations caused by human errors involving Gamma stereotactic radiosurgery (Gamma knife) 2000.
10. Solberg TD, Medin PM. Quality and safety in stereotactic radiosurgery and stereotactic body radiation therapy: can more be done? J Radiosurg SBRT. 2011;1(1):13–9.
11. Bogdanich WR, Rebelo K. A pinpoint beam strays invisibly, harming instead of healing. The New York Times. 2010. https://www.nytimes.com/2010/12/29/health/29radiation.html. Accessed 27 May 2019.
12. (ASTRO). Safety is no accident: a framework for quality radiation oncology and care. 2012. https://www.astro.org/uploadedFiles/_MAIN_SITE/Daily_Practice/Accreditation/Content_Pieces/SafetyisnoAccident.pdf. Accessed 27 May 2019.
13. Ford EC, Fong de Los Santos L, Pawlicki T, Sutlief S, Dunscombe P. Consensus recommendations for incident learning database structures in radiation oncology. Med Phys. 2012;39(12):7272–90.
14. Cunningham J, Coffey M, Knoos T, Holmberg O. Radiation Oncology Safety Information System (ROSIS)–profiles of participants and the first 1074 incident reports. Radiother Oncol. 2010;97(3):601–7.
15. Huq MS, Fraass BA, Dunscombe PB, Gibbons JP Jr, Ibbott GS, Mundt AJ, et al. The report of Task Group 100 of the AAPM: application of risk analysis methods to radiation therapy quality management. Med Phys. 2016;43(7):4209.
16. British Institute of Radiology, the Institute of Physics and Engineering in Medicine, the National Patient Safety Agency, the Society and College of Radiographers and the Royal College of Radiologists. Towards safer radiotherapy. 2008.
17. Institute of Medicine (US) Committee on Quality of Health Care in America. In: Linda TK, Janet MC, Molla SD, editors. To err is human: building a safer health system. Washington, DC: The National Academies Press; 2000.
18. Cafazzo JA, St-Cyr O. From discovery to design: the evolution of human factors in healthcare. Healthc Q. 2012;15(April (Special Issue)):24–9.
19. Pronovost P, Needham D, Berenholtz S, Sinopoli D, Chu H, Cosgrove S, et al. An intervention to decrease catheter-related bloodstream infections in the ICU. N Engl J Med. 2006;355(26):2725–32.

20. Hales BM, Pronovost PJ. The checklist–a tool for error management and performance improvement. J Crit Care. 2006;21(3):231–5.

21. Masini L, Donis L, Loi G, Mones E, Molina E, Bolchini C, et al. Application of failure mode and effects analysis to intracranial stereotactic radiation surgery by linear accelerator. Pract Radiat Oncol. 2014;4(6):392–7.

22. Manger RP, Paxton AB, Pawlicki T, Kim GY. Failure mode and effects analysis and fault tree analysis of surface image guided cranial radiosurgery. Med Phys. 2015;42(5):2449–61.

23. Teixeira FC, de Almeida CE, Saiful HM. Failure mode and effects analysis based risk profile assessment for stereotactic radiosurgery programs at three cancer centers in Brazil. Med Phys. 2016;43(1):171.

24. Xu AY, Bhatnagar J, Bednarz G, Flickinger J, Arai Y, Vacsulka J, et al. Failure modes and effects analysis (FMEA) for Gamma knife radiosurgery. J Appl Clin Med Phys. 2017;18(6):152–68.

25. Morrow DG, Leirer VO, Andrassy JM, Hier CM, Menard WE. The influence of list format and category headers on age differences in understanding medication instructions. Exp Aging Res. 1998;24(3):231–56.

26. Fong de Los Santos LE, Evans S, Ford EC, Gaiser JE, Hayden SE, Huffman KE, et al. Medical Physics Practice Guideline 4.a: development, implementation, use and maintenance of safety checklists. J Appl Clin Med Phys. 2015;16(3):5431.

27. Seung SK, Larson DA, Galvin JM, Mehta MP, Potters L, Schultz CJ, et al. American College of Radiology (ACR) and American Society for Radiation Oncology (ASTRO) Practice Guideline for the Performance of Stereotactic Radiosurgery (SRS). Am J Clin Oncol. 2013;36(3):310–5.

28. Halvorsen PH, Cirino E, Das IJ, Garrett JA, Yang J, Yin FF, et al. AAPM-RSS medical physics practice guideline 9.a. for SRS-SBRT. J Appl Clin Med Phys. 2017;18(5):10–21.

29. Klein EE, Hanley J, Bayouth J, Yin FF, Simon W, Dresser S, et al. Task Group 142 report: quality assurance of medical accelerators. Med Phys. 2009;36(9):4197–212.

30. Palmans H, Andreo P, Huq MS, Seuntjens J, Christaki KE, Meghzifene A. Dosimetry of small static fields used in external photon beam radiotherapy: summary of TRS-483, the IAEA-AAPM international Code of Practice for reference and relative dose determination. Med Phys. 2018;45(11):e1123–45.

31. Lightstone AW, Benedict SH, Bova FJ, Solberg TD, Stern RL. Intracranial stereotactic positioning systems: report of the American Association of Physicists in Medicine Radiation Therapy Committee Task Group No. 68. Med Phys. 2005;32(7Part1):2380–98.

32. Brock KK, Mutic S, McNutt TR, Li H, Kessler ML. Use of image registration and fusion algorithms and techniques in radiotherapy: report of the AAPM Radiation Therapy Committee Task Group No. 132. Med Phys. 2017;44(7):e43–76.

33. Langen KM, Willoughby TR, Meeks SL, Santhanam A, Cunningham A, Levine L, et al. Observations on real-time prostate gland motion using electromagnetic tracking. Int J Radiat Oncol Biol Phys. 2008;71(4):1084–90.

34. Bissonnette JP, Balter PA, Dong L, Langen KM, Lovelock DM, Miften M, et al. Quality assurance for image-guided radiation therapy utilizing CT-based technologies: a report of the AAPM TG-179. Med Phys. 2012;39(4):1946–63.

35. Willoughby T, Lehmann J, Bencomo JA, Jani SK, Santanam L, Sethi A, et al. Quality assurance for non-radiographic radiotherapy localization and positioning systems: report of Task Group 147. Med Phys. 2012;39(4):1728–47.

36. Pawlicki T, Whitaker M, Boyer AL. Statistical process control for radiotherapy quality assurance. Med Phys. 2005;32(9):2777–86.

37. Palaniswaamy G, Scott Brame R, Yaddanapudi S, Rangaraj D, Mutic S. A statistical approach to IMRT patient-specific QA. Med Phys. 2012;39(12):7560–70.

38. Letourneau D, Wang A, Amin MN, Pearce J, McNiven A, Keller H, et al. Multileaf collimator performance monitoring and improvement using semiautomated quality control testing and statistical process control. Med Phys. 2014;41(12):121713.

39. Chung JB, Kim JS, Ha SW, Ye SJ. Statistical analysis of IMRT dosimetry quality assurance measurements for local delivery guideline. Radiat Oncol. 2011;6:27.

40. Breen SL, Moseley DJ, Zhang B, Sharpe MB. Statistical process control for IMRT dosimetric verification. Med Phys. 2008;35(10):4417–25.

41. Able CM, Baydush AH, Nguyen C, Gersh J, Ndlovu A, Rebo I, et al. A model for preemptive maintenance of medical linear accelerators-predictive maintenance. Radiat Oncol. 2016;11:36.

42. Barnes MP, Pomare D, Menk FW, Moraro B, Greer PB. Evaluation of the TrueBeam machine performance check (MPC): OBI X-ray tube alignment procedure. J Appl Clin Med Phys. 2018;19(6):68–78.

43. Barnes MP, Greer PB. Evaluation of the TrueBeam machine performance check (MPC) beam constancy checks for flattened and flattening filter-free (FFF) photon beams. J Appl Clin Med Phys. 2017;18(1):139–50.

44. Barnes MP, Greer PB. Evaluation of the TrueBeam machine performance check (MPC) geometric checks for daily IGRT geometric accuracy quality assurance. J Appl Clin Med Phys. 2017;18(3):200–6.

45. Barnes MP, Greer PB. Evaluation of the TrueBeam machine performance check (MPC): mechanical and collimation checks. J Appl Clin Med Phys. 2017;18(3):56–66.

46. Eckhause T, Al-Hallaq H, Ritter T, DeMarco J, Farrey K, Pawlicki T, et al. Automating linear accelerator quality assurance. Med Phys. 2015;42(10):6074–83.

Quality Assurance for Small Fields

22

Richard A. Popple

Introduction

The measurement of dose from small fields is challenging. Incorrect measurement practices have been implicated in several radiosurgery misadministrations. In France, output factors of small MLC fields (<3 cm²) required for commissioning of the treatment planning system were measured using a Farmer chamber [1]. Consequently, 145 patients received an overdose. The error was detected a year after commissioning when the vendor conducted an intercomparison of the output factors in use at a number of clinics. A similar error occurred in Missouri [2]. For many years, the output of the 4 mm collimator of the Gamma Knife was underestimated by 9% in the treatment planning system [3].

Because the consequences of errors arising from improper measurement of small field dosimetry, it is critically important that physicists responsible for commissioning and quality assurance of stereotactic radiosurgery (SRS) have SRS-specific expertise and training, and adequate resources for the measurement of small fields. There are several comprehensive documents that provide in-depth guidance for small field dosimetry, including report 91 of the International

Commission on Radiation Units and Measurements (ICRU) [4], the International Atomic Energy Agency (IAEA) technical report series number 483 (TRS-483) [5], and the American Associate of Physicists in Medicine (AAPM) summary of TRS-483 [6]. This chapter will provide an overview of the key concepts, but physicists should be thoroughly familiar with these documents prior to initiating a radiosurgery program.

There is not a well-specified definition of a small radiation field. However, there is consensus that a field can be considered small when at least one of three conditions are met at the point of interest on the beam axis. A photon field is defined as small if there is a loss of lateral charged particle equilibrium (LCPE) on the central axis, if the field collimation partially blocks the photon source from the viewpoint of the detector position, or if the detector response changes as a function of the field size.

Loss of LCPE on the central axis occurs when the range of secondary electrons is larger than the half-width of the field. From Monte Carlo calculations, the secondary electron range r_{LCPE} as a function of beam quality, specified as %dd$(10,10)_x$, is given by

$$r_{LCPE}(\text{cm}) = 0.07797\%\text{dd}(10,10)_X - 4.112$$

The secondary electron range can also be expressed in terms of TPR$_{20,10}$(10) [6]. For beam energy between 6 and 10 MV, this results in loss of LCPE for field sizes less than 2–3 cm.

R. A. Popple (✉)
Department of Radiation Oncology, The University of Alabama at Birmingham, Birmingham, AL, USA
e-mail: rpopple@uabmc.edu

© Springer Nature Switzerland AG 2020
Y. Yamada et al. (eds.), *Radiotherapy in Managing Brain Metastases*,
https://doi.org/10.1007/978-3-030-43740-4_22

Shielding of the primary photon source by the collimator is due to the finite size of the source. For accelerator-produced x-rays, the size of the source is typically one to several millimeters, defined as the full width at half maximum of the bremsstrahlung radiation exiting the target. A sufficiently small collimator aperture will block the periphery of the finite source, resulting in a smaller output on the beam axis than would the same collimator for an ideal point source. This effect is significant when the field size is comparable or less than the source size. Consequently, field sizes that result in shielding of the source by the collimator will also exhibit loss of charged particle equilibrium, whereas the reverse is not always the case.

The dominant cause of changes in detector response in small fields is volume averaging. If the dose distribution is non-uniform over the sensitive volume, the detector response will be a convolution of the detector shape with the dose distribution. In addition to volume averaging, the perturbation of the charged particle fluence by the presence of the detector results in break-down of Bragg-Gray cavity theory. Therefore, small-field measurement conditions exist when the edge of the detector is less than r_{LCPE} from the field edge. An additional contribution to the change in detector response is the change in the energy spectrum for small fields. Because the phantom scatter is reduced relative to broad beams, and because the low-energy scatter from the linear accelerator head is reduced by the collimation, the spectrum of small fields is harder (has more high-energy photons) than broad beam fields. Spectrum hardening results in changes in the mass-energy absorption coefficients and the stopping-power ratios for the detector material. This effect is particularly significant for silicon-based diode detectors and for ionization chambers with high-Z electrodes [6].

Relative Dosimetry

The configuration of a treatment planning system typically requires the output relative to the calibration condition (the output factor), central axis depth dose, and beam profiles at specified depths. For fixed collimator (cone)-based radiosurgery, values are required for each collimator size. For multileaf collimator-based SRS, the output factors, depth doses, and beam profiles are for treatment planning system-specific field sizes, which may or may not be defined by the MLC.

Protocols for the calibration of linear accelerators specify the output at the reference depth in a 10 cm × 10 cm field. Other machine types, such as the Gamma Knife or Cyberknife, cannot create a 10 cm × 10 cm field. Therefore, formalisms have been developed that extend the linear accelerator protocols to non-standard field sizes. For a given machine type, the reference field is designated the machine-specific reference (msr) field. The msr is typically the largest field that machine can produce. The output factor, $\Omega_{Q_{\text{clin}}, Q_{\text{msr}}}^{f_{\text{clin}}, f_{\text{msr}}}$, is the ratio of absorbed dose in water for the field of interest to the absorbed dose in water for the machine-specific reference field.

The output factor is measured at a specified SSD and depth, typically 5 or 10 cm, to eliminate the effect of electron contamination. The output factor is obtained from measurement by

$$\Omega_{Q_{\text{clin}}, Q_{\text{msr}}}^{f_{\text{clin}}, f_{\text{msr}}} = k_{Q_{\text{clin}}, Q_{\text{msr}}}^{f_{\text{clin}}, f_{\text{msr}}} \frac{M_{Q_{\text{clin}}}^{f_{\text{clin}}}}{M_{Q_{\text{msr}}}^{f_{\text{msr}}}}$$

where $M_{Q_{\text{clin}}}^{f_{\text{clin}}}$ is the detector signal in the field of interest, $M_{Q_{\text{msr}}}^{f_{\text{msr}}}$ is the detector signal in the reference field, and $k_{Q_{\text{clin}}, Q_{\text{msr}}}^{f_{\text{clin}}, f_{\text{msr}}}$ is an output correction factor. For broad beams, the correction factor is unity. The correction factor is dependent on the detector design, the beam quality, and the field size. Experimental determination of the correction factor for a given detector requires a second detector having a known correction factor. Correction factors can also be computed using Monte Carlo simulations. The IAEA TRS-483 provides correction factors for a number of detectors [5]. For detectors not listed in TRS-483, users should search the literature – the correction factors for most commercial detectors suitable for small-field dosimetry have been reported (see, for example, [7–11]).

The orientation of the detector has an effect on the output factor measurement, with the preferred orientation dependent on the type and design of the detector. The length of cable in the field should be minimized to limit the leakage-induced signal. Particular care should be given to positioning the detector at the beam axis. This can be done by scanning the detector along both axes orthogonal to the beam axis for a very small field and placing the detector at the position of maximum signal. Because the output factor has a significant dependence on field size for small fields, output factor measurements should be accompanied by beam profile measurements to confirm the field size. This is particularly important for variable collimators, such as MLCs.

Percent Depth Dose and Beam Profiles

The depth dependence of both field size and energy spectrum contributes to the measurement accuracy of percent depth dose (PDD) in small fields. Because the lateral extent of the field increases with depth, so does the magnitude of volume averaging. This issue is most pronounced for microionization chambers. For example, for a 0.007 cm^3 spherical volume, the volume averaging correction for a 5 mm^2 MLC-defined field decreases by approximately 1% from 2 to 20 cm in a 6 MV beam. For diodes, the change in energy spectrum as a function of depth has a significant effect on measured PDD because of the high-Z materials used in their construction. Ionization chambers with high-Z electrodes will also have depth-dependent response [12]. When measuring PDD, the detector axis should be mounted parallel to the beam axis to minimize the effect of increasing field size with increasing depth and the detector should first be scanned across the beam to ensure that it is aligned with the beam axis at all of depths of interest.

Some planning systems require tissue-phantom ratios (TPRs) rather than percent depth dose. The methods for the conversion of depth dose to PDD used for broad beams are not accurate small fields [13]. Although other methods to convert PDD to TPR have been investigated [14–16], evidence for their accuracy in small fields is limited. Therefore, when TPR is required, direct measurement is recommended [4].

For profile measurements, energy dependence is not a consideration because the energy spectrum does not change significantly with off-axis distance. A high-resolution detector size is important to minimize the blurring of the lateral penumbra, which results from volume averaging. The detector orientation for scanning beam profiles should be selected to optimize spatial resolution and to ensure that the volume averaging is minimized. The effect of extra-cameral signal (stem effect) should be evaluated and considered in the detector orientation, particularly for microionization chambers.

Detector Types

Ionization Chamber

Standard ionization chambers, such as Farmer chambers, have been associated with output-related radiosurgical errors [1] and should not be used in small fields under any circumstances. Microionization chambers (volume less than approximately 0.02 cm^3) are designed for use in small fields, however, for fields smaller than about 2 cm × 2 cm microionization chambers nevertheless under respond by up to 15%. For example, for one commercially available chamber with volume 0.015 cm^3, the correction factor $k_{Q_{clin},Q_{10 \times 10}}^{f_{clin},f_{10 \times 10}}$ is 1.005, 1.025, and 1.128 for field sizes 1.5 × 1.5 cm^2, 1.0 × 1.0 cm^2, and 0.5 × 0.5 cm^2, respectively [17]. Because of volume averaging and energy dependence, ionization chambers are the least suitable detectors for use in small fields and should be avoided [18].

Note that the correction factor $k_{Q_{clin},Q_{msr}}^{f_{clin},f_{msr}}$ for a micro-ionization chamber is, like all other detectors, dependent on the design details and so the correction factor should be obtained for the specific chamber model. Correction factors for micro-chambers of similar design or volume are not suitable. For output factor measurement, a microionization chamber should be oriented perpendicular to the beam axis to minimize extra-cameral signal.

For beam scanning, the small volume results in sensitivity to extracameral irradiation. To reduce this effect, for beam profiles the chamber should be oriented parallel to the beam axis and the cable should be positioned to minimize the irradiated length. Despite being designed for small fields, the dimensions of microionizations chambers are typically several millimeters and will result in penumbra blurring. For percent depth dose measurements, the field size change with depth results in change in the volume averaging effect. Furthermore, the effective point of measurement is not well known, particularly when the detector is parallel to the beam axis, as recommended for the scanning of beam profiles [12].

Diode

Diode detectors are comprised of a silicon p-n junction in which radiation produces electron-hole pairs. The typical dimensions of the active volume are 1 mm^2 and ~1 μm to several hundred micrometers thick. Because silicon has an atomic number ($Z = 14$) higher than water, diodes have a significant energy-dependent response, over-responding to low energy photons. Some detector designs (shielded) include filtration to mitigate the energy dependence; however, it cannot be eliminated. The high-Z materials used in shielded diodes result in increased perturbations of the radiation fluence distribution, and consequently shielded diodes over-respond in small fields relative to unshielded diodes. For example, for one commercially available unshielded diode the correction factor $k_{Q_{clin},Q_{10\times10}}^{f_{clin},f_{10\times10}}$ is 1.005, 0.995, and 0.968, whereas that for a shielded diode is 0.983, 0.966, and 0.933 for field sizes 1.5 × 1.5 cm^2, 1.0 × 1.0 cm^2, and 0.5 × 0.5 cm^2, respectively [17]. Because of the perturbation by the high-Z shielding and since a variety of unshielded diodes designed specifically for small fields are commercially available, shielded diodes should be avoided for small-field dosimetry.

Unshielded diodes designed for use in small fields (stereotactic field diodes) are ideal for the measurement of beam profiles. The small size of the active volume provides high-resolution measurement with minimal penumbra blurring. These detectors have been shown to produce relative beam profile measurements nearly identical to Monte Carlo calculations. Because the photon spectrum does not change significantly as a function of off-axis distance, the energy dependence of the diode response is not a factor. Diodes have a disk-shaped active volume, which should be oriented perpendicular to the beam axis [19]. This orientation typically corresponds to the stem of the detector parallel to the beam axis; however, this is not universally true. Manufacturers usually mark the detector with the orientation of the active volume. Documentation provided by the vendor should be consulted to confirm the recommended orientation of the detector.

The energy dependence of diodes is a concern for the measurement of percent depth dose. However, changes in response as a function of depth are not significant and consequently unshielded diodes are well suited for the measurement of small-field PDDs [18]. The orientation of the diode should be the same as that used for profile scanning, with the area of the detector perpendicular to the beam axis. This orientation places the smallest dimension of the detector, typically several micrometers, parallel to the beam axis which results in extremely high spatial resolution and negligible volume averaging for PDD measurement.

Diamond

Commercially available diamond detectors are comprised of a layer of synthetic diamond deposited using chemical vapor deposition. The active volume is similar in dimensions to a diode, about 2 mm in diameter and 1 μm thick. Diamond is near-water equivalent, having $Z = 6$ compared to the effective $Z = 7.4$ for water and consequently having minimal energy dependence. Diamond detectors over-respond in small fields, similar to unshielded diodes. For a commercially available synthetic diamond detector, the correction factor $k_{Q_{clin},Q_{5\times5}}^{f_{clin},f_{5\times5}}$ was reported to be 0.991, 0.986, and 0.975, whereas that for a shielded diode was

0.994, 0.983, and 0.964 for fields of diameter 2.00, 1.08, and 0.76 cm, respectively [20]. Because diamond detectors are larger than diodes, the volume averaging effect is non-negligible in fields $<\sim1$ cm, partially compensating for the over-response. There is a disagreement in the literature regarding the correction factor for very small (<8 mm) field sizes that is likely due to this effect [20].

Diamond detectors are well suited for the measurement of beam profiles and percent depth dose. Similar to diodes, the active area should be perpendicular to the beam axis. Diamond detectors are modestly larger than diodes, having diameter approximately 2 mm compared to approximately 1 mm for stereotactic field diodes. When scanning beam profiles, a stereotactic field diode will have better resolution and less penumbra blurring.

Plastic Scintillator

Plastic scintillator detectors are comprised of a small organic plastic scintillator bonded to an optical fiber. The light produced in the scintillator is coupled by the fiber to a photodetector. The advantage of plastic scintillator detectors is their near-water equivalence and small volume. Consequently, the correction factors for scintillator detectors are very close to 1 [21]. The only significant effect on the correction factor is volume averaging. Commercially available scintillator detectors are 1 mm diameter and 1–3 mm long. For detectors longer than 1 mm, the long axis of the detector should be oriented parallel to the beam axis. In addition to the scintillation light produced in the detector volume, Cerenkov light is also produced in the optical fiber. The amount of Cerenkov light is related to the dose received by the fiber and thus is proportional to the amount of the fiber in the field. The contribution of Cerenkov signal is to the light output at the detector is dependent on irradiation conditions and must be corrected for. Several approaches have been investigated to remove the Cerenkov background [22], but only one, spectral discrimination, is in use for commercially available detectors. The scintillation spectrum is relatively narrow, whereas the Cerenkov spectrum is broad. To determine the dose received by the scintillator, the optical signal is split between two photodetectors having different optical filtration. One detector passes wavelengths in the scintillation spectrum, and the other passes only wavelengths longer than the scintillation spectrum. Consequently, the signal of the first detector (s_{Blue}) is primarily due to scintillation light, whereas the signal in the second (s_{Green}) is primarily due to Cerenkov light. The dose in the scintillator is given by

$$D = k_{gain} \times \left(s_{Blue} - k_{CLR} \times s_{Green} \right)$$

By irradiating the detector to known doses but with different lengths of fiber in the field, the constants k_{CLR} and k_{gain} can be determined. With careful correction for the Cerenkov background, plastic scintillator detectors are well suited to the measurement of output factors, percent depth dose, and profiles [23].

Radiochromic Film

Radiochromic film is comprised of a thin film of material that changes color upon exposure to ionizing radiation without any further development. The commercially available radiochromic film for medical use is based on an organic molecule. Exposure to ionizing radiation induces a polymerization reaction that causes the film to turn blue. Advantages of radiochromic film include near-water equivalence, minimal energy sensitivity [24], and high spatial resolution.

The most common method in current use for evaluating the optical density of radiochromic film is using a red-green-blue (RGB) scanner operated in transmission mode. In analogy to silver-halide radiographic film, the signal of the most responsive channel (typically the red channel) is used to determine the dose absorbed. This approach has several limitations. The first is that thickness variations of the polymer film results in a spatial variation in response [25]. Second is dependence of the scanner signal on the lateral distance from the center of the scan bed. This effect is minimal for distances less than about 5 cm but can result in an increasing overestimation of the dose as the position approaches the edge of the scan area. For small fields, this effect is minimized if sequential films are positioned consistently on the scanner bed. Both of these effects are mitigated using a multiple channel approach in which all three color channels are used to determine the dose [26].

Radiochromic film is suitable for output factor, percent depth dose, and beam profiles. However, it can have significant uncertainties arising from the film and scanner characteristics and consequently requires a careful processing protocol [27]. Another disadvantage of radiochromic film is that it is not a "real time" dosimeter.

Case Vignette – Case 1

Commissioning of Small Field Sizes for a Linear Accelerator

The output factors for the 10 MV flattening filter free beam of a linear accelerator were measured for field sizes ≥ 3 cm using a 0.125 cm^3 ionization chamber. For VMAT planning, the treatment planning system required only output factors for the secondary collimator jaws. To determine the output factor for field size 2 cm, three detectors were used: a 0.007 cm^3 micro-ionization chamber, a stereotactic diode having diameter 1 mm, and a synthetic diamond detector having diameter 2.2 mm. Each detector was placed in a 3D scanning water phantom at 10 cm depth and 90 cm SSD. The detector was scanned through the beam in both the transverse and radial direc-

tions and placed at the point of maximum signal for output factor measurements. Readings were obtained for 4 cm × 4 cm, 3 cm × 3 cm, 2 cm × 2 cm, and a range of rectangular 2 cm × Y and X × 2 cm field sizes, up to a maximum field size of 40 cm. Readings were referenced to a 4 cm × 4 cm field, and the output factor relative to 10 cm × 10 cm was obtained using the 4 cm × 4 cm output factor previously measured using the 0.125 cm^3 chamber. The correction factor for all three detectors was minimal (<0.8%) for fields larger than 1.5 cm × 1.5 cm [5, 10].

The measurements for each detector were compared and are shown in Table 22.1. The treatment planning system can extrapolate to smaller field sizes. Published values for the same model linear accelerator at 95 cm SSD and 5 cm depth were used to check the treatment planning system calculation, summarized in Table 22.2.

Treatment Planning System Commissioning and End-to-End Testing

In addition to the correct measurement of small fields for input into the treatment planning system (TPS), it is important to close the loop by verifying that the treatment planning system calculates small fields with acceptable accuracy. AAPM Medical Physics Practice Guideline 5.a (MPPG 5) provides extensive guidance on the commissioning and quality assurance of dose calculations; however, MPPG 5 explicitly excludes small fields from the scope of the report [29]. Despite the exclusion of small fields, the workflow of dose calculation algorithm commissioning, validation, and routine QA presented by

Table 22.1 Output factors at 90 cm SSD, 10 cm depth measured using three detectors calculated by the treatment planning system

X	Y	Microionization chamber	Stereotactic diode	Diamond	Treatment planning system calculation
3	3	0.887	0.886	0.888	0.888
2	2	0.832	0.835	0.837	0.835
2	5	0.875	0.878	0.878	0.877
5	2	0.870	0.870	0.871	0.869

Table 22.2 Output factors at 95 cm SSD, 5 cm depth measured by the treatment planning system and reported by Wen et al. [28]

X	Y	Treatment planning system calculation	Wen et al. [28]
3	3	0.926	0.925
2	2	0.880	0.880
1	1	0.737	0.731
2	5	0.915	0.916
5	2	0.906	0.908
1	5	0.815	0.821
5	1	0.808	0.800

MPPG 5 should be followed. Basic validation tests should include verification that the treatment planning system reproduces the input data within acceptable tolerance. Where applicable, additional measurements of output factors, depth dose, and beam profiles should be acquired for fields not included in the commissioning data set for comparison with treatment planning system calculations.

End-to-end testing is a critical component in the commissioning and on-going quality control of a radiosurgery program. The scope of end-to-end testing is much broader than evaluating the accuracy of small field delivery; however, dosimetric accuracy is an important component of end-to-end testing. An end-to-end test is comprised of obtaining imaging for a phantom, constructing a treatment plan similar to one for an actual patient, delivering the treatment plan to the phantom, and evaluating the resulting dose distribution. End-to-end tests can be done with simple water-equivalent plastic phantoms or anthropomorphic phantoms. A variety of phantoms are commercially available that can be instrumented with a variety of detectors, including film. A particularly valuable end-to-end test is to use a phantom provided and evaluated by an external entity, providing an independent audit of the accuracy of delivery. The M.D. Anderson Dosimetry Laboratory provides a head phantom containing a 20 mm diameter target, as well as phantoms for testing the output of cones. There is also at least one company that offers 3D printed phantoms containing a polymer gel dosimeter that can also be used for end-to-end testing.

Case Vignette – Case 2

End-to-End Testing of a VMAT SRS System

For a VMAT SRS system using a frameless immobilization system, two end-to-end tests were done. The first test was completed internally and the second used an external auditor.

The internal test used a commercial acrylic phantom placed in the frameless system as shown in Fig. 22.1. The phantom had two interchangeable inserts. The first contained a 20 mm diameter target sphere with sufficient contrast for identification on a CT image. The second contained a channel for the placement of a microionization chamber of volume 0.007 cm^3 at the same location as the center of the target sphere. A CT scan was obtained with the target sphere insert. The CT scan was imported into the treatment planning system and the 20 mm sphere was

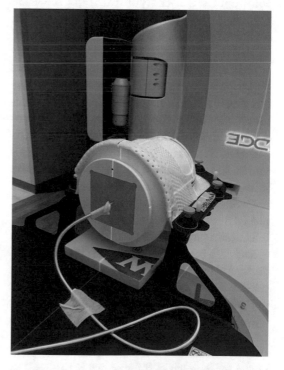

Fig. 22.1 Phantom in frameless positioning system with microionization chamber inserted at center of target volume

contoured as a planning target volume (PTV). An additional 5 mm diameter spherical volume was contoured concentric with the PTV to control the homogeneity of the dose distribution around the location of the ionization chamber. A treatment plan was created using the inverse planning system following the standard clinical protocol. The objective for the 5 mm central volume was dose uniformity in the central portion of the target sphere. Following planning, the treatment plan was transferred to the linear accelerator. The phantom was set up with the ionization chamber insert and positioned using the same image guidance protocol as for patients. The phantom was aligned to place the effective measurement point of the chamber at the center of the target sphere. The treatment plan was delivered and the chamber dose was 21.05 Gy, compared to 20.73 Gy calculated by the treatment planning system.

Following the in-house end-to-end test, an external test was done using an anthropomorphic Stereotactic Radiosurgery head phantom available from The University of Texas M.D. Anderson Dosimetry Laboratory (http://rpc.mdanderson.org/mdadl) (MDADL). The phantom is designed to test the ability to locate and treat an intracranial target to a high degree of precision. The phantom has two interchangeable inserts. The imaging insert is used for treatment volume definition, and the dosimetry insert contains radiochromic film and TLD. The instructions from the MDADL were to image, plan, and treat the phantom as an actual patient with the maximum dose in the target 30 Gy (to match the range of the radiochromic film insert). The phantom was placed in a custom mask for the frameless immobilization system and a CT obtained. The target sphere was contoured, and a treatment plan was created using the inverse planning system for a prescription dose of 20 Gy to the PTV. After optimization and dose calculation, the plan normalization was adjusted such that the maximum dose was 30 Gy (the adjustment was 1.5%). Quality assurance measurements were completed for the plan as if for an actual patient. The plan was delivered to the phantom, which was positioned on the treatment unit using the same image guidance protocol as for patients. The phantom was returned to the MDADL, where the dose to the film and TLDs was analyzed and compared to the treatment plan. The TLD results were 3% higher than the values calculated by the treatment planning system. The profiles are shown in Fig. 22.2.

Patient-Specific Quality Assurance

When a treatment plan is modulated, measurements should be done to verify the dose delivery [30]. Unfortunately, there is minimal guidance available for the measurement of small, modulated patient-specific dose distributions. Because it is water-equivalent and has minimal energy dependence, radiochromic film is a suitable detector for patient-specific QA. With careful calibration it can be used for absolute dosimetry [31]. Radiochromic film is labor intensive and requires adherence to a carefully designed processing protocol, and therefore, there is a strong incentive to use real-time dosimeters. However, the suitability of other detector types should be carefully evaluated. Although the field size is not well defined for a modulated plan and so correction factors calculated for output factor measurements cannot be applied, the dimensions of the dose distribution, as defined by the diameter of the 50% isodose volume (where 100% is the maximum dose), can be used to evaluate whether a given detector is appropriate. In addition to the response as a function of the size of the dose distribution, the directional dependence should be evaluated. Microionization chambers are suitable for dose distributions larger than approximately 15 mm. Plastic scintillator detectors are appropriate for radiosurgery distributions [32, 33], but volume averaging must be considered for dose distribution dimensions similar to the detector length.

Future Directions

Standardization of data in treatment planning systems will reduce the probability that an error in the measurement of small fields will impact

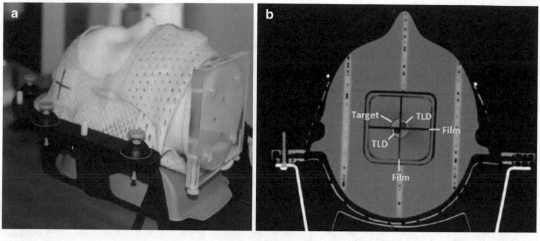

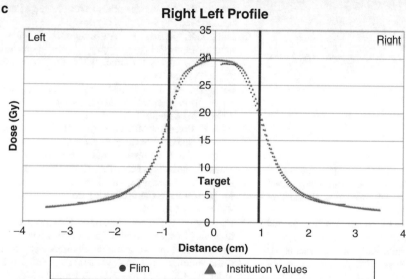

Fig. 22.2 The IROC Houston/M.D. Anderson Dosimetry Laboratory SRS head phantom positioned in a frameless system (**a**). A CT image (**b**) shows the target, thermoluminescent dosimeters (TLDs), and film in coronal and sagittal planes. An excerpt from the report (**c**) shows a dose profile through the center of the target. A summary of the report results is shown in Fig. 21.3 of Chap. 21

patient outcomes. One radiosurgery incident was revealed because the vendor of the treatment planning system compared commissioning data between institutions and discovered outliers. However, standardized beam data is not always correct as evidenced by the change in the output for the smallest collimator size on a Gamma Knife unit. It is important for individual physicists responsible for commissioning pre-configured planning systems to independently verify that the systems are operating as expected

and that the calculations match independent measurements. It is also important for user groups to share data and do multi-institutional evaluations of pre-configured planning systems.

For modulated delivery systems, patient-specific quality assurance measurements remain the standard of practice. However, system-level tests coupled with independent patient-specific dose calculations and data integrity tests will likely replace patient-specific QA in the future.

Key Points – Recommendations

- For output factor measurements, select detectors having correction factors for small field measurement <5%.
- For output factor measurements, use two or more detectors of different types and compare results.
- For depth dose and beam profile measurements, use a stereotactic field diode, synthetic diamond, or a plastic scintillator detector.
- Prior to clinical use, verify data against reference values obtained from the vendor, literature, and/or other users.
- Prior to clinical use, do an independent end-to-end test such as The M.D. Anderson Dosimetry Laboratory SRS head phantom.

References

1. Derreumaux S, Etard C, Huet C, Trompier F, Clairand I, Bottollier-Depois JF, et al. Lessons from recent accidents in radiation therapy in France. Radiat Prot Dosim. 2008;131(1):130–5.

2. Bogdanich WR, Rebecca R. Radiation errors reported in Missouri. New York Times. February 25, 2010.

3. Goetsch S. 4-mm Gamma Knife helmet factor. Int J Radiat Oncol Biol Phys. 2002;54(1):300; author reply 301.

4. International Commission on Radiation Units and Measurements. Prescribing, recording, and reporting of stereotactic treatments with small photon beams. Oxford: Oxford University Press; 2017.

5. International Atomic Energy Agency. Dosimetry of small static fields used in external beam radiotherapy: an IAEA–AAPM international code of practice for reference and relative dose determination. Technical Report Series No. 483. Vienna; 2017.

6. Palmans H, Andreo P, Huq MS, Seuntjens J, Christaki KE, Meghzifene A. Dosimetry of small static fields used in external photon beam radiotherapy: summary of TRS-483, the IAEA-AAPM international Code of Practice for reference and relative dose determination. Med Phys. 2018;45(11):e1123–45.

7. Veselsky T, Novotny J Jr, Pastykova V, Koniarova I. Determination of small field synthetic single-crystal diamond detector correction factors for CyberKnife, Leksell Gamma Knife Perfexion and linear accelerator. Phys Med. 2017;44:66–71.

8. Huet C, Moignier C, Barraux V, Loiseau C, Sebe-Mercier K, Batalla A, et al. Study of commercial detector responses in non-equilibrium small photon fields of a 1000MU/min CyberKnife system. Phys Med. 2016;32(6):818–25.

9. Francescon P, Kilby W, Satariano N. Monte Carlo simulated correction factors for output factor measurement with the CyberKnife system-results for new detectors and correction factor dependence on measurement distance and detector orientation. Phys Med Biol. 2014;59(6):N11–7.

10. Papaconstadopoulos P, Tessier F, Seuntjens J. On the correction, perturbation and modification of small field detectors in relative dosimetry. Phys Med Biol. 2014;59(19):5937–52.

11. Garnier N, Amblard R, Villeneuve R, Haykal R, Ortholan C, Colin P, et al. Detectors assessment for stereotactic radiosurgery with cones. J Appl Clin Med Phys. 2018;19(6):88–98.

12. Tessier F, Kawrakow I. Effective point of measurement of thimble ion chambers in megavoltage photon beams. Med Phys. 2010;37(1):96–107.

13. Ding GX, Krauss R. An empirical formula to obtain tissue-phantom ratios from percentage depth-dose curves for small fields. Phys Med Biol. 2013;58(14):4781–9.

14. Bjarngard BE, Zhu TC, Ceberg C. Tissue-phantom ratios from percentage depth doses. Med Phys. 1996;23(5):629–34.

15. Xiao Y, Altschuler MD, Bjarngard BE. Quality assurance of central axis dose data for photon beams by means of a functional representation of the tissue phantom ratio. Phys Med Biol. 1998;43(8):2195–206.

16. Sauer OA. Determination of the quality index (Q) for photon beams at arbitrary field sizes. Med Phys. 2009;36(9):4168–72.

17. Francescon P, Cora S, Satariano N. Calculation of k(Q(clin),Q(msr)) (f(clin),f(msr)) for several small detectors and for two linear accelerators using Monte Carlo simulations. Med Phys. 2011;38(12):6513–27.

18. Tyler M, Liu PZ, Chan KW, Ralston A, McKenzie DR, Downes S, et al. Characterization of small-field stereotactic radiosurgery beams with modern detectors. Phys Med Biol. 2013;58(21):7595–608.

19. Beddar AS, Mason DJ, O'Brien PF. Absorbed dose perturbation caused by diodes for small field photon dosimetry. Med Phys. 1994;21(7):1075–9.

20. O'Brien DJ, Leon-Vintro L, McClean B. Small field detector correction factors kQclin,Qmsr (fclin,fmsr) for silicon-diode and diamond detectors with circular 6 MV fields derived using both empirical and numerical methods. Med Phys. 2016;43(1):411.

21. Wang LL, Beddar S. Study of the response of plastic scintillation detectors in small-field 6 MV photon beams by Monte Carlo simulations. Med Phys. 2011;38(3):1596–9.

22. Liu PZ, Suchowerska N, Lambert J, Abolfathi P, McKenzie DR. Plastic scintillation dosimetry: comparison of three solutions for the Cerenkov challenge. Phys Med Biol. 2011;56(18):5805–21.

23. Gagnon JC, Theriault D, Guillot M, Archambault L, Beddar S, Gingras L, et al. Dosimetric performance and array assessment of plastic scintillation detectors

for stereotactic radiosurgery quality assurance. Med Phys. 2012;39(1):429–36.

24. Butson MJ, Cheung T, Yu PK. Weak energy dependence of EBT gafchromic film dose response in the 50 kVp-10 MVp X-ray range. Appl Radiat Isot. 2006;64(1):60–2.

25. Hartmann B, Martisikova M, Jakel O. Homogeneity of Gafchromic EBT2 film. Med Phys. 2010;37(4):1753–6.

26. Micke A, Lewis DF, Yu X. Multichannel film dosimetry with nonuniformity correction. Med Phys. 2011;38(5):2523–34.

27. Paelinck L, De Neve W, De Wagter C. Precautions and strategies in using a commercial flatbed scanner for radiochromic film dosimetry. Phys Med Biol. 2007;52(1):231–42.

28. Wen N, Li H, Song K, Chin-Snyder K, Qin Y, Kim J, et al. Characteristics of a novel treatment system for linear accelerator-based stereotactic radiosurgery. J Appl Clin Med Phys. 2015;16(4):5313.

29. Smilowitz JB, Das IJ, Feygelman V, Fraass BA, Kry SF, Marshall IR, et al. AAPM medical physics practice guideline 5.a.: commissioning and QA of treatment planning dose calculations – megavoltage photon and electron beams. J Appl Clin Med Phys. 2015;16(5):14–34.

30. Halvorsen PH, Cirino E, Das IJ, Garrett JA, Yang J, Yin FF, et al. AAPM-RSS medical physics practice guideline 9.a. for SRS-SBRT. J Appl Clin Med Phys. 2017;18(5):10–21.

31. Devic S, Tomic N, Lewis D. Reference radiochromic film dosimetry: review of technical aspects. Phys Med. 2016;32(4):541–56.

32. Dimitriadis A, Patallo IS, Billas I, Duane S, Nisbet A, Clark CH. Characterisation of a plastic scintillation detector to be used in a multicentre stereotactic radiosurgery dosimetry audit. Radiat Phys Chem. 2017;140:373–8.

33. Qin Y, Gardner SJ, Kim J, Huang Y, Wen N, Doemer A, et al. Technical note: evaluation of plastic scintillator detector for small field stereotactic patient-specific quality assurance. Med Phys. 2017;44(10):5509–16.

Techniques of Whole Brain Radiation Therapy Including Hippocampal Avoidance

23

Sean S. Mahase, Diana A. R. Julie, and Jonathan Knisely

Case Vignettes

Case 1

A 65-year-old man with a history of hypertension and right-sided stage IIIB adenocarcinoma of the colon status-post colectomy 1 year ago and adjuvant xeloda and oxaliplatin presented to the emergency department with new onset seizures. Imaging revealed a large hemorrhagic mass in the right frontal hemisphere, as well as over 20 smaller lesions of varying sizes. A number of the lesions are vasogenic and two punctate metastases are within his brainstem. The dominant mass was resected with pathology revealing metastatic adenocarcinoma consistent with his colon primary. Systemic imaging reveals multiple lesions consistent with metastases in the lungs and liver.

Given the widespread extent of his metastatic disease, and the distribution and number of metastases that are not amenable to SRS or resection, WBRT is an appropriate option to minimize further growth or possibly induce the regression of these brain metastases, with the goal of inducing a durable palliative response and offsetting symptomatic progression.

Case 2

A 32-year-old woman who palpated a mass in her right breast while breastfeeding her newborn, on subsequent workup for this mass, was initially diagnosed with stage IIIB triple positive invasive ductal carcinoma. Genetic testing was unremarkable. She underwent neoadjuvant chemotherapy with doxorubicin, cyclophosphamide, paclitaxel, and trastuzumab, followed by a right-sided mastectomy and adjuvant pertuzumab and trastuzumab. Two years later, imaging revealed multiple small brain and lung metastases for which she was treated with lapatinib and capecitabine, and SRS to the brain metastases. Six months later, surveillance imaging revealed a complete response in the lungs, but several new parenchymal brain metastases were seen, as well as focal leptomeningeal disease in the posterior fossa. Lumbar punctures did not detect cancer cells in the CSF. Her medical oncologist changed her systemic therapy to trastuzumab-emtansine, and all of her brain metastases (including the focal leptomeningeal

S. S. Mahase · D. A. R. Julie
Department of Radiation Oncology, New York-Presbyterian Hospital, Weill Cornell Medicine, New York, NY, USA

J. Knisely (✉)
Department of Radiation Oncology, Weill Cornell Medicine, New York–Presbyterian Hospital, New York, NY, USA
e-mail: jok9121@med.cornell.edu

© Springer Nature Switzerland AG 2020
Y. Yamada et al. (eds.), *Radiotherapy in Managing Brain Metastases*,
https://doi.org/10.1007/978-3-030-43740-4_23

disease) were again treated with SRS. Follow-up imaging demonstrated the progression of lepto-meningeal enhancement in the posterior fossa as well as in both internal auditory canals and along gyri in the high left parietal lobe, with sustained extracranial disease control. She is currently asymptomatic on examination.

The presence of leptomeningeal tumor involvement in the context of an overall inability to control her CNS disease despite multiple lines of systemic therapy and SRS courses warrants non-emergent WBRT to mitigate further disease progression. However, given her overall good performance status, young age, and well-controlled extracranial disease, every attempt should be made to minimize the long-term sequelae of WBRT.

Case 3

A 55-year-old male former 40-pack-year smoker presented with persistent cough. He is otherwise in good health, with excellent performance status. Upon complete work-up, including an unremarkable brain MRI, he is diagnosed with limited stage small cell lung cancer (SCLC) of the right lung, Stage IIB, T3N0M0. He is now status post-chemotherapy with cisplatin and etoposide, as well as concurrent thoracic radiation. Upon the completion of his definitive therapy, work-up reveals a complete response of his thoracic disease, and MRI brain was without evidence of metastases.

Standard of care for limited stage SCLC with a complete or partial response to concurrent chemoradiotherapy includes prophylactic cranial irradiation (PCI); therefore, this patient is a candidate for prophylactic WBRT. However, given his young age, excellent performance status, and complete response to therapy, attempts should be made to limit neurocognitive sequelae of treatment, with approaches such as are being tested in NRG Oncology CC003 (HA-WBRT and concurrent and adjuvant memantine). Alternatively, he could be observed, and if he eventually presents with a limited number of metastases in non-eloquent regions in the context of overall good performance status, SRS could be considered with WBRT held as a salvage option.

Introduction

Whole brain radiation (WBRT) is employed in the treatment of brain metastases, leukemia [1], germ cell tumors, and multicentric CNS lymphomas [2] and as part of a more comprehensive craniospinal irradiation protocol for pediatric malignancies, including medulloblastoma [3]. Brain metastases, the most common intracranial neoplasms in adults [4], occur in almost one-third of all cancer patients and are the cause of death in up to 50% of these individuals [5]. The rising proportion of cancer patients diagnosed with brain metastases parallel the development of progressively effective systemic agents that increase systemic progression-free survival and may confer an overall survival benefit in select cases. However, many of these agents possess a limited ability to bypass the blood-brain barrier [6]. Additionally, as only 10% of patients with brain metastases are diagnosed secondary to symptomatic presentations, incidence rates continue to increase with more common use of routine surveillance imaging [5]. The symptomatic management of brain metastases entails corticosteroids and other supportive care measures [7]. Validated definitive therapeutic options are limited as surgical resection is reserved for specific circumstances, many chemotherapeutic agents are unable to enter the central nervous system, and the efficacy of newer targeted agents and immunotherapy are under investigation. WBRT became the initial therapeutic standard for brain metastases and continues to be the predominant treatment choice in the setting of multiple lesions, recurrent metastases, and/or leptomeningeal disease. Accurate planning and treatment delivery are essential to delivering adequate tumor control and palliation of symptoms. Understanding and taking measures to minimize toxicities is of upmost importance as patients treated with WBRT live longer with the aid of increasingly effective systemic therapies.

Rationale and Initial Experiences

Radiotherapy as a treatment modality can provide rapid palliation of symptoms and possesses several favorable advantages over surgical resection and systemic therapy [8, 9]. It effectively penetrates chemotherapeutic sanctuary sites such as the brain, and its delivery is independent of vascular supply, hepatic and renal function, and other systemic agents. These considerations, combined with its non-invasive nature, promote its use in those with poor performance status, or who have impaired kidney or liver function. There is also flexibility in tailoring the treatment if additional disease in the spine needs to be covered, or if the treatment course must be expedited.

One of the earliest series using brain irradiation was documented in 1931 by Lenz and Fried, who treated symptomatic brain lesions in three "pre-terminal" patients with metastatic breast cancer. The symptoms were ascribed to increased intracranial pressure, characterized as headache in the first two patients, with the third patient also experiencing vomiting and convulsions. They reported radiotherapy resulted in temporary resolution of each patient's symptoms over several months, with an overall survival of 11, 18, and 20 months following symptomatic presentation. Additionally, several "terminal" patients with symptomatic brain metastases secondary to breast cancer received cranial irradiation, resulting in effective symptom palliation lasting for weeks to months [10]. In 1948, Richmond reported durable symptomatic improvement in eight patients receiving radiotherapy for brain metastases (four breast primaries, three lung primaries, one renal primary). He stressed the importance of uniformly treating a larger region of the brain than is indicated by x-ray and clinical examination given the infiltrative nature of brain metastases [11].

A larger single-institution series from Memorial-Sloan Kettering Cancer Center (MSKCC) published in 1954 demonstrated 24 of 38 patients with symptomatic brain metastases improved following brain irradiation (15 of 23 treated lung primaries, 4 of 7 breast primaries, 1 prostate cancer, 1 endothelioma, 1 teratoma, 1 esophageal cancer, and 1 leukemia). This translated to an average 8.2-month survival among those who responded to radiation, while non-responders, and those who didn't complete treatment, had a 4.6-month average survival time. The authors reported brain irradiation appeared effective in palliating neurological symptoms irrespective of tumor histology or intracerebral location. Furthermore, while the duration of symptoms prior to intervention did not affect the ability to provide effective palliation, the subset of responders that had shorter symptomatic intervals had quicker functional recovery. The authors concluded WBRT provides a benefit in those with multiple brain metastases, and with residual tumor following surgery, given its ability to palliate symptoms in the context of the overall poor prognosis of this population [8].

Chu and colleagues subsequently reported 77.8% of an apparently prospectively followed cohort of 158 patients receiving WBRT at MSKCC experienced sustained palliation of their symptoms, defined as lasting over 1 month. Those responding to treatment had an average 4.7-month symptom control duration and 6.6-month survival, while non-responders had a 2.3-month average survival time. Among this cohort, 86% of 64 breast cancer patients and 83.3% of 54 lung cancer patients responded to WBRT. Seventeen patients underwent a second course of WBRT for symptomatic recurrences, of which twelve responded with an average symptom control duration of 4.6 months, and an average 8.1-month survival, whereas non-responders had an average 1.4-month survival. The majority of patients in this series died of non-CNS-related causes [12].

Clinical Trials Evaluating WBRT

Early Radiation Therapy Oncology Group (RTOG) randomized trials validated WBRT as an effective treatment for those with well-controlled primary disease and favorable performance status, albeit these studies reported that many patients only survived a few months after completing treatment [13]. Patchell and colleagues subsequently conducted a trial that randomized patients with a single radiographically detected brain metastasis to WBRT alone or surgical resection followed by post-operative WBRT. They showed that a combination of surgery and post-operative WBRT improved overall survival to 40 weeks, compared to 15 weeks if WBRT was administered alone [14]. Patchell et al. followed up these findings by randomizing 95 patients who underwent resection of a brain metastasis to either observation or post-operative WBRT. While they reported no significant difference in overall survival among the cohorts, recurrence rates were reduced from 46% in the observation group to 10% in the WBRT group. WBRT also reduced the incidence of new brain metastases and death due to neurological causes, thereby establishing post-operative WBRT as the standard of care for brain metastases [15].

Evolution of Technique, Dose and Fractionation

Early Kilovoltage Era

Lenz and Fried used 200 kilovoltage (kV) X-rays with a 0.5 mm copper filter, 50 cm from the patient's skin or radium packs at a distance of 2–3 cm from the patient's skin surface. Treatment duration was based on the ability to elicit an erythematous reaction on the skin overlying the region of interest such that one, two, and more than two "erythema dose(s)" were considered a small, moderate, and large dose, respectively. They reported that the majority of patients experiencing symptomatic improvement in their series received a moderate radiation dose [10]. WBRT techniques have slowly but substantially evolved from this point over the following decades.

In the 1940s, photon energies used for treatment ranged from 180–250 kV. Given the likelihood of multiple metastases, many physicians elected to radiate the whole brain using simple AP-PA or opposed lateral fields, but by the 1960s, WBRT delivery had largely transitioned to using two opposed lateral fields, averaging 14 × 20 cm in size (Figs. 23.1 and 23.2). Clinical setups determined by a plane formed by the supraorbital ridge and the external auditory meatus and ending at the foramen magnum served as the inferior

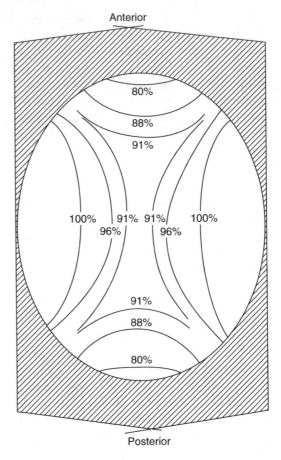

Fig. 23.1 Isodose distribution for WBRT using 250 kV x-rays with a 2.0 mm Cu HVL and 70 cm TSD (from Chao et al. [8]). The effects of scatter and of bone absorption of low-energy x-rays are ignored in this representation. Bolus bags surrounding the head and in contact with the scalp (in gray) were used in the treatment setups described. (From Chao et al. [8]. Reprinted with permission from John Wiley and Sons)

margin, while the anterior, superior, and posterior field edges were defined as 2 cm beyond ("flashing") the forehead, cranial vertex, and occiput, respectively. Bolus was often used during treatment, despite the fact that orthovoltage x-rays with a half value layer of 2.0 mm of copper were commonly employed with a short target-to-skin distance of only 50–70 cm because of low photon outputs with this equipment. Some physicians used lead blocks to shield the eye from the primary beam and to protect structures below the inferior border of the treatment field [8, 12, 16].

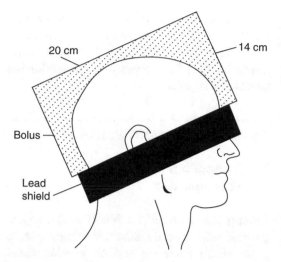

Fig. 23.2 Setup illustration for WBRT using parallel opposed lateral fields using equipment as described for Fig. 23.1. (From Chu and Hilaris [12]. Reprinted with permission from John Wiley and Sons)

It became convention among treating physicians to initiate therapy with smaller doses in an attempt to avoid further increasing intracranial pressure from treatment-related edema. Fractionation choice was also based on the patient's performance status, starting with 50–100 centiGray (cGy) for the initial 3–4 days and gradually increasing the dose by 50 cGy increments to 350–400 cGy in the absence of any worsening signs or symptoms (increased headache, vomiting, and papilledema) [12]. While some reports demonstrate effective palliation of metastases from solid tumor primaries using 2000 cGy or less, the majority of radiation oncologists administered 3000 cGy over 3 weeks as some anecdotally reported patients treated at lower doses recurred more quickly [17]. Chao et al. noted 9 of their 14 treatment failures received total doses under 3000 cGy. Conversely, increasing the total dose beyond 3000 cGy increased the occurrence of moist desquamation and permanent alopecia, without observable improvements in the duration of palliation [8]. Chu et al. reported longer remission rates among those receiving at least 2750 cGy, with no lung patients and 11% of breast patients receiving less than this threshold dose exhibiting durable palliation at 5 and 6 months, respectively [12].

2-Dimensional Treatment Planning Era

The 1960s ushered in the use of fluoroscopy-guided imaging during simulations to guide shaping the treatment field and block design. However, WBRT was often carried out without a formal simulation, with clinical setups arranged using external landmarks as described above. This method often did not cover the most inferior aspects of the brain.

As clinicians became more aware of skull-base recurrences in diseases such as medulloblastoma or leukemia in the region of the cribriform plate, and of lens toxicity from WBRT portals that were poorly designed and did not fully encompass the cribriform plate, greater care was devoted to portal design [3]. To avoid missing the portion of the brain extending inferiorly between the posterior aspect of the eyes, the cranial vault was treated with two opposed parallel lateral beams including the retro-orbital space, with the inferior border extending from the superior orbital ridge through the tip of the mastoid and including the first two cervical vertebrae. The treatment fields continued to extend 1–2 cm beyond the scalp superiorly and posteriorly. While a mask was used for immobilization, these adjustments provided inferior landmarks that could be delineated on the patient's face by radiation oncologists [1, 3]. Alternatively, immobilization was often performed by stretching a piece of adhesive tape across the forehead that was attached to the sides of the treatment couch. Using this method ensured the lens received ≤10% of the prescribed dose, keeping the total lens dose under 400 cGy [3]. It was realized that setting the central axis of the beams at the lateral canthi accounted for unwanted divergence into the contralateral eye while avoiding any need to adjust the couch or gantry positions to minimize divergence into the contralateral eye that would be needed if the isocenter were placed in a different location [18].

3-Dimensional Treatment Planning Era

Concerns grew about the aforementioned planning methods' liability to incompletely cover the target volume and thus promote subsequent treatment failure, particularly in the temporal and subfrontal regions [19]. Several studies attributed observed high subfrontal failure rates to incorrect eye block positioning [20, 21]. The advent and widespread utilization of computerized tomography (CT) scanning delivered a more accurate spatial approximation of the relevant anatomy with reference to beam placements, and any shielding required and provided a means of developing 3-dimensional (3D) computer-assisted radiotherapy treatment designs intended to generate more comprehensive planning than prior 2-dimensional (2D) methods. Planning CT data could be used to derive an image, referred to as a digitally reconstructed radiograph (DRR), which would have a role similar to conventional radiographic films used in fluoroscopic simulators, such as verifying beam placement during treatment [22–24]. Modern radiotherapy planning software enables the projection of contours of anatomic structures from CT scans, projection of collimator edges, custom blocks, and crosshairs onto the DRR, as well as the ability to create adequately scaled physical or virtual films for the purposes of simulation and beam placement verification [25].

Gripp and colleagues prospectively evaluated CT-based versus plain radiograph-based simulations in 5 patients with primary brain tumors and 15 patients with brain metastases. They used a face mask to immobilize each patient's head and various slice thicknesses ranging from 3 to 5 mm. CT-based planning reduced geographic misses from 8% to 0.6%, reducing incomplete coverage of the subfrontal region from 10% to 1%, while reducing exposure to the ipsilateral lens from 3% to 0%, and contralateral lens exposure from 22% to 11% [21]. Mah et al. demonstrated that CT-based 3D simulations improved accuracy in field placement and shielding through better localization of critical and target structures, as well requiring significantly less time than 2D simulations, an especially important consideration when simulating pediatric patients [26]. Andic et al. dosimetrically compared 2D and 3D WBRT using the scans of 30 patients. The same field center and angles were shared by the 2D and 3D plans. The mean value of minimum brain doses was significantly higher for 3D plans in which all patients received a minimum of 95% of the prescribed dose while improving dose homogeneity and protecting the ocular lenses [27].

Contemporary WBRT Practices

Treatment Planning, Dose and Fractionation

Patients are simulated for WBRT in the supine position using a head holder and a thermoplastic mask which conforms to their specific facial anatomy for immobilization. The creation of these masks takes approximately 15 minutes. Radiographically opaque setup marks can be placed on the mask rather than on the patient's skin. A non-contrast CT scan using a maximum 3–5 mm slice thickness from the vertex to the upper cervical spine is recommended for treatment planning. The two opposed lateral fields are slightly rotated off-axis, generally two to three degrees in the anterior oblique orientation, to create coplanar anterior field edges that do not diverge into the lenses of the contralateral eyes. An isocentric treatment technique is almost always employed, in which the patient's midline is aligned with the sagittal alignment line. The central axis may be defined by the lateral canthi (Fig. 23.3a, b), but this is not critical, as appropriate adjustments in couch and gantry angulation are possible that will achieve the same goal of avoiding divergence of radiation beams into the contralateral eye and still covering the entire cranial contents, paying particular attention to the cribriform plate (Fig. 23.3c, d). This flexibility is important as patients are not always symmetrically positioned at the time of simulation. In either case, the field is then opened until the entire brain is encompassed with the beam extending beyond the skull by several centimeters in all directions. The lower border of the field is commonly set at the caudal aspect of the first or second cervical vertebrae. Shielding can then be designed to protect normal tissues of the face outside the brain. While not essential for WBRT

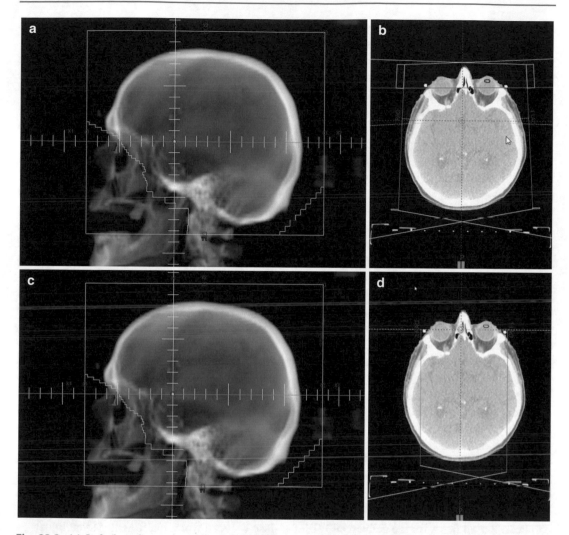

Fig. 23.3 (**a**) Left (lateral) anterior oblique field DRR with WBRT MLCs for WBRT plan shown in (**b**). Lenses are shown in color. (**b**) WBRT axial plane at the level of bony canthi, with isocenter at setup points defined by radio-opaque markers on immobilization mask at laser setup points. Gantry rotations are employed to ensure anterior beam edges are coplanar and do not diverge into contralateral lenses. (**c**) Left lateral DRR showing the setup of isocenter at radio-opaque markers placed on bony lateral canthi. Radiotherapy field is not shown. (**d**) WBRT axial plane at the level of bony canthi, with isocenter set at mid-separation between markers. This image illustrates posterior beam divergence to prevent inadvertent lens irradiation

planning, MRI anatomical information can be transferred to the CT planning imaging using image coregistration algorithms.

When the patient is positioned for treatment, the verification of setup accuracy is needed to confirm that treatment will be accurately delivered. This has been traditionally performed by checking MV or kV radiologic films to confirm isocenter location accuracy and block positioning. Surface-guided radiation therapy (employing open-faced masks that permit facial features to be tracked) may complement these approaches by optically monitoring patient position throughout each treatment [28, 29].

There are currently a range of accepted dose and fractionation schemes for WBRT or PCI, including 50 Gray (Gy) in 20 fractions, 40 Gy in 20 fractions, 40 Gy in 15 fractions, 37.5 Gy in 15 fractions, 36 Gy in 18 fractions, 30 Gy in 10 or 15 fractions, 25 Gy in 10 fractions, 24 Gy in 12 fractions, 20 Gy in 5 fractions, or 8Gy in 1 fraction [13]. The RTOG have evaluated several of these regimens in clinical settings [30]; however, no particular fractionation scheme to date has demonstrated a significant difference in the frequency of symptomatic improvement, time to progression, or overall survival following WBRT. Investigators have also explored altered fractionation regimens. One such study evaluating WBRT delivered in 2 Gy fractions three times a day to 30–36 Gy in 1 week demonstrated durable palliation of symptoms in 45% of patients 6 months after treatment with no significant adverse effects [31]. However, while alternate fractionation allows rapid treatment completion, delivering multiple fractions in 1 day can be taxing on the staff and also accelerate the emergence of adverse effects with insufficient data to demonstrate superiority over conventional fractionation. A recent Cochrane analysis demonstrated no improvements in overall survival or symptomatic improvement with higher biologically altered fractionation schedules, as compared with conventional regimens of 30 Gy in 10 fractions or 20 Gy in 5 fractions [32]. Thus, most physicians adhere to their respective institutional guidelines when selecting a particular WBRT course, with 30 Gy in 10 fractions as the most frequently used regimen in the United States [33].

Traditional 2D or 3D treatment planning with parallel opposed fields for the delivery of WBRT can result in large dose heterogeneity, as high as +/− 20% [34, 35]. To our knowledge, there is no data specifically regarding the effect of this dose inhomogeneity during WBRT, but areas of increased dose in the brain, as well as using doses above 3 Gy per fraction to large volumes, are associated with increased toxicity [36, 37]. Therefore, efforts have been made to deliver WBRT with less dose inhomogeneity. Most often, WBRT is planned with 6 MV photons, but 10 MV photons can improve dose homogeneity, reduce hotspots, and deliver a lower integral dose without compromising target coverage [38] (Fig. 23.4). At our institution, we retrospectively re-planned conventional WBRT patients with 6 and 10 MV photon energy and conducted a dosimetric analysis of the plans. 10 MV plans significantly improved the target volume receiving 98% of prescribed dose, reduced target volume receiving 105% of prescribed dose, and reduced the maximum dose delivered. Treatment plan homogeneity was significantly improved with 10 MV photons [unpublished data]. Field-in-field treatment planning has also been demonstrated to increase homogeneity and reduce hotspots [34].

In 3D conformal radiotherapy, each treatment field's aperture conforms to the target projection in its beam's eye view, creating uniform radiation intensity throughout the field. Conversely, using intensity-modulated radiotherapy (IMRT), the portion of a radiation beam directed to an organ at risk in a single field can be blocked with the dose to the corresponding target being compensated using other fields. This can be accomplished using MLCs with dynamic MLCs entailing the leaves being in motion at all times during delivery, or segmented MLC with static or step-and-shoot-based delivery whereby the leaves are fixed at various locations and time points for each individual beam and gantry angle [39].

IMRT can also be used to significantly reduce WBRT heterogeneity. Yu et al. performed a dosimetric evaluation of 3DRT versus IMRT WBRT in 10 patients with a nominal prescribed dose of 30 Gy in 10 fractions using 6 MV photons. They reported IMRT improved dose uniformity with the mean percentage of brain receiving >105% of dose reduced from 29.3% with 3D radiotherapy to 0.03% with IMRT. The mean maximum dose was reduced from 113% with 3D to 105% with IMRT while the mean volume receiving at least 98% of the prescribed dose was 99.5% for the 3D and 100% for IMRT. With conventional WBRT, hotspots were located in the superior and median frontal regions, and these were eliminated with IMRT. These improvements were attained without sacrifice in target coverage, although IMRT requires an approximately three-fold increase in monitor units for plan delivery. The authors estimated that IMRT treatment planning required only 20–25 minutes longer than conventional planning, with additional time required for target contouring and plan optimization. Additional time would also be required for IMRT QA [36]. The clinical implications of these reductions in

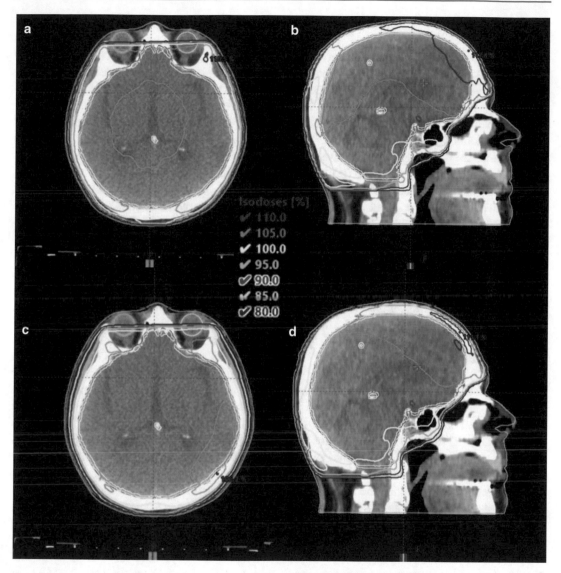

Fig. 23.4 (**a**) Axial WBRT dosimetry at isocenter using 6 MV photons. (**b**) Sagittal WBRT dosimetry at isocenter using 6 MV photons. (**c**) Axial WBRT dosimetry at iso- center using 10 MV photons. (**d**) Sagittal WBRT dosimetry at isocenter using 10 MV photons

dose inhomogeneity, especially within the frontal lobes responsible for higher cognitive functions, are currently unknown and may merit further investigation.

Volumetric modulated arc therapy (VMAT) is a form of IMRT where radiation is delivered in multiple arcs around the patient, potentially improving conformality of dose delivery. By using dynamic arcs, VMAT can allow for more rapid treatment delivery relative to IMRT. Shortened treatment time can improve patient comfort and decreased

intrafraction patient movement during treatment delivery. Studies evaluating VMAT for WBRT report excellent target coverage and plan homogeneity, as well as acceptable toxicity rates, perhaps lower than those observed with historic controls. Reported treatment times with VMAT WBRT are only 3–4 minutes [35]. As with any IMRT, VMAT planning does increase workload with regard to treatment planning and treatment QA.

Hippocampal avoiding whole brain radiation therapy is discussed below.

Tumor Histology

An increased understanding of radiobiology influenced physicians' decision to incorporate the relative radiosensitivity of a tumor in their selection of WBRT regimen. One study demonstrated improved palliation of brain metastases secondary to melanoma with higher total doses [40], while another study demonstrated improved outcomes using higher doses per fraction (≥500 cGy) albeit with increased toxicity [41]. Rades et al. retrospectively demonstrated that 6-month local control rate of brain metastases from renal cell carcinoma was improved from 21% using 30 Gy in 10 fractions to 57% using a higher dose of 40 Gy × 20 fractions or 45 Gy in 15 fractions. The overall 1-year survival was 13% with 30 Gy in 10 fractions and 47% with higher dose [42].

WBRT Plus SRS Boost

The use of an SRS-mediated tumor boost following WBRT has been explored in an effort to improve clinical outcomes. An early study evaluating WBRT to 35 Gy followed by a 15 Gy SRS boost of a solitary brain metastasis demonstrated no benefit over WBRT alone [43]. A prospective trial of 27 patients with multiple brain metastases randomized to WBRT alone (14 patients) or WBRT + SRS (13 patients) demonstrated a superior one 1-year local control of 100% in the WBRT + SRS cohort, compared to 8% in the WBRT alone cohort. The median time to local failure was 6 months after WBRT alone in comparison to 36 months after WBRT + SRS, and was independent of histology or number of tumors, but was related to the extent of extracranial disease. Furthermore, there was no increased morbidity observed in the WBRT + SRS group [44].

RTOG 9508 conducted the largest prospective trial on this topic to date, randomizing 167 patients with 1–3 brain metastases to WBRT + SRS and 164 to WBRT alone. The WBRT + SRS cohort had a significantly improved median survival of 6.5 months, compared to 4.9 months in the WBRT group. The WBRT + SRS cohort also demonstrated stable or improved KPS scores, improved local control rates, and a better complete response rate at 6 months in all patients. Of note, no survival benefit was seen in patients with multiple brain metastases receiving WBRT + SRS, but these patients reported improved performance status and decreased steroid dependence [45]. Thus, WBRT + SRS boost appears beneficial to those with a single brain metastasis; however, it is unclear whether SRS or surgery leads to better outcomes, or whether there is a benefit to surgery followed by WBRT and SRS. Finally, a recent Cochrane analysis reported that the hazard ratio of 1-year overall brain control of WBRT + SRS versus WBRT alone was 0.39, favoring the WBRT + SRS [32].

Although WBRT and SRS may be delivered in a sequential manner, they can be given simultaneously with VMAT on a linear accelerator [36, 39]. One group evaluated delivering WBRT to 20 Gy in 5 fractions with a simultaneous integrated SRS boost (SIB) to 20 Gy in 5 fractions, resulting in 40 Gy in 5 fractions delivered to the center of the metastases. The mean number of monitor units and the mean "beam on" time needed to deliver both arcs were 1600 MU and 180 seconds, respectively [46]. Borghetti et al. performed a comparative dosimetric and technical analysis of SRS versus a SIB, and of helical IMRT versus VMAT. For each of the 10 cases, 4 treatment plans were calculated and optimized, and one was actually delivered: WBRT (30 Gy/10 fractions) + SRS boost (15 Gy/1 fraction) with helical IMRT or VMAT or WBRT with SIB (45 Gy/10 fractions) using helical IMRT or VMAT. They reported that helical IMRT provided better target coverage than arc-based plans and that mean treatment time was 210 seconds, 467 seconds, 440 seconds, and 1598 seconds, respectively, for arc-based-SIB, arc-based-SRS, helical IMRT-SIB, and helical IMRT-SRS [47].

Post-operative WBRT

The intent of post-operative WBRT is to treat residual tumor in the resection bed while controlling distant microscopic and macroscopic disease in the remainder of the brain. Several phase III trials in addition to the aforementioned Patchell study [15] have evaluated the utility of postoperative WBRT. Muacevic et al. randomized 64 patients with a single brain metastasis ≤3 cm in diameter, KPS ≥ 70, and stable extracranial disease to Gamma Knife SRS alone versus surgical resection plus post-operative WBRT. WBRT was started within 14 days of tumor resection to a dose of 40 Gy in 20 fractions. The mean SRS dose applied to the tumor margin was 21 Gy, ranging from 20 to 27 Gy for radioresistant tumors such as melanomas and 14–20 Gy for radiosensitive tumors such as breast cancer. While there were no differences in 1-year local control, quality of life (QoL) at 6 months following radiotherapy, median survival (9.5 months in WBRT and 10.3 months in SRS patients), or neurological death among the cohorts, a worse 1-year distant control was seen in the SRS group (3% vs 25.8%) [48].

Kocher et al. evaluated the outcomes of 359 patients with 1–3 brain metastases, stable extracranial disease, and good performance status who either underwent upfront SRS (199 patients) or surgical resection (160 patients) and were subsequently randomized to observation or WBRT. While overall survival was similar in the WBRT and observation arms (10.9 vs 10.7 months), WBRT reduced the 2-year relapse rate both at initial sites (surgery: 59% to 27%; SRS: 31% to 19%) and at new sites (surgery: 42% to 23%; SRS: 48% to 33%) [49]. Brown et al. randomized patients with one resected brain metastasis and a resection cavity less than 5 cm in maximal extent to either postoperative SRS (12–20 Gy in 1 fraction) or postoperative WBRT (30 Gy in 10 fractions or 37.5 Gy in 15 fractions). SRS was associated with a shorter time to intracranial progression than WBRT (6.4 vs 27.5 months), and an inferior 6-month surgical bed control (80.4% vs 87.1%). While local and distant brain control were both worse in patients receiving SRS, there was no difference in the incidence of leptomeningeal disease among the cohorts. Of note, 20% of the patients in the SRS cohort eventually received WBRT as a component of their salvage therapy [50]. However, the emphasis of this trial was on the improved cognitive-deterioration-free survival in the SRS cohort, which will be discussed in detail below.

Repeat WBRT

A second course of WBRT can be considered in patients who develop growing or new brain symptomatic metastases after an initial course of WBRT [12]. Wong et al. retrospectively evaluated the outcomes of 86 patients who underwent repeat WBRT to a median of 20 Gy for progressive brain metastases following initial WBRT to 30 Gy. Resolution of presenting neurological symptoms was reported in 27%, with 45% experiencing a partial response and 29% having stable or worsened symptoms following repeat WBRT. On multivariate analysis, the absence of extracranial metastases was prognostic of response [51]. Another study entailed 17 patients receiving an initial WBRT course with a median dose of 35 Gy and a repeat WBRT to a median dose of 21.6 Gy following the development of neurological symptoms and radiological evidence of new or progressive brain metastases. Eight of ten patients with complete follow-up data demonstrated complete or partial symptomatic improvement. The cohort had a 5.2-month median overall survival following reirradiation, with 19.8-month median survival among those with stable extracranial disease and 2.5-month median survival among those with progressive extracranial disease. Side effects during reirradiation were all acute and limited to grade 1 or 2 in severity, including fatigue (35.5%), headache (23.5%), nausea and emesis (23.5%), ataxia (5.9%), skin irritation (5.9%), and dizziness (5.9%) [52]. Thus, a dose of 20 Gy can be safely given with the intention of providing effective palliation of symptoms or decreasing steroid dependence in those with limited expected survival.

Sparing of Organs at Risk

Since the prognosis of patients with brain metastases has traditionally been considered limited, sequelae of WBRT have been largely disregarded. However, a subset of patients, especially young patients, with a small number of metastases, good performance status, and favorable primary site, can experience prolonged survival. As diagnostic modalities advance, allowing for earlier detection of metastatic disease, and as systemic therapies improve, patients with brain metastases are experiencing longer overall survivals. As a result, an increasing emphasis is now being placed on minimizing sequelae of treatment.

Hippocampus

It is well documented that WBRT can result in neurocognitive and memory deterioration [36, 53–57]. It is difficult to distinguish the effects of radiotherapy from those of chemotherapy, surgery, and intracranial progression of disease in patients requiring WBRT. However, when WBRT patients subsequently complete rigorous neurocognitive testing, approximately half demonstrate significant abnormalities, and some studies have reported rates of dementia of 11–52% following WBRT [36, 55, 57]. The subgranular zone of the hippocampal dentate gyrus has been associated with the formation of new memories. It is hypothesized that injury to stem cells in this location contributes to radiation-induced impairments in memory and cognitive decline. There is evidence of a dose-response relationship between hippocampal radiation and decline in cognitive function, such as recall [53, 54, 56].

To test this, efforts have been made to minimize radiation dose to the hippocampi during WBRT, with the aim of reducing the incidence and severity of neurocognitive sequelae (Fig. 23.5). In recent years, IMRT techniques have been developed to conformally avoid the hippocampi, so-called hippocampal avoidance WBRT (HA-IMRT). Employing this technique, the authors have reported reductions in mean dose to the hippocampal neural stem-cell compartment of at least 80%, without compromising target coverage or homogeneity [53]. There are several ways to plan HA-WBRT, including helical tomotherapy, IMRT, and VMAT. Dosimetric comparisons of these techniques have concluded that helical tomotherapy most reduces mean, median, and maximum hippocampal dose. This treatment modality also improves target homo-

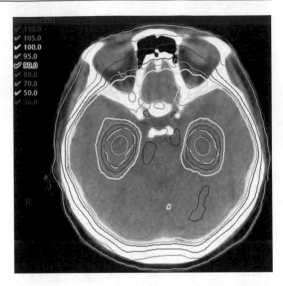

Fig. 23.5 Axial Hippocampal-avoiding WBRT dosimetry through anterior hippocampi using 6 MV photons

geneity by reducing hotspots, while not compromising target coverage. Helical tomotherapy may be the optimal method for the delivery of HA-WBRT, and that when this is not available, VMAT can be employed, with IMRT being a less favorable alternative [58, 59]. As noted earlier, in our experience, the use of 10 MV photons, rather than 6 MV, can reduce hippocampal radiation dose for conventional WBRT treatment planning.

RTOG 0933, a Phase II international, multi-institution trial, assessed neurocognitive outcomes with HA-WBRT. In this protocol, patients with brain metastases at least 5 mm from the hippocampi were treated with HA-WBRT to 30 Gy in 10 fractions. The hippocampi were contoured on co-registered MR imaging, and a 5 mm uniform expansion was applied, creating a hippocampal avoidance structure. The PTV was the brain parenchyma (excluding the hippocampal avoidance structure). The maximal point dose in the hippocampi was not to exceed 16 Gy, and no more than 9 Gy could be given to the 100% of the hippocampi. Patients experienced a mean relative decline in short-term memory, as measured by the Hopkins Verbal Learning Test-Revised Delayed Recall (HVLT-R DR), of 7%, compared to 30% for historical controls. The authors concluded that HA-WBRT for brain metastasis patients was associated with the significant preservation of memory function and QoL compared to conventional WBRT [53]. Other prospective trials have demonstrated consistent results. Tsai et al. delivered prophylactic or therapeutic HA-WBRT to 40 patients and evaluated neurocognitive function, including memory, executive functioning, and psychomotor speed and reported stable neurocognitive function at 4 months' follow-up. Hippocampal D0, D10, D50, and D80 less than 12.6 Gy, 8.81 Gy, 7.45 Gy, and 5.83 Gy, respectively, were associated with the preservation of neurocognitive functioning [56].

We performed HA-WBRT planning with VMAT delivery for 20 consecutive WBRT patients using 6 and 10 MV photon energies, using target structures, avoidance structures, and dose constraints as defined in RTOG 0933. Minimum and maximum hippocampal doses were significantly worse with 10 MV photons, and a greater number of plans met pre-defined constraints without deviations. Additionally, 6 MV photons improved target coverage and homogeneity [unpublished data]. Based upon our institutional experience, we recommend 6 MV photon energies be employed for the delivery of VMAT HA-WBRT.

An obvious concern with dose reduction to the hippocampi is increased risk of disease progression in this region. However, published literature suggests low rates of brain metastases within or near the hippocampus. Very large studies of patients with intracranial metastatic disease have revealed rates of metastases within 5 mm of the hippocampus in fewer than 3% of patients [53, 60–62]. Studies completed to date employing HA-WBRT have reported low rates of hippocampal failure and no evidence of isolated hippocampal recurrences [53, 63, 64]. In RTOG 00933, HA-WBRT was not associated with the significant development of new brain metastases in or near the hippocampi, with fewer than 5% of patients experiencing progression of disease in this region [53].

Memantine

Memantine is an *N*-methyl-D-aspartate (NMDA) receptor antagonist used in the management of

dementia associated with Alzheimer disease [56]. Two phase III placebo-controlled, randomized trials demonstrated tolerability and efficacy of memantine in the management of vascular dementia [57, 65]. Memantine may also be neuroprotective following radiotherapy, delaying the onset of neurocognitive decline, and decreasing impairments in memory, executive function, and processing speed [57]. RTOG 0614 is a double-blind, randomized, placebo-controlled trial of patients treated with WBRT to 37.5 Gy in 15 fractions, evaluating the neuroprotective effects of memantine versus placebo. Neurocognitive function was evaluated with a wide variety of validated assessment tools. Oral memantine (with an escalating dose schedule) was administered concurrently and adjuvantly with WBRT, for a total of 24 weeks.

Patients receiving memantine had significantly longer time to cognitive decline and lower probability of cognitive function failure. Patients receiving memantine also had significantly greater executive function, processing speed, and delayed recognition compared to patients receiving placebo. In the memantine arm compared to placebo, a trend toward significantly less decline in delayed recall was reported ($p = 0.059$). The authors attribute this failure to reach significance to poor compliance and resultant limited statistical power. The authors reported that memantine was well tolerated, with no difference in grade 3 or 4 adverse effects between the trial arms. Of note, 80% of the patients enrolled in RTOG 0614 had a documented neurocognitive decline by 6 months following the completion of WBRT, underscoring the great importance of mitigating treatment-related sequelae in this patient population [56].

Based upon the promising results of RTOG 0933 and RTOG 0614, two active NRG Oncology trials are further evaluating HA-WBRT and memantine for the preservation of neurocognitive functioning. NRG CC003 (NCT02635009) is a phase II/III trial of small cell lung cancer patients receiving PCI, who will be randomized to HA-WBRT or conventional WBRT. In the phase II portion of this trial, investigators will assess intracranial relapse, while the phase III portion will assess cognitive decline, employing the

HVLT-R DR instrument. NRG CC001 (NCT02360215) is a phase II trial of brain metastases patients receiving WBRT and memantine (administered as per RTOG 0614), randomized to HA-WBRT versus conventional WBRT [66]. This study identified that the risk of cognitive failure was significantly lower after HA-WBRT plus memantine versus WBRT plus memantine due to less deterioration in executive function at 4 months (23.3% v 40.4%; P = .01) and learning and memory at 6 months (11.5% v 24.7% [P = .049] and 16.4% v 33.3% [P = .02], respectively). Treatment arms did not differ significantly in OS, intracranial PFS, or toxicity. At 6 months, using all data, patients who received HA-WBRT plus memantine reported less fatigue (P = .04), less difficulty with remembering things (P = .01), and less difficulty with speaking (P = .049) and less interference of neurologic symptoms in daily activities (P = .008) and fewer cognitive symptoms (P = .01). Their conclusion was that HA-WBRT plus memantine better preserves cognitive function and patient-reported symptoms, with no difference in intracranial PFS and OS, and should be considered a standard of care for patients with good performance status who plan to receive WBRT for brain metastases with no perihippocampal metastases.

Parotids

The parotids and other salivary glands are particularly sensitive to radiation, and there is compelling evidence that even relatively low doses can decrease their function [67–70]. Parotid irradiation can result in xerostomia, which can ultimately lead to poor dental hygiene, caries, oral infections, oral discomfort, dysphagia, and malnutrition [68, 70, 71]. Significant xerostomia can have a marked negative impact on QoL [69, 70]. Xerostomia has been reported within 1–2 weeks of radiotherapy and has been noted to persist for 6–12 months beyond the completion of treatment [70, 72]. Often cited parotid dose constraints are mean dose of <24–26 Gy, at least one parotid mean dose <20 Gy, and V15 < 66% [69, 70, 73, 74].

Significant parotid gland volumes fall within traditional WBRT treatment fields, and parotid constraints may easily be exceeded unless efforts are made to spare these structures. There is a limited literature regarding parotid radiation dose and resultant toxicity for WBRT patients, and the parotids are not routinely contoured as OARs in WBRT treatment planning [68–71, 75]. The parotid glands are variable in volume and in position relative to bony anatomy. However, with 3D treatment planning now commonly employed, the parotids are easily visualized in relation to the treatment field, and the dose they receive is readily calculated [69, 70, 76].

Several investigators have evaluated parotid radiation with conventional WBRT and reported significant doses delivered, with approximately one third of patients receiving a mean parotid dose above 20 Gy [69, 70, 72]. To our knowledge, no studies have specifically evaluated the correlation between parotid dose-volume histograms and subsequent salivary function or xerostomia in WBRT treatments. A prospective trial evaluating xerostomia following WBRT has completed accrual, although results are not yet published (NCT02682199).

Fortunately, several simple treatment techniques have been demonstrated to reduce radiation dose to the parotid glands, with the goal of toxicity reduction. Conventional WBRT is often delivered to CNS with the caudad extent set at the inferior border of C1 or C2. Several investigators have demonstrated reduced parotid dose when the inferior border of the treatment field is reduced, either to the inferior border of C1 or such that only the brain parenchyma with a margin is treated [67, 74, 76]. Of course, clinical judgment must be used regarding the need to treat the upper cervical spine, such as in the cases of leptomeningeal disease. Published literature also demonstrates that parotid dose can be significantly reduced with simple collimator rotation to 70° or 110°, or with the careful use of MLCs to block the parotids without compromised brain coverage [74, 77, 78]. In our experience, the use of 10 MV photon energy, rather than 6 MV, for conventional WBRT treatment planning can reduce parotid dose (Fig. 23.6).

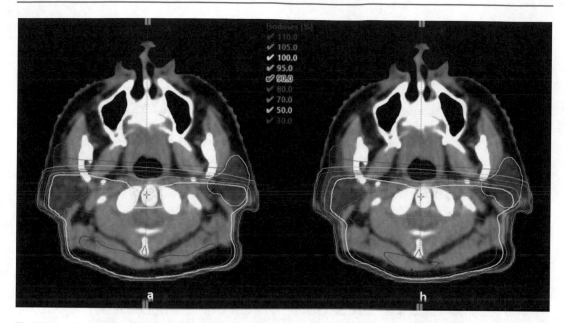

Fig. 23.6 (a) Axial WBRT dosimetry at the level of the parotids, using 6 MV photons. Nearly all of the irradiated parotids are covered by the yellow 100% isodose surface. (b) Axial WBRT dosimetry at the level of the parotids, using 10 MV photons. The more superficial portions of the parotids are spared full-dose irradiation

We retrospectively re-planned WBRT patients with 6 and 10 MV photon energies, demonstrating that with 10 MV photons, mean and maximum radiation dose to the parotids was significantly reduced (unpublished data). Additional beams can also be employed to reduce parotid dose. Park et al. demonstrated a significant reduction of parotid gland dose, while maintaining brain coverage, with the addition of a superior anterior field [79]. The same group has also used a four-field box for WBRT treatment planning, and tilted patients' heads 40°. A field-in-field technique was employed to minimize hotspots, and dynamic wedges were used to compensate for skull convexity. Parotid mean dose, V5, V10, V15, and V20 were significantly improved with this treatment planning technique [79].

Some investigators have also evaluated the ability of IMRT treatment planning to reduce parotid dose. In two similar studies, Pokhrel et al. and Sood et al. retrospectively evaluated the feasibility of HA-WBRT, as per RTOG 0933, in reducing parotid dose compared to conventional fields. These studies reported significant reduction in parotid mean dose, maximum dose, and V15 with HA-WBRT, without sacrifices in target coverage [80, 81]. A prospective randomized trial evaluating standard WBRT versus parotid sparing WBRT at the University of North Carolina at Chapel Hill is currently enrolling patients (NCT03595878).

Scalp Sparing

In conventional WBRT, the entire scalp, including hair follicles, is included within the treatment field. Hair follicles are very susceptible to RT, with tolerance as low as 2–3 Gy in 1 fraction [82, 83]. Unfortunately, almost total hair loss is experienced by nearly all patients undergoing conventional WBRT, and alopecia is a significant source of declines in patient QoL [80–85]. The duration of RT-induced alopecia appears to be dose-dependent and may be reduced with efforts at scalp sparing [80–83, 85]. Hair regrowth generally occurs 2–4 months following the completion of radiation. Unfortunately, there is limited robust evidence regarding the dose-response relationship of temporary alopecia in fractionated RT [82, 83].

Despite these limitations in our knowledge, efforts have been made to reduce WBRT scalp dose, and resultant alopecia with varied success. In our experience, the use of 10 MV photon energy rather than 6 MV for conventional WBRT treatment planning significantly reduces mean and maximum radiation dose to the scalp [unpublished data]. With advances in radiation technology, such as the use of IMRT, scalp sparing may be increasingly feasible [82–84]. There is evidence that using IMRT to limit the mean scalp dose of fractionated RT to 16–18 Gy may shorten the duration of temporary alopecia and reduce the risk of permanent alopecia [81, 84]. Several investigators have reported statistically significant reductions of calculated and measured scalp dose with IMRT WBRT. Unfortunately, these reported scalp dose reductions may be insufficient to result in significant clinical improvements in alopecia [82, 83]. A patient trial of scalp sparing IMRT WBRT was halted due to futility, as a meaningful reduction in alopecia scores was not observed [83]. Several studies have also evaluated the scalp sparing effect of HA-WBRT as per RTOG 0933 and have reported significant reductions in mean scalp dose, maximum scalp dose, and scalp V24 and V30 [80, 81, 85].

Areas of Uncertainty and Future Directions

Omitting WBRT

The QUARTZ trial, a phase 3 multi-institutional study, randomized 538 non-small cell lung cancer patients with brain metastases unsuitable for surgical resection or SRS to either to optimal supportive care (OSC) plus WBRT (20 Gy in 5 fractions) or OSC alone. There was no difference in the rate of serious adverse events, overall survival, or QoL between the two groups [7]. While the QUARTZ trial suggests OSC is a non-inferior option to WBRT in lung cancer patients with brain metastases not amenable to resection or radiosurgery, it is important to consider the study cohort largely comprised patients with a very poor prognosis, with both groups having a

median survival below 2 months. Thus, although WBRT may confer a survival benefit to specific populations including those under 60 years of age, a good performance status, and controlled extracranial disease [86, 87], these patients may be better served with SRS as an initial therapy, deferring WBRT for salvage, as their survival may be protracted, and any post-WBRT sequelae will be potentially present for the rest of their lives.

Role of Prophylactic Cranial Irradiation in Small Cell Lung Cancer

Prophylactic cranial irradiation (PCI) entails the use of WBRT in patients with primary malignancies that demonstrate proportionally high neurotropism rates, such as small-cell lung carcinomas (SCLC) [88]. Delivering PCI preceding radiographic diagnosis of brain metastases in patients with SCLC has been an ongoing topic of debate. PCI was initially shown to decrease the incidence of developing brain metastasis and improves disease-free and overall survival in those who responded to systemic therapy without developing brain metastases [89]. Slotman et al. prospectively randomized 283 patients with extensive stage SCLC with a response to systemic treatment to PCI or observation. Imaging of the brain was not mandatory prior to enrollment. The incidence of brain metastases at 1 year was reduced from 40.4% in the observation group to 14.6% in the PCI group, with an increase in median overall survival from 5.4 months in the observed group to 6.7 months in the PCI group. However, there was no radiologic verification that patients did not have brain metastases prior to chemotherapy or PCI. Additionally, a variety of PCI doses were allowed: 20 Gy/5 fractions or 8 fractions, 24 Gy/12 fractions, 25 Gy/10 fractions, 30 Gy/10 fractions or 12 fractions [90]. These findings are supported by a recent meta-analysis showing small-cell lung cancer patients completing PCI, demonstrating a significant survival benefit with a pooled relative risk of 0.92 [91]. However, a phase 3 multi-institutional Japanese trial randomized extensive stage SCLC patients with a response to chemotherapy and no evidence of brain metastases on post-chemotherapy brain MRI to PCI (25 Gy in 10 fractions) or observation and failed to show a survival benefit [92]. Explanations for these contrasting outcomes include (to varying degrees) differences in eligibility criteria and patient selection, PCI fractionation, chemotherapy, and patient genetics and demographics. While the field is still elucidating the role and benefit of PCI in SCLC, morbidity may be reduced by integrating HA and memantine during PCI, although this has not yet been shown to be the case in clinical trials.

Reduction of Treatment-Related Sequelae

As the prognosis for WBRT patients improves, attention is increasingly being turned to the adverse effects of treatment. Efforts have and continue to be made to reduce radiation dose to critical organs at risk with the aim of reducing toxicity and improving QoL. The use of 10 MV photons for treatment planning, or of IMRT and VMAT for HA-WBRT, have been demonstrated convincingly to reduce dose to the hippocampi. Evidence is mounting that HA-WBRT reduces neurocognitive decline relative to WBRT. Additionally, there is preliminary prospective evidence of the neuroprotective effects of memantine. Phase III studies to confirm the efficacy of memantine and determine its optimal dosing and duration of administration would be of great benefit. The ongoing NRG trials mentioned above will further our understanding of the effect of HA-WBRT, memantine, and their combination, in mitigating the undesirable neurocognitive decline observed with WBRT.

Numerous techniques of various complexities can be used to reduce potential morbidity for organs-at-risk outside the CNS such as the scalp and parotid glands, but the primary goal of controlling brain metastases cannot be forgotten as attempts are made to make WBRT less morbid. Prospective trials will need to demonstrate that these dosimetric advances result in clinically significant improvements in patient outcomes following WBRT.

Key Points

- WBRT is the treatment of choice for patients with leptomeningeal disease, or with brain metastases in eloquent brain regions, numerous brain metastases, and/or metastases that are too large for resection or SRS.
- Corticosteroids and anti-seizure medications should be considered when administering WBRT to aid with rapid symptomatic palliation and potentially improve neurological function.
- Conventional WBRT entails a nominal dose of 3000 cGy delivered in 10 fractions of 300 cGy each.
- The most common WBRT plan entails two opposed lateral fields slightly rotated off-axis two to three degrees in the anterior oblique orientation, to create coplanar anterior field edges that don't diverge into the lenses. The lower border of the field is commonly set at the caudal aspect of the first or second cervical vertebrae with two centimeters of flash posteriorly and superiorly.
- Choosing 10 MV photons as the treatment energy will improve dose homogeneity within the brain and improve parotid sparing relative to 6 MV photons for conventionally delivered WBRT without any compromise in target coverage.
- Common significant adverse effects of conventionally planned WBRT include neurocognitive decline, xerostomia, and alopecia.
- Advanced treatment planning techniques can be used to deliver WBRT with the avoidance of the hippocampi, which has been demonstrated to be safe, and to result in reductions in neurocognitive sequelae.
- Hippocampal-avoidance is better achieved with 6 MV photons than 10 MV photons when hippocampal-avoiding WBRT is planned.

- Advanced treatment planning techniques have also been demonstrated to reduce radiation dose to the parotid glands and scalp, although resultant clinically relevant reductions in xerostomia and alopecia, respectively, remain to be shown.

References

1. Hustu H, Aur R, Verzosa M, Simone J, Pinkel D. Prevention of central nervous system leukemia by irradiation. Cancer. 1973;32(3):585–97.
2. Jenkin D. The radiation treatment of medulloblastoma. J Neurooncol. 1996;29(1):45–54.
3. Uozumi A, Yamaura A, Makino H, Miyoshi T, Arimizu N. A newly designed radiation port for medulloblastoma to prevent metastasis to the cribriform plate region. Childs Nerv Syst. 1990;6(8):451–5.
4. Gavrilovic I, Posner J. Brain metastases: epidemiology and pathophysiology. J Neurooncol. 2005;75(1):5–14.
5. Halperin E, Wazer D, Perez C, Brady L. Perez & Brady's principles and practice of radiation oncology. 6th ed. Philadelphia: Lippincott Williams & Wilkins; 2013.
6. Steeg P, Camphausen K, Smith Q. Brain metastases as preventive and therapeutic targets. Nat Rev Cancer. 2011;11(5):352–63.
7. Mulvenna P, Nankivell M, Barton R, Faivre-Finn C, Wilson P, McColl E, et al. Dexamethasone and supportive care with or without whole brain radiotherapy in treating patients with non-small cell lung cancer with brain metastases unsuitable for resection or stereotactic radiotherapy (QUARTZ): results from a phase 3, non-inferiority, randomised trial. Lancet. 2016;388(10055):2004–14.
8. Chao J, Phillips R, Nickson J. Roentgen-ray therapy of cerebral metastases. Cancer. 1954;7(4):682–9.
9. Order S, Hellmän S, Von Essen C, Kligerman M. Improvement in quality of survival following whole-brain irradiation for brain metastasis. Radiology. 1968;91(1):149–53.
10. Lenz M, Freid J. Metastases to the skeleton, brain and spinal cord from cancer of the breast and the effect of radiotherapy. Ann Surg. 1931;93(1):278–93.
11. Jackson Richmond J. Cerebral tumours. J Fac Radiol. 1949;1(1):23–7.
12. Chu F, Hilaris B. Value of radiation therapy in the management of intracranial metastases. Cancer. 1961;14(3):577–81.
13. Borgelt B, Gelber R, Kramer S, Brady L, Chang C, Davis L, et al. The palliation of brain metastases: final results of the first two studies by the radiation therapy oncology group. Int J Radiat Oncol Biol Phys. 1980;6(1):1–9.
14. Patchell R, Tibbs P, Walsh J, Dempsey R, Maruyama Y, Kryscio R, et al. A randomized trial of surgery in the treatment of single metastases to the brain. N Engl J Med. 1990;322(8):494–500.
15. Patchell R, Tibbs P, Regine W, Dempsey R, Mohiuddin M, Kryscio R, et al. Postoperative radiotherapy in the treatment of single metastases to the brain. JAMA. 1998;280(17):1485–9.
16. Merriam G, Focht E. A clinical study of radiation cataracts and the relationship to dose. Am J Roentgenol Radium Therapy, Nucl Med. 1957;77(5):759–85.
17. Holmes G, Schulz M. Therapeutic Radiology. 1st ed. Philadelphia: Lea & Febiger; 1950.
18. Woo S, Donaldson S, Heck R, Nielson K, Shostak C. Minimizing and measuring lens dose when giving cranial irradiation. Radiother Oncol. 1989;16(3):183–8.
19. Dhellemmes P, Demaille M, Lejeune J, Baranzelli M, Combelles G, Torrealba G. Cerebellar medulloblastoma: results of multidisciplinary treatment. Report of 120 cases. Surg Neurol. 1986;25(3):290–4.
20. Jereb B, Sundaresan N, Horten B, Reid A, Galicich J. Supratentorial recurrences in medulloblastoma. Cancer. 1981;47(4):806–9.
21. Gripp S, Doeker R, Glag M, Vogelsang P, Bannach B, Doll T, et al. The role of CT simulation in whole-brain irradiation. Int J Radiat Oncol Biol Phys. 1999;45(4):1081–8.
22. Cheng C, Chin L, Kijewski P. A coordinate transfer of anatomical information from CT to treatment simulation. Int J Radiat Oncol Biol Phys. 1987;13(10):1559–69.
23. Goitein M, Abrams M, Rowell D, Pollari H, Wiles J. Multi-dimensional treatment planning: II. Beam's eye-view, back projection, and projection through CT sections. Int J Radiat Oncol Biol Phys. 1983;9(6):789–97.
24. Mohan R, Barest G, Brewster L, Chui C, Kutcher G, Laughlin J, et al. A comprehensive three-dimensional radiation treatment planning system. Int J Radiat Oncol Biol Phys. 1988;15(2):481–95.
25. Sherouse G, Novins K, Chaney E. Computation of digitally reconstructed radiographs for use in radiotherapy treatment design. Int J Radiat Oncol Biol Phys. 1990;18(3):651–8.
26. Mah K, Danjoux C, Manship S, Makhani N, Cardoso M, Sixel K. Computed tomographic simulation of craniospinal fields in pediatric patients: improved treatment accuracy and patient comfort. Int J Radiat Oncol Biol Phys. 1998;41(5):997–1003.
27. Andic F, Ors Y, Niang U, Kuzhan A, Dirier A. Dosimetric comparison of conventional helmet-field whole-brain irradiation with three-dimensional conformal radiotherapy: dose homogeneity and retro-orbital area coverage. Br J Radiol. 2009;82(974):118–22.

28. Freislederer P, Reiner M, Hoischen W, Quanz A, Heinz C, Walter F, et al. Characteristics of gated treatment using an optical surface imaging and gating system on an Elekta linac. Radiat Oncol. 2015;10(1):68.

29. Pham N, Reddy P, Murphy J, Sanghvi P, Hattangadi J, Kim G, et al. Frameless, real time, surface imaging guided radiosurgery: clinical outcomes for brain metastases. Int J Radiat Oncol Biol Phys. 2015;93(3):E105.

30. Mehta M, Khuntia D. Current strategies in whole-brain radiation therapy for brain metastases. Neurosurgery. 2005;57(Supplement):S4–33–44.

31. Biti G, Santoni R, Ponticelli P, Magrini S, Mungar V. Multiple daily fractionation in cerebral metastases. In: Proceedings of the third European conference on clinical oncology and cancer nursing. Stockholm: Federation of European Cancer Societies; 1985.

32. Tsao M, Xu W, Wong R, Lloyd N, Laperriere N, Sahgal A, et al. Whole brain radiotherapy for the treatment of newly diagnosed multiple brain metastases. Cochrane Database Syst Rev. 2018;1:CD003869.

33. Coia L, Hanks G, Martz K, Steinfeld A, Diamond J, Kramer S. Practice patterns of palliative care for the United States 1984–1985. Int J Radiat Oncol Biol Phys. 1988;14(6):1261–9.

34. Lo SS, Sahgal A, Ma L, Chang EL. Advances in radiation therapy of brain metastasis. In: Kim DG, Lunsford LD, editors. Current and future management of brain metastasis. Basel: Karger; 2012.

35. Andrevska A, Knight KA, Sale CA. The feasibility and benefits of using volumetric arc therapy in patients with brain metastases: a systematic review. J Med Radiat Sci. 2014;61(4):267–76.

36. Yu J, Shiao S, Knisely J. A dosimetric evaluation of conventional helmet field irradiation versus two-field intensity-modulated radiotherapy technique. Int J Radiat Oncol Biol Phys. 2007;68(2):621–31.

37. Lee A, Foo W, Chappell R, Fowler J, Sze W, Poon Y, et al. Effect of time, dose, and fractionation on temporal lobe necrosis following radiotherapy for nasopharyngeal carcinoma. Int J Radiat Oncol Biol Phys. 1998;40(1):35–42.

38. Zhang I, Yamamoto M, Knisely JPS. Multiple brain metastases. In: Chang EL, Brown PD, Lo SS, Sahgal A, Suh JH, editors. Adult CNS radiation oncology. Cham: Springer International Publishing; 2018.

39. Jin J, Wen N, Ren L, Glide-Hurst C, Chetty I. Advances in treatment techniques arc-based and other intensity modulated therapies. Cancer J. 2011;17(3):166–76.

40. Konefal J, Emami B, Pilepich M. Analysis of dose fractionation in the palliation of metastases from malignant melanoma. Cancer. 1988;61(2):243–6.

41. Katz H. The relative effectiveness of radiation therapy, corticosteroids, and surgery in the management of melanoma metastatic to the central nervous system. Int J Radiat Oncol Biol Phys. 1981;7(7):897–906.

42. Rades D, Heisterkamp C, Schild S. Do patients receiving whole-brain radiotherapy for brain metastases from renal cell carcinoma benefit from escalation of the radiation dose? Int J Radiat Oncol Biol Phys. 2010;78(2):398–403.

43. Hoskin P, Crow J, Ford H. The influence of extent and local management on the outcome of radiotherapy for brain metastases. Int J Radiat Oncol Biol Phys. 1990;19(1):111–5.

44. Kondziolka D, Patel A, Lunsford L, Kassam A, Flickinger J. Stereotactic radiosurgery plus whole brain radiotherapy versus radiotherapy alone for patients with multiple brain metastases. Int J Radiat Oncol Biol Phys. 1999;45(2):427–34.

45. Andrews D, Scott C, Sperduto P, Flanders A, Gaspar L, Schell M, et al. Whole brain radiation therapy with or without stereotactic radiosurgery boost for patients with one to three brain metastases: phase III results of the RTOG 9508 randomised trial. Lancet. 2004;363(9422):1665–72.

46. Lagerwaard F, van der Hoorn E, Verbakel W, Haasbeek C, Slotman B, Senan S. Whole-brain radiotherapy with simultaneous integrated boost to multiple brain metastases using volumetric modulated arc therapy. Int J Radiat Oncol Biol Phys. 2009;75(1):253–9.

47. Borghetti P, Pedretti S, Spiazzi L, Avitabile R, Urpis M, Foscarini F, et al. Whole brain radiotherapy with adjuvant or concomitant boost in brain metastasis: dosimetric comparison between helical and volumetric IMRT technique. Radiat Oncol. 2016;11(1):59.

48. Muacevic A, Wowra B, Siefert A, Tonn J, Steiger H, Kreth F. Microsurgery plus whole brain irradiation versus Gamma Knife surgery alone for treatment of single metastases to the brain: a randomized controlled multicentre phase III trial. J Neurooncol. 2008 May;87(3):299–307.

49. Kocher M, Soffietti R, Abacioglu U, Villà S, Fauchon F, Baumert B, et al. Adjuvant whole-brain radiotherapy versus observation after radiosurgery or surgical resection of one to three cerebral metastases: results of the EORTC 22952-26001 study. J Clin Oncol. 2011;29(2):134–41.

50. Brown P, Ballman K, Cerhan J, Anderson S, Carrero X, Whitton A, et al. Postoperative stereotactic radiosurgery compared with whole brain radiotherapy for resected metastatic brain disease (NCCTG N107C/CEC·3): a multicentre, randomised, controlled, phase 3 trial. Lancet Oncol. 2017;18(8):1049–60.

51. Wong W, Schild S, Sawyer T, Shaw E. Analysis of outcome in patients reirradiated for brain metastases. Int J Radiat Oncol Biol Phys. 1996;34(3):585–90.

52. Son C, Loeffler J, Oh K, Shih H. Outcomes after whole brain reirradiation in patients with brain metastases. Int J Radiat Oncol Biol Phys. 2010;78(3):S170–1.

53. Gondi V, Pugh S, Tome WA, et al. Preservation of memory with conformal avoidance of the hippocampal neural stem-cell compartment during whole-brain radiotherapy for brain metastases (RTOG 0933): a phase II multi-institutional trial. J Clin Oncol. 2014;32(34):3810–6.

54. Gondi V, Hermann BP, Mehta MP, Tome WA. Hippocampal dosimetry predicts neurocognitive function impairment after fractionated stereotactic radiotherapy for benign or low-grade adult brain tumors. Int J Radiat Oncol Biol Phys. 2013;85(2):348–54.

55. Tsai PF, Yang CC, Huang TY, et al. Hippocampal dosimetry correlates with the change in neurocognitive function after hippocampal sparing during whole brain radiotherapy: a prospective study. Radiat Oncol. 2015;10:253.

56. Brown PD, Pugh S, Laack NN, et al. Memantine for the prevention of cognitive dysfunction in patients receiving whole-brain radiotherapy: a randomized, double-blind, placebo-controlled trial. Neuro-Oncology. 2013;15(10):1429–37.

57. Gondi V, Tolakanahalli R, Mehta MP, et al. Hippocampal-sparing whole-brain radiotherapy: a "how-to" technique using helical tomotherapy and linear accelerator-based intensity-modulated radiotherapy. Int J Radiat Oncol Biol Phys. 2010;78(4):1244–52.

58. Rong Y, Evans J, Xu-Welliver M, et al. Dosimetric evaluation of intensity-modulated radiotherapy, volumetric modulated arc therapy, and helical tomotherapy for hippocampal-avoidance whole brain radiotherapy. PLoS One. 2015;10(4):e0126222.

59. Ghia A, Tome WA, Thomas S, et al. Distribution of brain metastases in relation to the hippocampus: implications for neurocognitive functional preservation. Int J Radiat Oncol Biol Phys. 2007;68(4):971–7.

60. Marsh JC, Gielda BT, Herskovic AM, Abrams RA. Cognitive sparing during the administration of whole brain radiotherapy and prophylactic cranial irradiation: current concepts and approaches. J Oncol. 2010;2010:198208.

61. Zhao R, Kong W, Shang J, Zhe H, Wang YY. Hippocampal-sparing whole brain radiotherapy for lung cancer. Clin Lung Cancer. 2017;18(2):127–31.

62. Oehlke O, Wucherpfennig D, Fels F, et al. Whole brain irradiation with hippocampal sparing and dose escalation on multiple brain metastases: local tumour control and survival. Strahlenther Onkol. 2015;191(6):461–9.

63. Lin SY, Yang CC, Wu YM, et al. Evaluating the impact of hippocampal sparing during whole brain radiotherapy on neurocognitive functions: a preliminary report of a prospective phase II study. Biom J. 2015;38(5):439–49.

64. Orgogozo JM, Rigaud AS, Stoffler A, et al. Efficacy and safety of memantine in patients with mild to moderate vascular dementia: a randomized, placebo-controlled trial (MMM 300). Stroke. 2002;33:1834–9.

65. Wilcock G, Mobius HJ, Stoffler A, et al. A double-blind, placebo-controlled multicentre study of memantine in mild to moderate vascular dementia (MMM500). Int Clin Psychopharmacol. 2002;17:297–305.

66. Brown PD, Gondi V, Pugh S, Tome WA, Wefel JS, Armstrong TS, et al. for NRG Oncology. Hippocampal avoidance during whole-brain radiotherapy plus memantine for patients with brain metastases: Phase III trial NRG Oncology CC001. J Clin Oncol. 2020;38:1019–29.

67. Wu CC, Wuu YR, Jani A, et al. Whole-brain irradiation field design: a comparison of parotid dose. Med Dosim. 2017;42(2):145–9.

68. Trignani M, Genovesi D, Vinciguerra A, et al. Parotid glands in whole-brain radiotherapy: 2D versus 3D technique for no sparing or sparing. Radiol Med. 2015;120(3):324–8.

69. Noh OK, Chun M, Nam SS, et al. Parotid gland as a risk organ in whole brain radiotherapy. Radiother Oncol. 2011;98(2):223–6.

70. Park J, Yea JW. Whole brain radiotherapy using four-field box technique with tilting baseplate for parotid sparing. Radiat Oncol J. 2019;37(1):22–9.

71. Burlage FR, Coppes RP, Meertens H, Stokman MA, Vissink A. Parotid and submandibular/sublingual salivary flow during high dose radiotherapy. Radiother Oncol. 2001;61(3):271–4.

72. Eisbruch A, Ten Haken RK, Kim HM, Marsh LH, Ship JA. Dose, volume, and function relationships in parotid salivary glands following conformal and intensity-modulated irradiation of head and neck cancer. Int J Radiat Oncol Biol Phys. 1999;45(3):577–87.

73. Deasy JO, Moiseenko V, Marks L, Chao KSC, Nam J, Eisbruch A. Radiotherapy dose-volume effects on salivary gland function. Int J Radiat Oncol Biol Phys. 2010;76(3 Suppl):S58–63.

74. Cho O, Chun M, Park SH, et al. Parotid gland sparing effect by computed tomography-based modified lower field margin in whole brain radiotherapy. Radiat Oncol J. 2013;31(1):12–7.

75. Roesink JM, Terhaard CH, Moerland MA, van Iersel F, Battermann JJ. CT-based parotid gland location: implications for preservation of parotid function. Radiother Oncol. 2000;55(2):131–3.

76. Fiorentino A, Caivano R, Chiumento C, et al. Technique of whole brain radiotherapy: conformity index and parotid glands. Clin Oncol (R Coll Radiol). 2012;24(9):e140–1.

77. Fiorentino A, Chiumento C, Caivano R, et al. Whole brain radiotherapy: are parotid glands organs at risk? Radiother Oncol. 2012;103(1):130–1.

78. Loos G, Paulon R, Verrelle P, et al. Whole brain radiotherapy for brain metastases: the technique of irradiation influences the dose to parotid glands. Cancer Radiother. 2012;16(2):136–9.

79. Park J, Park JW, Yea JW. Non-coplanar whole brain radiotherapy is an effective modality for parotid sparing. Yeungnam Univ J Med. 2019;36(1):36–42.

80. Pokhrel D, Sood S, Lominska C, et al. Potential for reduced radiation-induced toxicity using intensity-modulated arc therapy for whole-brain radiotherapy with hippocampal sparing. J Appl Clin Med Phys. 2015;16(5):131–41.

81. Sood S, Pokhrel D, McClinton C, et al. Volumetric-modulated arc therapy (VMAT) for whole brain radiotherapy: not only for hippocampal sparing, but also for reduction of dose to organs at risk. Med Dosim. 2017;42(4):375–83.

82. Roberge D, Parker W, Niazi TM, Olivares M. Treating the contents and not the container: dosimetric study of

hair-sparing whole brain intensity modulated radiation therapy. Technol Cancer Res Treat. 2005;4(5):567–70.

83. De Puysseleyr A, Van De Velde J, Speleers B, et al. Hair-sparing whole brain radiotherapy with volumetric arc therapy in patients treated for brain metastases: dosimetric and clinical results of a phase II trial. Radiat Oncol. 2014;9:170.

84. Kao J, Darakchiev B, Conboy L, et al. Tumor directed, scalp sparing intensity modulated whole brain radiotherapy for brain metastases. Technol Cancer Res Treat. 2015;14(5):547–55.

85. Mahadevan A, Sampson C, LaRosa S, et al. Dosimetric analysis of the alopecia preventing effect of hippocampus sparing whole brain radiation therapy. Radiat Oncol. 2015;10:245.

86. Sperduto P, Kased N, Roberge D, Xu Z, Shanley R, Luo X, et al. Summary report on the graded prognostic assessment: an accurate and facile diagnosis-specific tool to estimate survival for patients with brain metastases. J Clin Oncol. 2012;30(4):419–25.

87. Gaspar L, Scott C, Rotman M, Asbell S, Phillips T, Wasserman T, et al. Recursive partitioning analysis (RPA) of prognostic factors in three radiation therapy oncology group (RTOG) brain metastases trials. Int J Radiat Oncol Biol Phys. 1997;37(4):745–51.

88. Arriagada R, Le Chevalier T, Borie F, Riviere A, Chomy P, Monnet I, et al. Prophylactic cranial irradiation for patients with small-cell lung cancer in complete remission. J Natl Cancer Inst. 1995;87(3):183–90.

89. Aupérin A, Arriagada R, Pignon J, Le Péchoux C, Gregor A, Stephens R, et al. Prophylactic cranial irradiation for patients with small-cell lung cancer in complete remission. N Engl J Med. 1999;341(7):476–84.

90. Slotman B, Faivre-Finn C, Kramer G, Rankin E, Snee M, Hatton M, et al. Prophylactic cranial irradiation in extensive small-cell lung cancer. N Engl J Med. 2007;357(7):664–72.

91. Zhang W, Jiang W, Luan L, Wang L, Zheng X, Wang G. Prophylactic cranial irradiation for patients with small-cell lung cancer: a systematic review of the literature with meta-analysis. BMC Cancer. 2014;14(1):793.

92. Takahashi T, Yamanaka T, Seto T, Harada H, Nokihara H, Saka H, et al. Prophylactic cranial irradiation versus observation in patients with extensive-disease small-cell lung cancer: a multicentre, randomised, open-label, phase 3 trial. Lancet Oncol. 2017;18(5):663–71.

Index

Printed in the United States
by Baker & Taylor Publisher Services